Introduction to the
Cellular and Molecular Biology of Cancer

Third Edition

Edited by

L. M. Franks and N. M. Teich

Imperial Cancer Research Fund, London

Oxford   New York   Tokyo
OXFORD UNIVERSITY PRESS

Oxford University Press, Great Clarendon Street, Oxford OX2 6DP

Oxford   New York

Athens   Auckland   Bangkok   Bogotá   Buenos Aires   Calcutta
Cape Town   Chennai   Dar es Salaam   Delhi   Florence   Hong Kong   Istanbul
Karachi   Kuala Lumpur   Madrid   Melbourne   Mexico City   Mumbai
Nairobi   Paris   São Paulo   Singapore   Taipei   Tokyo   Toronto   Warsaw

and associated companies in
Berlin   Ibadan

Oxford is a trade mark of Oxford University Press

Published in the United States
by Oxford University Press Inc., New York

© The contributors listed on pp. xv–xvi, 1997
First published 1997
Reprinted 1998

A catalogue record for this book is available from the British Library

Library of Congress Cataloging in Publication Data
(Data available)

ISBN 0 19 854855 9 (Hbk)
ISBN 0 19 854854 0 (Pbk)

Printed in Great Britain by Bath Press Ltd., Bath

Preface to the third edition

Successive editions of this book have mirrored developments in cancer research and we hope that this new edition will achieve our original objective of providing a relatively brief but comprehensive introduction to the initiation, development, and treatment of cancer. On this background we have tried to provide an introduction to the results and new developments in the field using the current techniques of cell and molecular biology. A fuller understanding of the detail in some chapters needs a basic knowledge of molecular biology which can be found in several textbooks (e.g. Lodish *et al.* 1995) but the general principles in each chapter should be comprehensible without this. This edition has allowed us to bring up-to-date information in fields in which there has been great activity and even some achievement. In particular, the chapters concerned with epidemiology, genetic and chromosome changes, oncogenes, chemical and radiation carcinogenesis, growth factors, the biology of human leukaemia, and hormones and cancer, and the Glossary have been rewritten or extensively revised. Other chapters have been brought up-to-date and new chapters on cytokines and cancer, the molecular pathology of cancer, cancer prevention, and screening have been added.

Gene nomenclature may cause some confusion since although there is now a standardized format it is not yet generally accepted by all workers in the field. Many of the genes and oncogenes described by some earlier workers have retained their original format for historical reasons. Some genes were discovered in mouse cells, others in humans, and still others in viruses, and different names were given to genes which are now known to be essentially the same. Genes described for human cells are now usually written in upper case, italic type and their protein products in roman type. Mouse genes are often given in lower case italic type, their products as for those of human genes; those from *Drosophilia* are italicized with only the first letter capitalized. Specific oncogenes may be cited by a lower case first letter (c for cellular, v for viral), followed by a hyphen, and then the gene name in italic type. However, there may be further modifier terms. For the most part, we have tried to maintain some degree of consistency but in some chapters we have retained the original format if this is still used by many workers.

The apparently inevitable increase in girth that seems to accompany middle age has had its effect on the book which is somewhat larger than its predecessors but we hope that the increase in information will compensate.

As one of the philosophers in The Crock of Gold (Stephens 1931) commented 'Perfection is finality; finality is death. Nothing is perfect. There are lumps in it.'* No doubt there are lumps, and errors, and omissions in this new edition. We should be pleased to have comments and suggestions for their correction.

References

Lodish, H., Baltimore, D., Berk, A., Zipursky, S. L., Matsudaira, P., Darnell, J. (1995). *Molecular Cell Biology*. Scientific American Books, W. H. Freeman, New York.

Stephens, J. (1931). *The Crock of Gold*. Macmillan, London.

London   *L. M. F.*
June 1996   *N. M. T.*

---

*He was complaining to his wife about his porridge. She hit him on the head.

Preface to the second edition

The second edition of this book—prepared sooner than we had expected—has given us an opportunity to correct some of the faults and errors pointed out by our readers and reviewers, as well as allowing us to bring the book up-to-date in a number of areas in which there have been rapid developments. In particular the chapters on the genetic and chromosomal changes, growth factors, immunotherapy, and epidemiology have been expanded and more information on viral and chemical carcinogenesis added to the appropriate sections. We have also clarified and added new information to most of the other chapters.

At some stage all authors and editors of introductory textbooks are faced with the awful choice of deciding what to leave out. When does completeness conflict with comprehension? Is the omission of this and that piece of information really a mortal sin or could the distinguished reviewer who pointed it out just happen to have been told about it by a passing graduate student? In the end of course we did what all editors must do and made our own choice.

We hope that this second edition will continue to be of use to its readers as an introduction to cancer studies and as a source of further information either in key references or in specialized reviews such as *Cancer Surveys*.

We should still appreciate comments and suggestions for further improvement.

London
January 1990

L. M. F.
N. M. T.

Preface to the first edition

Cancer holds a strange place in modern mythology. Although it is a common disease and it is true to say that one person in five will die of cancer, it is equally true to say that four out of five die of some other disease. Heart disease, for example, a much more common cause of death, does not seem to carry with it the gloomy overtones, not always justifiable, of a diagnosis of cancer. This seems to stem largely from the fact that we had so little knowledge of the cause of a disease which seemed to appear almost at random and proceed inexorably. At the turn of the century, when the ICRF was founded (in 1902), the clinical behaviour and pathology of the more common tumours was known but little else. Over the years clinicians, laboratory scientists and epidemiologists established a firm database. The behaviour patterns of many tumours, and in some cases even the causal agents, were known but how these agents transformed normal cells and influenced tumour cell behaviour remained a mystery.

The development of molecular biology opened up a major new approach to the molecular analysis of normal and tumour cells. We can now ask and begin to answer questions particularly about the genetic control of cell growth and behaviour that have a bearing on our understanding not only of the family of diseases that we know as cancer but of the whole process of life itself. It is this, as much as finding a cause and cure for the disease, that gives cancer research its importance.

The initiating event which ultimately led to the publication of this book was the realization that many graduate students and research fellows who came to work in our Institute, although highly specialized in their own fields, had relatively little knowledge of cancer and there were few suitable textbooks to which they could be referred. Consequently, regular introductory courses were organized for new staff members at which 'experts' were asked to give a general introduction to their particular field of study. The talks were designed to give a background for the non-expert, as for example, molecular biology for the morphologist or cell biology for the protein chemist. The courses proved to be very popular. This book follows a similar pattern and has many of the same contributors—hence the fact that most are, or have been, connected with the Imperial Cancer Research Fund.

After a general introduction describing the pathology and natural history of the disease, each section gives a more detailed, but nevertheless general, survey of its particular area. We have tried to present principles rather than a mass of information, but inevitably some chapters are more detailed than others. Each chapter gives a short list of recommended reading which provides a source for seekers of further knowledge.

The topics covered have been selected with some care. Although some, particularly those concerned with treatment, may not at first glance appear to be directly related to cell and molecular biology, we feel that a knowledge of the methods used must give a wider understanding of the practical problems which may ultimately prove to be solvable by the application of modern scientific technology. On the other hand, knowledge of inherent cell behaviour (e.g. radiosensitivity, cell cycling, development of drug resistance, etc.) is important for the design of novel therapeutic approaches that rely less on empirical considerations.

Despite differences in the levels of technical details presented in some chapters, we hope that all are comprehensible. We have provided a fairly comprehensive glossary so that if some terms are not explained adequately in the text, do try the glossary. Finally, the editors would appreciate any comments, suggestions or corrections should a second edition prove desirable.

London
December 1985

L. M. F.
N. M. T.

Contents

Contributors

G. E. ADAMS — MRC Radiobiology Unit, Chilton, Didcot OX11 0RD, UK.

FRANCES R. BALKWILL — Imperial Cancer Research Fund, PO Box 123, London WC2A 3PX, UK.

ALLAN BALMAIN — The Beatson Institute, Garscube Estate, Switchback Road, Bearsden Glasgow, G61 1BD, UK.

PETER BEVERLEY — The Edward Jenner Institute for Vaccine Research, Compton, Newbury RG20 7NN, UK.

S. R. BLOOM — Department of Medicine, Royal Postgraduate Medical School, Hammersmith Hospital, London W12 0HS, UK.

W. F. BODMER — Principal, Hertford College, Cane Street, Oxford OX1 3BW, UK.

FRANCIS J. BURROWS — Chiron Technologies, Center for Gene Therapy, 11075 Roselle Street, San Diego, CA 92121, USA.

R. COX — MRC Radiobiology Unit, Chilton, Didcot OX11 0RD, UK

JACK CUZICK — Imperial Cancer Research Fund, PO Box 123, London WC2A 3PX, UK.

IAN FENTIMAN — ICRF Clinical Oncology Unit, UMDS, London SE1 9RT, UK.

D. FORMAN — Centre for Cancer Research, University of Leeds, Arthington House, Cookridge Hospital, Leeds LS16 6QB, UK.

L. M. FRANKS — Imperial Cancer Research Fund, PO Box 123, London WC2A 3PX, UK.

MEL GREAVES — The Leukaemia Research Fund Centre, Institute of Cancer Research, Fulham Road, London SW3 6JB, UK.

BEVERLY E. GRIFFIN — Department of Virology, Royal Postgraduate Medical School, Hammersmith Hospital, London, W12 0HS, UK.

I. R. HART — ICRF Richard Dimbleby Cancer Research Labs., St. Thomas' Hospital, Lambeth Palace Road, London SE1 7EH, UK.

T. KEY — ICRF Cancer Epidemiology Unit, The Gibson Building, Radcliffe Infirmary, Oxford OX2 6HE, UK.

NICHOLAS R. LEMOINE — Molecular Pathology Lab, ICRF, Royal Postgraduate Medical School, Hammersmith Hospital, Du Cane Road, London W12 0HS, UK.

J. S. MALPAS — ICRF Medical Oncology Unit, St. Bartholomew's Hospital, London EC1 7BE, UK.

GEORGE PANAYOTOU — The Ludwig Institute, Courtauld Building, 91 Riding House Street, London W1P 8BT, UK.

M. G. PARKER — Imperial Cancer Research Fund, PO Box 123, London WC2A 3PX, UK.

M. C. PIKE — Department of Preventive Medicine, USC School of Medicine, 1441 Eastlake Avenue, Los Angeles, CA 90033-0800, USA.

J. M. POLAK — Department of Histochemistry, Royal Postgraduate Medical School, Hammersmith Hospital, London W12 0HS, UK.

ALASTAIR D. REITH — The Ludwig Institute, Courtauld Building, 91 Riding House Street, London W1P 8BT, UK.

DENISE SHEER — Imperial Cancer Research Fund, PO Box 123, London WC2A 3PX, UK.

GORDON STAMP — Department of Histopathology, Royal Postgraduate Medical School, Hammersmith Hospital, Du Cane Road, London W12 0HS, UK.

NATALIE M. TEICH — Imperial Cancer Research Fund, PO Box 123, London WC2A 3PX, UK.

RAYMOND TENNANT — Laboratory of Environmental Carcinogenesis, National Institute of Environmental Health Sciences, Research Triangle Park, NC 27709, USA.

PHILIP E. THORPE — Department of Pharmacology and Hamon Center for Therapeutic Oncology Research, U. T. Southwestern Medical Center, 5323 Harry Hines Boulevard, Dallas, TX 75235, USA.

H. S. WASAN — Imperial Cancer Research Fund, PO Box 123, London WC2A 3PX, UK.

EDWARD J. WAWRZYNCZAK — Institute of Cancer Research, Haddow Laboratories, 15 Cotswold Road, Sutton SM2 5NG, UK.

ROBIN A. WEISS — Institute of Cancer Research, Fulham Road, London SW3 6JB, UK.

CAROLINE WIGLEY — Department of Anatomy UMDS (Guy's Campus), London Bridge, London SE1 9RT, UK.

JOHN WYKE — The Beatson Institute, Garscube Estate, Switchback Road, Glasgow G61 1BD, UK.

Abbreviations

5-MeC	5-methyl cytosine
AAF	acetylaminofluorene
AAV	adenovirus-associated virus
ABMT	autologous bone marrow transplant
ACTH	adrenocorticotrophic hormone
ADCC	antibody-dependent cell-mediated cytotoxicity
ADEPT	antibody-directed enzyme–prodrug therapy
AEV	avian erythroblastosis virus
AFP	α-fetoprotein
AGM	aorta, gonad, mesonephros region
AIDS	acquired immunodeficiency syndrome
AIG	anchorage-independent growth
AL	acute leukaemia
ALL	acute lymphoblastic leukaemia
ALV	avian leukaemia virus
AMF	autocrine motility factor
AML	acute myeloid leukaemia
AP	activator protein
APC	adenomatous polyposis coli
APL	acute promyelocytic leukaemia
APUD	amine precursor uptake and decarboxylation
ASCUS	atypical squamous cells of undetermined significance
AT	ataxia telangiectasia
ATL	adult T cell leukaemia
ATP	adenosine triphosphate
AUC	area under the curve
bHLH	basic helix–loop–helix
bp	base pair
BSE	breast self examination
C cell	calcitonin-producing cell
CALLA	common acute lymphoblastic leukaemia
CAM	cell adhesion molecule
cAMP	cyclic adenosine monophosphate
CBF	core-binding factor
CDC	complement-dependent cytotoxicity
CDK	cyclin-dependent kinase
CDKN2	cyclin-dependent kinase-4 inhibitor
cDNA	complementary DNA
CEA	carcinoembryonic antigen
CGRP	calcitonin gene-related peptide
CHO	Chinese hamster ovary
CIN	cervical intraepithelial neoplasia
CKI	CDK inhibitors
CLL	chronic lymphocytic leukaemia

CML	chronic myeloid leukaemia
CMV	cytomegalovirus
CPE	cytopathic effects
CRH	corticotropin releasing hormone
CSF	cerebrospinal fluid
CSF	colony-stimulating factor
CT	computerized tomography
CTLs	cytotoxic T lymphocytes
DCC	deleted in colon carcinoma (gene)
DHFR	dihydrofolate reductase
DHT	dihydrotestosterone
DM	double minute chromosome
DNA	deoxyribonucleic acid
EBV	Epstein–Barr virus
EGF(R)	epidermal growth factor (receptor)
ENU	ethylnitrosourea
ERE	oestrogen response element
ES	embryonic stem cells
Fab	antigen-binding fragment of antibody
FAK	focal adhesion kinase
FAP	familial adenomatous polyposis
Fc	crystallizable fragment
FGF(R)	fibroblast growth factor (receptor)
FISH	fluorescence *in situ* hybridization
FITC	fluoroscein isothiocyanate
FMTC	familial medullary thyroid carcinoma
FNAC	fine needle aspiration cytology
FSH	follicle stimulating hormone
G6PD	glucose-6-phosphate dehydrogenase
GAP	GTPase-activating protein
GdDTPA	gadolinium diethylenetriamine pentacetic acid dimeglumine
GDEPT	gene-directed enzyme–prodrug therapy
GNRF	guanine nucleotide releasing factors
GnRH	gonadotropin releasing hormone
GPAT	gene–prodrug activation therapy
GRE	glucocorticoid response element
GRF	growth hormone-releasing factor
GRP	gastrin-releasing peptide
GTAC	Gene Therapy Advisory Committee (UK)
GTP	guanosine 5'-triphosphate
GVHD	graft versus host disease
H&E	haematoxylin and eosin (stain)
HAT	Hypoxanthine, aminopterin, and thymidine (medium)
HCC	Hepatocellular carcinoma
HCG	human chorionic gonadotropin
HCL	hairy cell leukaemia
HDF	Hirschsprung's disease
HGF	scatter factor/hepatocyte growth factor
HGSIL	high grade squamous intraepithelial lesions
HIV	human immunodeficiency virus
HLA	human leukocyte antigen

HPRT	hypoxanthine phosphoribosyl transferase
HPV	human papillomavirus
HSR	homogeneously staining regions
HTLV	human T cell leukaemia virus
HVA	homovanillic acid
IARC	International Agency for Research on Cancer
ICRP	International Commission on Radiological Protection
Id	idiotype
IFN	interferon
Ig	immunoglobulin
IHC	immunohistochemistry
IL	interleukin
IRF-1	Interferon regulatory factor
IRS	insulin receptor substrate
ISCN	International System for Human Cytogenetic Nomeclature
ISH	*in situ* hybridization
kb	kilobase
kDa	kilodalton
KRAB	Kruppel-associated box
LAK	lymphokine-activated killer (cells)
LET	low energy transfer
LFA	lymphocyte function-associated antigens
LFS	Li–Fraumeni syndrome
LGSIL	low grade squamous intraepithelial lesions
LH	luteinizing hormone
LIF	leukaemia inhibitory factor
LOH	loss of heterozygosity
LT	lymphotoxin
LTR	long terminal repeat
MAGE	melanoma antigen gene
MAP kinase	mitogen-activated protein kinase
MAPKK	mitogen-activated protein kinase kinase
MCC	mutated in colon carcinoma (gene)
MDR	multidrug resistance (gene)
MDS	myelodysplastic syndrome
MEN	multiple endocrine neoplasia
MFO	mixed function oxidases
MHC	major histocompatibility complex
Min	multiple intestinal neoplasia
MLL	myeloid–lymphoid leukaemia
MMP	matrix metalloproteinases
MMSP	malignant melanoma of soft parts
MMTV	murine mammary tumour virus
MOM-1	modifier of Min
MPD	myeloproliferative disease
MRI	magnetic resonance imaging
mRNA	messenger RNA
MSF	migration stimulating factor
MT	methyltransferase
MTC	medullary thyroid carcinoma
MuLV	murine leukaemia virus

NGF	nerve growth factor
NHL	non-Hodgkin's lymphoma
NK	natural killer
NPC	nasopharyngeal carcinoma
NSAID	non-steroidal anti-inflammatory drug
NSE	neurone-specific enolase
PAGE	polyacrylamide gel electrophoresis
PCR	polymerase chain reaction
PDGF	platelet-derived growth factor
PEG	polyethylene glycol
PEM	polymorphic epithelial mucin
PET	positron emission tomography
PH	pleckstrin homology
PI	phosphatidylinositol
PKC	protein kinase C
PLA2	secretory phospholipase A2
PLL	prolymphocytic leukaemia
PLZF	promyelocytic zinc finger
PML	promyeloctyic leukaemia (gene)
PP	pancreatic polypeptide
pPNET	peripheral primitive neuroectodermal tumours
PSA	prostate-specific antigen
PTB	phosphotyrosine binding domain
pTyr	phosphotyrosine
r	recombination fraction
RAC	Recombinant DNA Advisory Committee (US)
RadLV	radiation leukaemia virus
RAID	radioimmunodetection
RAR	retinoic acid receptor
RARA	retinoic acid regulator (gene)
RB	retinoblastoma
RBE	relative biological efficiency
RER	replication error
RFLP	restriction fragment length polymorphism
RNA	ribonucleic acid
RSV	Rous sarcoma virus
RTK	receptor protein tyrosine kinase
RXR	retinoid X receptors
SH	Src homology
SIV	simian immunodeficiency virus
SOD	superoxide dismutase
SPECT	single photon emission computer tomography
SRE	serum response element
SRF	serum response factor
SSV	simian sarcoma virus
SUV	single unilamellar vesicles
TACAs	tumour-associated carbohydrate antigens
TCR	T cell receptor
TGF	transforming growth factor
TIL	tumour-infiltrating lymphocytes
TIMP	tissue inhibitor of metalloproteinase

TK	thymidine kinase
TMP	thymidine monophosphate
TNF	tumour necrosis factor
topo II	topoisomerase II
TPA	tumour promoting agent activator
TRH	thyrotropin
tRNA	transfer ribonucleic acid
TSH	thyroid-stimulating hormone
TTP	thymidine triphosphate
UNSCEAR	United Nations Scientific Committee on the Effects of Atomic Radiation
VDJ	variable diversity and joining segments
VEGF	vascular endothelial growth factor
VIP	vasoactive intestinal polypeptide
VMA	vanillylmandolic acid
XP	xeroderma pigmentosum
YAC	yeast artificial chromosome
ZIP	leucine zipper

1

What is cancer?

L. M. FRANKS

1.1 Introduction

Cancer has been known since human societies first learnt to record their activities. It was well known to the ancient Egyptians and to succeeding civilizations, but, as we shall see, most cancers develop late in life so that until the expectation of life began to increase from the middle of the nineteenth century onwards, the number of people surviving into the 'cancer age' was relatively small. Now that the common diseases of childhood and infectious diseases, the major causes of death in the past, have been controlled by improvements in public health and medical care, the proportion of older people at risk has increased dramatically. Although diseases of the heart and blood vessels are still the main cause of death in our ageing population, cancer is a major problem. At least one in three will develop cancer and one in four men and one in five women will die from it. For this reason alone

its control, or even better, its prevention, are important. But cancer research has an even wider significance. Cancer is not confined to humans and the higher mammals but may affect almost all multicellular organisms, plant as well as animal. Since it involves disturbances in cell growth and development, a knowledge of the processes underlying the disease will help us to understand the basic mechanisms concerned with life itself.

About 140 years ago a German microscopist, Johannes Mueller, showed that cancers were made up of cells, a discovery that began the search for changes that would help to pin-point the specific differences between normal and cancer cells. Although we know a great deal about the structure and behaviour of tumour cells, the main questions remain unanswered. The rapid advances in biological technology, particularly in cell and molecular biology, now allow us to try to answer questions which even 10 years ago could not be approached.

Even the most advanced technology, however, is of no value if it is not applied to the appropriate area. The cancer biologist must ask the right questions and to do this he must be aware of the biological background of the disease process he is studying. In this book we try to provide a brief background to the epidemiology and clinical aspects of the group of diseases we describe as 'cancer', and try to interpret changes in the structure and behaviour of normal and tumour cells at the biological and molecular levels, against this background. We also try to indicate the areas in which new and exciting discoveries are being made. This introductory chapter provides a brief account of the general biology, cellular pathology, and aetiology of cancer and some general definitions. The succeeding chapters deal with specific aspects in more detail.

Cancer is a disorder of cells and although it usually appears as a tumour (a swelling) made up of a mass of cells, the visible tumour is the end result of a whole series of changes which may have taken many years to develop. In this Chapter, I discuss what is known about the changes that take place during the process of tumour development and consider tumour diagnosis and nomenclature. To understand this, we need to know a little about the structure of normal cells and tissues and the mechanisms that control their growth.

1.2 Normal cells and tissues

The tissues of the body can be divided into four main groups; the general supporting tissues, collectively known as mesenchyme; the tissue-specific cells—epithelium; the 'defence' cells—the reticuloendothelial system; and the nervous system. The mesenchyme consists of connective tissue, fibroblasts which make collagen fibres and associated proteins, bone, cartilage, muscle, blood vessels, and lymphatics. The epithelial cells are the specific cells of the different organs, e.g. skin, intestine, liver, glands, etc. The reticuloendothelial system consists of a wide group of cells, mostly derived from precursor cells in the bone marrow which give rise to all the red and white blood cells; in addition some of the cells (lymphocytes and macrophages) are distributed throughout the body, either as free cells or as fixed constituents of other organs, e.g. in the liver, or as separate organs such as the spleen and lymph nodes. Lymph nodes are specialized nodules of lymphoid cells that are distributed throughout the body and act as filters for cells, bacteria, and other foreign matter. The nervous system is made up of the central nervous system (the brain and spinal cord and their coverings), and the peripheral nervous system of nerves leading from these central structures. Thus, each tissue has its own specific cells, usually several different types, which maintain the structure and function of the individual tissue. Bone, for example, has one group of cells responsible for bone formation and a second group responsible for bone resorption when the need arises, as in the repair of fractures. The intestinal tract has many different epithelial cell types responsible for the different functions of the bowel; and so on.

The specific cells are grouped in organs which have a standard pattern (Fig. 1.1). There is a layer of epithelium, the tissue-specific cells, separated from the supporting mesenchyme by a basement membrane. The supporting tissues (or stroma) are made up of connective tissue (collagen fibres) and fibroblasts (which make collagen), which may be supported on a layer of muscle and/or bone depend-

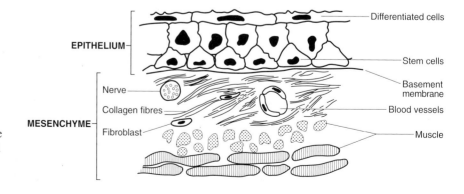

Fig. 1.1 A typical tissue showing epithelial and mesenchymal components.

ing on the organ. Blood vessels, lymphatic vessels, and nerves pass through the connective tissue and provide nutrients and nervous control, among other things, for the specific tissue cells. In some instances, e.g. the skin and intestinal tract, the epithelium, which may be one or more cells thick depending on the tissue, covers surfaces. In others it may form a system of tubes (e.g. in the lung or kidney), or solid cords (e.g. liver), but the basic pattern remains the same. Different organs differ in structure only in the nature of the specific cells and the arrangement and distribution of the supporting mesenchyme.

1.3 Control of growth in normal cells

The mechanism of growth control is one of the most important and least understood areas in biology. In normal development and growth there is a very precise mechanism that allows individual organs to reach a fixed size, which, for all practical purposes, is never exceeded. If a tissue is injured, the surviving cells in most organs begin to grow and replace the damaged cells. When this has been completed, the process stops, i.e. the normal growth-controlling mechanism persists throughout life. Although most cells in the embryo can proliferate (increase in number), not all adult cells retain this ability. In most organs there are special reserve or stem cells which are capable of growing in response to a stimulus, e.g. an injury, and of developing into the organ-specific cells. The more highly differentiated (developed) a cell is, e.g. muscle or nerve, the more likely it is to have lost its capacity to grow. In some organs, particularly the brain, the most highly differentiated cells, the nerve cells, can only proliferate in the embryo, although the special supporting cells in the brain continue to be able to grow. A consequence of this, as we shall see later, is that tumours of nerve cells are only found in the very young and tumours of the brain in adults are almost invariably derived from the supporting cells.

In other tissues there is a rapid turnover of cells, particularly in the small intestine and the blood and immune system cells. A great deal of work has been done on the factors controlling stem cell growth in the red and white cells (haemopoietic system), and the relationships of those factors to tumour development (see Chapter 12). Strangely enough, for reasons still unknown, rapid cell growth itself is not necessarily associated with an increased risk of tumour development; e.g. tumours of the small intestine are very rare.

From what little is known about growth control, it would appear that there are stimulatory and inhibitory factors that are normally in balance until a growth stimulus is required, either for repair or because extra work is required from a particular organ. These objectives may be achieved by hypertrophy, i.e. an increase in size of individual components, usually of structures that do not normally divide. An example is the increase in size of particular muscles in athletes. The alternative is the increase in number of the cells of the organ involved—hyperplasia. This may be in response to a physiological stimulus, e.g. some hormones, or in repair. These processes are all subject to normal growth control. When the stimulus is removed the situation returns to the *status quo*.

We now know that there is a close relationship between growth factor production and tumour growth and that their production may be controlled by some genes (protooncogenes) that are genetically similar to some tumour-producing viruses. A number of different growth factors have now been identified and it is clear that they are widely distributed, that many do not act alone, and that they have many different functions. For example, one such factor TGF-β under different conditions may act as a growth stimulator, a growth inhibitor, or a regulator of gene activity in many different cell types. These findings have opened up whole new areas in cancer research. They are discussed in detail in Chapters 8–12.

1.4 The cell cycle

The method by which cells increase in number is similar in all somatic cells, and involves the growth of all cell components, leading eventually to division of the cell into two new cells. Although the structural changes that take place have been known for many years, our knowledge of the molecular basis of the process is far from complete. Four stages are usually recognized: G1-S-G2-M; G1 is a gap or pause after stimulation where little seems to be happening although there is much biochemical activity; S is the phase of synthesis, particularly of DNA, to double the normal amount, although other components also increase; G2 is a second gap period; and M is the stage of mitosis in which the nucleus breaks down to form chromosomes, which, in the normal cell, separate into two identical groups, the nuclear membranes reform about each group and the whole cell then divides into two identical cells. Cells may be blocked at particular stages in the cycle by drugs (see Chapter 18) or by physiological agents, or they may move out of the division cycle into a resting phase known as G0. Other more complicated patterns of the cell cycle have been described but the one given here is sufficient for the purposes of this book.

One of the more interesting recent findings in this field was the discovery that there are two major control points in the cell cycle: one towards the end of G1, known as the restriction point, and the other at the initiation of mitosis. G2 cells deprived of growth factors before the restriction point will leave the cycle and enter G0.

From work on yeast a gene, *cdc*2/CDC28, concerned with the production of a specific protein that is involved with both the passage through the restriction point and the initiation of mitosis has been identified. The protein—a threonine or serine kinase (an enzyme that adds phosphate groups to amino acid residues—does not act directly but is thought to activate other key proteins that initiate S in G1 and initiate mitosis in G2. Some human cells have now been found to contain a similar gene. This work illustrates the complexity of the process of growth control but also shows how studies on simple organisms may help to explain changes in more complex individuals (see Beach *et al.* 1991, pp. 187–190 and 206–7, and Kastan 1997 for details).

1.5 Tumour growth or neoplasia

It is not possible to define a tumour cell in absolute terms. Tumours are usually recognized by the fact that the cells have shown abnormal growth, so that a reasonably acceptable definition is that tumour cells differ from normal cells in that they are no longer responsive to normal growth-controlling mechanisms. Since there are almost certainly many different factors involved, the altered cells may still respond to some but not to others. A further complication is that some tumour cells, especially soon after the cells have been transformed from the normal, may not be growing at all. In the present state of knowledge any definition must be 'operational'.

Given these qualifications we can classify tumours into three main groups:

1. Benign tumours may arise in any tissue, grow locally, and cause damage by local pressure or obstruction. However, the common feature is that they do not spread to distant sites.

2. *In situ* tumours usually develop in epithelium and are usually, but not invariably, small. The cells have the morphological appearance of cancer cells (see p. 9 *et seq.*) but remain in the epithelial layer. They do not invade the basement membrane and supporting mesenchyme. Some authorities recognize a stage of dysplasia (epithelial irregularity) which is not absolutely identifiable as cancer *in situ* but which may sometimes precede cancer *in situ*. Theoretically, cancers *in situ* may arise also in mesenchymal, reticuloendothelial, or nervous tissue, but they have not been recognized.

3. Cancers are fully developed (malignant) tumours with a specific capacity to invade and destroy the underlying mesenchyme—local invasion. The tumour cells need nutrients that are provided through the blood stream in normal tissues. Some tumour cells produce a range of proteins that stimulate the growth of blood vessels into the tumour, thus allowing continuous growth to occur. The new vessels are not very well formed and are easily damaged so that the invading tumour cells may penetrate these, and lymphatic vessels. Tumour fragments may be carried in these vessels to local lymph nodes or to distant organs, where they may produce secondary tumours (metastases). Cancers may arise in any tissue. Although there may be a progression from benign to malignant, this is far from invariable. Many benign tumours never become malignant.

Some of these problems of definition may be more easily understood if we consider the whole process of tumour induction and development (carcinogenesis)—see Chapters 5–11 for a further discussion).

1.6 The process of carcinogenesis

Carcinogenesis is a multistage process (Fig. 1.2). The application of a cancer-producing agent (carcinogen) does not lead to the immediate production of a tumour. There are a series of changes after the initiation step induced by the carcinogen. The subsequent stages—tumour promotion—may be produced by the carcinogen or by other substances (promoting agents) which do not themselves produce tumours. Initiation, which is the primary and essential step in the process, is very rapid, but once

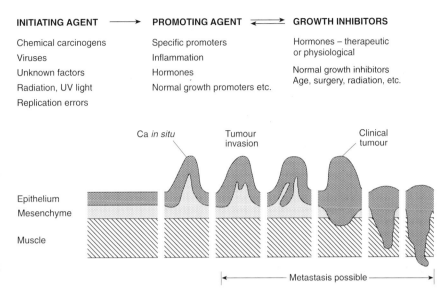

INITIATING AGENT ⟶ PROMOTING AGENT ⇌ GROWTH INHIBITORS

Chemical carcinogens   Specific promoters   Hormones – therapeutic
or physiological
Viruses   Inflammation
Unknown factors   Hormones   Normal growth inhibitors
Radiation, UV light   Normal growth promoters etc.   Age, surgery, radiation, etc.
Replication errors

Ca *in situ*   Tumour invasion   Clinical tumour

Epithelium
Mesenchyme

Muscle

Metastasis possible

Fig. 1.2 Factors influencing tumour development showing progression from normal to invasive tumour.

the initial change has taken place the initiated cells may persist for a considerable time, perhaps the life span of the individual. The most likely site for the primary event is in the genetic material (DNA), although there are other possibilities. The carcinogen is thought to damage or destroy specific genes probably in the stem cell population of the tissue involved (see Cairns 1975 for a review).

Initiated cells remain latent until acted upon by promoting agents. Many of these 'transformed' cells may not grow at all or grow very slowly. It is at this stage that the influence of growth appears. Promoting agents are not carcinogenic in themselves but they do induce initiated cells to divide. Many agents will induce cell division, but only promoters will induce tumour development, so that although cell growth is necessary for tumour development there must also be other factors involved. The suggestion is that promoting agents may interfere with the process of differentiation that normally takes place when cells move from the dividing stem cell population into functioning, and usually non-dividing, cells. Even though these growth-promoting stimuli are acting on the cells, they may still be sensitive to the normal growth-inhibiting factors in the body so that the final outcome depends on the balance between the factors and the extent of the changes in the initiated cells. This explains why preneoplastic, or even apparently fully transformed tumours, can be found but do not appear to be growing, and sometimes even regress.

The whole sequence of events in the process of tumour formation is almost certainly a consequence of gene changes, although gene expression may be influenced by the host. We are now beginning to understand some of these changes, although there are still many problems unsolved. The discovery that oncogenes of tumour-producing viruses are related to genes (protooncogenes) (see Chapter 9) in normal, as well as some tumour, cells has led to intensive research into the relationship of these genes to normal development and tumour growth and development. These genes have been localized to specific chromosomes and some to sites of chromosome abnormalities (see Chapter 10) in tumours. Much speculation now centres on the question of whether the initiation, progression, and maintenance of some tumours depends on overexpression through gene amplification (an increase in the number of copies of a particular gene), or inappropriate expression (i.e. at the wrong time) of normal genes, or whether mutations in a critical region of a gene are necessary. A possible hypothesis is that a mutation may be necessary for the initiation event but that some or all of the later stages may depend on over or inappropriate expression. These possibilities are discussed in the sections on carcinogenesis (Chapters 5–11).

One theory, for which there is now increasing evidence, was proposed by Knudson (described in more detail in Chapters 4 and 10). He suggested that at least two independent mutations are needed before tumours can develop. In cases of inherited (familial) tumour predisposition, the first mutation is present in the germ cells (sperm or ovum) and is therefore inherited by every cell. Only one further mutation is required in these cases. In the more common, non-familial cases two mutations (which may include gene deletions) in the same cell are required and the chances of this happening are consequently much smaller. It now seems certain that the changes must occur at the same site in each of the pair of homologous chromosomes, and in some cases the exact chromosome has been identified (see Chapter 10). An attractive hypothesis for some tumours is that the deleted or altered genes normally produce a product that suppresses the expression of trans-forming growth factors (see Chapter 11) by another pair of genes. The term tumour suppressor gene has been used to describe DNA sequences (genes) that act as dominant suppressors of malignancy and the identification of such genes, e.g. *p53* (see Chapter 9), and their relationship to the genes identified by Knudson and others in familial tumours is a field in which there is now much activity (see Chapters 4, 9, and 10 and Levine 1992).

Another major and unexplained area is concerned with the time-scale of carcinogenesis. The latent period between initiation and the appearance of tumours is one of the least understood aspects of tumour development. In humans, after exposure to industrial carcinogens, it may take over 20 years before tumours develop. Even in animals given massive doses of carcinogens, it may take up to a quarter or more of the total life span before tumours appear. The time for the reduction in risk after removing the carcinogen is equally long. Alcohol induces cancer of the oesophagus but the risk is reduced by stopping drinking. For former moderate drinkers the risk returns to normal after 10–14 years, but for heavy drinkers high risk remains for 15 years or more. Yet another unexplained fact is that only a very small number of cells 'initiated' by a carcinogen will eventually produce tumours; perhaps only one or two from many millions of treated cells.

1.7 Factors influencing the development of cancers

Many different factors are involved in the development of tumours. A cancer-producing agent or carcinogen, and presumably promoting agents, must be present. Carcinogens may be chemical or physical, e.g. radiation or ultraviolet light which causes skin cancer in Caucasians exposed to tropical sunlight but rarely in dark-skinned races. Identified chemical carcinogens include hydrocarbon carcinogens present in coal tar and a series of chemicals used in the rubber industry. Several specific promoting agents have now been identified and work on the mechanism of action of the different types is in progress (see Chapter 6). Animal experiments suggest that viruses may be associated with the initiation of some cancers, mainly the leukaemic group; viruses also seem to be associated with some types of human cancer. The role of oncogenes has already been mentioned. It is also becoming obvious that there is often an interaction between chemical carcinogens and viruses in tumour induction. A good example of this is seen in the association between hepatitis B virus and environmental chemicals in the development of liver cancer (see Chapters 6 and 8) and there is suggestive evidence in other tumours, particularly in cancer of the cervix (see Chapter 8). In other cases, such as with cigarette smoking, no single agent has been isolated but cigarette smoke is a very complex mixture of chemicals many of which may contribute to the carcinogenic effect of smoking. We know that cigarette smoking leads to the development of lung cancer and that the more an individual smokes the greater his (or her) chance of developing lung cancer, but all cigarette smokers do not develop lung cancer. There is considerable individual variation in response. We know from animal experiments and epidemiological studies (see Chapters 3, 4, and 6) that there is a genetic (DNA-associated) basis for this. Analysis of these changes are now being done at a cellular and molecular level (see Chapters 9 and 10). Some genetically homogeneous, inbred strains of mice are particularly susceptible to tumour induction by particular viruses or chemicals; some species are more susceptible than others to particular chemicals. In human populations some families and some races are more prone to develop certain cancers. This may be owing to genetic or environmental factors. The chance of a particular individual developing cancer depends on the balance between the various factors concerned. For example, exposure to a massive dose of a carcinogen may override an inherent genetic resistance, or genetic susceptibility may be so high that the development of specific tumours is invariable. With some tumours, particularly lung cancer and some industrial cancers, exposure to the carcinogen alone is sufficient to almost override other factors, but for the so-called spontaneous tumours, i.e. those that develop without a so-far recognizable cause, we have little idea of the relative importance of the various factors. Some of these factors are considered in more detail in Chapters 3–6.

Another factor that influences the type of cancer that develops is age. One of the few definite facts we have about cancer is that there is an age-associated, organ-specific tumour incidence. Most cancers in humans and experimental animals can be divided into three main groups depending on their age incidence. (i) Embryonic, e.g. neuroblastoma (tumours of embryonic nerve cells), embryonal tumours of kidney (Wilms' tumours), retinoblastomas, etc. (ii) Those predominantly in the young, e.g. some leukaemias, tumours of the bone, testis, etc. (iii) Those with an increasing incidence with age, e.g. tumours of prostate, colon, bladder, skin, breast, etc.

The incidence of human tumours is considered in more detail in Chapter 3. There are at least three possible explanations for this last group of age-associated tumours which includes the most frequently occurring human tumours. (i) There is a continuous exposure throughout life to low levels of a cumulative carcinogen. (ii) With age, humoral changes are induced, i.e. in the cellular environment, by alterations in the immune or hormonal systems, which allows or encourages neoplastic change to take place. (iii) There are age-associated changes in some cells, which increase their susceptibility to neoplastic transformation. There is some evidence for each of these possibilities. The first is the most likely for many tumours. The relationship between tumour development in endocrine-sensitive organs, such as the breast or prostate, to age-associated hormonal changes in the patient is still to be defined, but seems likely to be involved in the rate of growth of these tumours. The relationship between the immune system and cancer is discussed in Chapter 16. Finally, there is some experimental evidence for an increased sensitivity to neoplastic change in tissue culture and in transplants after the application of carcinogens to cells from some organs, such as bladder from old animals (see Franks and Wigley 1979 for a review of this topic).

We still do not know which of these explanations is correct or whether more than one process is involved.

1.8 The natural history of cancer or tumour progression

A series of changes takes place after a tissue cell is 'initiated' but the rate at which this occurs depends on changes in the cell and on changes in the host. Most chemical and physical cancer-inducing agents are very highly reactive and when they react with DNA in the affected cell they usually damage many other sites as well as the relatively few that are thought to control neoplastic transformation. Thus, the same agent may produce tumours in a given organ that differ greatly from each other, depending on the specific genes that have been altered or lost. At one extreme, if only the 'transforming' sites have been altered, the resulting tumour cells will still retain much of the normal differentiated structure and function of the cell from which they have arisen. In the skin, for example, the tumour cell will still resemble a skin cell (Fig. 1.3) and may still produce normal skin products and be responsive to normal growth-controlling factors. If the genes responsible for normal structure are more severely damaged, the resulting tumour cells have fewer normal properties. At the other extreme, the cells may have lost almost all the normal properties of the cell from which they have arisen. The loss of normal characteristics is known as dedifferentiation or anaplasia. The pathologist can grade tumours by making an approximate assessment of the degree of structural dedifferentiation by examining sections of tumours under the microscope. As a rule, there is an approximate correlation between the tumour grade and the growth rate. The most differentiated tumours (low grade, i.e. Grade I) tend to be more slow growing, and the most anaplastic (high Grade III or IV) more rapidly growing. Unfortunately, this relationship is not absolute but it does give a useful guide to tumour behaviour. Human breast cancers have been graded in this way and it has been shown that about 80 per cent of patients with well-differentiated Grade I breast cancers will be alive and well at five years (and much longer), but only 20 per cent of patients with Grade IV tumours will survive for this time. It is of course equally obvious from these figures that although 80 per cent of patients with Grade I cancers survive, 20 per cent with the same structural type of tumour do not, hence tumour growth is influenced by factors other than tumour structure, particularly the reaction by the patients own

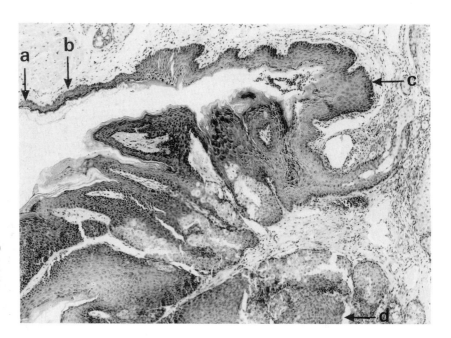

Fig. 1.3 Section (stained with haemotoxylin and eosin) if the edge of a squamous carcinoma of skin, with normal skin (a) on the left and increasing dysplasia (b) and (c) leading into the main mass of the tumour (d) below right. (×50)

defence mechanisms. Unfortunately, we have few ideas about the nature of these mechanisms. In hormone-responsive tissues such as the breast, the tumour cells may still retain some of the normal responsiveness to hormones (see Chapters 14 and 15). The pathologist's assessment of tumour grade is based only on alterations in structure and these are not invariably related to changes in function. Some cells may have lost their specific structural characters but still retain differentiated biochemical characters, and others may still appear structurally differentiated but have lost many normal functional attributes.

Another practical problem in the assessment of tumours is that tumours are not homogeneous (see Chapter 2 for a fuller discussion) and some may contain areas with more than one tumour grade. Note that in the tumour shown in Figs 1.3 and 1.4, there is a progression from benign to malignant resembling that illustrated in Fig. 1.2, but the progression is in space rather than necessarily in time. It used to be thought that tumours arose from a single altered cell, i.e. were clonal in origin, but there is now some evidence to suggest that this may not be invariably true. Even if it were true, there is no doubt that by the time a tumour is detectable clinically, whether it has arisen from one or many cells, it has been present for a long

time and the cells have had to go through a large number of cell divisions so that variation and selection of different cell populations have occurred. A tumour about 0.5 cm in diameter, which is just detectable, may contain over 500 million cells. The developed tumour usually consists of a mixed population of cells, which may differ in structure, function, growth potential, resistance to drugs or X-rays, and ability to invade and metastasize. Many of these characteristics may not be stable and may be influenced by the host response or by treatment. An obvious example is the destruction of X-ray-sensitive cells by X-ray treatment. If the tumour also contains X-ray-resistant cells, the cancer cells that are left after treatment will be X-ray resistant. Any individual character may vary independently.

Tumour progression is the development by a tumour of changes in one or more characters in its constituent cells. Although progression is usually towards greater malignancy, this is not invariably so. There are a number of cases (unfortunately small) in which rapidly growing tumours have ceased to grow, or have even disappeared completely. Although we do not yet have any explanation for this, it does show that there are natural mechanisms still to be discovered that will eventually allow us to control tumour growth.

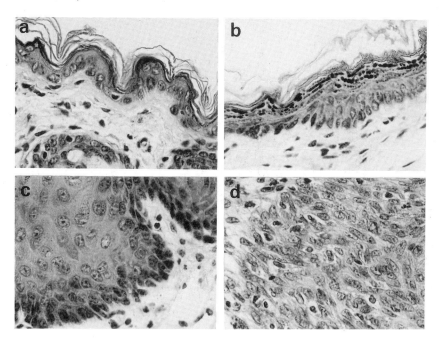

Fig. 1.4 Shows the areas marked in Fig. 1.3 but at a higher magnification. (a) Normal skin (compare with Fig. 1.1) showing mesenchyme below, covered by normal epithelium with basal cells and more differentiated superficial cells, covered by layers of keratin formed from the superficial cells. (×360) (b) Dysplastic skin. There is an increase in the basal cells, which are more irregular than the normal, and there is a disturbance in the formation of keratin, which is clumped into an irregular dark mass in the surface layer instead of the normal flattened sheets seen in Fig. 1.4a, i.e. differentiation is disturbed. (×360) (c) Cell overgrowth. The cells themselves are abnormal:

they vary in shape and size, the nuclei are much larger than normal, and some are more deeply stained. The usually distinct separation between epithelium and stroma is not seen, suggesting that invasion may be taking place. The cells are still recognizable as skin cells. This would be diagnosed as a moderately well-differentiated, squamous carcinoma. (×360) (d) The centre of the tumour is made up of a mass of irregular spindle-shaped cells with no recognizable skin features. This would be diagnosed as an anaplastic (undifferentiated) carcinoma. (×360)

1.9 The diagnosis of tumours

There are no absolute methods for diagnosing and assessing the degree of malignancy of tumours. Although many laboratories are trying to establish methods for doing this, none are entirely satisfactory. Microscopic examination of tissue is still the most reliable method for routine use. The function of the pathologist is to decide whether the structure of the cells in the tissue is sufficiently removed from the normal to allow a diagnosis of neoplasia to be made, and, if so, whether the tumour is likely to be benign or malignant, its probable cell of origin, its degree of malignancy, and its extent of spread. For

practical purposes the two techniques used are tumour grading and tumour staging. Tumour grading attempts to measure the degree of dedifferentiation in tumours and is based on histological and cytological criteria (Figs 1.3 and 1.4). Histological differentiation is concerned with alterations in the structure of the tissue, i.e. the relationship of cells to each other and to their underlying stroma. Cytological grading is based on the application of similar criteria to the structure of the specific tumour cells. Tumour staging assesses the extent of spread of tumours. Many investigators in the laboratory and the clinic have tried to find absolute markers of malignancy but, as I have already indicated, carcinogenesis is a multistage process. We should like to have markers for each stage of the process, but, unfortunately, apart from histology, which as we have seen is not entirely satisfactory, we do not have such markers. This is a major deficiency in studying cancer. Many workers are now trying to identify tumour-specific or tumour-associated proteins, either by direct measurement or by developing specific antibodies to these proteins. This seems to be a promising approach, not only in diagnosis (see Chapters 13 and 16), but also as a vehicle for carrying drugs or other agents that destroy cancer cells to their specific targets (see Chapter 19).

Thus, at present there are few true diagnostic tests for malignancy except for the genetic and chromosome-associated changes discussed in Chapters 4 and 10. The production of abnormal hormones, or normal hormones in abnormal amounts, may, in some instances, be a useful guide to the presence of tumours (see Chapter 14), but these are not true markers of malignancy. The experimental methods used for tumour identification are discussed on pages 17 *et seq.*

For the moment the most commonly used method of diagnosis depends on histology. Many millions of words have been written on tumour diagnosis and the World Health Organization has so far published 21 volumes on the structure and classification of tumours by an international panel of tumour pathologists. The following brief survey will only give a guide. I have chosen some of the examples, not because they are common, but because they illustrate some points more clearly than the more common tumours.

1.9.1 Benign tumours

Benign tumours usually resemble their tissue of origin but every tissue component need not be involved and the cells may or may not be in their normal relationship. Benign tumours arise in most tissues, increase in size, but do not invade. They are usually separated from the surrounding normal tissue by a capsule of connective tissue. Cytologically the specific tumour cells do not differ substantially from the structure of the normal organ cells. Benign tumours of bone or cartilage may produce nodules of bone or cartilage indistinguishable from normal tissues. In epithelial tissues, groups of cells

may also form local benign tumours made up of all tissue components. The covering or lining tissues of skin, intestinal tract, bladder, etc. may produce wart-like outgrowths containing all the tissue components, but closely packed to form a solid nodule. The common wart is a local outgrowth of all skin components. In other situations only one constituent cell may give rise to a benign tumour. The pituitary, for example, is a small gland at the base of the brain which produces many different hormones, each produced by a different type of cell, arranged in solid cords. Benign tumours of one cell type may develop and these tumours may then produce an excess of the particular hormone normally produced by that cell. Other benign tumours of the pituitary may contain more than one cell type, or produce more than one hormone, and some may be derived from non-hormone-producing cells. The cells in all these tumours are arranged in solid cords as in the normal gland. The benign tumours do not invade the surrounding tissue, but, if they increase in size, they may press on and damage the remaining normal cells or overlying nervous tissue or press on the optic nerves, which pass nearby, and lead to blindness. So, although the tumours themselves are benign they may cause serious disturbances by local pressure, or they may continue to produce excessive amounts of their normal product, which may in itself cause severe symptoms. Benign tumours of any other hormone-producing gland, such as the thyroid, adrenal, etc., may have similar effects. Alternatively, benign tumours may damage the remaining normal cells and cause a loss of normal function.

Benign epithelial tumours arise in many other organs. There is a different pattern of tumour growth in organs with a tubular structure. Both the kidney and breast, for example, are made up of tubular structures with the epithelial tubules lined by several different epithelial cell types and surrounded by connective tissue. Benign tumours in these organs are made up of tubules usually with one or, less commonly, two different epithelial cell types, together with a variable amount of connective tissue.

1.9.2 Malignant tumours

Malignant tumours show two characteristic features—cellular abnormalities (dyskaryosis), sometimes slight, and invasion of surrounding tissues. When both are present diagnosis is easy. The standard cellular criteria include a local increase in cell number, loss of the normal regular arrangement of cells, variation in cell shape and size, increase in nuclear size and density of staining (both of which reflect an increase in total DNA), an increase in mitotic activity (increased cell division), and the presence of abnormal mitoses and chromosomes (see Chapter 10). The diagnosis of carcinomas (malignant epithelial tumours) *in situ* depends on the recognition of these cellular changes in an area of epithelium, usually on a surface, the cervix of the uterus, or skin, but it may occur in the bladder or other organs. The changes only involve the epithelium and there is no invasion of underlying tissues, i.e. the neoplastic cells remain where they began—*in situ*. The only definite evidence of malignancy is invasion of underlying tissues. In most cases this is easily recognized since the tumour cells destroy and replace the normal tissues. Sometimes tumour cells may be found invading blood or lymphatic vessels; they may then be carried to other parts of the body in blood or lymph and develop into secondary tumours (metastases) in these distant sites. This type of spread is characteristic of malignant tumours and is the major problem in treatment since a tumour that remains localized to its site of origin can usually be removed surgically or destroyed by radiation. The problem of metastasis is discussed in Chapter 2. Malignant tumours have no well-defined capsule and the tumour cells grow in a much more disorganized form than is found in benign tumours. The same criteria apply to all malignant tumours, whatever their tissue of origin.

1.10 The names of tumours (nomenclature) and the need for tissue diagnosis

Although the precise naming of tumours may seem to be an academic exercise, it is of great practical importance in deciding on the treatment of each individual patient (see Chapters 17 and 18). Obviously, it is important for each pathologist and surgeon to use the same name for the same type of tumour. Even after many years of effort by international organizations, there is still some confusion about names although, fortunately, more or less agreed versions are now coming into general use.

But a more important point is that a knowledge of the type of tumour cell and the extent of spread are essential in planning treatment. Some tumours are known to be sensitive to drugs, hormones, or X-rays but others are resistant. Knowing the extent of spread will help to define the area for treatment by radiation or surgery, or even whether surgery is possible. For these reasons, the surgeon will usually remove a piece, or the whole tumour if it is readily accessible, for examination by a pathologist. The tissue removed (a biopsy) is preserved by a chemical fixative and thin sections are prepared for examination under an optical or electron microscope (see Chapters 13 and 17).

Although the names given to tumours seem to be confusing, there is a simple, logical basis to tumour nomenclature. The terms tumour, growth, or neoplasm can be used to describe a malignant tumour. Tumours are described by a generic name which specifies the general tissue of origin, i.e. mesenchyme, epithelium, or reticuloendothelial, and whether the tumour is benign or malignant. This generic name is qualified by the specific tissue of origin, e.g. kidney, breast, and this too may be qualified by further terms describing the cell of origin (if identifiable) and the pattern of growth. Some examples will make this clearer; a list is given in Table 1.1.

1.10.1 Tumours of epithelium

Benign tumours Benign tumours of epithelium are usually described by their growth pattern and their tissue of origin. Benign tumours of skin may be papillary (a warty outgrowth or papilloma) or solid. A benign skin tumour derived from squamous (flattened) epithelium could be described as a squamous cell papilloma of skin. Benign tumours of glandular tissues are called adenomas and may be solid or papillary, e.g. solid or papillary adenoma of thyroid.

Malignant tumours The generic name for malignant tumours of epithelium is carcinoma, e.g. carcinoma of skin. The common skin carcinomas may arise from the differentiated squamous cells or from the less differentiated basal cells, so that skin carcinomas may be described as squamous cell carcinomas or basal cell carcinomas. They may grow as flat (sessile) plaques or as warty (papillary) outgrowths. So a tumour may, for example, be described as a papillary squamous cell carcinoma of skin. Its grade and the extent of invasion may also

Table 1.1 Nomenclature of common tumours

Tissue	Basic cell type	Benign tumour	Malignant tumour
Skin	Squamous epithelium	Papilloma	Squamous carcinoma
	Basal cell		Basal cell carcinoma[1]
	Pigment cell	Melanoma (naevus)	Malignant melanoma
Alimentary tract			
Lips, mouth, tongue, oesophagus	Squamous epithelium	Papilloma	Squamous carcinoma
Stomach / Small bowel (rare) / Large bowel	Columnar epithelium	Papillary adenoma	Carcinoma
Nasopharynx, larynx, lungs[2]	Bronchial (respiratory) epithelium	Adenoma (rare)	Carcinoma
Urinary system			
Bladder	Urothelium (transitional epithelium)	Papilloma	Carcinoma
Solid epithelial organs Liver, kidney, prostate, thyroid, pancreas, pituitary, etc.	Specific epithelium	Adenoma	Carcinoma
Gonads			
Ovary	Surface epithelium	Serous cystadenoma	Serous cystadenocarcinoma
		Mucinous cystadenoma	Mucinous cystadenocarcinoma
	Germ Cells	Teratoma	Teratocarcinoma
			Choriocarcinoma
Testis	Germ cells	Teratoma	Seminoma
			Embryonal carcinoma
			Choriocarcinoma
			Malignant teratoma (rare)
Mesenchyme			
Fibrous tissue	Fibrocytes	Fibroma	Fibrosarcoma
Fat	Adipocytes	Lipoma	Liposarcoma
Bone	Osteocytes	Osteoma	Osteosarcoma
Cartilage	Chondrocytes	Chondroma	Chondrosarcoma
Smooth muscle[3]	Smooth muscle cells	Leiomyoma	Leiomyosarcoma
Striated muscle[4]	Muscle cells	Rhabdomyoma	Rhabdomyosarcoma
Blood vessels	Endothelium	Haemangioma	Haemangiosarcoma
Lymph vessels	Endothelium	Lymphangioma	Lymphangiosarcoma
Nervous system			
Nerve cells[5]			Neuroblastoma[5]
			Retinoblastoma
Supporting cells	Astrocytes		Astrocytoma[6]
	Oligodendrocytes		Oligodendrocytoma[6]
Covering cells (Central nervous system)	Meningeal cells	Meningioma	
Covering cells (Peripheral nervous system)	Perieneurium / Endoneurium	Neurofibroma	Neurofibrosarcoma
Reticuloendothelial system[7]			
White blood cells[8]	Myeloid cells		Myeloid leukaemia
	Monocytes		Monocytic leukaemia
	Granulocytes		Granulocytic leukaemia
	Lymphocytes		Lymphatic leukaemia

Table 1.1 Nomenclature of common tumours (contd.)

Tissue	Basic cell type	Benign tumour	Malignant tumour
Red blood cells	Erythrocytes		Erythroleukaemia
Lymph nodes	Lymphocytes Fixed reticulo- endothelial cells		Non-Hodgkin's lymphoma Hodgkin's disease
Embryonic type tissues	Mixed tissues	Teratoma	Teratocarcinoma

[1] Invades locally; does not metastasize.

[2] Lung tumours usually arise from lining epithelium of bronchi.

[3] Muscle of intestine, bladder, blood vessels, etc.

[4] Muscles under volunary control, e.g. limb muscles; tumours very rare.

[5] Nerve cell tumours in the very young only.

[6] No absolute distinction between benign and malignant tumours possible; do not metastasize.

[7] See p. 14.

[8] See Chapter 12.

be given. The final pathologist's report may read 'moderately well-differentiated (Grade II) squamous carcinoma of skin. The structure is mainly papillary but there is invasion of the underlying connective tissue; muscle is not involved'. This report tells the oncologist that the tumour is made up of squamous cells which are known to be sensitive to X-irradiation and that the extent of spread is limited, i.e. that it could easily be removed by local surgery. The final decision on treatment would then depend on the exact position of the tumour and, among other factors, whether surgery or irradiation would be easier or leave less scarring.

Malignant tumours of glandular tissues are also carcinomas but are sometimes described as adenocarcinomas, e.g. adenocarcinoma of breast, implying that the tumour has a glandular structure. As with the skin tumours, the cell type can be described (e.g. columnar cell or cuboidal) and if the cell of origin is known, this too can be added (e.g. ductal cuboidal cell adenocarcinoma of breast). The gross pattern of growth (sessile or papillary) and extent of spread can also be defined. Adenocarcinomas have a wider range of cellular patterns than tumours of covering epithelium. The cells may be arranged as large or small tubules or solid cords (trabeculae) or masses, and this pattern will also be described. In some cases the tumour grade can be assessed.

Most tumours still retain some of the structural features of the cells from which they have arisen, and, as we have seen, this allows the pathologist to make a rough assessment of the degree of malignancy, by means of the extent to which the tumours have departed from the normal (grading); it also may allow the source of a secondary tumour to be established. But there are still problems. Some

tumours may be so dedifferentiated that they no longer retain any structure that indicates the tissue of origin. In others, some cells may develop in an abnormal way. A common event is that tumour cells from a glandular organ such as the breast, which are normally columnar in structure, may develop into squamous cells resembling those in skin tumours. This process is known as metaplasia and, although confusing to the pathologist, does not as a rule influence the degree of malignancy. A final point is that in many tumours the structure is not homogeneous and more than one cell type, growth pattern, or grade of tumour may be present. All these features will be indicated in the pathologist's report.

1.10.2 Tumours of mesenchyme

Benign tumours Benign tumours of mesenchyme are described by the cellular tissue from which they arise (see Table 1.1), although confusion may be induced if Latin or Greek roots are introduced. Benign tumours of fibrous tissue are fibromas, benign tumours of bone may be described as osteomas, and benign tumours of blood vessels as angiomas, but, as can be seen from Table 1.1, the principles are simple.

Malignant tumours The generic name for malignant tumours of mesenchyme is sarcoma, and, as with carcinomas, this is qualified by the cell of origin and growth patterns. Thus, a malignant tumour of bone cells is called a bone sarcoma or osteosarcoma, but this can be qualified to describe behaviour. A tumour made of cells forming bone could be described as an osteogenic sarcoma and one with bone-destroying cells as an osteolytic sarcoma. Tumours derived from blood vessels are angiosarcomas, and so on. The extent of spread of sarcomas can also be defined and, in principle, sarcomas may also be graded in the same way as carcinomas, depending on the degree of dedifferentiation. In practice this is rarely done since most of the sarcomas are in fact very rapidly growing.

1.10.3 Tumours of the reticuloendothelial system

This is a very complicated field. Benign tumours of the reticuloendothelial system do occur but, since tumours in this system vary considerably in their degree of malignancy and since the tumours may affect the whole system which is widely distributed throughout the body, it is difficult if not impossible to distinguish between a malignant tumour that has spread and a benign tumour that has originated in several different sites, i.e. has a multicentric origin.

Malignant tumours may arise from any of the cells of the reticuloendothelial system. These cells develop from a population of multipotential stem cells in the bone marrow and give rise to families of differentiated cells with widely differing structures and functions (see Chapter 12). They include circulating red and white cells, including T and B lymphocytes and other cells of the immune system (see Chapter 12), as well as fixed cells of the system in the spleen, lymph nodes, and other organs. The tumours that arise from these cells may retain some or all (or none!) of the functions of the parent cells.

The tumours can be conveniently divided into two main groups, those arising from blood-forming cells (leukaemia), and those forming solid tumours (lymphomas), but the distinction is not clear-cut. In the first group, the tumour cells develop from precursor cells in the bone marrow and pass into the blood stream in the same way as normal blood cells so that the blood is filled with abnormal cells (leukaemic). Any of the stem cells of the bone marrow may give rise to leukaemias which may show any degree of differentiation, so that there may be undifferentiated stem cell leukaemias, or leukaemias with cells that retain some differentiated characters of normal white blood cells—myeloid (granulocytic), monocytic, lymphoid, or very rarely from red blood cell (erythroid) precursors. Although the striking feature of the leukaemias is that most of the tumour cells are in the blood stream, the cells may also penetrate normal tissues and form metastatic deposits in almost any organ. The biology of the leukaemias is described in Chapter 12. The solid tumours form a very mixed group. Their identification depends on the cell from which they are derived and the functions that they still express, particularly whether they are of T cell, B cell, or other origin. This distinction can now be made more precisely by using molecular markers (see Chapter 12).

One group of tumours, Hodgkin's lymphoma, identified by its clinical presentation and histological structure, is usually separated off from the non-Hodgkin's lymphomas, for which there is now a more or less agreed classification (the Keil Classification). The reader is advised not to dabble in this area without expert guidance, but pick your expert carefully (see Knowles 1992 for a review).

1.10.4 Tumours of the nervous system

Benign and malignant tumours arise in the nervous system, but, most remarkably, malignant tumours hardly ever spread outside the brain or spinal cord. Tumours of the nerve cells proper (neurones) only appear in the embryo or very shortly after birth. These are called neuroblastomas, or, if they arise from the specialized nerve cell layer in the eye (the retina), retinoblastomas. Almost all other tumours in the brain and spinal cord arise from the supporting cells, e.g. astrocytes which give rise to astrocytomas, etc. or from the coverings of the brain (the meninges) which give rise to meningiomas. More details are given in Table 1.1. As with tumours of other sites, tumours of the nervous system can be graded by assessing the degree of differentiation.

1.10.5 Tumours of mixed tissues

Very rarely tumours that contain a whole range of different tissues may be found. These tumours, known as teratomas, are thought to arise from primitive cells of embryonic type and are usually found in the testis or ovary, but may occur elsewhere. They are sometimes benign but very often malignant change occurs in one component tissue.

1.11 Tumour staging and the spread of tumours—metastasis

Tumour metastasis is the major practical problem, and a common cause of death, in clinical cancer. Tumours invade the surrounding tissues and may grow out of the organ in which they arise and involve surrounding tissues (Fig. 1.2). During this local invasion, tumour cells may penetrate the lymphatics and be carried to the regional lymph nodes where they are arrested. Some are destroyed but others may grow and produce new tumours. If tumour cells get into blood vessels, they may be carried to any organ in the body. Again, many are destroyed but others grow into secondary tumours. There are many unexplained problems. Carcinomas often involve lymph nodes but sarcomas rarely do. Some tumours give rise to secondary deposits more frequently in particular organs than in others. Metastasis in the lungs, liver, and bone are common since these organs have many small blood vessels in which tumour cells in the blood become trapped, yet other organs like muscle and spleen, which also have many small blood vessels, are rarely the site of tumour deposits. The relative importance of the seed (the tumour cells) and the soil (the organs involved) are still to be explained. Some of these problems are discussed in more detail in Chapter 2.

Tumour staging is used to give an assessment of the extent of spread of tumours. One of the more commonly used systems is that established by the International Union Against Cancer. This 'TNM' system is based on an assessment of the primary tumour (T), the regional lymph nodes (N), and the presence or absence of metastases (M). Each of these categories is qualified by a number which indicates the precise extent of involvement according to clearly defined criteria.

1.12 How tumours present—some effects of tumours on the body

Tumours are usually diagnosed if they produce some effects (see Chapter 17). Tumours of the skin or of organs that can be easily examined, such as breast, often present as a lump. Many cells in tumours die and these dead cells release enzymes that damage the overlying tissues so that a non-healing ulcer may form. Blood vessels at the base of the ulcer are damaged so that bleeding occurs. In the bowel or the urinary system, blood may be present in the stools, or in the urine, so that bleeding is a common presenting symptom in these organs. Many of the effects produced by tumours are a result of the position of the tumour, which may press on or destroy surrounding tissues or affect nerves and cause pain.

Tumours in the bowel, for example, may cause obstruction either because the tumour mass grows into the cavity of the bowel, or because it grows into the wall and destroys the muscle that normally moves the contents down the intestine. Tumours of the brain may present with headache caused by increased pressure inside the skull; tumours involving the bile ducts leading from the liver may cause jaundice; and so on. The physical effects obviously depend on the exact site of the tumour. Some tumours, particularly those that arise from hormone-producing organs, may cause excess production of the hormones that the normal organ produces, or a hormone deficiency through damage to the remaining normal gland cells. Less commonly, tumours may produce abnormal hormones, or hormones may be produced in tumours of organs that do not normally produce these substances (ectopic expression), e.g. some lung tumours may produce hormones normally produced by the pituitary gland. Anaemia caused by bleeding from the tumour or some toxic effects on the bone marrow is a not uncommon presenting symptom. As well as these effects, many tumours may cause general wasting and loss of appetite (tumour cachexia), sometimes even though the primary tumour is still fairly small. The cause is unknown but it is thought to be owing to some toxic product of the tumour.

As well as these harmful effects, some tumours may stimulate the defence systems of the body so that they react against the tumours. Unfortunately, we know very little about the way in which this occurs, but it seems very likely that some of the unexplained differences in the growth and development of tumours in different individuals may be due, in part, to this host defence reaction. This is an important area in which research is still in its early stages, but promising results are beginning to appear (Chapter 16). For many years it has been known that the body sometimes produces substances that destroy cancer cells. Two of these substances, tumour necrosis factor (TNF), derived from macrophages, and lymphotoxin (LT), derived from lymphocytes, have now been identified and their genes isolated. Using modern gene technology, it is possible to produce these substances in large enough quantities for clinical trials as a treatment. We now know that TNF, like other growth factors, is one of a family of cell regulatory proteins called cytokines which have many different functions. It seems that local, transient production of the factor may benefit the host, but that sustained production may be harmful. For example, one type of TNF, TNF-α, is probably largely responsible for tumour cachexia, while another type, TNF-β, is one of a family of completely different proteins associated with the induction of differentiation (see Chapters 11 and 20 for a review of this group and similar factors now known as biological response modifiers).

1.13 How does cancer kill?

As we have seen, many cancers develop in older people and a substantial number of patients do not die as a consequence of the disease but of some unrelated condition such as heart disease, incidental infections, or even as a result of an accident. Tumour-related events may cause death directly or indirectly depending on the site of the tumour and the extent of spread. A common cause of death is the involvement of vital organs, either by direct local invasion or from distant metastases, for example, in the brain, lung, or liver. Rarely, death may be owing to haemorrhage. More often, anaemia and unexplained wasting may lead to decreased resistance to infection so that terminal bronchopneumonia or infection of the urinary tract (pyelonephritis) is common. In many cases it is not possible to establish the immediate cause of death.

1.14 Treatment of cancer

The aim of an ideal cancer treatment is the removal or destruction of all cancer cells and, ideally, of areas already predisposed to tumour development. In many cases this may not be possible because the tumour has involved vital organs or has spread throughout the body. Although theoretically unsatisfactory since many believe that tumour spread takes place at a very early stage in the disease, local surgical removal of the primary tumour remains a very effective method of treatment in many cases. The scalpel remains the surgeon's best weapon but attempts to improve on this are being developed using laser-induced energy or cryosurgery, using liquid nitrogen probes, to coagulate tumour cells *in situ*. One experimental technique is to give photosensitizing drugs that may be concentrated in the tumour and activated by the local application of laser energy of the appropriate wavelength.

Radiation therapy is another widely used method for destroying tumour cells but there are often problems in applying a high dose to kill tumour cells without destroying the surrounding normal tissues. Some tumour cells are also resistant to radiation-induced damage. Radiation risks and dosage are discussed in Chapter 7. Because of these difficulties cytotoxic drugs (see Chapter 18) or methods for stimulating the body's own immune system (see Chapters 16 and 19) are in use and have the added advantage of potentially being able to destroy tumour cells that have already spread away from the primary tumour. Since, as we have seen, neoplastic change in cells is associated with DNA changes (either mutations or the incorporation of oncogenes or tumour viruses) attempts are being made to correct these changes by incorporating normal genes, or inhibitors to the abnormal gene products responsible for tumour cell growth into the cell. The replacement of defective tumour suppressor genes (p53) or the insertion of a gene (*myc*) that is thought to control cell death in normal cells are good examples of this. An even more exciting possibility is the suggestion that the insertion of genes controlling cell adhesion may prevent tumour metastasis. Unfortunately, it is unlikely that a single gene change is responsible for the whole pattern of cell behaviour that we identify as a clinical cancer. Ultimately gene therapy may be the most satisfactory method for tumour control. These points are discussed in Chapter 22. Two major problems for gene therapy, as well as for cytotoxic drug treatment and immunotherapy, are delivery of the therapeutic agents to the tumour cells and specificity, i.e. restricting the toxic agent to tumour cells only, without damage to normal tissues. The identity of absolute tumour-specific markers would allow an approach to this and may allow the development of specific antitumour antibodies. Even if absolute markers are not available it may still be possible to use antibodies against normal tissues if the tissue-specific determinants are only exposed if the tissue architecture is disturbed, as in tumours (see Chapter 19). Molecular biological research is beginning to indicate a way forward in these fields.

1.15 Cancer prevention and screening

Since at least one in three people will develop cancer at some time in their lives prevention seems an obvious approach. However, 70 per cent of all cancers develop in people over 60 years old and even the prevention of all cancers would not have a substantial effect on the total life span, since those saved would inevitably die of some other disease. The rationale for prevention and effective treatment is to improve the quality of life. Prevention is based mainly on the avoidance of cancer-producing agents. Since lung cancer alone is responsible for about a quarter of all cancer deaths the avoidance of smoking and other tobacco products would make a more dramatic reduction in cancer than almost any other measure known at present. The reduction of other environmental hazards and the effects of diet would play a lesser role. Research in these areas is discussed in Chapter 3.

Common sense also suggests that early treatment should lead to a better end result and for this reason massive (and expensive) screening programmes have been set up to try to identify tumours before they produce symptoms in organs, such as the uterine cervix, breast, colon, ovary, and prostate, and in areas of high incidence, such as the stomach (Japan and China) and the liver (southern Africa). Unfortunately, common sense may not be a good guide to the value of screening and early treatment because of the nature of the disease. Some claim that screening may detect small tumours that would never cause any symptoms of disease or that early diagnosis may not influence the total life span and that the increased survival is a spurious effect and only demonstrates that the physician has known that the tumour has been there for a longer time. This is an area in which beliefs are held with an almost religious fervour and convincing facts are still to be established. Screening is thought to reduce mortality for cancers of the breast and cervix. Its value in cancers of the colon, ovary, prostate, liver, or stomach, although widely discussed, has yet to be determined. Before screening has any general relevance we need reliable methods for assessing the malignant potential of the tumours discovered and a rational method of treatment—if treatment is required. Some of these problems are discussed in Chapter 21.

1.16 Experimental methods in cancer research

Much of our knowledge of the development and growth of tumours is derived from a close study of cancers in patients by clinicians and pathologists. This has allowed us to define many of the problems for which we should like to find answers, and, although the application of new techniques in cell and molecular biology to human tumours continues to provide us with valuable information, other methods have to be used to study changes that cannot be easily observed in humans. These include, for example, observations on cell behaviour in the very early stages of carcinogenesis, the direct effects of carcinogens on the genome, the direct effects of drugs on tumours, and so on. Although cancer is a disorder of cells, it is influenced by changes in the environment in the host, so that for experimental analysis we need methods that allow us to study the changes that occur in isolated cells as well as in the whole animal. We also need standardized methods for producing tumours, and for some purposes we need to transplant tumours into a new host to study the effects of a different environment on growth and behaviour.

1.16.1 Tumour induction and transplantation

The induction of tumours by giving or applying carcinogenic agents to animals is an essential experimental tool, not only for studying the process of carcinogenesis (see Chapters 6–8), but also for screening drugs or chemicals before use in humans or for industrial processes. For some purposes one needs samples of the same tumour for testing. The usual way to do this is to transplant the tumour into another animal. In ordinary populations there are large differences between individuals so that transplanted tumours (or normal tissues) are recognized as foreign by the new host and destroyed by the immune system. To avoid this, scientists have developed many 'pure line' (inbred) strains of mice. These mice have been selected and inbred for many generations so that each individual in the colony is essentially genetically identical with any other (syngeneic). Tumours and normal tissues in these animals can be transplanted easily. A further refinement is that tumours can now be specially prepared and stored frozen in ampoules in liquid nitrogen at $-193°C$ until needed for retransplantation into mice. Inbred strains particularly prone to develop a particular type of cancer, or with a particular sensitivity to carcinogens, have also been developed, so that the genetic basis for some tumours can be studied. For human tumours or tumours from species in which no inbred strains are available, transplants can be made into animals in which the immune system has been impaired by treatment or in which there is a congenital defect in the immune system. One group of mice that have a congenital defect of this type also show loss of hair. These 'nude' mice (*nu*) are used to maintain transplants of human and other tumours. Tumour or normal tissue grafts between individuals of the same species are allografts, between genetically identical individuals (e.g. identical twins or inbred strains) are isografts, and between foreign species (e.g. human tumour in nude mice) are xenografts. Unfortunately, not all tumours can be transplanted for reasons that are, so far, unknown.

1.16.2 Tissue culture techniques

For direct observation of tumour and normal cells isolated from their normal environment, tissue culture techniques are used. These methods allow studies on the direct effects of agents on living cells and the separation of different cell types from a mixed cell population, as well as the characterization of cell products. The most commonly used technique is cell culture, in which fragments of tissue, tumour, or separated cells are put into sterile glass or plastic containers in a fluid nutrient medium and maintained at body temperature in an incubator, in an atmosphere of air and carbon dioxide (usually 5 per cent) similar to that *in vivo*. If the cultures are successful, cells grow out from the explants and fill the container. They can then be removed and transplanted to other containers or treated for storage in liquid nitrogen. These populations are mixed, but single cells can be isolated and large numbers of genetically identical daughter cells (a clone) can be grown up from it and used for a more detailed study. Many tumour cell lines have been established and stored although only a small population of tumours will give rise to cell lines that can be maintained indefinitely. So far, normal cells can only be maintained for relatively short periods, but they have been used to study the induction of neoplastic transformation under closely controlled conditions. Cell culture can also be used to study the effects of drugs and of cells on each other (cell interactions). A modification of the technique allows pieces of tumour or normal tissue to be maintained in an organized form ('organ cultures'). This method is particularly useful for looking at the effects that involve more than one cell type, e.g. some hormone effects. Cell culture has proved to be an essential

basic technique for the development of modern cell and molecular biology, as will be seen later.

1.17 Experimental methods for tumour identification

Although the tissue diagnosis of most established tumours is usually straightforward using standard histological methods (see p. 9), there are still no absolute markers for malignant or premalignant cells, or methods for assessing the malignant potential (i.e. capacity for growth and spread) of tumours.

1.17.1 Histochemical methods

Refinements in microscopic techniques are sometimes of value. Histochemistry, in which chemical reactions are carried out on histological sections, is a technique that has still to be fully exploited. The precise cellular localization of enzyme reactions or tissue products can be established, and by using sensitive microfluorimeters or microspectrophotometers the amount of the end-product can be measured.

Tumour-specific and tumour-associated proteins can be identified by immunohistochemistry (see Chapters 13, 15, and 19) in which a specific antibody to a particular protein can be applied to cells or to tissue sections and the bound antibody visualized by a second reaction specific to the antibody itself. These methods have been of great value in identifying the cell types in tumours, particularly of the lymphoid system, and in identifying structural components in cells, such as the cytokeratins found in epithelial cells, vimentin and desmin found mainly in mesenchymal cells, and specific proteins found mainly in cells of the nervous system. A technique that is similar in principle, *in situ* hybridization, is also available for nucleic acids, using labelled probes specific for segments of nucleic acids or viruses (see Chapter 15). Histochemical techniques and *in situ* hybridization can be applied to light or electron microscope sections and the great virtues of these methods are that they allow the identification of small numbers of positive cells in a large mass of tissue, and also allow the precise intracellular localization to be established.

1.17.2 Other methods

Many other techniques for tumour identification are still being explored. Oncogene products are being studied as potential tumour markers. Nuclear magnetic resonance (NMR) is being used to study membrane changes in tumour cells (proton NMR) and for tumour detection in the clinic.

1.17.3 Methods for genetic analysis

Methods for family and population genetics are considered in Chapters 3 and 4, but a number of special techniques are needed for the analysis of genetic changes in cells. The development of these methods is responsible for the rapid increase in our knowledge of the structure of the mammalian genome. The ultimate aim is to define the chemical structure, order, and spacing of genes along the double helix that makes up the DNA, which contains the whole genome (see Chapter 5), and to identify alterations that are associated with abnormal function. Low resolution physical maps can be made by determining the appearance of individual chromosomes (karyotyping and banding), and specific genes can be localized to particular areas on individual chromosomes (see Chapter 10). Higher resolution maps can be determined by molecular analysis (see Chapters 5 and 9).

DNA function can be studied by transferring DNA (transfer or transfection) from one cell to another and observing any changes in function. The whole genome can be transferred by fusing two cells together (whole-cell fusion). Smaller amounts can be transferred by fragmenting the nucleus of the donor cell with chemicals and fusing the 'micro' cells that are produced (microcell fusion). Individual chromosomes can also be separated and transferred to other cells (chromosome-mediated gene transfer), as can pieces of separated DNA (DNA-mediated gene transfer). The methods used in gene mapping are reviewed by Bentley *et al.* (1988). The influence of the cytoplasm on cell functions is studied by a reciprocal technique, i.e. cytoplasm from which the nucleus has been removed is fused with another whole cell (cytoplast fusions).

1.18 Conclusions

It must be obvious from this survey that there are many gaps in our understanding of the phenomena that are concerned with the initiation and development of tumours. The succeeding chapters consider the present state of our knowledge and try to identify areas in which current research suggests that further studies may be profitable.

References and further reading

Alberts, B., Bray, D., Lewis, J., Raff, M., Roberts, K., and Watson, J. D. (ed.) (1994). *Molecular biology of the cell*, (4th edn). Garland Publishing, New York.

Ausubel, F. M., Brent, A., Kingston, R. E., Moore, D. D., Seidman, J. C., Smith, J. A., Struhel, K. (ed.) (1987). *Current protocols in molecular biology*. Wiley, New York. (A loose-leaf manual of techniques updated four times a year.)

Barker, D. J. P. (ed.) (1993). *Fetal and infant origins of adult disease*. British Medical Journal Books, London.

Beach, D., Stillman, B., and Watson, J. (ed.) (1991). *The cell cycle*. Cold Spring Harbor Symposia of Quantitative Biology, Vol. 56. Cold Spring Harbor Press, New York.

Bentley, K. L., Ferguson-Smith, A. C., and Ruddle, F. H. (1988). A review of genomic physical mapping. In *Somatic cell genetics and cancer*. Cancer Surveys, Vol. 7, No. 2, pp. 267–294. Oxford University Press, Oxford.

Cairns, J. (1975). The cancer problem. *Scientific American*, **233**, 64–78.

Cotran, R. S., Kumar, V., and Robbins, S. L. (1994). *Pathologic basis of disease*, (5th edn). W.B. Saunders, Philadelphia. (A good general text on pathology.)

DeVita, T., Hellman, S., and Rosenberg, S. A. (ed.) (1997). *Cancer*, (5th edn). J. B. Lippincott, Philadelphia. (A good general text on clinical aspects.)

Erlandson, R. A. (1994). *Diagnostic transmission electron microscopy of tumors*. Raven Press, New York.

Franks, L. M. and Wigley, C. B. (ed.) (1979). *Neoplastic transformation in differentiated epithelial cell systems in vitro*. Academic Press, London.

Freshney, R. I. (ed.) (1994). *Culture of animal cells*, (3rd edn). Alan R. Liss, New York. (A manual of basic techniques.)

Ghadially, F. N. (1988). *Ultrastructural pathology of the cell and matrix*, (3rd edn). Butterworth, London.

Knowles, D. (ed.) (1992). *Neoplastic hemopathology*. Williams and Wilkins, Baltimore.

Levine, A. J. (ed.) (1992). *Tumour suppressor genes, the cell cycle and cancer*, Cancer Surveys, Vol. 12. Cold Spring Harbor Press, New York.

Lodish, H., Baltimore, D., Berk, A., Zipursky, S. L., Matsudaira, P., and Darnell, J. (ed.) (1995). *Molecular cell biology*, (3rd edn). W.H. Freeman, New York.

Varmus, H. and Weinberg, R. A. (1993). *Genes and the biology of cancer*. Scientific American Library, New York.

Watson, J. D., Hopkins, N. H., and Roberts, J. W. (1987). *Molecular biology of the gene*, (4th edn). Benjamin-Cummings Publishers, San Francisco.

Watson, J. D., Gilman, M., Witkowski, J., and Zoller, M. (1992). *Recombinant DNA*. W.H. Freeman, New York.

Willis, R. A. (1967). *Pathology of tumours*, (4th edn). Butterworth, London. (Over 25 years old but still the best general text on tumour pathology.)

Specialized reviews

De Vita, V. T., Hellman, S., and Rosenberg, S. A. (ed.) *Important advances in oncology*. J. B. Lippincott/Harper & Row/Gower Medical Publishing. Published annually. Shorter reviews covering basic research and clinical aspects.

Hesketh, R. (1994). *The oncogene handbook*. Academic Press, London. A useful listing of known oncogenes.

Kastan, M. B. (ed.) (1997). *Checkpoint controls and Cancer*, Cancer Surveys, Vol. 29. Cold Spring Harbor Press, New York

Klein, G. and Weinhouse, S. (ed.) *Advances in cancer research*. Academic Press, San Diego. Published annually. Detailed reviews on individual topics.

Tooze, J. (ed.) *Cancer surveys*. Cold Spring Harbor Laboratory Press, New York. Published quarterly. Each issue provides an up-to-date review on a specific topic and covers clinical, experimental, and epidemiological aspects.

2

The spread of tumours

I. R. HART

2.1 Introduction

2.1.1 Significance of tumour spread

Metastasis is 'the transfer of disease from one organ or part to another not directly connected with it. It may be caused by the transfer of pathogenic organisms or the transfer of cells as in malignant tumours'. This transfer of cells is one of the fundamental problems of clinical oncology. Surgical removal, often combined with irradiation, is frequently successful in the treatment of primary tumours, but widespread dissemination often defeats this mode of treatment. Cancer spread is responsible for a large proportion of cancer deaths and the relentless and seemingly intractable movement from primary site to distant organs is a major factor in people's fear of neoplastic disease.

2.1.2 Pathogenesis of the process

Tumour dissemination is a complex process where the eventual outcome depends on the result of a number of interactions between the tumour cells and host cells. There are five major steps involved in metastasis, although it should be realized that the process is a dynamic one which may pass from one step to another without interruption, and a number of the steps will be operating concurrently. Following tumour development and growth there must be:

(1) invasion and infiltration of surrounding normal host tissue with penetration of small lymphatic or vascular channels;

(2) release of neoplastic cells, either as single cells or small clumps, into the circulation;

(3) survival in the circulation;

(4) arrest in the capillary beds of distant organs; and

(5) penetration of the lymphatic or blood vessel walls followed by growth of the disseminated tumour cells (Fig. 2.1).

If all these steps are completed, the result will be formation of a secondary tumour in a distant organ.

2.1.3 Tumour progression/evolution

As mentioned in Chapter 1, tumours do not necessarily come into being with all their characteristics already developed. This view of cancer as a static population of cells has been replaced by one in which they are seen as much more dynamic entities, where there is gradual acquisition of new characters as the tumour develops. This process has been termed tumour progression and, while there are exceptions, the general trend is for tumours to go from bad to worse. Thus, with tumour progression there is a movement towards a more aggressive behavioural pattern and the ability to invade and metastasize may not be manifested until relatively late in the course of neoplastic development. Some

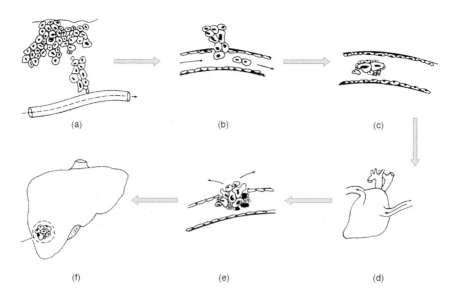

Fig. 2.1 The spread of malignant tumours. (a) Primary tumour invades and spreads into adjacent normal tissue, eventually coming into contact with small blood vessels or lymphatics. (b) These small vessels are penetrated by tumour cells which are released into the circulation. (c) In the circulation a number of interactions occur between the released tumour cells and circulating host cells, such as platelets, lymphocytes, and monocytes. (d) The passage of individual neoplastic cells or small emboli throughout the body is made possible by a number of junctions between the lymphatics and blood vessels; few tumour cells survive this passage. (e) Those tumour cells that survive must arrest in distant organs, possibly in mixed clumps containing both neoplastic cells and platelets or lymphocytes, breach the integrity of the vessel wall, and move out into the surrounding normal tissues. (f) Growth of such extravasating tumour cells gives rise to secondary tumour deposits (here shown growing in the liver) and the process may be repeated.

of the possible mechanisms involved in this process of evolution and progression will be discussed later in this chapter, but, for the present, it should be remembered that the fully malignant tumour cell, i.e. one that is able to invade and metastasize, may differ considerably in its character from a cell in the early stages of the transformation process.

2.2 Tumour angiogenesis

Growth of solid tumours beyond a size of approximately 2-mm diameter means that nutritional requirements of the cancer cannot be met solely by the process of diffusion. New capillary blood vessels, derived from pre-existing capillaries or venules, must be elicited from surrounding host tissue in what is termed the process of tumour angiogenesis, or neo-vascularization. The impetus for this ingrowth of columns of aligned endothelial cells, which anastamose with adjacent columns to form loops and a patent lumen, are so-called angiogenic peptides, which stimulate endothelial cell motility and proliferation. Many of these angiogenic peptides are produced and released by the neoplastic cells themselves, including vascular permeability factor or vascular endothelial growth factor (VEGF), while other peptides, such as transforming growth factor-α (TGF-α), may be produced by either the tumour cells or by infiltrating host cells like macrophages. Blocking or abrogation of the activity of these angiogenic peptides may well provide a novel approach to cancer therapy in future years. Indeed, it has been shown that antibodies specific to the VEGF peptide will inhibit the growth of different human tumour cell lines in recipient athymic mice, while having no such inhibitory effects on the cells under *in vitro* conditions (Kim *et al.* 1993).

Since the likelihood of metastasis occurring increases with increasing size of tumour mass in approximately 80 per cent of cancers, and since tumour growth is dependent in large measure on the provision of new blood vessel formation, it seems likely that a correlation exists between the occurrence of tumour spread and angiogenesis. Indeed, the counting of microvessel number in histological sections of tumour tissue has proven to be a strongly predictive marker of the probability of metastatic disease in breast cancer (Weidner *et al.* 1991; Gasparini *et al.* 1994). These findings suggest that the correlation between angiogenesis and metastatic risk is a strong one and that, if the causality of this relationship were understood better, interference with this association might prove to be one way of developing antimetastatic therapies.

2.3 Mechanisms of tumour invasion

Two of the five steps outlined in the pathogenesis of cancer spread depend on the ability of tumour cells to invade or infiltrate into areas of normal tissue. There is no evidence to show that the mechanisms used to gain access to the circulation are any different from the mechanisms used by the cells in moving out from the vessels in which they have become arrested, so that both steps will be considered together here.

In general, the mechanisms of tumour invasion are poorly understood, although the three most likely possibilities are that it occurs as a result of:

(1) mechanical pressure;

(2) release of lytic enzymes; and

(3) the increased motility of individual tumour cells.

Obviously, these mechanisms are not mutually exclusive and it is possible that in a given tumour any combination of the three may be involved and that the relative importance of each may vary depending on both the tumour type and its anatomical location. Equally, it should be noted that many normal cells, including leucocytes, trophoblasts, fibroblasts, and endothelial cells as mentioned above, are also invasive and can share many of these presumed mechanisms with tumour cells. The rapid proliferation of neoplastic cells may build up pressure which forces sheets, or fingers, of tumour cells along lines of least mechanical resistance in a manner somewhat analogous to the way that plants force their roots through the soil. Invasion, resulting from this phenomenon, is thus just a direct consequence of uncontrolled growth;

pressure from the growing mass occludes (blocks) local blood vessels, leading to local tissue death and a reduction in mechanical resistance, which further aids the process. While it is true that the gross appearance of many malignant tumours conforms with this picture, with finger-like projections of tumour cells emanating from the main growth, it is also true that there are many observations that cannot be explained solely by this suggested mechanism. Some highly invasive tumours grow more slowly than their benign counterparts; histological examinations often reveal clumps of neoplastic cells, which, in serial sections, reveal no connection with the main tumour, and cancer cells often invade and penetrate loose tissues where it would not seem to be possible to build up any pressure effect.

Areas of normal host tissue adjacent to areas of tumour invasion are often severely disrupted and show considerable amounts of lytic damage. Because many animal and human tumours have higher levels of proteases and collagenases than do corresponding benign or normal tissue, the concept that malignant tumours produce and secrete lytic enzymes that degrade normal tissue has become firmly established in the literature. However, technical difficulties have made any correlation between malignant behaviour and increased proteolytic enzyme activity difficult to interpret. Direct sampling of tissue (biopsy) may damage tissue and this may give rise to elevated levels of enzyme activity. Furthermore, tumours are not composed solely of neoplastic cells but contain both stromal and infiltrating reticuloendothelial cells. Many of the infiltrating cells, such as polymorphonuclear leucocytes and monocytes, contain high levels of those enzymes most likely to be involved in tissue degradation; indeed, their presence may well contribute to the eventual invasive behaviour of the tumour, either by releasing their own lytic enzymes or by behaving as inadvertent 'guides' for infiltrating neoplastic cells. Since the number of these infiltrating cells varies from tumour to tumour, or even between different parts of the same tumour, their contribution to overall enzyme activity also varies considerably.

Immunohistochemical staining for different collagenases and proteases has located many of these enzymes at the periphery of growing tumours, frequently at the sites of overt tissue damage and tumour cell invasion. However, the central portions of tumours are often necrotic and the peripheral staining observed may reflect the production of these enzymes by living cells rather than direct involvement in invasion. For these reasons, perhaps the most compelling evidence on the role of proteolytic enzymes in tumour invasion has come from experimental studies where it has proved possible to examine enzyme production by tumour cells grown in tissue culture and then to correlate this capacity with the subsequent invasive behaviour of the cells after transplantation into animals. Using this approach it was possible to establish positive correlations between invasion and high levels of the enzymes cathepsin B, type IV collagenase, and plasminogen activator. These correlations are not universal in as much as different researchers have found conflicting results depending on the tumour types used. While this lack of a simple answer may owe much to the use of different model systems and different tumour types, it may also reflect the fact that proteolysis is not the consequence of protease expression alone. Tumour cells not only produce proteolytic enzymes, like the members of the metalloproteinase family, but, at the same time, also produce inhibitors of these molecules, such as the so-called TIMPs (tissue inhibitors of metalloproteinases). These glycoprotein inhibitors bind to and inactivate both latent and active enzymes so that the net destructive activity of the cancer cell is the result of a balance between these opposing activities. and might vary not just from tumour type to tumour type but also within various microanatomical compartments. Recently clinical trials have begun in cancer patients using synthetic inhibitors of matrix metalloproteinases in the hope that these agents will block tumour cell invasion.

Whilst, as discussed above, immunochemistry has usually shown localization of proteolytic enzymes to nests of tumour cells, the results with *in situ* hybridization for the production of messenger RNA have revealed a very different picture. With many of the proteases examined to date it appears that the message is produced, not in the neoplastic cells, but in the adjacent stromal fibroblasts (Basset *et al.* 1990). These cells, presumably under the influence of proteins produced and secreted by the cancer cells, synthesize and secrete the proteolytic enzymes, which then are sequestered by the malignant tumour cells. How all this relates to our rather simplistic ideas derived from the analysis of only tumour cells in tissue culture awaits resolution, but it points

out the difficulty of trying to analyse these complex pathophysiological processes.

Evidence for the role of tumour cell motility in invasion is also equivocal. The finding of individual tumour cells or small clumps of tumour cells separate from the main tumour mass is difficult to explain without invoking the concept of tumour cell motility. Cinematography has been used to show that tumour cells in the body, as in tissue culture, are capable of active movement and migration. To what extent this ability is used in tumour invasion is unknown but it seems highly likely that the neoplastic cells do move through normal tissues by active locomotion. If motility does play a role in invasion, the next step is to determine to what extent such movement is directional in nature. Tumour cells in tissue culture can move towards substances that attract them (chemotactic factors), and changes in the surfaces on which they move may also affect the direction of movement. It is tempting to speculate that such mechanisms operate *in vivo*, but, because of the difficulties in assessing such responses in the whole animal, firm evidence is lacking. However, it is possible that this situation could be improved in the next few years because of some recent biochemical investigations. Liotta *et al.* (1986) at the National Cancer Institute in the United States have described the isolation and purification of a cell motility-stimulating molecule, which they have termed autocrine motility factor (AMF). This 54-kilodalton (kDa) protein, first isolated from human melanoma cell lines, stimulates random motility of transformed cells but does not stimulate the motility of their untransformed counterparts. Further studies have shown that AMF is produced by, and stimulates a response in, a variety of neoplastic cells and it has even been detected in the urine of patients with transitional cell carcinoma of the bladder. Thus it is likely that the production of a motility factor by a tumour cell could play a major role in the local invasive behaviour of cancer. Certainly, with the availability of complementary DNA (cDNA) probes for *in situ* hybridizations, and monoclonal antibodies for immunohistochemistry, there will be opportunities to examine material from a wide range of invasive tumours to determine the extent of any correlation between AMF production and infiltrative behaviour. An even more exciting prospect is the possibility that blocking the response to AMF, or inhibiting the production of AMF, could lead to an inhibition of the invasive process, with resultant therapeutic gains. Liotta (see Hart 1988) has reported that just such an inhibitor has profoundly affected the number of spontaneous metastases arising from a murine sarcoma. The generality, or indeed the likely significance of this observation, remains to be verified, but it illustrates the underlying rationale for many investigations into the mechanisms of cancer spread; i.e. an improved understanding of the pathogenesis of the process at the molecular level will lead to the design of new methods of treatment.

AMF is not the only 'motility factor' known to be produced by or to act upon tumour cells. Where the mitogenic molecules AMF, migration-stimulating factor (MSF), and scatter factor/hepatocyte growth factor (HGF) act, and how they regulate tumour cell movement, requires careful and prolonged investigation but it seems probable that they control an important part of tumour cell activity.

It should be pointed out that tissues vary considerably in their ability to withstand tumour invasion. Tumours rarely penetrate the walls of arteries, arterioles, or even the larger veins, while they readily invade capillaries and lymphatics. Such resistance is due, in part, to the greater mechanical strength of the larger vessels but there is also a suggestion that certain of the tissues resistant to invasion, such as cartilage or the elastic fibres that surround the larger vessels, are resistant because they release antiproteolytic factors which inhibit proteases.

Such a mechanism is thought to be involved in the well-known, although not universally accepted, observation that cirrhotic livers are more resistant to metastatic involvement than are the normal organs. It has been reported (Barsky and Gopalakrishna 1988) that myofibroblasts (the cells involved in the collagenous bands found in cirrhosis) secrete a metalloproteinase inhibitor which not only inhibits the activity of type I and type IV collagenases, but also prevents the invasive behaviour of human tumour cells in an *in vitro* assay of tumour cell invasion. This, it is argued, is why cirrhotic livers exhibit a strong resistance to metastasis as evident in post-mortem analyses. The presence of these factors in tissues with a natural resistance to invasion provides further support for the idea that proteolytic enzymes may play a role in mediating tumour spread.

2.4 Dissemination of tumour cells via lymphatics and/or blood vessels

Once tumour cells enter the lumen of lymphatic or blood vessels, either they remain at the site of penetration and grow there, with consequent occlusion of the vessel, or they release cells which are carried away in the lymph or blood. The release of individual cells or small emboli (clumps) has led to the suggestion that the cells of malignant tumours are less strongly attached to each other than cells of benign tumours and are more readily detached from the primary mass. The molecular basis of this reduction in tumour cohesiveness is thought to relate to the down regulation of active homotypic (i.e. like binding to like) cell adhesion molecules (CAMs), which is often observed in metastatic cells (Reeves 1992). For example, E-cadherin, a member of the cadherin family of calcium-dependent CAMs, has been shown to be expressed to a much reduced extent in more aggressive, less differentiated, colorectal tumours, which have a poorer prognosis (Dorudi *et al.* 1993). This reduction in cell to cell adhesion activity need not be a result solely of down regulation at the messenger RNA level. For example, mutations in the cadherin ligand-binding sites, or even in the catenins, proteins that connect the cytoplasmic domains of the cadherins to the internal cellular cytoskeleton, could also cause loss of function in these cell–cell adhesion molecules.

It is a common clinical observation that carcinomas, which are epithelial in origin, generally spread in the lymphatic system as well as in the blood, while sarcomas of mesenchymal origin appear to spread by the haematogenous route. However, this may be an arbitrary division. There are connections between the lymphatics and the blood vessels, and radiolabelled, circulating tumour cells have been shown to be capable of moving between these two systems, either through direct venolymphatic communications (anastomoses) or from the lymphatics into the thoracic duct, which empties into the jugular vein and the venous circulation. The preferential involvement of the lymph nodes with metastatic carcinoma may be a reflection of organ-specific growth rather than a tendency to infiltrate specifically one system only. Alternatively, it may be that there is a greater concentration of lymphatics in epithelial structures and a greater increase in the likelihood that these vessels, rather than blood vessels, will be penetrated.

In this chapter, the spread of tumours either by the lymphatics or by the haematogenous route will be considered as a common process. From clinical observations and from experimental studies it is known that the mere presence of neoplastic cells in the circulation does not constitute metastasis. The process is inefficient and most of the cells released into the circulation die without forming a metastatic deposit. The death of many of the released cancer cells may be attributable to the controlling influence of the host's immune response but much may simply be the result of non-specific factors such as turbulence. The environment in the circulation is generally thought of as being hostile to disseminating tumour cells, but some of the interactions to which cells are exposed may aid their survival. Aggregation, either with other tumour cells or with host cells such as lymphocytes and platelets, may result in the formation of larger emboli (particles in the bloodstream), which are more easily filtered out in distant capillary beds. Surrounding the tumour cells by aggregating blood cells may also provide a protective outer layer, which prevents damage to the central tumour cells.

To leave the circulation, cells must be arrested and implant in the capillary bed of an organ. Generally, tumour cells do not adhere to the walls of the large vessels, where, presumably, blood flow is sufficiently vigorous to sweep away attaching cells. Even though tumour cells can be deformed (are not rigid) and can pass through capillaries of narrower bore than their resting diameter, it is in the capillary bed that the cells are generally arrested. This arrest may be owing to passive filtering, as in the case of emboli rather than individual cells, or it may represent an active process. It can be shown that tumour cells, like platelets, do not adhere well to intact, quiescent endothelium, but attach preferentially to exposed basement membrane. Tissue culture studies suggest that the tumour cells themselves might stimulate endothelial cell retraction and loss, although the shedding of endothelial cells from the wall is a normal physiological process and the basement membrane is frequently being exposed at various sites in the vascular system. Some proteins, such as fibronectin and laminin, are involved in the attachment of normal cells to each other and to basement membrane and may also play a part in determining both the specificity and the kinetics of tumour cell attachment. Endothelial damage leads to platelet adherence and the tumour cell–platelet clumps may attach passively to the areas of endothelial retrac-

tion; arrest of the circulating neoplastic cell could then occur in the absence of any active ability or proclivity to attach to basement membrane. Equally, it is possible that disseminating tumour cells might leave endothelial cells in an unretracted state but, through the release of cytokines which cause increased expression of a variety of cell surface-located adhesion molecules, modify their capacity to interact with and arrest these migrating cells.

A family of cell surface receptors termed the integrins (involved in a variety of functions including cell adhesion, migration during embryogenesis, thrombosis, and lymphocyte function) (see Juliano 1987) has been identified based on the ability of these receptor molecules to recognize glycoprotein ligands (see Glossary) bearing the amino acid sequence Arg–Gly–Asp, known as the RGD motif. Many tumour cells express integrin-like receptors at their cell surface, and it is considered likely that a good fraction of the tumour cell–basement membrane interactions are mediated by these molecules. The integrins may, on occasion, also serve as cell–cell adhesion molecules and in this respect it is interesting that $\alpha_4\beta_1$, an integrin that is expressed at a higher level by more malignant, compared with more benign, melanoma tumours, serves to mediate cell binding to V-CAM. This latter molecule is an inducible member of the immunoglobulin superfamily expressed on the surface of 'activated' endothelium and therefore the $\alpha_4\beta_1$–V-CAM interaction may be responsible for attachment of metastatic melanoma cells in distant capillary beds. Much interest has been generated by the demonstration that Arg–Gly–Asp-containing synthetic peptides can block both invasion *in vitro* and the formation of lung tumour nodules in mice coinjected with tumour cells and the inhibitory peptides (Gehlsen *et al.* 1988). It is unlikely that this represents a possible therapeutic approach since it is true that such peptides have a very short half-life in the circulation, that attachment sites other than the RGD site may be utilized by disseminating cancer cells, that the peptides have to be used at very high plasma levels, and that, at the time of presentation, many cancer patients will already have established micrometastases and so have passed the stage at which such treatments might be beneficial. None the less, as with the abrogation of AMF activity discussed earlier in this chapter, these types of approaches highlight the value of an understanding of the mechanisms of tumour spread in trying to design novel therapeutic agents.

The binding of solid cancer cells to endothelium or to basement membranes underlying endothelium is a phenomenon very reminiscent of the way in which lymphocytes/leucocytes bind to and pass through endothelium at sites of inflammation. Not surprisingly, therefore, it is thought that those molecules that regulate this process in normal situations might also be involved in the pathological events of tumour spread. Evidence confirming such a comparability was provided by the elegant work of Gunthert and her colleagues (1991) in studies on the molecule called CD44. This lymphocyte-homing receptor was found to exist as a different isoform, resulting from the process of RNA splicing, in rodent tumours possessing the capacity to metastasize. Subsequent work has shown that similar isoform expression occurs in human tumours and it has even been suggested that the presence of this alternatively spliced molecule may be diagnostic of those human cancers with the propensity for metastatic behaviour (Matsumura and Tarin 1992). Whether or not this association is shown to be a consistent finding in a larger series of tumours, these results point out the probable importance of cell adhesion receptors in tumour cell arrest, and possibly underscore their role in determining patterns of metastatic spread (see below).

2.5 Patterns of metastatic spread

Some tumours often metastasize to particular organs. Thus osteosarcomas normally give rise to pulmonary metastases, whereas neuroblastomas most commonly spread to the liver. The reason for this organ selectivity is unknown but two hypotheses have been proposed In the 'mechanistic theory' the eventual site of metastasis development is a consequence of the anatomical location of a primary tumour; the number of viable tumour cells delivered to the capillary bed in the first organ encountered is a consequence of the pattern of blood flow. For example, the venous blood flow from the large bowel goes to the liver through the portal veins and, perhaps as a consequence, the liver is the commonest site for secondary deposits from bowel tumours. Whilst this is undoubtedly true for some tumours, it does not explain all patterns of tumour spread. Muscle is well vascularized and the kidney receives up to 25 per cent of cardiac blood output, yet both these organs are infrequently involved in metastasis formation.

Almost one hundred years ago, Paget suggested the 'seed and soil' hypothesis, wherein the provision of a fertile environment (the soil) in which compatible tumour cells (the seed) could grow was the determining factor in deciding metastatic sites. Failure of an organ to develop metastases was not a consequence of the failure of disseminating cells to reach that site, but was because of the inability of the organ to provide a favourable environment for growth. This hypothesis, perfectly suited to the Victorian era, with its biblical overtones of seeds falling on stony ground, has received strong support in recent years both from experimental results and clinical studies on the use of shunts to relieve extensive exudation of fluid in the peritoneal cavity (ascites) in terminally ill patients with abdominal cancers. Many of these patients produce considerable volumes of fluid in the abdomen leading to marked distress and discomfort; relief can be obtained by withdrawal of this fluid (paracentesis), but the procedure often needs to be repeated, often almost daily. To provide such patients with relief from this unpleasant consequence of their tumours, it has proved possible to insert an artificial shunt from the abdomen into the jugular vein; fluid is thus continually returned to the venous circulation and the uncomfortable build up of ascites is avoided. Within the ascitic fluid are large numbers of viable tumour cells and returning them to the jugular veins means the first capillary bed encountered is that located in the lungs. In spite of this, many patients who survive with this treatment for a number of weeks or more show no evidence of pulmonary metastases, even though many millions of viable cells have been passed into their lungs where, according to the mechanistic theory of metastasis development, they should have been filtered out of the circulation. Whilst these results are most compatible with the 'seed–soil' hypothesis, there is no information on the number of cells retained in the lung and thus the evidence, although suggestive, is not confirmatory.

In recent years considerable attention has focused on the possible role of autocrine/paracrine (see Chapter 11) control of tumour cell proliferation in the development of neoplasia. Certainly, it is possible that the local production of paracrine factors by specific organs, either mitogens or inhibitors of cell proliferation, or the stimulation of autocrine growth factor production and release by the tumour cells themselves in response to organ-derived signals, could have profound effects on patterns of metastatic involvement. The likely complexity of this type of growth regulation is underscored by the fact that peptide growth factors may inhibit or stimulate proliferative activity of different cell types, or may even have conflicting activities on a single cell type depending on the nature of other signal molecules present. Unravelling the factors involved in the metastatic patterns of specific tumours is likely to be a difficult task, but with the availability of increasing numbers of recombinant-derived peptide growth factors considerable insight into this aspect of tumour biology should be gained in the next few years.

One adjunct to this direct regulation of tumour cell growth, which could also be involved in determining metastatic patterns, is organ-related control of angiogenesis (see Section 2.2). It is possible that organ-specific variations exist in levels of some of these angiogenic factors, although evidence to confirm such an hypothesis is lacking at the present time. Many of the angiogenic factors, such as the fibroblast growth factors (FGFs), are distributed so ubiquitously throughout the body that, at first sight, they appear to be unlikely candidates for organ-related activity. However, some of these factors appear to be maintained in a functionally inactive state, either sequestered within the cells of origin or stored in the extracellular matrix, and the activation signal, possibly provided by the tumour cells themselves, might be organ specific and so account for preferential growth. It is also possible that a third mechanism may be responsible for determining site-specific metastasis. It has been suggested that there are specific interactions between cell surface proteins of tumour cells and organ-specific proteins on the endothelial cells lining the capillaries or the exposed basement membrane in the capillary beds of different organs (see Section 2.4). Metastasis in this instance would not be the result of the increased delivery of tumour cells to the organ but of enhanced retention by selective adhesion. Certainly, lymphocyte recirculation, a process that might be considered analogous to many of the steps in the dissemination pathway, is dependent on just such a specific interaction between cell surface molecules on the peripatetic lymphocyte and the endothelial cells lining the vessels of the lymphoid system. It is possible that variations in specificity of expression of the various matrix receptors of the integrin family (see above) in response to

signals from the cell's environment could modulate the attachment behaviour of metastatic cells. Again, results are likely to come from experimental model systems and their significance has to be assessed by the difficult process of extrapolating to clinical observations.

2.6 The role of the immune system in modulating metastasis

The immune system reacts against foreign proteins either by direct attack by cells of the system or by the production of soluble antibodies against the proteins. The influence of the immune system on tumour growth is complicated and is discussed in detail in Chapter 16. As far as metastasis is concerned, it must be noted that the process occurs in the presence of a mass of antigenic material, i.e. the primary tumour, so that this phenomenon might be thought to be highly susceptible to immune modulation. Results from experimental systems have confirmed this idea and have shown that the immune system can exert a profound influence on the eventual outcome of the metastatic process. Interestingly, the immune system does not always exert an inhibitory effect on tumour spread but acts as a 'double-edged' sword. Thus, lymphocyte aggregation with circulatory tumour cells can increase the size of emboli and assist in their arrest and lodgement. Furthermore, lymphocytes are capable of inducing angiogenesis and may facilitate the provision of nutrients to a proliferating secondary tumour.

A subpopulation of lymphocytes, termed NK (natural killer) cells (see Chapter 16), has been implicated as being of great importance in regulating metastatic spread in experimental animals. Athymic nude mice have high levels of these cells and it has been suggested that the known infrequency of metastatic spread of allogeneic and xenogeneic tumours implanted into these mice might be attributable directly to the efficacy of the NK cell system. Suppression of NK cell activity by various techniques has led to enhanced metastasis of certain tumours; although, to repeat a refrain that is becoming very familiar in this chapter, there appear to be no simple generalizations that can be drawn from such experiments, since in other experimental systems the effect of NK cell depletion on metastasis seems to be minimal. It is a reasonable assumption that those tumour cells that have managed to survive the circulation have successfully avoided, or subverted, immune surveillance mechanisms. The molecular basis of such avoidance strategies has received increasing attention in recent years.

Cytotoxic T lymphocytes recognize foreign antigens only in association with major histocompatibility (MHC) class I cell surface antigens. Consequently, one way in which metastatic cells could avoid a T cell immune response is by a selective deficiency in MHC class 1 antigen expression. Much work has been aimed at examining this question in murine transplantable tumours but there are also some limited immunohistochemical studies on human material that support this concept. However, suppression of MHC class I gene expression is not likely to be the sole determinant in the balance between tumour cells and host immunity.

Recent work has shown that two types of signal are required to initiate a T cell response, and while one signal is provided by interaction of the T cell receptor with peptides presented by the MHC, the second signal is generated by a costimulator molecule, such as B7, which interacts with other receptors on the T cell. Tumour cells may evade an immune response, therefore, not only through a lack of expression of the MHC class 1 genes, but also through a lack of expression of the costimulatory molecules.

Class I antigens and costimulatory molecules are not the only cell surface molecules involved in determining immune cell–cell interactions. Thus a variety of surface proteins on both lymphocytes and the target cell, termed lymphocyte function-associated antigens (LFAs) (see Chapter 16), which have been assigned membership of the integrin superfamily of adhesion molecules discussed above, serve to stabilize the adhesion reactions necessary for conjugate formation, which leads to cell lysis. It is conceivable, therefore, that aberrations in the expression of such molecules, or the ligands for such molecules, by the tumour target cells will lead to alterations in cytotoxicity which could be reflected by increased survival of disseminating cells. Again, the availability of molecular probes should go a long way to answering such questions in the next few years.

Mononuclear phagocytes also appear to play a role in determining metastatic spread. Correlations have been established between the macrophage content of a series of tumours of similar histological origin and an inability to metastasize. Differences in absolute numbers of macrophages found in metastasizing or non-metastasizing tumours may be matched by differences in the functional capacity of such infiltrating cells. Thus, there are reports that macrophages isolated from non-metastasizing or regressing tumours are cytotoxic, whereas macrophages from progressing/metastasizing tumours are non-cytotoxic or may even stimulate tumour growth. Additionally, circulating monocytes are cytotoxic to various tumour cells *in vitro* and if these cells are capable of exerting such effects *in vivo* it is possible that, in conjunction with NK cells, they may make a significant contribution to the elimination of circulating tumour cells.

The exact role of humoral (antibody-mediated) immunity in the modulation of metastasis is no clearer than that of the cell-mediated arm of the immune system. Once again it would seem evident that any tumour capable of evoking a humoral immune response would be more susceptible to such a response while circulating as individual cells or as small emboli. Antibodies directed against tumour antigens have been identified in many experimental tumour systems and against a few naturally occurring human tumours. In cases of human melanoma there is a strong suggestion that the presence of circulating antibody correlates with the absence of metastasis. Antibody plus complement (see Glossary) may lead to direct lysis of circulating cells or may facilitate removal of such cells by mononuclear phagocytes. Physical coating of the cells with antibody might interfere with certain of the steps in the metastatic sequence, such as aggregation or adherence. Much more work remains to be done before any definite conclusions can be drawn. Recent work identifying and cloning specific tumour antigens has focused on the use of cloned T cell lines to isolate these molecules, thus suggesting that the cell-mediated arm of the immune system may be the more important one in modifying tumour behaviour. However, the availability of these antigens should now go a long way towards resolving these questions.

2.7 Tumour cell heterogeneity

2.7.1 Differences between primary and secondary tumours

Not all cells in a single tumour are identical, but there is a range of population of cells expressing many different characters (phenotypes). Cells in a tumour may show differences in structure, e.g. morphology, growth rate, karyotype (chromosome pattern), or behaviour (e.g. invasion and metastasis). This diversity is a consequence of tumour progression and some of the possible mechanisms involved in generating this diversity will be discussed below. The concept of heterogeneity is accepted by most pathologists, biologists, and clinical oncologists. What is far more contentious is the idea, developed from experiments with transplantable rodent tumours, that metastases are derived from pre-existing subpopulations of cells in the primary tumour. Metastasis is an inefficient process and the majority of tumour cells released into the circulation do not give rise to secondary tumours. Do those few cells that survive do so fortuitously in a completely random manner, or is metastasis a selective process that allows the emergence of a pre-existent subpopulation of cells? Presumably, such cells would possess certain characteristics that differ from those of the majority of cells. If only a few cells are capable of metastasizing then therapy should be targeted against those cells; the vast mass of cells in the tumour would not be life threatening. Again, evidence for and against this concept comes from experimental studies because of the difficulties of analysing such characteristics in human tumours.

Some workers have been able to show that cells derived from metastases are more metastatic than cells from the primary tumour, whereas others, working with different tumour systems, have been unable to demonstrate this phenomenon. It seems highly likely that the process is a combination of both elements. If metastasis was entirely selective then it could be demonstrated in animal systems by the repeated selection of metastatic cells until 100 per cent efficiency was obtained; the injection of 100 metastatic cells should then lead to an eventual tumour burden of 100 metastatic nodules. This has never been achieved, even after selection; metastasis remains inefficient probably because it is largely a random event where the destruction and elimination of circulating tumour cells is haphazard, regardless of whether cells are capable of forming metastatic tumours or not. There is, however, a selective aspect to the process, which is why metastatic variants can be isolated from heterogeneous populations of cells both by selection techniques and by cloning procedures. This could help to explain why there are many examples in the litera-

ture of differences between primary tumours and their metastases in terms of enzyme levels, karyotypes, drug sensitivity, and cellular oncogenes. Alternatively, since tumours are known to be heterogeneous, it is possible that the selection for these differences is fortuitous and is not associated with the process of metastasis *per se*. Whether metastatic deposits in cancer patients are the result of the proliferation of selected subpopulations of cells would seem to be the most important question in the pathogenesis of cancer spread.

2.7.2 Epigenetic and genetic mechanisms for generating phenotypic diversity

Since tumours are so obviously heterogeneous for a wide variety of characteristics, what is the source of this diversity? Studies based on individual markers in leukaemias and lymphomas have shown that these cancers appear to be almost universally monoclonal in origin, i.e. descended from a single transformed cell; the situation in the solid tumours is less clear-cut and there is a certain amount of evidence to suggest that some carcinomas might be multicellular in origin. Even if such tumours are monoclonal in origin, by the time of presentation in the clinic tumour progression and the generation of diversity has occurred. To explain this diversity Nowell (1976) suggested that the transition from normal to transformed cell carried with it the acquisition of inherent genetic instability. This genetic instability, he suggested, allowed transformed cells to mutate at a higher rate than normal cells so that new variants were being produced continuously (see Chapter 10). Many of these variants would be eliminated by metabolic or immunological mechanisms, but certain of these variants would possess selective growth advantages and these clones would grow to dominate the tumour populations. Sequential selection over time would lead to the emergence of sublines, which would be increasingly abnormal both genetically and biologically. Genetic alterations occurring in progressing tumours could range from point mutations to gross aberrations such as loss or gain of complete chromosomes. These topics are discussed in more detail in Chapter 10. Certainly the malignant solid human cancers, which are able to metastasize, commonly show a degree of aneuploidy (variation in chromosome number) and mitotic variation. The hypothesis that neoplastic cells have greater genetic instability and mutate at a faster rate than normal cells has been tested experimentally. The measurement of mutation rates at different sites (loci) in the cellular genetic material (genome) has shown that, in experimental tumours, transformed cells are more genetically unstable than their normal counterparts. A similar change appears to accompany the transition from low to high metastatic activity. This last observation may help to explain how metastatic cells develop from the original tumour cell population, but, as with many findings in cancer research, it raises many new questions.

The mechanisms by which these alterations in gene activity may influence tumour growth and metastasis may include overexpression of normal gene products, gene amplification, or mutation (aberration in gene structure and function). Alternatively, epigenetic (non-genetic mechanisms altering gene expression) factors may be responsible for changes in metastatic behaviour. These mechanisms are discussed in detail elsewhere (Chapters 9 and 10) but active research in this field is opening up exciting possibilities, not only in the general area of tumour growth, but also, possibly, in understanding the process of metastasis.

2.8 Experimental models/approaches to metastasis

It is apparent that, in concrete terms, relatively little is known about the exact molecular mechanisms underlying tumour spread. In part this is a reflection of the complexity of the process and the fact that tumours of all types may not use identical mechanisms. It also reflects the difficulties involved in studying a dynamic process by means of essentially static observations. There is a wealth of data gathered on naturally occurring tumours in humans from histological, surgical, and autopsy procedures. Many of the mechanisms likely to be involved have been inferred from these observations rather than by direct demonstration through experimental analysis. Biochemical studies on material from primary and secondary tumours obtained at the same time is often difficult because of problems in obtaining the material, so considerable reliance has to be placed on the use of transplantable tumours in experimental animals to study the process of metastasis.

There are many advantages, and not a few disadvantages, associated with these animal models. The advantages arise from the ability to standardize procedures and the ease with which tumour cells growing as implants or as cell lines in tissue culture can be manipulated. The major disadvantage of the models is that the majority of the tumours represented are of mesenchymal origin, since these cells grow more readily in tissue culture, whereas, as pointed out in Chapter 1, the vast majority of human solid cancers are epithelial in origin. Information derived from studies on mesenchymal cells may not be directly applicable to epithelial cells and there is a great need for the development of more realistic models of tumour spread (see Chapter 6). It may be that the use of epithelial lines of human tumour cells injected into athymic nude mice will provide such models. Notwithstanding these reservations about currently available transplantable tumour systems, it is true that a considerable amount of information has been derived from experimental studies and much of this has come about because of awareness of the cellular heterogeneity existing in tumours. While there has been some controversy over whether or not metastatic subpopulations of cells do pre-exist in the parental tumour, there is no doubt that general acceptance of this concept has led to the development of some powerful experimental tools. From a single parental tumour one can isolate sublines or variants that exhibit different metastatic capacities. When these differences are relatively stable, comparisons can be made between the variants to determine factors responsible for these phenotypic differences. Comparisons between metastatic and non-metastatic tumours of different origin, a situation somewhat akin to comparing apples and oranges, are thus avoided.

These matched lines of varying metastatic capacity have been used in the preparation and differential screening of cDNA libraries. This technique, which is limited to the detection of mRNA transcripts constituting > 0.01 per cent of the total mRNA population, has resulted in the identification of a number of genes which are either up or down regulated in expression between the variants. Such an approach has identified the variant CD44 isoform discussed earlier (see p. 27), metalloproteinases, and the adhesive glycoprotein fibronectin. However, perhaps the most interesting and exciting gene implicated in regulating tumour spread, which has been identified by this differential hybridization procedure, is the *nm23* gene identified by Steeg and her colleagues (Steeg *et al.* 1988). This gene, *nm23*, codes for a protein that has sequence homology with a developmentally regulated protein in *Drosophila* (the abnormal wing disc or *awd* gene). Mutations in *awd* cause abnormal tissue morphology in *Drosophila* and lend credence to the idea that loss of genes like *nm23/awd*, which normally regulate development rather than the acquisition of expression, is the mechanism underlying the achievement of the metastatic state (Rosengard *et al.* 1989). Clinical support for the relevance of this gene comes from the demonstration of low levels of *nm23* RNA in human breast carcinomas of more aggressive behaviour (Bevilacqua *et al.* 1989). Future studies that focus upon these differences between metastatic and non-metastatic tumours are likely to shed increasing light on this area of tumour behaviour.

2.9 Summary

Tumour metastasis is the aspect of cancer biology responsible for the majority of tumour-related deaths. Understanding the molecular basis of the mechanisms underlying this phenomenon is important, not only in terms of intellectual satisfaction, but also because it may offer new approaches to therapy.

References and further reading

Barsky, S. H. and Gopalakrishna, R. (1988). High metalloproteinase inhibitor content of human cirrhosis and its possible conference of metastasis resistance. *Journal of the National Cancer Institute*, **80**, 102–8.

Basset, P., Bellocq, J. P., Wolf, C., Stoll, I., Hutin, P., Limacher, J. M., Podhajcer, O. L., Chenard, M. P., Rio, M. C., Chambon, P. (1990). A novel metalloproteinase gene specifically expressed in stromal cells of breast carcinomas. *Nature*, **348**, 699–704.

Bevilacqua, G., Sobel, M. E., Liotta, L. A., and Steeg, P. S. (1989). Association of low nm23 RNA levels in human primary infiltrating ductal breast carcinomas with lymph node involvement and other histopathological indicators of high metastatic potential. *Cancer Research*, **49**, 5185–90.

Dorudi, S., Sheffield, J. P., Poulsom, R., Northover, J. M., Hart, I. R. (1993). E-cadherin expression in colorectal cancer. An immunocytochemical and in situ hybridization study. *American Journal of Pathology*, **142**, 981–6.

Fearon, E. R., Cho, K. R., Nigro, J. M., Kern, S. E., Simons, J. W., Ruppert, J. M., Hamilton, S. R. *et al.* (1990). Identification of a chromosome 18q gene that is altered in colorectal cancers. *Science*, **247**, 49–56.

Fidler, I. J., Gersten, D. M., and Hart, I. R. (1978). The biology of cancer invasion and metastasis. *Advances in Cancer Research*, **28**, 149–205.

Gasparini, G., Weidner, N., Bevilacqua, P., Maluta, S., Dalla-Palma, P., Caffo, O., Barbareschi, M., Boracchi, P., Marubini, E., Pozza, F. (1994). Tumor microvessel density, p53 expression, tumor size and peritumoral lymphatic invasion are relevant prognostic markers in node-negative breast carcinoma. *Journal of Clinical Oncology*, **12**, 454–66.

Gehlsen, K. R., Argraves, W. S., Piersbacher, M. D., and Ruoslahti, E. (1988). Inhibition of in vitro tumor cell invasion by ArgGlyAsp-containing synthetic peptides. *Journal of Cell Biology*, **106**, 925–30.

Gunthert, U., Hofmann, M., Rudy, W., Reber, S., Zoller, M., Haussmann, I., Matzku, S., Wenzel, A., Ponta, H., Herrlich, P. (1991). A new variant of glycoprotein CD44 confers metastatic potential to rat carcinoma cells. *Cell*, **65**, 13–24.

Hart, I. R. (ed.) (1988). Tumour progression and metastasis. *Cancer Surveys*, Vol. 7, No. 4. Oxford University Press, Oxford.

Hart, I. R. and Saini, A. (1992). Biology of tumour metastasis. *Lancet*, **339**, 1453–7.

Juliano, R. L. (1987). Membrane receptors for extracellular matrix macromolecules: relationship to cell adhesion and tumour metastasis. *Biochimica et Biophysica Acta*, **907**, 261–78.

Kim, K. J., Li, B., Winer, J., Armanini, M., Gillett, N., Phillips, H. S., Ferrara, N. (1993). Inhibition of vascular endothelial growth factor-induced angiogenesis suppresses tumour growth in vivo. *Nature*, **362**, 841–4.

Liotta, L. A. and Hart, I. R. (ed.) (1982). *Tumour invasion and metastasis*. Martinus Nijhoff, The Hague.

Liotta, L. A., Mandler, R., Murano, G., Katz, D. A., Gordon, R. K., Chiang, P. K., Schiffmann, E. (1986). Tumor cell autocrine motility factor. *Proceedings of the National Academy of Sciences, USA*, **83**, 3302–6.

Matsumura, Y. and Tarin, D. (1992). Significance of CD44 gene products for cancer diagnosis and disease evaluation. *Lancet*, **340**, 1053–8.

Nowell, P. C. (1976). The clonal evolution of tumour cell populations. *Science*, **194**, 23–8.

Prehn, R. T. (1976). Do tumors grow because of the immune response of the host? *Transplantation Reviews*, **28**, 34–42.

Reeves, M. E. (1992). A metastatic tumour cell line has greatly reduced levels of a specific homotypic cell adhesion molecule activity. *Cancer Research*, **52**, 1546–52.

Rosengard, A. M., Krutzsch, H. C., Shearn, A., Biggs, J. R., Barker, E., Margulies, I. M., King, C. R., Liotta, L. A., Steeg, P. S. (1989). Reduced NM23/awd protein in tumour metastasis and aberrant *Drosophila* development. *Nature*, **342**, 177–80.

Steeg, P. S., Bevilacqua, G., Kopper, L., Thorgeirsson, U. P., Talmadge, J. E., Liotta, L. A., Sobel, M. E. (1988). Evidence for a novel gene associated with low tumor metastatic potential. *Journal of the National Cancer Institute*, **80**, 200–4.

Weidner, N., Semple, J. P., Welch, W. R., and Folkman, J. (1991). Tumour angiogenesis and metastasiscorrelation in invasive breast carcinoma. *New England Journal of Medicine*, **324**, 1–8.

Willis, R. A. (1972). *The spread of tumours in the human body*. Butterworth, London.

3

Epidemiology of cancer

T. KEY, D. FORMAN, AND M. C. PIKE

3.1 Introduction

Cancer epidemiology is the study of the pattern of cancer in populations and is predominantly statistical, its methods and conclusions being expressed in terms of probabilities; for example, 'Japanese women have less than a quarter the breast cancer risk of US women' or 'women who have a baby before age 20 have only half the chance of getting breast cancer of women without children'. Its primary objective, in the area of public health, is to identify preventable (avoidable) causes of cancer, but it also has an important role in other areas of cancer research; for example, in the evaluation of screening tests to detect cancer at an early stage and in aiding the understanding of the mechanistic basis of cancer.

The most basic task of cancer epidemiology is simply to describe the occurrence of human cancer, noting differences between, for example, males and females, people of different ages, different socioeconomic classes, people in different occupations, different time periods, different areas of a country, and different countries. This descriptive epidemiology has been a most fruitful source of ideas as to the possible causes of various cancers. For example, the enormous rise of lung cancer in men, but not in women, between 1920 and 1945 suggested that some recently introduced habit of men, but not of women, must be responsible, and cigarette smoking

became the prime candidate. More recently the finding of large differences in the occurrence of colorectal cancer between different countries has led to intense investigation of the possible roles of various aspects of the normal diet (such as fat or fibre content) as factors in the aetiology of this cancer.

3.2 Descriptive epidemiology

3.2.1 Incidence rates

To describe the differences in occurrence of a particular cancer between different groups the most useful concept is that of an incidence rate—the probability of an individual in a particular group being newly diagnosed as having the particular cancer within a year. In epidemiological studies these probabilities are usually expressed as a rate usually 'per 100 000' or 'per million'. For example, the incidence rate of breast cancer in females in England and Wales in 1989 was 107.2 per 100 000; this was estimated by noting that there were 25 893 400 females in England and Wales on 30 June 1989 and that 27 768 new breast cancer cases were diagnosed in females in that year: $27\,768/25\,893\,4000 = 0.001072$ or 107.2 per 100 000.

3.2.2 Age-specific incidence rates

For most forms of cancer the incidence rate increases rapidly with increasing age. For aetiologically meaningful comparisons, incidence rates must be worked out separately for groups of people of a similar age. The collection of such incidence rates over a span of age groups is referred to as an age-specific incidence curve.

Table 3.1 and Fig. 3.1 show the age-specific incidence rates for cancer of the colon in females in England and Wales in the period 1983–7. These particular age-specific incidence rates display a more than 100-fold increase between age 25 and age 70. It is most useful to plot both incidence rate and age on logarithmic scales, because the 'log–log' plot thus obtained is, for cancers at many different sites, very close to a straight line (Fig. 3.2). Deviations from the straight line pattern provide important insights into the aetiology of a number of cancers; in particular, the major hormone-associated cancers of women (breast, endometrium, and ovary).

The age-specific incidence curve for breast cancer in females in England and Wales in 1983–7 is shown in Fig. 3.3; there is a roughly linear relationship of the logarithm of incidence with the logarithm of age until about age 50. Then, the rate of increase of incidence with increasing age clearly slows down. This incidence curve therefore strongly suggests that something occurs around age 50 in women that acts as a brake on the rate of increase of breast

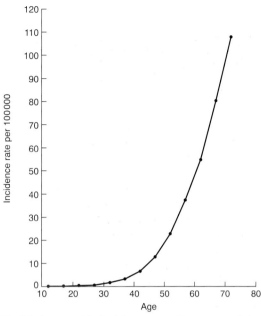

Fig. 3.1 Age-specific incidence rates for cancer of the colon in females in England and Wales, 1983–7.

cancer incidence with age—the obvious candidate is menopause. The protective effect of menopause (either natural or resulting from removal of the

Table 3.1 Age-specific incidence of cancer of the colon in females in England and Wales (1983–87)[1]

Age	Rate per 100 000
0–4	0.0
5–9	0.0
10–14	0.0
15–19	0.1
20–24	0.3
25–29	0.4
30–34	1.5
35–39	3.0
40–44	6.3
45–49	12.5
50–54	22.5
55–59	37.2
60–64	54.5
65–69	79.9
70–74	107.5

[1] From Parkin *et al.* (1992).

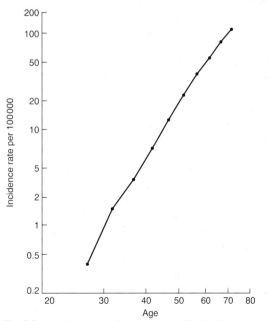

Fig. 3.2 Log–log plot of the age-specific incidence rates for cancer of the colon in females in England and Wales, 1983–7.

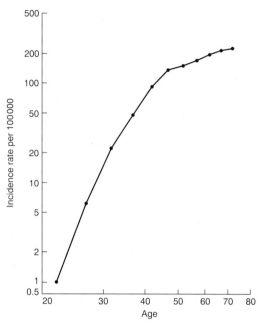

Fig. 3.3 Log–log plot of the age-specific incidence rates for cancer of the breast in females in England and Wales, 1983–7.

ovaries) has now been definitely established (see Section 3.4.4), and this observation plays a central role in research into the causes and prevention of breast cancer.

If the incidence rates for a particular cancer are changing rapidly in time, then the log–log plot of incidence against age for a particular calendar period will not show the true relationship between incidence and age. If incidence rates are increasing, as they did for lung cancer when cigarette smoking became common, then the incidence at old age will be lower than the incidence that the population providing the incidence at young ages will have when they reach old age (see later, Table 3.5). The log–log plot will therefore have too shallow a slope and may even reach a peak before old age and then decline. The opposite phenomenon will be observed if the incidence rates are decreasing. The correct interpretation of an age-specific incidence curve, therefore, also requires an understanding of its changes over calendar time.

3.2.3 Age-standardized incidence rates

Comparisons of age-specific incidence curves between different groups for a particular cancer usually show that the pattern of change with age is

very similar and it is only the level of incidence that varies. For example, Fig. 3.4 shows the age-specific incidence of stomach cancer in men in Japan and in the US in 1983–7. For these situations, comparisons between the different populations can most simply be made by giving a summary statistic representing the incidence rate for each population. The statistic chosen is usually either the sum of the incidence rates at each single year of age between, for example, 0 and 74 years (the cumulative incidence rate) or a weighted average of the age-specific incidence rates (the age-standardized incidence rate). The cumulative incidence rate is the probability that a person gets the specific cancer within the age range considered (if he or she does not die from any other cause), while the age-standardized rate gives the incidence in a standard group whose age structure is represented by the weights used in calculating the weighted average; both methods give similar comparative information.

If the pattern of change of incidence with age is not similar in the groups being compared, then summary statistics cannot, of course, adequately represent the differences between the groups. Cumulative incidence rates or age-standardized rates will still

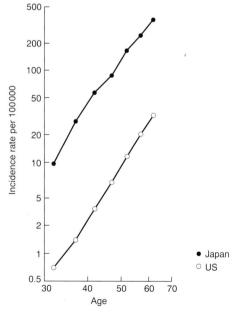

Fig 3.4 Log–log plot of the age-specific incidence rates for cancer of the stomach in males in Miyagi Prefecture, Japan and in the US, the Surveillance, Epidemiology, and End Results programme, 1983–7.

provide valuable information on the occurrence of cancer in the different groups, but they need to be supplemented with a description of the age-specific patterns in the different groups.

3.2.4 Comparisons between populations

Table 3.2 shows the cumulative incidence rates (ages 0–74) of breast cancer in different populations around 1970 and around 1985; the rates vary more than sixfold. Japan, China, India, and black Africa have the lowest rates, while the highest rates are observed in North American whites. It should also be noted that 16 out of the 17 populations shown in the table for which rates are available at both points in time show an increase during the 15 years consid-

ered; in most cases this occurred at a rate in excess of 1 per cent per year. Some of this increase is a result of more complete cancer registration, but it is likely that, at least in some populations, there has been a real increase in incidence.

Table 3.3 shows that Japanese, Chinese, and African immigrants to the US have breast cancer rates intermediate between those of their country of origin and the US white population (the rates in Africa are based on only one relatively small registry and should be interpreted with some caution). Japanese in Japan have a rate less than one-quarter that of US whites, whereas those in the US have over three-quarters that rate. These dramatic effects of migration on breast cancer rates show that environmental and/or behavioural factors are major determinants of breast cancer risk. The fact that Japanese American women now have rates of breast cancer closer to those of white Americans than to

Table 3.2 Cumulative incidence rates (ages 0–74 of breast cancer in different populations

Populations	Cumulative incidence rate (%)	
	ca. 1970[1]	ca. 1985[2]
US, San Francisco, white	8.9	12.0
Canada, British Columbia	8.8	8.7
Israel, Jews, Europe/US born	6.5	8.2
US, San Francisco, black	6.4	9.1
New Zealand, non-Maori	5.8	7.0
Sweden	5.8	7.0
New Zealand, Maori	5.7	7.2
US, Hawaii, Japanese	5.3	7.6
England and Wales	5.3[3]	6.2
Norway	4.9	6.1
Finland	3.7	5.7
Columbia, Cali	2.9	3.8
Israel, Jews, Africa/Asia born	2.9	5.1
India, Bombay	2.2	2.8
China, Shanghai	2.2[4]	2.3
Singapore, Chinese	2.2	3.4
Nigeria, Ibadan	1.7	N/A[5]
Japan, Osaka	1.3	2.4
Senegal, Dakar	1.3[4]	N/A[5]

[1] From Waterhouse et al. (1976).

[2] From Parkin et al. (1992).

[3] Calculated from England and Wales Cancer Registration Statistics for 1971 (Office of Population Censuses and Surveys 1979).

[4] These rates are ca. 1975 (Waterhouse et al. 1982).

[5] N/A, not available.

Table 3.3 Cumulative incidence rates (ages 0–74) of female breast and male colon cancer in different populations (ca. 1985)[1]

	Population	Cumulative incidence rate (%)
Female breast cancer	US, white	10.6[2]
	US, Japanese	8.2[3]
	Japan	2.5[4]
	US, Chinese	6.4[3]
	China	2.3[5]
	US, black	8.1[6]
	Africa, black	1.1[7]
Male colon cancer	US, white	3.6[2]
	US, Japanese	4.6[3]
	Japan	1.9[4]
	US, Chinese	2.6[3]
	China	0.9[5]
	US, black	3.8[6]
	Africa, black	0.3[7]

[1] From Parkin et al. (1992).

[2] Weighted means of rates from eight US Registries (Alameda, Bay Area, Los Angeles, Connecticut, Atlanta, New Orleans, Detroit, Hawaii).

[3] Weighted means of rates from two US Registries (Los Angeles, Hawaii).

[4] Weighted means of rates from four Japanese Registries (Hiroshima, Miyagi, Nagasaki, Osaka).

[5] Weighted means of rates for two Chinese Registries (Shanghai, Tianjin).

[6] Weighted means of rates from seven US registries (Alameda, Bay Area, Los Angeles, Connecticut, Atlanta, New Orleans, Detroit).

[7] Rates from one African Registry (Mali).

those in Japan shows that the low rates of breast cancer in Asia are not simply due to a difference in genetic susceptibility. Breast cancer is not unusual in showing large differences between incidence rates in different populations; for most cancer sites, the pattern of disease in migrants comes to resemble that of their host country in a few generations as they adopt the local life style. A similar effect is observed for colon cancer in men (Table 3.3), and, in this case, the rates in Japanese-Americans exceed those in white Americans.

Table 3.4 shows the cumulative incidence rates for the common cancers in England and Wales, and the lowest incidence rate observed among populations in Europe, or of European origin; restricting the comparison to European populations reduces the possibility that any of the variation is a result of major genetic differences. For each site, the potential reduction in the rate has been estimated assuming that the lowest observed European rate could be achieved in the UK—the reductions are over 50 per cent for most of the major sites, although some of the reductions may be overestimates as a result of under-recording of cancers in some of the low incidence areas. There is clearly tremendous potential for preventing cancer if the environmental and/or behavioural factors responsible for the extreme variations in site-specific cancer rates could be identified and people were prepared to adopt the low risk behaviour patterns.

3.3 Analytical epidemiology

In the previous section we explained how epidemiology is used to describe the occurrence of cancer and to describe associations that can lead to specific hypotheses concerning the aetiology of cancer. In this section we outline the main epidemiological methods used to test hypotheses by analysing the relationships between putative risk factors and the development of cancer in individuals.

There are two fundamentally different designs for analytical epidemiological studies: (i) retrospective studies, in which people who have already developed

Table 3.4 Comparison of England and Wales cumulative incidence rates (ages 0–74) for common cancer sites with the lowest incidence population among populations in Europe or of European origin (*ca.* 1985)[1]

Primary site of cancer	Cumulative incidence rate (%)			
	England and Wales rate	Lowest incidence rate	Lowest incidence population	Potential reduction (%)
Males				
Lung	8.2	3.2	Sweden	61
Stomach	2.0	0.7	USA, Atlanta	65
Prostate	2.4	1.0	Spain, Granada	58
Bladder	2.1	1.0	Poland, Warsaw 'Rural'	52
Colon	1.9	0.4	Poland, Nowy Sacz	79
Rectum	1.6	0.7	Spain, Granada	56
Pancreas	0.9	0.4	Spain, Granada	56
Females				
Breast	6.2	2.3	Poland, Nowy Sacz	63
Lung	2.7	0.3	Spain, Murcia	89
Colon	1.6	0.4	Poland, Nowy Sacz	75
Ovary	1.3	0.5	Italy, Latina	62
Cervix	1.2	0.5	Finland	58
Endometrium	1.0	0.7	Portugal, V N de Gaia	30
Rectum	0.9	0.6	Romania, County Cluj	33
Stomach	0.7	0.2	USA, Atlanta	71

[1] Parkin *et al.* (1992).

cancer are identified and their exposures before diagnosis are estimated; (ii) prospective studies, in which information relating to exposures is collected from a large number of healthy people who are then followed until some of them develop cancer.

The main type of retrospective study is the retrospective case–control study, in which information from cancer patients is compared with a group of controls (usually people without cancer) randomly selected to be representative of the same population from which the cases were identified. The advantages of this method are that it is relatively quick and cheap, it can be used to study a large number of exposures in considerable detail, and it can be used to study rare cancers. The two main disadvantages are: selection bias—not all potential cases and controls identified agree to participate, and those who do may be a biased sample of the total population; and recall bias—participants are frequently asked to remember exposures in the past and this recall may be systematically better (or worse) in people with cancer, especially if they are aware of the hypothesis being tested or if they are unwell. These sources of bias should be quite small in well-conducted studies, but can be a major problem when studying small relative risks. A further disadvantage of retrospective studies is that measurements on biological samples such as blood cannot always be interpreted in relation to the aetiology of the disease, because any differences found in people with cancer may be a consequence (rather than a cause) of the disease.

In prospective studies, also called cohort studies, information (questionnaires, blood samples, etc.) is collected from a large number of people without cancer and the whole population (cohort) is then followed. Measurements made on people who develop cancer subsequent to recruitment are compared with measurements made on the rest of the cohort (or a sample of these people) who remain cancer free. The advantages of prospective studies are that they do not suffer from selection bias or recall bias, that measurements made in biological samples precede the diagnosis of cancer by a known time, and that several types of cancer can be studied during prolonged follow-up. The disadvantages are that they are relatively slow and expensive, it is not usually practical to collect very detailed information concerning exposure, and the information collected may precede diagnosis by many years and thus may miss important

later exposures (unless there is a mechanism for continuous updating).

3.4 Identifying the causes

In this section we consider the nature of the research findings that underlie our current understanding of the causation of the five commonest types of cancer in the UK: lung, stomach, colorectal, breast, and prostate. In the subsequent section we give a brief description of the known, and strongly suspected, risk factors for the complete range of cancer sites.

3.4.1 Lung cancer

Lung cancer is by far the most frequent cancer world-wide and the most common form of cancer in men in the UK. After breast cancer, it is the second most common cancer in women in the UK. In the UK there are approximately 44 000 new cases and 40 000 deaths from this cancer each year, with a five-year relative survival of about 7 per cent. This cancer occupies a unique position among the important cancers in that tobacco smoking has been known for at least 40 years to be the cause of some 90 per cent of it.

Figure 3.5 shows the trends in male and female lung cancer mortality in England and Wales from 1931 to 1992. The size of the male risk and its continuing increase persuaded scientists and public health officials in the years immediately after the Second World War that the reason for the increase warranted urgent study. That cigarette smoking could be the cause of the increase was suggested by a number of people, and by the end of 1950 eight case–control studies had been published; these studies compared the cigarette smoking history of lung cancer cases to that of similar men without the disease and all showed a clear relationship between increasing risk and increasing exposure.

There was, naturally, a great deal of reluctance to accept the findings of the early case–control studies (cigarette smoking was an almost universally accepted habit) and many further epidemiological studies were soon initiated, partly to answer criticisms that had been made of the case–control studies, but also to investigate whether smoking was associated with cancers of other sites. A number of these epidemiological studies were cohort studies, i.e. studies in which large numbers of people with

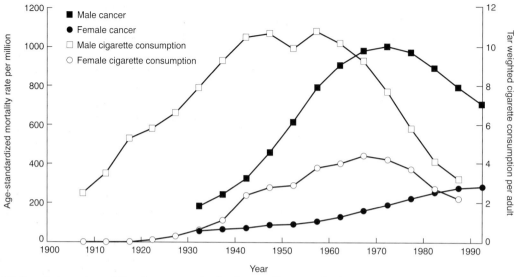

Fig 3.5 Trends in male and female age-standardized mortality rates for lung cancer in England and Wales, 1931–92, and tar-weighted cigarette consumption per adult.

different smoking habits were identified and their subsequent mortality monitored. In the UK, the smoking habits of a large number of doctors were recorded and, after 40 years of follow-up, the lung cancer mortality rates in smokers of 1–14, 15–24, and 25 or more cigarettes per day were 8-, 15-, and 25-fold higher, respectively, than those of lifelong non-smokers (Doll *et al.* 1994). Cohort studies not only confirmed the lung cancer cigarette smoking association, but established that smoking was also causally associated with cancers at many other sites (see later, Table 3.7).

Further studies of the relationship between cigarette smoking and lung cancer also showed that stopping smoking has an almost immediate effect on lung cancer risk. The absolute difference between the ex-smoker's lung cancer risk and the lung cancer risk of a non-smoker effectively stays constant with length of time after stopping, rather than continuing to increase as it does for the continuing smoker. These studies showed, moreover, that the age-specific incidence rates of lung cancer in people in late-middle or old age depend on lifelong cigarette smoking habits, so that age-standardized lung cancer rates depend not only on current cigarette consumption but also on the consumption as young adults, 40 or more years before. Furthermore, reductions in population cigarette consumption will take decades to show up in reduced lung cancer rates in older people.

The tobacco industry responded to the ever mounting evidence of the carcinogenic effects of cigarette smoke by reducing the tar and nicotine content of cigarettes, first by introducing filters and later by modifying the tobacco. The tar content of the cigarettes is probably the relevant constituent with regard to lung cancer, and the average tar yield per cigarette has declined steadily, from approximately 32 mg/cigarette in 1960 to the current level of less than 14 mg/cigarette.

The average number of cigarettes smoked by men in Britain was approximately 10.5/day from 1950 to 1970, but has declined steadily since then and is now approximately 6.5/day. The average number of cigarettes smoked by women in Britain was less than 4/day up until 1960, rose to a maximum of 7/day in the mid 1970s, and then declined. It is now approximately 5/day.

Figure 3.5 shows the changes in tar-weighted cigarette consumption and age-standardized mortality rates for lung cancer in England and Wales this century. In men, cigarette consumption reached a peak in the 1940s and 1950s, and lung cancer peaked about 30 years later, in the early 1970s; since then rates have fallen considerably. The pattern is somewhat similar in women, but the peaks are lower and occurred later; cigarette consumption began to fall in the 1970s and by the early 1990s lung cancer rates had levelled off but had not yet begun to fall. Figure 3.5 obscures the differences in mortality trends in different age groups, which are shown in Table 3.5; in both men and women declines in mortality are seen first among the youngest age groups, because falls in cigarette consumption quickly reduce the life-time exposure of young people. Rates in men are now declining at all ages, except for those currently in their eighties. We can now look forward, in the UK, to an overall two-thirds reduction in the male lung cancer rate, even if no further reduction in tar content or cigarette smoking takes place. Female lung cancer rates are also showing a sharp decline at young ages, and although lung cancer rates for older women (over the age of 60 years) are still rising (because of the early adoption of smoking by the present cohort of older women), we can also confidently look forward to a substantial reduction in female lung cancer in the not too distant future.

Unfortunately, in many other countries smoking rates are now increasing, especially in young people, in a manner similar to that which took place in the UK between 1900 and 1950. As these populations age there will be a large increase in their lung cancer rates. It has been estimated that, world-wide, as many as three million smoking-related lung cancer deaths will occur each year by 2025, compared with about one million now, plus another seven million deaths from other diseases caused by smoking (Peto *et al.* 1994). For Europe, the 2025 figure has been estimated at 670 000 (480 000 men, 190 000 women), up from the current figure of 260 000 (230 000 men, 30 000 women); the relatively larger increase for women reflects the changes in the number of young women currently taking up smoking. This is a major public health challenge.

There are large differences between the age at onset of lung cancer in different people with the same smoking habits. These differences suggest that different people have different genetic suscept-ibilities to cigarette smoke-induced lung cancer. The host factors that have excited most interest are the genes coding for the cytochrome P450 enzymes which control the metabolic oxidative activation of various chemical carcinogens to an active cancer-inducing form (see Chapter 6). The different levels of such enzymes, which are known to be genetically controlled in many animal species, could give rise to significant between-person variation in the genera-tion of carcinogenic derivatives of the chemicals in cigarette smoke. Human studies have focused recently on the two gene systems *CYP1A1* and *CYP2D6*. There is some evidence that individuals with greater activity of the enzymes produced by these genes are at greater risk of developing lung

Table 3.5 Changes in lung cancer mortality rates in England and Wales, 1946–90

Age	Death rate per 100 000					Reduction from peak rate to 1986–90 (%)
	1946–50	1956–60	1966–70	1976–80	1986–90	
Males						
30–34	*3.6*	3.5	2.5	1.6	0.7	81
40–44	23.6	*25.1*	21.6	13.8	10.0	60
50–54	95.4	*124.8*	116.0	99.6	57.6	54
60–64	171.7	331.5	*369.5*	332.0	262.6	29
70–74	140.0	387.8	621.0	*662.5*	577.0	13
80–84	76.5	225.8	456.3	762.3	*785.7*	—
Females						
30–34	1.2	*1.4*	1.1	0.8	0.6	57
40–44	4.8	6.0	*8.1*	6.2	6.3	22
50–54	11.7	16.9	28.4	*35.9*	25.8	28
60–64	22.1	32.8	51.5	84.6	*109.6*	—
70–74	31.6	44.5	73.1	110.5	*170.5*	—
80–84	28.0	45.1	65.7	106.2	*164.9*	—

The highest rate for each age group is italicized and emboldened.

cancer caused by cigarette smoke, but the evidence is not yet conclusive.

Since cigarette smoke is carcinogenic, it is reasonable to assume that involuntary (passive) smoking will also cause a certain amount of lung cancer; the epidemiological question of interest is not really whether or not involuntary smoking causes lung cancer, but how much lung cancer does it cause. Epidemiological studies suggest that a never-smoker's risk of lung cancer may be increased by some 20 to 30 per cent from exposure to cigarette smoke from other people. This estimate has been disputed by a number of researchers who suggest rather that the increased risk of lung cancer seen among never-smokers exposed to passive smoking is largely the effect of a proportion of reported never-smokers having at some time been actual smokers. A figure of a 10 per cent increase in risk is suggested by studies of cotinine (a measure of absorbed nicotine) in active and passive smokers. The relationship between the amount of nicotine absorbed and the amount of tar deposited in the lungs is not necessarily the same in passive and active smoking, however, and this could influence the postulated risk in either direction. At present we conclude that it is most reasonable to regard the 30 per cent figure as an upper limit of risk.

Although cigarette smoking is by far the main cause of lung cancer, exposure to a number of other substances has created a significant added risk of lung cancer for workers in certain industrial occupations. The most important of these has been exposure to asbestos. A substantial number of men previously exposed to high levels of asbestos, particularly in the shipbuilding and insulation industries, have very high lung cancer rates. This risk is now universally recognized and the asbestos levels permitted in industry have been greatly reduced. Occupational exposure to polycyclic aromatic hydrocarbons from the combustion of fossil fuels has also been an important source of added lung cancer risk; high-level exposure has occurred particularly to men working in the fumes from coke ovens and in coal gas manufacturing. Other substantial risks to small groups of workers have resulted from exposure to some aspects of the use of chromates and arsenic and the refining of nickel, chromium, and copper (because of the arsenic associated with it), and from exposure to radiation from the radioactive gas radon in the air of certain mines.

Radon is not confined to underground areas, but is present in the air in some houses and other buildings where it is not free to diffuse away. Current estimates of exposure indicate that radon accounts for nearly half the average exposure of the UK population to ionizing radiation. In the UK, the primary determinant of the indoor radon concentration is the underlying geology. In parts of Cornwall and some other areas of the UK, the exposure of some individuals may be more than 15 times the national average, and exposures that would not be permitted for workers in the nuclear industry are not uncommon. In some other countries, radon exposure from building materials and the radon content of water also influences heavily the indoor radon concentration. Extrapolation from studies of uranium and iron ore miners in North America and Sweden indicates that approximately 5 per cent of all lung cancers may be caused by exposure to indoor radon. If these estimates are correct, radon would be the second most important cause of lung cancer, after smoking. Intensive investigation is underway to provide better quantitative information on these risks.

In the past the general population has also been exposed to significant amounts of polycyclic aromatic hydrocarbons in urban air, mainly from the uncontrolled burning of coal. Such general air pollution may have contributed to as much as 10 per cent of all lung cancer in heavily polluted cities, but with the introduction of clean air legislation over the years, air pollution of this type has been reduced dramatically and current levels are unlikely to be making more than a small contribution to lung cancer risk.

There is good evidence that diet has a modest effect on the risk for lung cancer. Numerous analytical epidemiological studies have shown, almost without exception, that people in any population who eat the most fruit and vegetables have about 50 per cent of the risk of developing lung cancer of those who eat the least fruit and vegetables. This finding has persisted after careful adjustments for cigarette smoking (smokers are known to eat less fruit and vegetables than non-smokers) and has also been observed among non-smokers. Similar protective associations have been seen for both dietary and serum levels of vitamin C and carotene, major antioxidant nutrients supplied largely by fruit and vegetables. However, the protective agent could be any of the large number of constituents of fruit and vegetables. A recent trial among middle-aged male smokers in Finland did not support the hypothesis that β-carotene supplements are protective; men who received β-carotene had a somewhat higher mortality from lung cancer than those who did not, but the interpretation of this finding is unclear owing to the relatively short follow-up in comparison with the presumed duration of carcinogenesis.

3.4.2 Stomach cancer

World-wide, stomach cancer is the second most important cancer after lung cancer. In the UK, there are approximately 13 000 new cases and 8 500 deaths from this cancer each year with a five-year relative survival of about 10 per cent. In most developed countries, incidence and mortality rates have been declining rapidly for much of the latter half of the twentieth century. Incidence rates vary approximately tenfold internationally, being highest in Japan and parts of South America and lowest in the United States, Australia, and parts of Africa. Migrant studies suggest that populations moving from high to low risk countries maintain the high risk of cancer in the generation that moves, while the second generation children have lower risks. Incidence rates are invariably higher in males than in females (by about 2:1) and in lower socioeconomic classes than in more affluent classes (by about 3:1).

The generally accepted model for carcinogenesis in the stomach, developed by Correa and co-workers (Correa, 1988), proposes that cancer is the end-result of a series of mutations and cell transformations that begin early in life. First, the normal stomach lining undergoes a chronic inflammatory process, "superficial gastritis", involving some cell injury. Although this might be caused by factors such as a high salt intake, it is now thought that infection with the bacterium *Helicobacter pylori* is the major causative factor in this process (see below). The next stage involves extensive cell loss and results in 'chronic atrophic gastritis'. With this condition, the gastric microenvironment changes mainly as a result of impaired acid secretion, and the pH increases to an extent that permits extensive colonization with many species of bacteria. Several of these species can reduce nitrate to nitrite and also catalyse the N-nitrosation reaction between nitrite and dietary proteins, resulting in the formation of *N*-nitroso compounds. These are both mutagenic and carcinogenic and may cause further transformations in the epithelial cells towards metaplasia, dysplasia, and, ultimately, cancer.

Several risk factors have been identified for stomach cancer including employment in dusty occupations, e.g. coal mining; various heritable conditions, e.g. pernicious anaemia; surgical procedures, e.g. partial gastrectomy; and a relatively minor influence of smoking. The most intensively investigated exposures, however, have been dietary factors.

Several studies have shown risks associated with a high intake of salt and preserved meat or fish, i.e. cured, salted, or smoked. Results for these risk factors are, however, not consistent from study to study, although difficulties in accurate assessment of intake may be a reason for some of the discrepancies, especially for salt. Pickled vegetables have been shown to increase cancer risk but only in Chinese and Japanese populations. Food storage *per se* appears to be an important factor, and a number of studies have shown that long-term use of domestic refrigeration is a protective factor. It is, however, unclear whether refrigerator use is simply a surrogate for diets with a low intake of preserved foods.

The strongest and most consistently observed dietary association is, however, that between the risk of stomach cancer and a diet with a relatively low level of fruit and/or vegetable consumption. This association has been observed in both retrospective and prospective studies, and in populations from several European countries, North and South America, and many parts of Asia. As with lung cancer (see Section 3.4.1), within any one population, those with the highest intake of fruit and vegetables have about half the risk of developing stomach cancer compared with those with the lowest intake levels. As a high consumption of fruit and vegetables is associated with reduced cancer risk at sites other than the stomach and reduced risk of several other diseases, and, as there are no known adverse consequences of increasing intake, advocating changes in this direction should be a key component of any public health dietary advice related to cancer.

As a consequence of the observed protective effects of fruit and vegetable intake, there has been considerable interest in attempting to identify the specific nutrients responsible. Most attention has been focused on the antioxidant vitamins, especially vitamin C and β-carotene. Conventional dietary epidemiological studies are relatively limited in their ability to disentangle which of the numerous constituents found in fruit and vegetables might have specific anticancer properties. Much interest has been given, therefore, to recent results from two large, randomized intervention trials in which daily vitamin supplements, or placebos, were given for 5–8 years to middle-aged adults. These took place in China and Finland and, whereas in China a supplement of β-carotene, selenium, and α-tocopherol in combination significantly reduced the incidence of stomach cancer, in Finland neither β-carotene or α-tocopherol supplements (or both combined) had any effect on incidence rates in comparison with placebo. The lack of consistency between the two studies could be due to selenium (present in China but not in Finland) or to the extremely low vitamin levels within China before the start of the trial. In China, another group of subjects received a daily ascorbic acid supplement, but this group did not show any significant difference in its incidence rate for stomach cancer in comparison with the placebo group. Taken together, these trials do not resolve the issue of which specific component of fruit and vegetables is protective, although continued follow-up of these subjects might help. In the absence of additional data, the taking of supplements containing antioxidant micronutrients as a means of preventing stomach cancer cannot be recommended.

Generally, a decrease in the dependency on preserved foodstuffs and salt, together with increased availability of fruit and vegetables, is consistent with the world-wide decline in stomach cancer. These four dietary factors are, however, insufficient to explain the full extent of the decline. In the UK, for example, stomach cancer has declined by almost an order of magnitude in the past 40–50 years, but changes in the consumption of fruit and vegetables, salt, and preserved food have been much smaller, even allowing for a 20–30-year lag period between dietary change and change in cancer mortality. The most important additional factor, which helps to complete the picture regarding the causes of stomach cancer and the reasons for its decline, is infection with *Helicobacter pylori*. This bacterium has specifically evolved to live in the highly acidic conditions of the human stomach where it is found adjacent or attached to the cell lining beneath the surface mucous layer. Many millions of people are infected with *H. pylori* (possibly half the world's population), mostly acquiring the infection during childhood. Although combinations of antibiotics can eradicate the infection, the bacteria are usually resistant to the normal host immunological defence

mechanisms. As infection is often asymptomatic, people will harbour the bacteria for decades and most will experience no adverse health effects. *Helicobacter pylori* does, however, rapidly cause a chronic inflammatory response leading to gastritis. In some individuals this may eventually result in peptic ulceration while in others the gastritis progresses to become atrophic. The latter situation predisposes to stomach cancer.

The strongest direct evidence for an association between *H. pylori* infection and the subsequent development of stomach cancer has come from three prospective studies. These made use of established cohorts to compare subjects who developed stomach cancer with matched controls who did not. Anti-*H. pylori* antibodies were measured in blood samples collected up to 24 years prior to the diagnosis of cancer. All studies reported significantly elevated relative risks (approximately fourfold) for the development of stomach cancer following *H. pylori* seropositivity. On the basis of these studies, it has been estimated that at least one-third, and possibly two-thirds or more, of stomach cancers could be attributable to *H. pylori* infection.

Parallels between the descriptive epidemiology of stomach cancer and of *H. pylori* infection are also compatible with a causal association. There is evidence to suggest that, like stomach cancer incidence rates, *H. pylori* infection rates have fallen over the last few decades. Improvements in living conditions and trends towards a smaller family size (risk factors for *H. pylori* acquisition) could explain this reduction, and could, in turn, help to explain the reduction in stomach cancer rates. Similarly, the two- or three-fold excess of stomach cancer seen in those of lower socioeconomic status is matched by a similar excess of *H. pylori* infection in the same socioeconomic groups. Finally, there are geographical correlations between populations with high stomach cancer rates and populations with high *H. pylori* infection rates.

There are also several experimental observations that lend support to the association, although it should be emphasized that there is no evidence that *H. pylori* infection is not directly genotoxic. There are a number of important properties of *H. pylori* infection that result from the ineffective immune response of the host to the bacteria. The stimulation of leucocytes should, theoretically, lead to the activation of immune defence mechanisms that would eventually cause limitation and resolution of the infection. It is characterized by the regulation of several cytokines, especially IL-8 (interleukin-8), and the induction of proteolytic enzymes, adhesion molecules, and reactive oxygen metabolites. What is of relevance, in the context of carcinogenesis, is that this intended bactericidal response is not short-lived but may continue indefinitely as the *H. pylori* infection avoids immune defences and becomes established. Thus, the toxic response may, over an extensive time period, cause structural and biochemical damage to the epithelium. One example of this abnormal host response is the excess production of reactive oxygen metabolites by stimulated leucocytes. These are highly reactive chemicals, capable of causing extensive DNA damage and molecular mutations.

There is also a substantial increase in epithelial cell turnover rates with an approximate doubling of cell turnover associated with *H. pylori* infection. Cell division is, of course, vital to the development of cancer and an elevated rate of mitosis increases the likelihood of a somatic DNA mutation avoiding the surveillance of DNA repair enzymes and becoming fixed. The role of *H. pylori* in cancer development is restricted to relatively early events as the bacterium will not colonize cancerous tissue, or the common precursor, intestinal metaplasia. Thus, events beyond metaplastic transformation are likely to be determined by other risk factors.

In comparison with the high prevalence of *H. pylori* infection, gastric cancer is a very rare event, and, as yet, it is unclear what additional factors are required for a bacterial gastritis to become malignant. Related to this is the question of why certain populations, notably in Africa, have low gastric cancer rates despite almost universal infection. Whether it is the host's genetic background, age at acquisition of infection, or the presence of other environmental and dietary cofactors that are of importance requires clarification.

From a public health perspective, we have the capability to identify and treat infected individuals, at least in developed countries, but there is no clear indication as to who should be screened for infection. Also, it is not yet known whether eradicating the infection in adult life will actually reduce future cancer risk. It is, however, encouraging to note that most of the *H. pylori*-induced changes that may be of relevance to carcinogenesis, e.g. development of gastritis, reactive oxygen metabolite formation, and

increased cell division, can be reversed following successful eradication of the bacterial infection.

In summary, several factors involved in the aetiology of stomach cancer have now been identified. It is highly likely that increasing fruit and vegetable consumption and decreasing salt intake will reduce risk, and one immediate task for epidemiology is to attempt to quantify the level of risk reduction more precisely. The role of *H. pylori* eradication in the prevention of stomach cancer also requires quantifying within the context of controlled studies.

3.4.3 Colorectal cancer

Ideally, colon cancer and rectal cancer should be considered separately, because the epidemiology of these diseases is somewhat different. However, classification of cancers as colonic or rectal may vary between studies, and much of the available data is for the two sites combined. It is most convenient, therefore, to consider them together.

Colorectal cancer is the second commonest cancer in developed countries, but is much rarer in most developing countries. In the UK, there are approximately 31 000 new cases and 18 000 deaths from this cancer each year, with a five-year relative survival of about 37 per cent. Incidence rates for colorectal cancer are increasing at all ages in most low risk populations for which data are available. The rise can be very rapid; in urban Shanghai, for example, age-adjusted incidence rates for colon cancer increased by more than 75 per cent between 1972 and 1979. As seen in Table 3.3, migrants from low risk to high risk countries have experienced particularly high rates of increase. In populations that currently have high rates of colorectal cancer, there were increases in incidence during the 1960s and 1970s, and there has generally been a further small increase in the age-adjusted incidence between the late 1970s and the late 1980s. However, recent trends have varied between age groups, with increases at older ages but some decrease at younger ages. In England and Wales, for example, colorectal cancer incidence at ages 25–49 years fell between 1971–3 and 1984–6 by 14 per cent in men and by 21 per cent in women. This could be a result of dietary changes, which, as with the effects of changes in cigarette consumption on lung cancer (see Section 3.4.1), would be expected to affect young people first.

Understanding of the aetiology of colorectal cancer has advanced considerably in recent years, but important gaps still remain. A small proportion of cases of colon cancer are due to inheritance of mutations in certain genes such as the adenomatous polyposis coli gene (see Chapter 4), but the majority of cases of colorectal cancer are sporadic (i.e. not due to inheritance of a mutated gene but to mutations arising in somatic cells). Studies of cells from sporadic colorectal cancers have shown that mutations of several genes (including that for adenomatous polyposis coli) are common and probably cause the neoplastic behaviour of the cells, but the causes of these mutations are not yet known (see Chapter 4).

Interest in the role of nutritional factors in the aetiology of colorectal cancer stems largely from the wide variation in disease rates between populations with different diets, plus the plausibility of the hypothesis that the contents of the colon and rectum could affect the risk of cancer. Burkitt originally suggested that dietary fibre may protect against colorectal cancer, while subsequent ecological analyses of diet and cancer rates suggested that meat or animal fat might increase risk and that starch as well as fibre may be protective. Analytical epidemiological studies have examined the roles of meat, animal fat, fibre, fruits and vegetables, and, more recently, antioxidant nutrients and folate.

The results of the analytical studies vary somewhat but in general are consistent with the hypothesis that meat and/or animal fat increase the risk for colorectal cancer and that fibre-containing foods (cereals, vegetables, fruits) are protective. For micronutrients, there is some evidence that folate is protective against colorectal adenomas, a known precursor of colorectal cancer, and perhaps against colorectal cancer, but the hypothesis that antioxidant micronutrients might be protective is only weakly supported by observational studies. A recent trial in the US found no evidence that supplements of β-carotene, vitamin C, or vitamin E could prevent the development of further colorectal adenomas amongst patients who had previously been diagnosed as having an adenoma.

Clinical and laboratory investigations have established plausible mechanisms that could explain the observed associations of diet with the risk for colorectal cancer. For example, high fat diets increase the production of bile acids, which may promote tumour growth; high meat, low fibre diets increase the faecal concentration of ammonia and N-nitroso compounds; while cooked meat and fish are sources of heterocyclic amines, which are potential carcinogens. Fibre and starch affect bacterial metabolism in the large bowel, increasing stool weight and butyrate production and decreasing pH, secondary bile acids, diacyl glycerol, free ammonia, and probably amines, amides, and N-nitroso compounds. In addition to being a source of fibre, fruit and vegetables could be beneficial because of the effects of antioxidant vitamins or of other non-nutrient chemicals (Potter, 1992). Alcohol consumption has been frequently considered as a risk factor for colorectal cancer, the evidence being slightly more compelling for cancer of the rectum. Inconsistency of results currently precludes a definitive assessment of this relationship.

Improving our knowledge of the effects of diet on the risk for colorectal cancer is perhaps the highest priority today in the field of diet and cancer. We know that dietary changes could prevent a large proportion of cases of this disease, and we have some idea of which dietary factors are relevant, but we do not yet know which aspects of diet are really important in determining risk and which are merely associated with risk, owing to correlation with other factors. Identification of the key factors could result in very different recommendations. For example, do we need to avoid meat or animal fat or total fat, and do we need to eat more starch and fibre or more fresh fruit and vegetables?

As well as the effects of diet, there is quite consistent evidence to suggest that the risk for colon cancer is reduced by two other factors. Increased physical activity appears to have a protective effect for colon, but not rectal, cancer. The mechanism for this has not been established, but it might be a result of a shortened time for the transit of food through the alimentary tract. Long-term use of aspirin and other non-steroidal anti-inflammatory drugs, as occurs in people with rheumatoid arthritis and similar conditions, also appears to be protective. This association is currently being evaluated in controlled intervention studies. The mechanism here probably involves inhibition of prostaglandin synthesis which would inhibit tumour growth and spread.

3.4.4 Breast cancer

Breast cancer is the third most common cancer in the world, and is the commonest cancer amongst women in the UK. There are approximately 30 000 new cases and 15 000 deaths each year, with a five-year relative survival of about 62 per cent. Breast cancer rates vary about sevenfold between populations world-wide, with high rates in Western countries, including the UK, and low rates in most poor countries and in east Asia, including Japan. Breast cancer rates rise in migrants from low to high risk populations; this rise is not as rapid as that seen for colorectal cancer, since rates in migrants typically do not approach those of the host population until the second generation, nevertheless some increase can occur quite quickly (increases of 80 per cent in breast cancer incidence have been observed in Asian migrants after 10 or more years residence in the US). Breast cancer mortality rates in the UK were increasing by about 1% per year until the late 1980s. Since then the mortality rates have fallen by over 10%, partly due to earlier diagnosis and partly due to improvements in treatment.

The aetiology of breast cancer is not yet well understood. A small proportion of cases—about 5 per cent over all ages, but more at young ages—are largely due to inheritance of mutations in certain genes such as *BRCA1*, *BRCA2*, and *TP53* (see Chapters 4 and 9). Analysis of cells in breast cancer tissue has shown frequent mutations in a number of genes, including tumour suppressor genes such as *TP53* and oncogenes such as *ras*, and it is likely that some of these genetic changes cause the malignant phenotype of the cells (see Chapter 9). However, it is not yet clear which genetic changes are most important and whether they generally arise in a particular order, and the causes of the genetic changes are not known.

Hormones appear to hold the key to the understanding of human breast cancer (Pike *et al.* 1993). Epidemiological research has established early menarche, late first birth, low parity, late menopause, and obesity as major risk factors for breast cancer (Table 3.6). A delay of three years in age at menarche has been found to reduce breast cancer risk by up to a half. Similarly, the earlier a woman has her menopause the greater the reduction in her breast cancer risk: women with natural menopause before age 45 have only one-half the risk of women whose menopause occurs after age 55. The earlier a woman has her first birth, the greater the reduction in her breast cancer risk; women with a first birth under age 20 have about one-half the risk of nulliparous women, but nulliparous women do not have as high a risk as women whose first birth is after age 35. This protective effect of first birth does not appear, however, until some years after the birth; before about age 32

Table 3.6 Effects of age at menarche, age at first birth, age at menopause, and postmenopausal weight on breast cancer risk[1]

Risk factor		Relative risk
Menarche (years)	≤ 11	1.0
	12	0.9
	≥ 13	0.5
First birth (years)	≤ 19	0.8
	20–24	1.0
	25–29	1.3
	30–34	1.6
	≥ 35	2.0
	Nulliparous	1.7
Menopause (years)	40–44	1.0
	45–49	1.3
	50–54	1.5
	55–59	2.0
Postmenopausal weight	≤ 59	1.0
	60–69	1.6
	≥ 70	1.8

[1] Pike and Ross (1984).

parous women as a group are in fact more at risk of breast cancer than nulliparous women. Full-term pregnancies after the first cause some further reduction in lifetime risk. The overall effect of obesity is to increase the risk of breast cancer, but this increased risk is restricted to older postmenopausal women.

These associations are probably all due to hormonal factors. The protective effect of early menopause—and the corresponding decrease in the slope of the age-incidence curve at about 50 years old—shows that exposure of the breasts to oestradiol and/or progesterone during normal menstrual cycles causes an increase in breast cancer risk. Thus, late menopause and early menarche increase breast cancer risk by increasing the duration of exposure of the breasts to the ovarian hormones, probably because ovarian hormones stimulate breast cell division. The relative roles of oestradiol and progesterone in this are still not certain, but it appears that oestradiol is the major stimulant of cell division and that this stimulation is not opposed by progesterone. This contrasts strikingly with the control of cell division in the cells lining the uterus, where oestradiol strongly stimulates cell division, but this stimulation is completely opposed by progesterone. Obesity in postmenopausal women probably increases breast cancer risk because it is associated with high levels of endogenous oestrogens, formed by aromatization of the adrenal androgen androstenedione in the adipose tissue. Full-term pregnancies cause some long-term changes in hormone levels, but it is likely that their protective effect is largely owing to the differentiation of the epithelial cells and thus the reduction in the number of undifferentiated stem cells at risk.

Both combination-type oral contraceptives (i.e. the common preparations comprising an oestrogen and a progestin together) and hormone replacement therapy with oestrogen cause some increase in breast cancer risk, but the increase is relatively small (about 20 per cent) and is largely confined to current and recent users of these preparations. The effects of combined hormone replacement therapy, with an oestrogen and a progestin, are not yet well established, but the available data suggest that these combinations increase breast cancer risk at least as much as oestrogens given alone. As with the reproductive factors discussed above, the simplest explanation for these effects is that these exogenous hormones increase risk by raising the total exposure of the breasts to oestrogens and/or progestins, thus increasing the rate of cell division.

Detailed study has been made of the extent to which differences in the four major risk factors (age at menarche, age at first birth, age at menopause, and weight) between Japanese and American women could explain the large differences in their breast cancer rates. Age at first birth has not differed greatly between the two populations, and the distribution of age at menopause appears to vary little between the populations, but Japanese females born around 1900 had an average age at menarche some two years later and they weighed some 22 kg less at age 70 than the 1900 cohort of white US women. These differences accounted for as much as two-thirds of the difference in the observed breast cancer rates in the two countries, but white US women still had 2.5 times the breast cancer risk of Japanese women even after allowing for these factors. This 2.5-fold difference might be explained by lower levels of oestradiol in premenopausal Japanese women. Under the hypothesis that oestrogens increase breast cancer risk by increasing the rate of breast cell division, it can be predicted that the 2.5-fold difference in breast cancer risks could be due to a 20 per cent lower breast cell mitotic rate in the premenopausal Japanese women. Such a reduction in premenopausal mitotic rate could result from an approximately 20 per cent

reduction in premenopausal hormone levels (averaged over the menstrual cycle). Recent studies, which paid special attention to obtaining samples from Oriental women who were maintaining their old life style, clearly show lower serum oestradiol concentrations in the Oriental women compared with women in the US or UK. Thus it is reasonable to conclude that the premenopausal oestradiol levels of the Japanese could easily have been 20 per cent lower than the levels in Western whites. We therefore appear to have a plausible hormonal explanation for the difference between Japanese and US breast cancer rates.

The late menarche and low body weight of Japanese women are partly determined by nutritional factors. General undernutrition can cause delay in menarche, although other factors such as exercise and chronic or recurrent infections may also be involved. General overnutrition in relation to energy expenditure is probably the main determinant of obesity. It is probable that the low oestrogen levels in Japanese and other east Asian premenopausal women are caused by dietary factors. There is some evidence that diets that are both low in fat and high in fibre cause a reduction in serum oestrogen concentrations, possibly by reducing the enterohepatic circulation of oestrogens, but more information on these relationships is required.

Total fat intake is strongly correlated with the international variation in breast cancer rates, and has been shown to increase the incidence of mammary tumours in some animal models; although at least some of this effect is a result of an increase in energy intake rather than a specific effect of fat. However, analytical epidemiological studies have not produced clear support for the fat hypothesis. Many of the case–control studies have produced weakly positive results, but these studies are susceptible to recall and selection biases, which could be sufficient to explain their positive results. The prospective studies have not supported the fat hypothesis. It now appears to be unlikely that total fat intake in adult women within the range of fat intakes studied (c. 25–40 per cent energy from fat) has an important effect on breast cancer risk, but it is still possible that fat intake during childhood and adolescence, fat intake at levels below the range studied, or the type of fat eaten could affect breast cancer risk.

In addition to fat, epidemiological studies have examined the possible associations of alcohol, antioxidant micronutrients, fibre, and phyto-oestrogens (plant-derived oestrogens) with breast cancer risk. Positive associations between alcohol and breast cancer risk have been observed in most studies. The associations have been weak but may represent a causal relationship, possibly mediated by hormonal effects. No clear relationships have been shown with carotene, vitamin C, or vitamin E, and several good prospective studies have shown no relationship between selenium levels and breast cancer risk. Some studies have found an inverse association between fruit and vegetable consumption and breast cancer risk, but these findings have been less consistent than those for either lung cancer or stomach cancer. Of the few studies on the association of fibre with breast cancer, some have suggested that there may be a protective effect. Two studies have reported an inverse association of risk with consumption of soya, a rich source of phyto-oestrogens, but other recent studies have not confirmed this.

Breast cancer mortality can be reduced by mammographic screening of women aged over fifty, but the greatest reduction in mortality achieved in trials has been about 30 per cent and there is therefore an urgent need to reduce incidence. Trials currently underway are evaluating the antioestrogenic drug tamoxifen as a potential preventative agent, mainly among postmenopausal women (see Chapter 21). Tamoxifen has been shown to reduce mortality in early breast cancer and to reduce the incidence of second primary cancers in the remaining breast among women who have had a mastectomy for unilateral breast cancer; the results of the current primary prevention trials will be available in about ten years. Another hormonal treatment under investigation as a possible means for the primary prevention of breast cancer is a contraceptive regimen containing a luteinizing hormone releasing hormone agonist to suspend ovarian production of oestrogen and progesterone. This is administered together with low doses of oestrogen and intermittent progestin, just enough to maintain normal blood lipids and bone integrity and to prevent endometrial hyperplasia. This regimen is designed for use in premenopausal women (among whom more uncertainties surround the use of tamoxifen) and would be expected to reduce breast cancer risk. A feasibility study has shown that this treatment can change the mammographic appearance of breast tissue from a pattern associated with high risk to a lower risk pattern (see also Chapters 14 and 21 for discussions on breast cancer).

3.4.5 Prostate cancer

Prostate cancer is the fourth most frequent cancer of men world-wide and the second most common cancer among men in the UK. There are approximately 14 000 new cases and 10 000 deaths in the UK each year, with a five-year relative survival of about 43 per cent. Between the early 1970s and the mid to late 1980s, the rates increased in the UK, with increases of incidence and mortality at ages 50–64 of 33 and 35 per cent, respectively.

Prostate cancer incidence rates vary 50-fold between populations world-wide, but part of this variation is due to differences in the extent of diagnosis of small cancers that have not caused clinical disease. The variation in mortality rates is smaller, but still substantial, at about tenfold. Mortality rates are highest in northern Europe and among non-whites in the US, intermediate in western Europe and among whites in the US, and lowest in the far east. Prostate cancer rates increase in migrants from low risk to high risk countries, such as Japanese men in the US, but these men still have lower rates than US whites. The international variation in prostate cancer rates is broadly similar to that for breast cancer, except for the particularly high rates of prostate cancer in African Americans and in northern Europe.

A unique feature of prostate cancer is the high prevalence of latent disease. While the incidence of clinically overt prostate cancer, and the prevalence of infiltrating latent cancer, vary widely between populations, the prevalence of non-infiltrating latent cancer is similar in different populations. It therefore appears that the factors that determine the international variation in incidence rates act mostly by promoting the growth of existing cancers rather than by initiating the disease.

Apart from age and population group, the only well-established, important risk factor for prostate cancer is a family history of the disease. Men with a father or brother affected with prostate cancer have about twice the risk of men without affected relatives. The risk is higher still for men with more than one affected relative and for men with a relative who developed the disease at a young age. Segregation analysis has suggested that the familial clustering might be explained by autosomal dominant inheritance of a rare high risk allele leading to early onset of prostate cancer and be responsible for about 9 per cent of cases of prostate cancer by age 85.

The large variation in prostate cancer rates between countries, together with the increase in rates in migrants from low risk to high risk areas, indicates that environmental factors are important determinants of risk. It should be noted, however, that, whereas for breast cancer the international variation and the migrant studies suggest that genetic differences between countries are, at the most, minor determinants of risk, the current impression for prostate cancer is that genetic factors may be a significant determinant of some of the population variation in risk; for example, the higher rates of this disease in blacks than in whites in the US. Recent research has suggested that the racial variation in risk may be partly determined by differences in the genes for the androgen receptor and for the enzyme 5-α-reductase which converts testosterone into the more potent dihydrotestosterone.

Current research into possible environmental effects on prostate cancer risk has largely concerned hypotheses related to either sexual activity or diet. For sexual activity, one hypothesis is that risk is increased by high serum concentrations of testosterone, because this hormone stimulates cell division among the prostatic epithelial cells; it is further suggested that high levels of testosterone may be indicated by high levels of sexual activity. The other main hypothesis is that risk is increased by exposure to a sexually transmitted infectious agent. There is some evidence in support of both of these hypotheses, but it is not conclusive for either. Several recent studies have reported a positive association between vasectomy and subsequent risk for prostate cancer, but other studies have found no evidence for this association and it is possible that some of the results may have been affected by detection bias. More research on this topic is urgently needed, but vasectomy is a procedure introduced quite recently and it could not be responsible for more than a small proportion of current cancers.

Epidemiological studies of diet and prostate cancer have concentrated on two main areas, the role of fat and the role of carotene. The fat hypothesis for prostate cancer is that risk is increased by a high intake of total fat, animal fat, or animal products. This hypothesis was generated by the observed correlations of average intakes of these foods with prostate cancer rates in different countries. The fat hypothesis has been tested by a number of (mostly small) case-control studies, and a few prospective studies. The results have not been entirely consistent but most of the studies have given some support to the hypothesis. Several recent studies in experimental animals have examined a modification of this hypothesis, namely that n-6 polyunsaturated fatty acids increase risk and that n-3 polyunsaturated fatty acids are protective, but there are virtually no human data on this question.

The original hypothesis concerning carotene was that risk is decreased by a high intake of carotene. Surprisingly, the results of some of the early studies generated an alternative hypothesis, that risk is increased by a high intake of carotene. The results of studies that have estimated risk in relation to total carotene consumption, or in relation to the consumption of the two major sources of carotene (carrots and dark green vegetables), have produced very varied results. Some have found a significant positive association with risk, some a significant negative association with risk, and some no association. Furthermore, several studies have examined their results subdivided by age group (e.g. less than or greater than about 70 years old) and have reported different associations according to age, but these possible interactions have not been consistent between studies. In aggregate, the data do not provide evidence for an association between carotene intake and prostate cancer risk . It is possible that, as for breast cancer, dietary factors such as fibre and phyto-oestrogens could influence prostate cancer risk by affecting sex hormone metabolism. These topics require further research.

Some cases of early prostate cancer can be detected by measuring the serum concentration of prostate-specific antigen. This has led to the introduction in some areas of screening programmes for the detection and treatment (usually by radical prostatectomy) of early prostate cancer (see Chapter 21). This is unfortunate because there is no information concerning the effect of this screening and treatment on the outcome for men with early prostatic cancer. Screening should not be offered to the general population before the completion of randomized controlled trials to test its effect.

A trial is currently underway in the US to test whether prostate cancer can be prevented by treating healthy men at relatively high risk for the disease with finasteride. This drug inhibits the conversion of testosterone into dihydrotestosterone, which is a much more potent androgen and is the hormone that stimulates cell division in the prostate. No other options for prevention are currently available.

3.5 Risk factors

Table 3.7 summarizes the known and major suspected risk factors for each cancer site in order of the percentage of all cancer deaths caused by the tumour in England and Wales in 1992. The incidence and mortality figures give a rough guide to the relative importance of the site as a source of cancer; the relation between the incidence and mortality figures is a measure of the fatality rate associated with the particular cancer; and the male to female ratio for sites common to both sexes suggests the importance of exposure to sex-specific risk factors. The established risk factors have been divided into major and minor categories in terms of their importance to the total cancer burden in England and Wales for the specific site. This division is somewhat arbitrary but a major risk factor, perhaps in combination with other factors, might account for more than 25 per cent of a particular cancer. Suspected risk factors have only been listed if they are likely to belong in the major category if proven. Table 3.7 also lists, in a separate column, the major established risk factors for cancers in countries other than the UK.

Several aspects of Table 3.7 are noteworthy. Over half of all cancer mortality is accounted for by cancers of the lung, large bowel, breast, prostate, and stomach. The other 29 specific sites in Table 3.7 together, therefore, contribute less to total cancer mortality than these five sites. Although, scientifically, there will be much to learn from understanding the aetiological factors for an uncommon cancer, preventing part or even all of the mortality from such a cancer will have only a small impact on total cancer mortality. Minor risk factors for a common cancer may have a much greater public health significance than major risk factors for rarer forms of cancer.

3.5.1 Smoking (and alcohol)

Lung cancer, by itself, accounts for about a quarter of total cancer mortality in the UK. The relationship between smoking and lung cancer has been discussed above (see Section 3.4.1). Table 3.7 shows that smoking is also a major established risk factor for cancers of the lip, mouth, tongue, pharynx, larynx, oesophagus, bladder, and pancreas. Smoking is, therefore, a direct and avoidable cause of an enormous cancer burden. No other known single factor has anything like the same degree of importance for cancer in the developed world.

Smoking-related cancers in the upper respiratory and digestive tracts (i.e. mouth, tongue, pharynx, larynx, and oesophagus) also share alcohol as an established major risk factor. For the larynx and oesophagus, it has been demonstrated that smoking and alcohol act synergistically, i.e. their effects are more than additive and are, in fact, close to multiplicative. The results of one large study of oesophageal cancer found that a non-drinking smoker of 20 cigarettes per day has a 1.7-fold increased risk, while a non-smoking drinker of 100 g of alcohol per day had a 7.2-fold increased risk, but a 20 cigarettes per day drinker of 100 g of alcohol per day had a 12.1-fold increased risk. Such synergism is not uncommon with cancer risk factors, and shows that control of one risk factor may have a larger effect than one might predict from studies in which people, or experimental animals, were only exposed to the single agent.

3.5.2 Diet

Dietary factors have been the subject of much epidemiological research in recent years and there is a general belief that modifications to the diet could have a major impact on cancer rates. Table 3.7 indicates that stomach cancer and colorectal cancer certainly have major causal dietary components that breast and prostrate cancers may have as well, and that dietary factors are a minor established risk factor for lung cancer. Thus, all five major sites of cancer in the UK could be affected by diet.

Research on diet and cancer has increased greatly in recent years, but progress in identifying dietary factors that alter risk has been slow. There are several reasons for this. Probably the most important is the difficulty in measuring diet accurately in epidemiological studies. In studies of small numbers of people, nutritionists use multiple days of weighed dietary intake to obtain reasonably accurate estimates of usual long-term diet. This method is not applicable in retrospective epidemiological studies because these aim to measure past diet, and it is not practical in prospective epidemiological studies because of the very large number of people involved. Epidemiological studies have therefore relied mostly on simpler methods of dietary assessment, especially food frequency questionnaires, which are relatively easy to use but which produce rather inaccurate estimates of usual diet. This inaccuracy makes it hard to detect relationships between dietary factors and cancer risk and, where significant relationships are

Table 3.7 The contribution to total cancer incidence and mortality, male to female mortality ratio, and epidemiological risk factors for major sites of cancer in the UK

Site of cancer (in order of decreasing contribution to mortality)	Proportion of all cancers—incidence[1] (%)	Proportion of all cancers—mortality[2] (%)	Male/female mortality ratio	Risk factors			
				Major[3] established	Minor[3] established	Likely (possibly major[3]) but unproven	Major established but not in the UK
Lung	15.5	23.1	2–5:1 at different ages	Smoking	Radon Asbestos Polycyclic aromatic hydrocarbons Arsenic Nickel refining Chromates Bischloromethyl ether Low intake of fresh fruit and vegetables[4]		
Large bowel	11.4	11.9	1:1	Western-type diet	Polyposis coli	Low fibre intake Low vegetable intake High fat intake High meat intake Sedentary lifestyle	Schistosoma japonicum
Breast	11.8	9.4	0.01:1	Early menarche Late menopause Late first birth Low parity Inherited susceptibility	Postmenopausal obesity Postmenopausal hormone replacement therapy Ionizing radiation[5]	Endogenous hormones Western-type diet	
Prostate	5.3	6.0	M	Black racial group		Endogenous hormones High fat intake	
Stomach	4.6	5.7	1.5:1	Low socioeconomic status Low intake of fresh fruit and vegetables[4] Helicobacter pylori	Blood group A Smoking		High intake of salt and preserved foods
Pancreas	2.6	4.1	0.9:1	Smoking	Diabetes		
Oesophagus	2.2	3.7	1.6:1	Smoking Alcohol			Vitamin deficiency

Bladder	4.8	3.5	2.2:1	Smoking	Aromatic amines Certain anticancer drugs		*Schistosoma haemotobium*
Ovary	2.1	2.7	F	Low parity Oral contraceptives (protective) Early menarche Late menopause			
Non-Hodgkin's lymphoma	2.5	2.6	1.1:1		Immune impairment (in conjunction with epstein–Barr virus)		Epstein–Barr virus (for Burkitt's lymphoma)
Leukaemia	2.1	2.5	1.2:1		Ionizing radiation[5] Benzene Certain genetic syndromes Certain anticancer drugs	Population mixing and transmission of infection (childhood only)	Human T-cell leukaemia virus
Brain and nervous system	1.4	2.0	1.4:1				
Kidney (including pelvis)	1.7	1.8	1.6:1		Smoking Aromatic amines Phenacetin		
Myelomatosis	1.1	1.4	1.0:1	Black racial group			
Cervix	1.7	1.1	F	Certain human papillomavirus strains Multiple sexual partners Low socioeconomic status	High parity	Genital hygiene	
Liver	0.5	1.1	1.3:1	Cirrhosis	Hepatitis B and C viruses Excessive intake of alcohol Anabolic steroids Oral contraceptives Vinyl chloride monomer Thorotrast Immunosuppression		Hepatitis B and C viruses Aflatoxin Liver fluke (*O.viverrini, C.siniensis*)

Table 3.7 The contribution to total cancer incidence and mortality, male to female mortality ratio, and epidemiological risk factors for major sites of cancer in the UK (contd)

Site of cancer (in order of decreasing contribution to mortality)	Proportion of all cancers—incidence[1] (%)	Proportion of all cancers—mortality[2] (%)	Male/female mortality ratio	Risk factors			
				Major[3] established	Minor[3] established	Likely (possibly major[3]) but unproven	Major established but not in the UK
Tongue, mouth, and pharynx (excluding naso-pharynx)	1.0	0.9	1.9:1	Smoking Alchohol	Oral tobacco		Betel quid chewing Inverted smoking
Endometrium	1.7	1.0	F	Early menarche Late menopause Low parity Exogenous oestrogens (in absence of progestogens) Combined oral contraceptives (protective) Obesity			
Skin (melanoma)	1.5	0.8	1.0:1	Sun or other ultraviolet light Benign melanocytic naevi White racial group	Xeroderma pigmentosa Immune impairment	Sunburn	
Larynx	0.8	0.6	3.7:1	Smoking Alchohol		Certain human papillomavirus strains	
Gall bladder and bile ducts	0.5	0.5	0.6:1	Obesity Gall stones	High parity		
Connective tissue	0.5	0.4	1.0:1				
Pleura and peritoneum	0.4	0.4	4.6:1	Asbestos (some types)			
Vagina and vulva	0.4	0.4	F		Immunosuppressive drugs Maternal use of diethylstilboestrol		
Hodgkin's disease	0.5	0.3	1.5:1		Infectious mononucleosis Jewish race		
Skin (non-melanoma)	13.3	0.3	1.3:1	Sun or other ultraviolet light White racial group AIDS virus—for Kaposi's sarcoma only	Immune impairment Arsenic Polycyclic aromatic hydrocarbons Xeroderma pigmentosa		Tropical ulcers

Site	Incidence[1]	Mortality[2]	M:F ratio[3]	Causes and associations
Thyroid	0.4	0.2	0.4:1	Ionizing radiation[5]
Bone	0.2	0.2	1.1:1	Paget's disease
Nose and nasal sinuses	0.2	0.1	1.6:1	Nickel refining; Hardwood furniture; Leather manufacture; Isopropyl alcohol production; Smoking
Testis	0.5	0.1	M	Undescended testis; Early puberty; White racial group
Nasopharynx	0.1	0.1	1.6:1	Salted fish; Epstein-Barr virus; HLA type
Salivary gland	0.1	0.1	1.4:1	
Penis	0.2	0.1	M	Circumcision (protective); Certain human papillomavirus strains
Lip	0.1	0.03	1.7:1	Smoking (esp. pipe); Sun or other ultraviolet light

[1] The incidence figure is for England and Wales cancer registrations in 1989 expressed as a proportion of all malignant cancer registrations.

[2] The mortality figure is for England and Wales in 1992 expressed as proportion of all malignant cancer deaths.

[3] The distinction between major and minor is inevitably somewhat arbitrary. A major risk factor may, in combination with other risk factors, account for more than 25 per cent of a particular cancer.

[4] Low intake of fresh fruit and vegetables may protect against several types of cancer, although most evidence relates to cancers of the lung and stomach (see text).

[5] Ionizing radiation can be a cause of nearly all cancers (excepting possibly chronic lymphatic leukaemia and Hodgkin's disease), but the proportional increases in risk are highest for leukaemia (except chronic lymphatic leukaemia) and for thyroid cancer (following exposure in childhood).

found, can cause profound underestimation of the size of the effect on risk; a tenfold increase in true risk associated with a dietary factor could be estimated as a less than twofold increase in risk by many of the dietary questionnaires used in epidemiological studies. Inaccurate measurement also makes it difficult to distinguish between the effects of different dietary factors, since intakes of many foods and nutrients are correlated with each other.

Other problems with epidemiological studies of diet and cancer include the relatively narrow range of dietary exposures within a population, the long period during which the disease develops, and the changes in diet during a lifetime. The best prospects for improving our understanding of the relationship between diet and cancer appear to lie with very large prospective studies now underway. Currently it is possible to make some general comments about diet and cancer risk, but few specific relationships have been established.

In very broad terms, epidemiological research to date has provided evidence that diets high in total fat or animal fat (or perhaps animal protein) may increase the risk for some types of cancer, whereas diets high in fibre or starch, and diets high in fruit and vegetables, may decrease the risk for some types of cancer. Some of this evidence has been discussed above in the sections on the five commonest cancers in the UK (Sections 3.4.1–3.4.5).

The mechanisms underlying the observed relationships between these dietary factors and cancer risk are not well understood. Diets high in total fat or animal fat may increase the risk for colorectal cancer by increasing the production of bile acids, but there is no obvious mechanism to explain their association with the risk for prostate cancer. Diets high in fibre or starch may reduce the risk for colorectal cancer by binding bile acids, reducing transit time, increasing faecal bulk, and by fermentation to beneficial volatile fatty acids. For fruit and vegetables, which are consistently associated with lower risks for lung cancer and stomach cancer, most research has concerned the possible protective effects of carotene and vitamin C, two dietary antioxidants. However, current epidemiological studies have limited ability to distinguish between associations with carotene, vitamin C, and fruits and vegetables themselves, because these factors are strongly correlated with each other. This problem applies both to estimates of dietary intake of carotene and vitamin C and to serum concentrations of these

nutrients. Randomized controlled trials can test the effects of individual nutrients. Of the four large trials published so far, the trials of lung cancer prevention in Finland and the US found no protective effect for β-carotene against lung cancer (indeed in two of the three trials mortality from lung cancer was significantly higher in the men given β-carotene than in the men not given β-carotene) or against stomach cancer, while the trial of oesophageal cancer prevention in China reported results for stomach cancer and found a small reduction in the risk for patients given supplemental β-carotene with vitamin E and selenium, but no protective effect for vitamin C with molybdenum. Thus, the protective factors in fruits and vegetables have not yet been identified.

The strongest evidence for a protective effect of micronutrients (vitamins and trace minerals) against cancer is for oesophageal cancer. In Western countries such as the UK, this cancer is caused largely by tobacco and alcohol; high use of both these items increases risk, with extremely high risk in people who both smoke and drink heavily. However, tobacco and alcohol do not explain the huge variation in oesophageal cancer rates between different populations worldwide; the variation in men in different regions is about 500-fold, which is much larger than the range for other common cancers. The very high risk populations, which include parts of Iran around the south of the Caspian Sea and also parts of China, have restricted diets which are low in fruit, vegetables, and animal products and consequently low in several micronutrients including retinol, β-carotene, riboflavin, vitamin C, and zinc. It is very likely that a substantial proportion of the high incidence of oesophageal cancer in the very high risk populations is due to dietary deficiencies of some of these micronutrients, but it has not yet been established which factors are most important, and the high risk in some populations may be partly due to other factors such as dietary N-nitroso compounds.

Cancer risk can be increased by dietary consumption of known chemical carcinogens. Examples of this mechanism have not been established in the UK, but dietary carcinogens are important in other areas. Aflatoxin, produced by fungal growth on grains, peanuts, and other foods stored in warm, humid conditions, is probably a major cause of liver cancer in several tropical countries. In the coastal region of south-east China, a type of salted fish is fed to infants at weaning, and this practice is associated with a large increase in the risk for nasopharyngeal cancer, probably because the salted fish contains various mutagens. In both these examples, the dietary carcinogens appear to act largely in association with viral infections (see Chapter 8).

3.5.3 Infection

After tobacco and diet, infectious agents are estimated to be the third most important cause of cancer in the UK. The concept of an infectious aetiology to human cancer is one that has passed in and out of fashion over the decades, although a number of well-characterized, virally induced cancers in animal models have provided one of the corner-stones for our current understanding of molecular carcinogenesis. There is now no doubt that many cancers can be caused by infections, especially in developing countries, and, in some circumstances, infections may be easier targets for public health interventions (by primary prevention or vaccination) than control of smoking or diet.

Epidemiological study design can be considerably simplified when considering exposure to infectious agents and the characterization of individuals as exposed or unexposed, using appropriate biological markers, and is relatively straightforward in comparison with assessment of, for example, exposures to dietary nutrients or ultraviolet light. For this reason, once a potential infectious agent has been suspected of causing cancer, establishing whether or not there is an association and estimating the size of the risk can be carried out quite quickly. In some instances, traditional epidemiological questionnaires can provide data indicative of an infectious aetiology in the absence of a specific infectious agent. Thus, cervical cancer was thought to be associated with a venereally acquired infection, as a result of its epidemiological relationships with sexual behaviour, a long time before the relevant papillomavirus strains were identified as the responsible agent. Similarly, there is now an impressive body of evidence to suggest that childhood leukaemia might be associated with recent introduction of common infections into unexposed populations but no candidate has as yet been found. In contrast, until *H. pylori* was identified, no one gave much credence to the hypothesis that stomach cancer had an infectious aetiology.

Although many infections that cause cancer are viral in origin and interact directly with DNA to cause genetic mutations, there are several non-viral infections which primarily act by inducing a persistent chronic inflammatory response in the host. This gives rise to an abnormal exposure to toxic and mutagenic biochemicals (notably free radical oxygen and nitrogen oxides) which derive from the host's immune response. *Helicobacter pylori* has been discussed from this perspective, but the same model would apply to cancers caused by chronic schistosomiasis (bladder and large bowel cancers) or liver fluke (liver cancer) infections in developing countries. It is also possible that the hepatitis B and C viruses have a similar effect although they are also known to integrate into the host's genome.

In the UK, the major cancers in which infectious agents play a role are stomach cancer (see Section 3.4.2) and cervical cancer. There is also interest in the role of viral infections in certain types of leukaemia and lymphoma. For cervical cancer, case-control studies have shown very large relative risks (of the order of 50) in association with infection with certain subtypes (especially 16 and 18) of the human papillomavirus. It is now certain that this virus is the major causative agent for cervical cancer, although the development of cancer following infection is affected by other factors which probably include hygiene and perhaps diet. A vaccine against the relevant subtypes of human papillomavirus could prevent a majority of cases of this disease and clinical trials evaluating such a vaccine are just commencing.

3.5.4 Occupation

Established carcinogens that occur mainly in occupational settings are nearly all categorized as minor risk factors in Table 3.7 (with the exception of asbestos in relation to cancer of the pleura and peritoneum). This does not mean that they are of minor importance for everyone; indeed for workers in the relevant industries, they may be of great importance. For example, bladder cancer has been shown to be caused by occupational exposure to a number of chemicals used in the dye and rubber industries. These chemicals (2-naphthylamine, benzidine, 3,3'-dichlorobenzidine, and 4-aminobiphenyl) belong   to a class of chemicals (the aromatic amines) that are now known to be animal carcinogens. 2-Naphthylamine is particularly carcinogenic; all 19 distillers in one factory developed bladder cancer, and it is no longer used in UK industry. There are several other occupational carcinogens which in the past would have constituted significant health hazards for specific groups of workers. At present, however, only a small proportion of the total cancer mortality experienced by the population as a whole can be attributed to occupational carcinogens.

3.5.5 Other risk factors

Several factors which are often thought to be associated with cancer are either not included in Table 3.7 or are categorized as minor factors. Industrial pollution, pesticide exposure, and psychological stress are not listed at all. A number of these omissions may reflect a failure of cancer epidemiology to investigate certain subjects adequately (e.g. stress) but these omissions also reflect the fact that, although many chemicals are reported as positive in animal carcinogenicity or *in vitro* tests, they appear to make a negligible contribution to human cancer. In some cases this is because the doses employed in testing are orders of magnitude above those to which people are exposed. It is now also apparent that the human body is continually confronted with genotoxic agents, not only from industrial chemicals, but also from a wide range of products found naturally in many foods. It may, therefore, prove to be the case that many genotoxic agents will be of much less importance to human cancer than, say, host DNA repair mechanisms or factors that stimulate cells to proliferate. Clearly, some genotoxins are of considerable importance, for example, ultraviolet light and the carcinogens present in tobacco smoke; others may be of limited relevance to human cancer.

3.5.6 Summary

A comprehensive overview of our current understanding of the causes of all types of cancer has been made by Doll and Peto and their conclusions are summarized in Table 3.8. Tobacco (more specifically, cigarette smoking) stands out in that it accounts for an estimated 33 per cent of all cancer mortality and it is the only factor for which all the associated deaths could undoubtedly be avoided by the implementation of known practical measures. Dietary modifications could perhaps prevent about the same number of cancer deaths as changes in smoking (maybe 30 per cent), but our ignorance of the specific changes required means that there is a lot of uncertainty in the estimate of what is possible (20–60 per cent). The contribution of occupa-

tional risk factors to the total population cancer burden is estimated as being no more than 4 per cent, and probably closer to 3 per cent. Occupational exposure to established carcinogens has been substantially reduced, e.g. asbestos, or entirely eliminated, e.g. 2-naphthylamine, in the UK, so that there are very few practical measures that could be implemented now which would guarantee a reduction in occupationally related cancer.

Further details of the calculations that underlie Table 3.8 can be found in Doll and Peto (1981) while their more recent publication (Doll and Peto 1996) expands on this discussion of risk factors on a site by site basis.

Acknowledgement

We would like to thank Richard Doll, Richard Peto, Leo Kinlen, and Sarah Darby for their contributions to specific sections of this chapter.

Table 3.8 Proportions of cancer deaths in the US[1] attributable to various factors

Factor or class of factors	Per cent of all cancer deaths		
	Best estimate (%)	Range of acceptable estimates (%)	
		Minimum	Maximum
Tobacco	33	25	40
Diet	30	20	60
Infection	9	5	15
Reproductive factors and hormones	7[2]	5	10
Ionizing radiation	6	4	8
Occupation	3	2	4
Alcohol	3	2	4
Ultraviolet light	1	0.5	1
Industrial products	<1	<1	2
Pollution	<1	<1	2
Medical drugs	<1	<1	2
Food additives	<1	−2[3]	1
Other and unknown	?		

[1] After Doll and Peto (1981, 1996). Similar figures would apply to the UK.

[2] Manipulation of some reproductive factors (e.g. age at first birth) to avoid cancer is clearly possible but not necessarily practical or acceptable.

[3] "Allowing for a possible protective effect of antioxidants and other preservatives" (Doll and Peto, 1981).

References and further reading

Ames, B. N., Magaw, R., and Gold, L.S. (1987). Ranking possible carcinogenic hazards. *Science,* **239,** 271–80.

Block, G., Patterson, B., and Subar, A. (1992). Fruit, vegetables and cancer prevention: a review of the epidemiological evidence. *Nutrition and Cancer,* **18,** 1–29.

Blot, W. J., Li, J.Y., Taylor, P. R., Guo, W., Dawsey, S., Wang, G. Q. *et al..* (1993). Nutrition intervention trials in Linxian, China: supplementation with specific vitamin/mineral combinations, cancer incidence, and disease-specific mortality in the general population. *Journal of the National Cancer Institute,* **85,** 1483–92.

Correa, P. (1988). A human model of gastric carcinogenesis. *Cancer Research,* **48,** 3554–60.

Doll, R. (1992). Are we winning the war against cancer? A review in memory of Keith Durrant. *Clinical Oncology,* **4,** 257–66.

Doll, R. and Peto, R. (1981). *The causes of cancer: quantitative estimates of avoidable risks of cancer in the United States today.* Oxford University Press, Oxford.

Doll, R. and Peto, R. (1996). Epidemiology of cancer. In *Oxford textbook of medicine* (ed. D. J. Weatherall, J. G. G. Ledingham, and D. A. Warrell). Oxford University Press, Oxford.

Doll, R., Peto, R., Wheatley, K., Gray, R., and Sutherland, I. (1994). Mortality in relation to smoking: 40 years' observations on male British doctors. *British Medical Journal,* **309,** 901–11.

Greenberg, E. R, Baron, J.A., Tosteson, T. D., Freeman, D. H. Jr., Beck, G. J., Bond, J. H. *et al.* (1994). A clinical trial of antioxidant vitamins to prevent colorectal adenoma. *New England Journal of Medicine,* **331,** 141–7.

Muñoz, N., Bosch, F. X., de Sanjose, S., Tafur, L., Izarzugaza, I., Gili, M. *et al.* (1992). The causal link between human papillomavirus and invasive cervical cancer: a population-based case-control study in Colombia and Spain. *International Journal of Cancer,* **52,** 743–9.

Nomura, A. M. Y. and Kolonel, L.N. (1991). Prostate cancer: a current perspective. *American Journal of Epidemiology,* **13,** 200–27.

Parkin, D. M, Muir, L. S., Whelan, S. L., Gao, Y.-T., Ferlay, J., and Powell, J. (1992). *Cancer incidence in five continents,* Vol. VI. International Agency for Research on Cancer and International Association of Cancer Registries (WHO), Lyon.

Parkin, D. M., Pisani, P., and Ferlay, J. (1993). Estimates of the worldwide incidence of eighteen major cancers in 1985. *International Journal of Cancer,* **54,** 594–606.

Peto, R., Lopez, A. D., Boreham, J., Thun, M., and Heath, C. Jr. (1994). *Mortality from smoking in developed countries 1950–2000: indirect estimates from national vital statistics.* Oxford University Press, Oxford.

Pike, M. C. and Ross, R. K. (1984). Breast Cancer. *British Medical Bulletin,* **40,** 351–4.

Pike, M. C., Spicer, D. V., Dahmoush, L., and Press M. F. (1993). Estrogens, progestogens, normal breast cell proliferation, and breast cancer risk. *Epidemiologic Reviews,* **15,** 17–35.

Potter, J. D. (1992). Reconciling the epidemiology, physiology, and molecular biology of colon cancer. *Journal of the American Medical Association,* **268,** 1573–7.

Schottenfeld, D. and Fraumeni, J. F., jun. (1990). *Cancer epidemiology and prevention,* (2nd edn). W.B. Saunders, Philadelphia.

Steinmetz, K.A. and Potter, J. D. (1991). Vegetables, fruit, and cancer. II. Mechanisms. *Cancer Causes and Control,* **2,** 427–42.

The Alpha-Tocopherol, Beta-Carotene Cancer Prevention Study Group. (1994). The effect of vitamin E and beta-carotene on the incidence of lung cancer and other cancers in male smokers. *New England Journal of Medicine,* **330,** 1029–35.

Waterhouse, J., Muir, C., Correa, P., and Powell, J. (1976). *Cancer incidence in five continents,* Vol. III. IARC Scientific Publication No. 15. International Agency for Research on Cancer, Lyon.

Waterhouse, J., Muir, C., Shanmugaratnam, K., and Powell, J. (1982*). Cancer incidence in five continents,* Vol. IV. IARC Scientific Publication No. 42. International Agency for Research on Cancer, Lyon.

4

Inherited susceptibility to cancer

H. S. WASAN AND W. F. BODMER

4.1 Introduction: the cellular genetic basis for cancer

Epidemiological studies, especially of variations in cancer incidence in different populations and their migrants (as discussed in Chapter 3) strongly suggest that at least 80 per cent of cancer incidence is attributable in the broadest sense to environmental factors. The response to such factors, may of course be dependent, to a variable extent, on the host's genetic composition. Studies on the incidence of cancer in the relatives of patients with the disease support the view that, overall, the direct contribution of inheritance to cancer susceptibility is not as large as compared with other major diseases, such as some of the cardiovascular, neurological, neuropsychiatric, and autoimmune disorders. At the cellular level, however, in the individual in whom cancer develops, genetic changes within the cells destined to form a malignant tumour are the key to the progression from a normal to a neoplastic cell.

In this chapter, the evidence for the importance of genetic changes at the cellular level in the development of a cancer will be briefly reviewed, and then discussed more extensively with respect to the situations where there is an inherited basis for cancer susceptibility. This also provides the basis for understanding the changes at a cellular level.

Most of the fundamental ideas on the causation of cancer were suggested in the early years of this century, while the idea that exposure to substances in the environment could be a cause of cancer goes back at least to the British surgeon Percival Pott in 1775. He pointed out that chimney sweeps tended to get cancer of the scrotum because they were chronically exposed to soot. Thus, not only was he the first person to clearly identify an environmental carcinogen, but also an occupational cancer. Indeed, this association led to the subsequent decline in incidence of this disease: a powerful example of successful cancer prevention!

The major fundamental ideas about the causes of cancer, which may be inherited or acquired, are as follows.

1. Genetic changes, or mutations, in somatic cells of the body are the main initiating events, and are responsible for tumour progression; these changes may be either inherited or acquired. If cells have a mutation in any of the pathways that have evolved to repair DNA damage, this may also

lead to an increased propensity for malignant progression.

2. The related idea that changes in the chromosomes, either in their number or organization, for example by deletion or translocation (see Glossary), are key events (see Chapter 10).

3. Some cancers are caused by viruses (see Chapter 8).

4. Cancers represent a form of dedifferentiation or, more generally, a perturbation of the differentiated state, which is associated with loss of growth control and disturbances of cell cycle regulation.

5. The immune system plays a role in combating or preventing cancer through recognition of novel antigens either in or on cancer cells (see Chapter 16).

In addition to these five general points, the concept of programmed cell death or apoptosis must now be added, which is normally an integral part of growth and development. Although not yet specifically attributable as a cause, the regulated control of cell death appears to be just as crucial as that of cell division and differentiation in determining the growth characteristics of any tissue. Indeed, programmed cell death could be thought of as part of a terminal differentiation process and can be shown to be perturbed through genetic changes in tumours. Resistance to programmed cell death could contribute to the progression of the malignant phenotype, by allowing already aberrant cells to survive when they otherwise should not, and perhaps also to accumulate further DNA damage, as will be discussed in more detail later. This concept can interrelate with any of the five points above. For example, both chromosomal translocation (e.g. leading to overexpression of bcl-2 in follicular lymphomas) and virus–host interactions (e.g. through p53 binding to transforming viral proteins such as the SV40 T antigen) can lead to fundamentally altered cells which also demonstrate resistance to apoptosis.

In recent years, modern developments in genetics, cell biology, and virology, especially at the molecular level, have made it possible to establish, in detail, the relative importance of these fundamental concepts for the development of many cancers. These six ideas can all be interrelated through the basic assumption that a cancer develops through a series of genetic changes progressing from a single initiated cell to the ultimate malignant cell, whose progeny eventually give rise to the cancer.

4.2 Evidence for a genetic basis

There are several major lines of evidence to support the view that cancer is a genetic disease at the somatic cell level. Cancers, as populations of cells, tend to breed true as far as their cell types are concerned. This is the fundamental basis for the histopathological diagnosis of a cancer, as, for example, a particular sort of lymphoma or carcinoma. Staying true to type, however, says little more than that the cells of a cancer reflect, on the whole, the properties of the tissue from which they originated. Normal differences between types of cells are based on differential gene expression. This emphasizes the possibility that some of the steps in tumour progression may not necessarily involve mutations directly, but rather aberrant control of gene expression by mechanisms, such as DNA methylation, which may be analogous to those that control cellular differentiation. The term 'epigenetic' is often used to describe this situation, to contrast it with the direct effects of genetic changes in the sense of mutations, namely alterations in the DNA sequence itself. However, the difference between genetic and epigenetic may turn out to be no more than semantic, in that, ultimately, epigenetic phenomena are also genetically regulated.

Genetic markers have been used to show that the majority of cancers are clonal in origin. That is, they are derived at some point by cell division from a single cell. The evidence for this depends on the fact that in females, cells contain two X chromosomes, of which only one is active, or fully functional. This ensures that males (XY) and females (XX) have the same level of X chromosome gene activity. The female receives one of her X chromosomes from her mother and the other from her father. Subsequently, random inactivation of one of the X chromosomes occurs in all embryonic somatic cells. This leaves roughly half the cells with the maternal X chromosome active, whereas in the other half it is the paternal X chromosome that remains operative. This process is called lyonization, after Mary Lyon. Thus, a female who is heterozygous for the two forms, or alleles, of a gene on the X chromosome represents a mosaic of cells, half of which, on average, express one allele, and the other half, the other allele. Glucose-6 phosphate dehydrogenase (G6PD), a metabolic enzyme involved in glycolysis, occurs in some populations (especially those of African origin), in at least two different forms, A and B, which can be distinguished by the technique of protein electrophoresis. A female who is heterozygous G6PD A/B, is thus a mosaic of cells with approximately half expressing G6PD A, and the rest expressing G6PD B. A tumour in such a heterozygous female, if clonal, should therefore not be a mosaic. That is, all the cells of the tumour will either be G6PD A or G6PD B, depending on which allele was active in the initiated cell from which the tumour was originally derived (Fig. 4.1). Such studies on tumours, which were pioneered by Gartler and Fialkow, among others, demonstrated that the vast majority of leukaemias in G6PD A/B heterozygotes are clonal in origin by this criterion. There are similar data in mice supporting the fact that the vast majority of experimentally induced liver tumours are also clonally derived, using another X chromosome enzyme marker.

Modern techniques demonstrating clonality, are generally still dependent on this principle of lyonization or X chromosome mosaicism but do not depend any longer on protein electrophoretic differences and so can analyse loci other than G6PD by assessing the degree of differential DNA methylation of two alleles on the X chromosome. Indeed, using this method, in apparently multifocal tumours in the urinary bladder, there is evidence by such methylation-restriction patterns in females that, perhaps surprisingly, even these might be clonal. This suggests that these seemingly disparate tumours have a common cell of origin and may therefore have arisen at separate (but probably nearby) sites through mucosal or surface seeding of one malignant clone. These X chromosome-dependent techniques have, however, some important limitations as to their significance. X chromosome clonality of a tissue structure, for example, colonic crypts, may be established long before initiation of a tumour, as lyonization occurs in the early embryo. In other words, even if a tumour was derived from several cells, if these all came from a localized 'patch' of epithelial tissue they would almost certainly all be expressing the same X chromosome already, that is, either all paternal or all maternal, at the time of tumour initiation. Furthermore, such studies are generally limited to female tissues only.

The analysis of clonality can now be taken even further by looking at the pattern of specific muta-

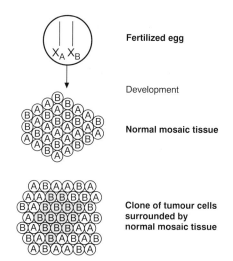

Fig. 4.1 Scheme to illustrate the use of the X-linked G6PD marker to show the clonal origin of tumours. The female heterozygote carries the allele A for G6PD A on one X chromosome, and B for G6PD B on the other X chromosome. The two forms of the enzyme can be distinguished by their different electrophoretic mobility on a gel. During development the fertilized egg divides to give rise to the somatic tissues. Each somatic cell has only one active X and since the mechanism of inactivation appears to be random, normal tissues will usually be a mosaic of two different sorts of cells with respect to G6PD activity, one expressing the A variant and the other expressing the B variant. If tumours arise from a single progenitor cell, then all the cells of the tumour will be derived by division from this progenitor and express the same G6PD type as the cell that initiated the tumour. Thus, tissue from a tumour will express only one of the two alleles (G6PD B in this figure), whereas samples of normal tissue will continue to express a mixture of the two.

tions in oncogenes and tumour suppressor genes in the primary tumour and demonstrating identical mutations in metastatic or recurrent tumour at a later stage. Infrequently, this may even be visible as a karyotypic abnormality (see below). This approach is not only of academic interest but is potentially an exquisitely sensitive way of aiding in tumour diagnosis and management. In specific circumstances, such as with the lymphomas, demonstration of clonality is often a diagnostic necessity in clinical practice to differentiate malignant from benign lymphoid proliferation, and is easily demonstrated for both B and T cells by surface antibody light-chain restriction and receptor gene rearrangements, respectively.

All this evidence, of course, only shows that at some point in the development of a tumour, it becomes clonal. It does not rule out the possibility that epigenetic influences, such as, for example, a persistent immune reaction or tissue repair to a specific insult, may create a multicellular environment that favours the initiation of a tumour or provides the conditions for the selection of a particular clone of cells from an originally multiclonal tumour. In such a situation, the tumour could potentially be derived from any one of a number of cells in this altered cellular milieu.

Chromosomal changes have been seen in tumours since they were first studied by Boveri and others in the early years of this century. However, as discussed in Chapter 10, it is only comparatively recently that quite specific chromosome changes have been identified that are often characteristic of a particular tumour. The initial and classical example is the Philadelphia chromosome found in chronic myeloid leukaemia (CML). Since 1973, this has been known to be a specific translocation, namely an exchange of particular parts between two chromosomes (in this case 9 and 22), and therefore represents a specific genetic event. The Philadelphia chromosome is almost always seen in all CML cells, and this in itself is evidence for at least one critical genetic step in the development of this particular tumour. Added to this is the observation that this specific change has never been seen in a normal cell, so that the frequency with which it is produced must be exceedingly low. Thus, the fact that the Philadelphia chromosome is found in almost all CML cells is further evidence for the clonality of this tumour, since the probability of that particular chromosomal mutation occurring independently two or more times in the same tissue must be negligible. The detailed genetic consequences of the Philadelphia chromosome translocation have now been elucidated most elegantly at the molecular level (see Chapters 10 and 12). The novel 'fused' gene formed by bringing together two different, normally unassociated, genes from chromosomes 9 and 22 in the translocation, now forms the basis for a remarkably sensitive test for the presence of residual leukaemic cells in the blood and bone marrow of CML patients after treatment. Many further examples of specific clonal chromosome changes in cancers are described in Chapter 10.

The majority of cancer-causing agents, or carcinogens, are also mutagens, that is, they cause genetic mutations (see Chapter 6). One of the most widely used simple carcinogen screening tests is a test for mutagenicity using bacterial strains, the so-called Ames test. Many agents act directly on DNA to cause genetic mutations and, in this case, there is often a good parallel between their mutagenic and carcinogenic activity. There are, however, at least three important limitations to this approach for the detection of carcinogens. The first is that many carcinogens are converted into active forms in the body by various enzymes, such as the cytochrome P450 mixed function oxidases of the liver. In these cases, unless the specific enzymes are provided, as additional reagents for the test (for example as a liver extract), the test will be negative. The second limitation is that some agents can cause genetic changes, for example by interfering with chromosome organization, in a way that cannot be detected by bacterial mutagenesis assays. The third limitation is that the tumour promoters, which are chemicals that on their own cannot initiate a cancer, but which enormously increase the probability of a cancer developing once a cell is initiated, work by different mechanisms that cannot be detected by bacterial or other mutagenesis assays (see Chapter 6).

There are a number of relatively rare but well-described inherited diseases that involve an inability to repair damaged DNA arising from specific insults and so consequently increase the mutation or chromosomal damage rates. These inherited syndromes are usually associated with a marked increase in the susceptibility to cancer, particularly lymphomas and leukaemias. There is now also accumulating evidence that, for at least a small subset of the more common solid cancers such as colon and breast, the inherited susceptibilities, which involve some form of incompetence in specific DNA repair pathways, may be more frequent than was originally thought (see Section 4.5.1).

A final piece of evidence for genetic changes in tumour cells comes from the exciting studies on oncogenes, mainly those identified in the oncogenic viruses. Using recombinant DNA techniques, specific genetic changes in the normal versions of the oncogenes have been demonstrated in a number of human and animal tumours, as discussed in several of the chapters in this book, especially Chapters 8, 9, and 10.

The general notion that changes in gene expression in somatic cells, mostly owing to mutation (which in the broadest sense includes, for example, chromosome translocation), underlie the origin of cancer, unites the major fundamental ideas about its causes. Mutation, chromosome changes, the effects of viruses, novel determinants on the surface of tumour cells, and changes in the pattern of expression of differentiated gene products are all subsumed, in one way or another, under this general hypothesis, for which there is increasing direct experimental evidence.

Many lines of evidence suggest that tumour progression is a multistep process, presumably involving several successive genetic changes (see Chapters 1, 6, and 14). In 1953, analysis of the increase in incidence of cancer as a function of age was used by Doll, Armitage, Peto, and others to provide approximate estimates for the number of steps involved, which comes to about four or five at least for the carcinomas. This, although no more than a very rough guess, has been shown experimentally to be remarkably accurate to date, as seen by the number of steps required for adenocarcinoma of the colon. Such estimates, however, cannot clearly distinguish between genetic and epigenetic changes. One problem in the interpretation of the multistep hypothesis is that a single genetic change, for example in the control of a series of genes involved in a differentiation pathway, may lead to multiple changes in gene expression in one step. A possible example of this is the occurrence of intestinal metaplasia in the gastric epithelium: intestinal metaplasia describes a focal region of the gastric epithelium which takes on, often almost completely, the phenotype of the intestine rather than the stomach. This occurs usually as a result of a continuous chronic insult, such as from inflammation secondary to chronic gastritis caused by colonization with the bacterium *Helicobacter pylori*, an ulcer, or smoking. It is as if a switch has been thrown which changes the pattern of epithelial differentiation in small areas of epithelium from that of the stomach to that of the intestine. This can be identified by a whole series of differences in gene expression associated with the intestinal phenotype. The clinical significance of these lesions is that some specific types of metaplasia appear to have an increased propensity for malignant change to a carcinoma. This is supported by epidemiological data, which suggests a strong association of smoking, but

a relatively weaker one for *Helicobacter*, and gastric cancer.

Each change in gene expression during the progression from the initial cell to the final malignant tumour must give rise to a selective advantage in terms of enhanced growth rate or independence of growth from the effects of the immediate environment of the tumour in at least a substantial fraction of the cells. Otherwise, the change would not be seen at all. In this sense tumour progression is an evolutionary process at the somatic level within the individual. Heterogeneity within a tumour can clearly arise both from different evolutionary sublines within any given tumour, and also from variations in expression, associated with environmentally determined differences in the stage of residual differentiation of the cells.

4.3 Genetic markers, DNA polymorphisms, and genetic linkage

The simplest family data providing evidence for inherited cancer susceptibility involve the patterns of inheritance expected for a clear-cut Mendelian trait due to a single recessive or dominant gene. A well-known example of a recessive inherited susceptibility is xeroderma pigmentosum (XP), an inherited DNA repair deficiency which predisposes nearly all deficient individuals to skin cancer. In this case, in its simplest form, affected individuals carry two defective copies of the relevant gene, one inherited from each of the parents, who will be unaffected carriers of the defective gene. The chance that an offspring of two such carriers is affected is the classical Mendelian ratio of one in four. The situation, however, is now known to be much more complex, as there is a complement of (rather than one) genes that are probably involved (discussed further in Section 4.5.1). In contrast, retinoblastoma is an example of a dominantly inherited susceptibility, in this case to tumours of the eye. A single defective gene is enough to give rise to the susceptibility, so that an affected parent will, on average, produce 50 per cent affected offspring. There are many such examples of individually rare instances of clear-cut inherited cancers. Each of these cases may in itself be of fundamental interest in understanding oncogenesis, as will be discussed in the next section. Collectively, however, their overall inherited contribution to the incidence of common cancers remains to be ascertained, but is unlikely to be more than a few per cent.

To understand the basis of these inherited susceptibilities we initially need to identify and isolate the corresponding genes and establish their functions, and through that their relationship to cancer susceptibility. In the absence of a clear-cut clue as to the functional basis of an inherited predisposition, an important first step in identifying the gene is to find out where it lies on the chromosomes.

There are now many techniques by which a defined protein product or, now more often, a specific human DNA sequence can be assigned to its position on a human chromosome. An important initial step to this was the development of techniques for the genetic analysis of cells in culture, called 'somatic cell genetics', based on hybridizing or fusing human cells with other cells to form somatic cell hybrids (Fig. 4.2). Humanmouse hybrid cells containing different combinations of human chromosomes can be used to associate a given human DNA sequence with a particular chromosome, or chromosome fragment, as a major step towards localization. Newer, more powerful techniques have generally superseded this method, as it is now possible to visualize directly the position of a DNA sequence on a chromosome spread using *in situ* hybridization coupled with autoradiography or a fluorescence-based techniques, as described in Chapter 10. [A more detailed description of the techniques for localizing human genes to their particular positions on the chromosomes can be found in various chapters in Franks (1988).] Once a gene has been localized on a chromosome, a selection of markers, as described below, facilitates the basis for its identification and subsequent functional analysis.

The estimated 70 000 or so human genes are distributed among 23 pairs of human chromosomes.

Genes on homologous chromosomes are combined and passed on at random from parent to offspring. If a heterozygous A1/A2 individual is also heterozygous B1/B2 at a second locus on a different chromosome, then the combinations A1B1, A1B2, A2B1, and A2B2 are each passed on with a frequency of, on average, a quarter to each offspring. Suppose, on the other hand, that the A and B loci are on the same chromosome, so that, for example, one of the pairs of homologous chromosomes in an individual carries A1B1 while the other carries A2B2. Then, if the genes are sufficiently close together, the combinations A1B1 and A2B2 will be passed on to the offspring more frequently than the 'recombinant' combinations A1B2 and A2B1. The frequency with which these recombinant, non-parental types are passed on is called the recombination fraction (r), and is an empirical measure of the distance between the A and B genes on the chromosome. The recombination fraction is thus less than half when genes are sufficiently close together on the same chromosome, and the genes are then said to be linked (Table 4.1). Suppose, for example, that the A1 and A2 allele difference is the one that determines an inherited susceptibility to cancer, while the B1 and B2 difference can be directly observed, as, for example, the inherited HLA tissue types. Then, the latter difference between B1 and B2 is said to be a marker difference, and will be distorted in its distribution among individuals in a family with cancer, owing to the linkage between the A and the B genes. Thus, the closer together the two genes are, the smaller is the recombination fraction r, and the greater will be the distortion in the distribution of the marker difference between B1 and B2 among individuals with cancer. Therefore, if A1 is a dominant susceptibility gene, when linkage is close and the recombination fraction r, is very small, almost all the

Table 4.1 Linkage and recombination

	Parent	Gametic (egg or sperm) combinations		
No linkage	A1 B1	A1B1, A2B2, A2B1, A1B2		
	A2 B2	passed on to offspring with equal frequencies of $\frac{1}{4}$		
		Parental	Recombinant	
Linkage	A1B1A*	A1B1	A2B2	A1B2	A2B1
	A2B2				
	frequencies	$\frac{1}{2}(1-r)$	$\frac{1}{2}(1-r)$	$\frac{1}{2}r$	$\frac{1}{2}r$

A1 A2 and B1, B2 are alleles at loci A and B respectively.

* The line separating A1B1 from A2B2 indicates that A1B1 are together on one cromosone and A2B2 on the other.

r is the 'recombination fraction'; the smaller f is the fewer recombinants are produced, and the closer together are the genes A and B. When, on the other hand, r is $\frac{1}{2}$, the result is as if there where no linkage.

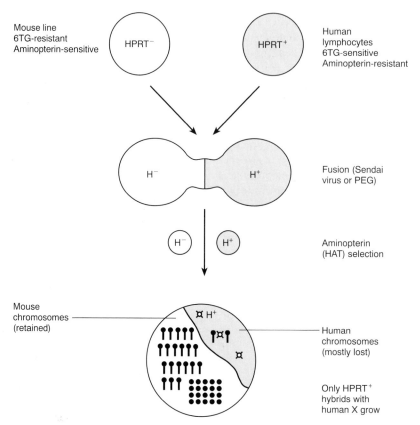

Fig. 4.2 Human–mouse cell fusion and hybrid selection. This figure illustrates the typical scheme for the production of human–mouse hybrids, using either Sendai virus or polyethylene glycol (PEG) to fuse the cells and a drug resistance marker to select for the hybrid. The mouse cells are a continuously growing cell line resistant to the drug 6TG (6-thioguanine) and as a result are sensitive to the drug aminopterin. Normal human lymphocytes are sensitive to 6TG, but resistant to aminopterin and cannot grow autonomously. After fusion of a mixed population of cells, only a small proportion will give rise to growing human–mouse hybrid cells and these must then be specifically selected out amongst a background of cells that have either failed to fuse, or have done so but are not hybrids (i.e. mouse–mouse or human–human). Hybrid cells that result from fusion between the two different parental cell types will be resistant to aminopterin, like the original human cells, but otherwise retain the growth properties of mouse cell lines. Since normal human lymphocytes do not grow in culture, if the fused mixture of cells is suspended in the presence of a selective medium containing aminopterin (called HAT, as it also contains hypoxanthine and thymidine), only the human–mouse hybrid cells will be able to grow. HPRT (hypoxanthine–guanine phosphoribosyl transferase) is the enzyme that is deficient (−) in 6TG-resistant (R), aminopterin-sensitive (S) cells, but present (+) in normal (6TG-S aminopterin-R) cells. Since the HPRT gene is on the human X chromosome, this chromosome must also be retained in those successful hybrids that grow in the HAT medium. These hybrid cells retain mouse chromosomes but lose most, but not all, of the human chromosomes. The specific combination of human chromosomes retained in a particular hybrid, forms the basis on which genetic segregation can be tested.

affected offspring of an A1B1/A2B2 individual will carry the B1 marker, whereas in the absence of linkage only one-half would be expected to.

Thus, the first step in locating a susceptibility gene is to find a marker that is genetically linked, preferably as physically close as possible to the disease gene in question. This is done by studying the pattern of inheritance of different markers in families of susceptible individuals and looking for a marker that associates in the family specifically with that susceptibility, owing to close genetic linkage. Often, data from several families need to be combined using special statistical techniques to assess the significance of a genetic linkage to a marker. Subsequently, candidate genes found in this way and identified by physical mapping, have to be screened for mutations to distinguish consistent changes within one gene in affected individuals. This approach, is known as positional cloning and contrasts with the classical genetic approach of identifying genes only through an initial understanding of their protein sequence and, often, function (Fig. 4.3).

In the past, such studies were only possible with linkage to easily ascertained differences in protein-determined phenotypes, such as the blood groups. Indeed, the first genetic linkage described in humans was between the ABO blood group locus and the nail–patella syndrome (a rare but easily identified medical disorder) in 1955. Later, electrophoretic variants between enzymes (isoenzymes) were exploited, but the number of such differences is limited. Now, however, using recombinant DNA techniques (see Chapter 9 and Appendix), a potentially unlimited source of genetic markers can be produced. Using a cloned DNA probe, differences in the sequence with which it is associated can be identified using restriction enzymes that cut the DNA at specific short sequences, in combination with the technique known as Southern blotting (Fig. 4.4(a)). The incidence of differences between individuals at the DNA level is such that there should be little difficulty in finding a set of genetic differences, called restriction enzyme fragment length polymorphisms or RFLPs, that cover all the chromosomes at a reasonable recombination interval. These differences, which have generally been superseded by those detected using the powerful PCR (polymerase chain reaction) technique (see below and Fig. 4.4(b)), can now be used systematically in cancer families to look for markers that

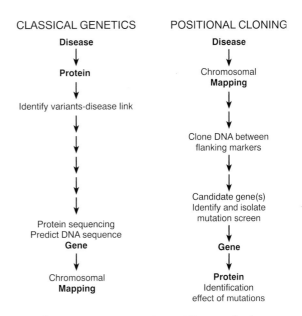

Fig. 4.3 Schematic outline of the differences in the two approaches to mapping and eventually cloning unknown genes. Positional cloning (also unfittingly referred to as 'reverse genetics'), allows the isolation of genes based solely on their chromosomal location, and relies on analysing families in which the disease segregates with known polymorphic markers (termed linkage). It is often coupled initially with cytogenetic studies, which may help accelerate localization, if gross abnormalities (e.g. interstitial deletions or rearrangements) are present. Positional cloning is now the preferred method because of the availability of increasingly dense genetic and physical maps of the genome, which contrasts with the relative scarcity of protein polymorphisms required for mapping via the classical approach.

are associated with, or closely linked to, genes giving rise to inherited susceptibilities to cancer.

Using such approaches, The Human Collaborative Research Group published the first 'linkage map' of the human genome in 1987. This map established 403 loci and such has been the pace of progress in this field that the density of markers of this map has now been increased over fivefold, representing an average recombination distance of under 3 centimorgans (or about 3 million base pairs) between markers. This has mainly been possible because eukaryotic genomes contain many sequences of nucleotides that occur repeatedly from a few to many thousand times. These repeats

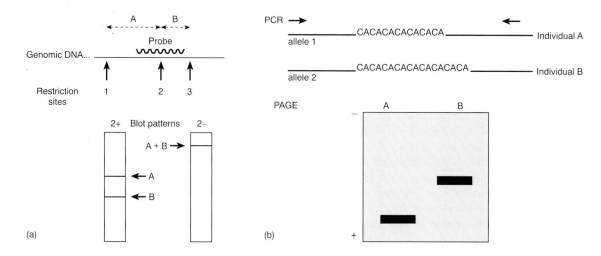

Fig. 4.4 (a) DNA variation on a Southern blot. Restriction fragment length polymorphism (RFLP). Genomic DNA cut by a given restriction enzyme (shown as restriction sites) is separated on a gel by an electric current according to its size (electrophoresis). The gel is then 'blotted' on to a suitable membrane (nylon or nitrocellulose paper) which is fixed so that the cut pieces of transferred DNA can be 'probed' with a radioactively labelled test sequence (Southern blot). The pattern is visualized by autoradiography which reveals the position(s) where the probe has hybridized to the blot by the radioactive emission from the label in the probe. Probe, here, refers to a DNA clone which overlaps segments A and B of the genome straddling site 2 where there is a difference between individuals for a restriction enzyme site. In 2+ individuals, the enzyme yields fragments A and B identified by the probe as on the blot on the left. In 2−individuals, the DNA is not cut at position 2 and so the probe detects only the segment A + B. This runs as a single band at a higher molecular weight as in the blot on the right.

(b) DNA variation in a dinucleotide repeat sequence. Genomic DNA from two individuals, A and B, is amplified by the polymerase chain reaction (PCR) using specific primers (shown as opposing arrows) near a known dinucleotide $(CA)_n$ repeat polymorphism. In individual A, n represents 7 repeats whereas in B n is 9. After amplification, the PCR products undergo polyacrylamide gel electrophoresis, or PAGE, under conditions capable of separating fragments differing in size by as little as two base pairs. The DNA fragments can then be visualized by direct staining (which avoids the use of radioactivity as in Southern blots). In this simple example, the individuals A and B are homozygous for the alleles 1 and 2, respectively, as shown. If, however, an individual was heterozygous and carried the two different alleles, these would show up as two different sized bands within that one individual upon PAGE.

vary in complexity from about three hundred base pair units (e.g. non-coding 'Alu', which recurs about 50 000 times in the human genome) to just one or two base pair units, called mononucleotide and dinucleotide repeats (e.g. cytosine–adenosine repeats: $[CACACA]_n$), respectively. In fact, the simplest represent the commonest type and is estimated to recur in over 100 000 locations. These repeat sequences, also referred to as microsatellites, are highly polymorphic with respect to the exact number of repeat units (n) among humans. It is specifically this variability in the number at each distinct site that allows us to order or map the relative positions of marked sequences (which may also include genes), on the basis of how often they are inherited together. These markers therefore provide the tools to initiate mapping of any Mendelian trait, and, in particular, monogenic human diseases, which includes some cancers. The importance of the susceptibility to change in these repeat sequences is also now established when they occur within, or very near to, coding sequences of genes, in that they are prone to mutation or specific replication errors called replication slippage, which often represents the functional equivalent of a nonsense mutation. This is discussed in more detail in Section 4.5.1.

To date, over 400 'disease' genes have been mapped in this way, with at least 40 of these actually cloned. Furthermore, these maps are also a prerequisite for studying more complex diseases which do not obviously follow Mendel's laws. Such disorders might include those that involve the interaction of two or more genes (either at a molecular *or* protein level), and also those that encompass the interaction between genes and our environment, which up to now has barely been possible. Indeed, it is likely that cancers will turn out to have some, however small, inherited predisposition which may represent the net effect of a variety of genes, and which will therefore vary as a continuum of risk across the population. The manifestation of this risk may then be determined by the host interaction with critical environmental triggers.

4.4 Dominant inherited susceptibility and recessive genetic changes in tumours

4.4.1 Basic mechanisms

Mechanisms underlying inherited susceptibilities to cancer must be consistent with the general views described in Sections 4.1 and 4.2 as to their nature at the cellular level. There are, in principle, two basic types of mechanisms that can underlie an inherited susceptibility. The first could be through an influence on the particular cells from which a certain type of tumour is derived, which can be thought of as essentially a tissue-specific influence. The second may be through systemic effects, examples being the frequency with which mutations arise as a result of environmental effects, or on the efficiency with which potential carcinogens are metabolized or activated. While the former mechanism should influence susceptibility to a particular form of cancer, the latter, in principle, which will be discussed later, may give rise to an inherited susceptibility to a wide range of cancers.

In 1971, Knudson pointed out that there should be some relationship between the genetic changes in a somatic cell that give rise to a cancer, and changes in these same genes in the germ line, which will be passed on in the usual way from parent to offspring following Mendelian laws of inheritance. This follows from the fact that, when one of the particular genetic changes involved in initiation or progression of a tumour occurs in the germ line, all the somatic cells of an individual who has inherited this particular change will already carry one of the steps required for malignant change. This should increase the chance that a tumour will develop in such an individual, and so lead to an inherited susceptibility to that particular cancer. Clearly, there could be such inherited changes that may involve, for example, genes for growth factors or their receptors in such a way that they influence the development of a variety of different tumours. In this sense, such a mechanism need not necessarily be tissue specific. Knudson emphasized that a corollary of these ideas was that identification of the gene involved in such an inherited susceptibility, would also pinpoint a gene that might be involved in somatic changes in the same type of tumour even when there was not an inherited susceptibility. We now know that this prediction is essentially true in more than one case, and some specific examples are discussed in detail.

4.4.2 Retinoblastoma

Retinoblastoma, a rare tumour of the eye that occurs overall in about 5 per 100 000 children, was the first and, still is the best, example of the application of Knudson's ideas. About 40 per cent of all cases of retinoblastoma occur as a clear-cut, dominantly inherited Mendelian disorder. The remainder are sporadic, in the sense that their first-degree relatives (parents, siblings, or grandchildren) have no increased risk of developing retinoblastoma over the general population. The inherited or familial cases are frequently bilateral, whereas sporadic cases are often unilateral and, therefore in this context, less severe. Knudson argued that in the familial cases of retinoblastoma, one of the genetic changes essential for the development of the tumour was already inherited through the germ line. He also reasoned that the change *within the tumour* was recessive, so that the relevant alleles on both homologous chromosomes had to be mutated or somehow changed to become inactive. Hence, in the inherited form, one of the genes was already mutated, and so only one further alteration in the remaining normal gene on the homologous chromosome was needed for the development of the tumour. In the sporadic cases, on the other hand, independent mutational events in both homologous genes are required, and this, therefore, has a much lower chance of occurring. This hypothesis can account for the difference in incidence between the inherited and sporadic forms.

The inherited susceptibility gene on the basis of Knudson's model is dominant because, having inherited one abnormal gene, the probability of a second event occurring is sufficiently high, giving the individual with the single aberrant gene an almost certain chance of developing at least one retinoblastoma (or complete penetrance of this tumour). At the cellular level, however, the relevant genetic change is recessive since it is assumed that both copies of the gene must eventually be inactivated as a prerequisite to tumour development.

These ideas have now received dramatic support from chromosomal, genetic, and molecular studies which have subsequently led to the cloning of the retinoblastoma gene. Thus, it was first observed that about 5–10 per cent of retinoblastoma patients have a small visible deletion of part of the long arm of chromosome 13 (at band 13q14). By using the fact that the isoenzymes of esterase D had been mapped by somatic cell genetic studies to chromosome 13, it was then shown, by linkage of the esterase D marker to retinoblastoma in familial cases, that these were all probably caused by a mutation at the position on chromosome 13 that was deleted in that small minority of retinoblastoma patients. These results were then extended to demonstrate, in a simple but elegant way, that the same gene also played a critical role in the sporadic or non-familial cases of retinoblastoma by Cavanee *et al.* (1983). They argued that, if Knudson's ideas were correct, markers that mapped to chromosome 13, when heterozygous in an individual, should become homozygous in a tumour because a common mechanism for the second somatic change could be chromosome loss or somatic recombination (Fig. 4.5). Indeed, DNA probes for chromosome 13 (again mapped using somatic cell hybridization techniques), revealed only one RFLP marker allele within the tumour, confirming that only the defective retinoblastoma allele was present. Thus, loss of the whole or part of the chromosome carrying the normal allele during tumour progression (which might sometimes be followed by reduplication of the remaining chromosome), would lead to a cell carrying only the defective retinoblastoma allele and at the same time only one of the RFLP marker alleles. Somatic recombination, in which there is an exchange between homologous regions in paired chromo-

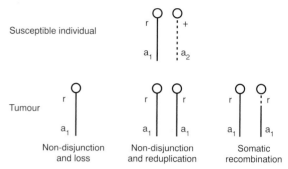

Fig. 4.5 Possible mechanisms for allele loss or homozygosity in retinoblastoma. In normal tissues of subjects that inherit the risk, r and + are the retinoblastoma (mutant) and corresponding normal heterozygous marker alleles a_1 and a_2, respectively, on chromosome 13. The tumours however, may be hemizygous a_1 r, or homozygous a_1a_1, rr. The latter can occur by at least four different mechanisms, two of which are shown. Gene conversion and two independent, but similar mutations are the two other possible, but less likely, mechanisms. It is not clear as yet which is the common or preferred mechanism for allele loss in tumours. See also Figs 4.8 and 4.11.

somes in somatic cells, can lead to a similar endeffect. Thus, either of these processes would be detected by the fact that in individuals who are heterozygous for the RFLP, as revealed, for example, by normal tissue surrounding a tumour, the tumour itself would express only one of the alleles detected by the chromosome 13 RFLP probe. In other words, while the individual is heterozygous for the marker, the tumour can be either homozygous or hemizygous, either of which constitute loss of heterozygosity (LOH) or allele loss. Using this approach, Cavanee and his colleagues demonstrated such changes in a high proportion of both sporadic and familial retinoblastoma. This provides dramatic confirmation of Knudson's ideas on the recessive basis for some genetic changes in tumours.

The precise localization and isolation by positional cloning of the actual retinoblastoma (*RB*) gene to chromosome 13q14.2 in 1987, has been followed by marked progress in elucidating the function of the RB gene product. Clues as to its function originally came from studies showing that the RB protein associates with the adenovirus E1A protein, which is itself a transforming product. The subsequent finding that the normal cDNA of RB, when transfected into retinoblastoma and osteosarcoma cells containing mutant endogenous RB, could cause reversion of the malignant phenotype, made this the first demonstration of a tumour suppressor gene (Lei *et al.* 1988). That is, a gene in which apparent *loss* of function is critical for tumour initiation or progression so that the normal alleles behave as dominant repressors of malignancy, which contrasts with their functional significance to oncogenes, which are frequently overexpressed.

It is now known that RB's normal function is intrinsically linked to cell cycle control and that it is normally phosphorylated during cell division. However, in its unphosphorylated form, it can block the passage of a cell from G_1 to S phase (see Chapter 1) by complexing with a factor known as E2F, which is then inactivated. Normally, E2F appears to be a key transcription component, which, when bound appropriately, can activate important cell cycle genes. Mutations that inactivate RB also appear to disable RB binding to E2F, allowing its continuous transcriptional activity and, thereby, unregulated stimulation of cell division. However, there remain some fundamental unexplained questions regarding RB. It is not clear why defects in such an apparently important protein, which is expressed in most tissues of the body, only predispose to a relatively small range of essentially rare malignancies such as retinoblastoma, osteosarcoma, and small-cell lung cancer, and not to the commoner solid tumours such as colon cancer. To complicate matters further, genetically engineered mice, which are constitutionally heterozygous for an inactivating or null allele of RB (homozygotes being embryonically lethal at 16 days), do not develop retinoblastoma but pituitary tumours instead (see Table 4.5 later).

The elucidation of the inherited basis for retinoblastoma at the molecular level is a remarkable example of the power of modern techniques of molecular biology when combined with classical family studies. These approaches now make it possible to localize, identify, and analyse functionally any disease susceptibility gene and its product at the molecular level, particularly when there are both sporadic and familial forms of the disease.

4.4.3 Familial adenomatous polyposis

Colonic tumours are among the commonest of all carcinomas, with an incidence of about 6 per 10 000 of the population in the Western world. They are generally thought to arise sequentially from precancerous polyps or adenomas. Familial adenomatous polyposis (FAP, often also called APC for adenomatous polyposis coli, its corresponding gene), is a dominantly inherited susceptibility to colon cancer occurring in about 1 per 8000 of the population. Although relatively rare, it is one of the commonest dominantly inherited diseases known. Affected individuals develop from a few hundred to over a thousand adenomatous polyps in their large intestine. Since the polyps may be precancerous growths, among such a large number there is a high probability that at least one, if not more, will give rise to a carcinoma by the age of 40. Thus, almost invariably, an individual with adenomatous polyposis will develop one or more colon carcinomas if left untreated, hence, the disease shows complete penetrance (Fig. 4.6). Early screening of individuals from affected families has been used to identify the polyps at a stage when prophylactic removal of the colon can prevent most of the risk of developing a carcinoma. FAP patients can also develop a wide variety of other clinical features which have a variable penetrance compared with the colonic polyps as listed in Table 4.2. There are other, rarer hereditary intestinal polyp syndromes described which also have a predisposition to malignant transformation, although invariably to a lesser extent than FAP. Some examples are shown within the classification listed in Table 4.3.

The initial clue to the localization of the gene for APC to chromosome 5 was in a case report of a

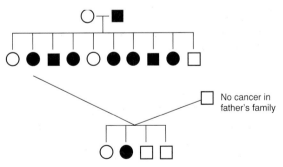

Fig. 4.6 Pedigree of the first clear-cut reported case of inherited polyposis coli (Lockhart-Mummery 1925). The disease is passed down through three generations from one affected parent. The pattern of inheritance is characteristic of a dominantly inherited trait. Symbols: ●/■ affected female/male; ○/□ unaffected female/male.

Table 4.2 Clinical manifestations of FAP

FAP: Gastrointestinal manifestations	Extra-gastrointestinal		
	Benign	*Vs.*	Malignant
Colorectal polyposis and carcinoma	Oestomas		
Duodenal polyps and carcinoma	Desmoids/fibromas		
Gastric polyps and carcinoma	Sebaceous or epidermoid cyst		
Peri-ampullary cancer	Lipomas		
Bile duct cancer	CHRPE (congenital hypertrophy of the retinal pigment epithelium)		
	Dental anomalies[1]		
Rare			
Carcinoma *in situ* of the gall bladder Hepatoblastoma	Adrenal cortical adenoma		Thyroid papillary carcinoma Adrenal cortical carincoma Brain tumours
?lymphoid polyposis[2] ?Caroli's disease[3]			

Once FAP is diagnosed most patients are now offered a prophylactic colectomy (removal of most of the large intestine) in early adulthood. Consequently desmoids (often intra-abdominal) and duodenal carcinoma now account for significant morbidity and mortality. Although classified as benign, desmoids can be life threatening through local growth and expansion into surrounding structures. Gardener's syndrome was originally described as a clinical syndrome of colonic polyposis, lipomas, and osteomas but should not be regarded as a separate entity (see text).

[1] These include impacted teeth, supernumerary teeth, congenitally missing teeth, and abnormally long and pointed roots on the posterior teeth.

[2,3] The significance of these lesions has yet to be ascertained. Caroli's has only been reported once in association with FAP and is a condition that presents with dilatation of the distal intrahepatic bile ducts with intrahepatic stone formation.

Table 4.3 Clinical familial syndromes predisposing to intestinal cancers

Preceded by multiple polyps	*or*	Few or no polyps
Adenomatous		
FAP (includes Gardner's/ Oldfield's)		HNPCC—cancer family/ LFS-1 and -2
?Turcot's		Muir-Torre
Non-adenomatous		
Peutz-Jeghers		Cowden's
Juvenile polyposis		Gorlin's
Gorlin's		

Gardner's and Oldfield's syndromes were previously clinically defined entities and thought separate from FAP but are now known to be encompassed by it. Turcot's is polyposis with malignant brain tumours, but generally there remains confusion between FAP associated with brain tumours as an extracolonic feature, and the rare, probably recessive, Turcot's syndrome. (In FAP the cerebral tumours tend to be of neuronal rather than neuroglial origin as in Turcot's syndrome). Muir–Torre syndrome represents cutaneous sebacious neoplasms, keratoacanthomas, colonic, and other neoplasms. At least some of the cases fall under the HNPCC umbrella. The polyps in the non-adenomatous syndromes generally tend to be hamartomatous (benign mixed-tissue tumours) and the risk of malignant change is much less than their adenomatous counterparts.

mentally retarded individual with multiple developmental abnormalities who also had colorectal carcinoma on a background of multiple polyps. He died of complications characteristic of those seen in individuals with adenomatous polyposis. This individual was shown to have a small deletion on the long arm of chromosome 5 (5q), suggesting that the polyposis gene might lie within this deleted region. A DNA probe which had been assigned to chromosome 5 revealed a polymorphism that was shown to be closely linked to *APC* (see Fig. 4.7; and Bodmer *et al.* 1987). This probe, called C11P11, localized to the region of the long arm of chromosome 5 called 5q21–q22, which was missing in this one, multiply abnormal, sporadic case of FAP. These observations were confirmed by other linkage analyses that demonstrated that 5q21 chromosome markers were tightly linked to the development of polyps in numerous FAP kindreds.

Following Knudson's arguments and the application of RFLP analysis to establishing the case for a recessive change in retinoblastoma, polymorphic DNA probes assigned to chromosome 5 were used to look for allele loss in sporadic colorectal carcino-

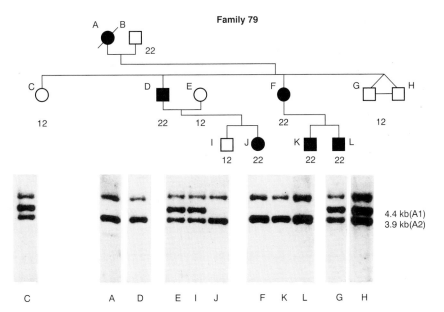

Fig. 4.7 Family 79 demonstrating segregation of FAP with a 3.9-kb fragment using the probe C11p11. The alleles are 1 at 4.4 kb and 2 at 3.9 kb and are denoted under each symbol. Symbols: ●/■ affected female/male; ○/□ unaffected female/male. A diagonal slash through the symbol represents death of the individual.

mas. Thus, using a highly polymorphic probe for chromosome 5, it was shown that at least 20–40 per cent of sporadic colorectal carcinomas become homozygous or hemizygous for chromosome 5 markers (Fig. 4.8). This indicates that the *APC* gene becomes recessive in a relatively high proportion of colorectal carcinomas, suggesting that only a mutant *APC* allele remains. This was the first clear example of such a recessive defect in one of the common cancers.

Using a yeast artificial chromosome (YAC) library screened with 5q21 markers, the *APC* gene was eventually identified in 1991 by positional cloning. Phenotypically, Gardner's syndrome represents a subset of FAP with a specific pattern of extracolonic manifestations. However, at the molecular level both these conditions were shown to be genetically similar in having *APC* mutations in the germ line, a powerful demonstration of how diseases may be reclassified with further understanding. The reasons for the manifest differences between the two remain to be explained but may be related in part to the presence of other modifying or 'interacting' genes and the specific sites of mutation within *APC*.

Detailed mutation analyses of colonic tumours in both FAP and sporadic cases has led to *APC* being one of the best studied genes at the molecular level. Virtually all *APC* mutations (germ line or sporadic) are nonsense or involve deletions causing a frameshift or other inactivating mutations, consistent with

the simple hypothesis that it is a tumour suppressor gene. Intriguingly, virtually no mutations are found beyond the middle of the gene (Fig. 4.9), which suggests that mutations that do occur in the 3′ half of the gene in humans do not cause functional inactivation. However, a paradox exists in that in transgenic mice designed with such a nonsense mutation in the 3′ half of the gene, the phenotype is akin to mice with the mutation at the 5′ end.

The genomic sequence of *APC* encompasses over 120 kilobases. The protein product contains 2843 amino acids with an intriguing combination of limited homologies to other proteins such as repetitive cytoskeletal elements and consensus zinc finger motifs. A tyrosine kinase phosphorylation site is also present (Fig. 4.9). Current evidence suggests that normal APC protein self-associates through amphipathic alpha-helical regions towards the N-terminus, forming a homodimer, which also has binding sites that allows it to complex with β-catenin, a molecule involved in the control of E-cadherin-mediated intracellular adhesion. In some way, therefore, mutations in *APC* may interfere with cell adhesion and the normal constraints that this puts on cell growth. It has, however, not yet been directly demonstrated whether such *APC* mutations alone confer transforming ability, any growth advantage, or the disregulation of cells.

Despite the fact that there is invariably some ascertainment bias both in patient selection methods

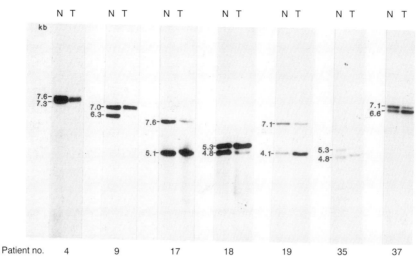

Patient no.　　4　　　9　　　17　　　18　　　19　　　35　　　37

Fig. 4.8 Allele loss in primary colorectal tumours. DNA from matched normal (N) and tumour (T) pairs was tested with a highly polymorphic DNA probe known to map to the tip of the long arm of chromosome 5. Patient no. 9 demonstrates a typical clear example of allele loss (band 6.3) from the tumour sample compared with its normal tissue pair.

In the other cases, the ratio of the intensity of one band in tumour tissue is much greater than another (for example, 5.1 versus 7.6 in patient no. 17's tumour). This usually also represents evidence for allele loss as the tumour DNA, when extracted, may be contaminated with normal DNA from surrounding tissues.

and techniques of mutational analysis used, the world-wide database of *APC* mutations is now sufficiently large and geographically varied enough to give not only some clues as to the functionally important domains of the protein, but also to begin correlating the specific sites of the mutations within the gene (or genotype) to the variable phenotype that the patients often display (Fig. 4.9).

In general, the pattern of types of mutation is similar for both germ line and sporadic colorectal tumours. Frameshift mutations, especially small deletions, account for over a half of all mutations. Over three-quarters of the remaining point mutations are of the nonsense type. Hence, over 95 per cent of mutations in both germ line and sporadic cases are predicted to truncate the APC protein product. This has important consequences both for the understanding of APC protein function and in the molecular methods chosen to screen for *APC* mutations. The sites of mutation reveal similar but not identical patterns between germ line-acquired or sporadic tumours. The germ line mutations found to date are fairly evenly distributed in the first half (3′-end) of the gene, whereas the somatic mutations, while generally within the same region, are clustered so that about two-thirds of them fall in a relatively

small area termed the mutation cluster region, which represents less than 10 per cent of the entire coding sequence (Fig. 4.9). This also happens to coincide with the site for about 20 per cent (and so the commonest) germ line mutations, although these are clustered in one very highly mutable site. The specific type of sporadic mutations (Fig. 4.10(a)) indicates that mutagenic carcinogens are probably not a major factor in the instigation of colorectal carcinogenesis with respect to these genes.

4.4.4 p53 and the Li–Fraumeni syndrome

In 1969, in a retrospective review of childhood rhabdomyosarcoma (a malignancy of skeletal muscle), Li and Fraumeni identified four families in which the incidence of breast cancer, soft-tissue sarcomas, and other tumours was also strikingly high. Subsequent studies confirmed this as a familial cancer syndrome now eponymously coined the Li–Fraumeni syndrome (LFS). It is rare, with an incidence estimated at 2–4 per 100 000 population, but the probability of one of a diverse spectrum of tumours occurring by age 30 is high, at about 50 per cent, compared with a population age-adjusted risk of 1 per cent. Furthermore, multiplicity of primary tumours is fre-

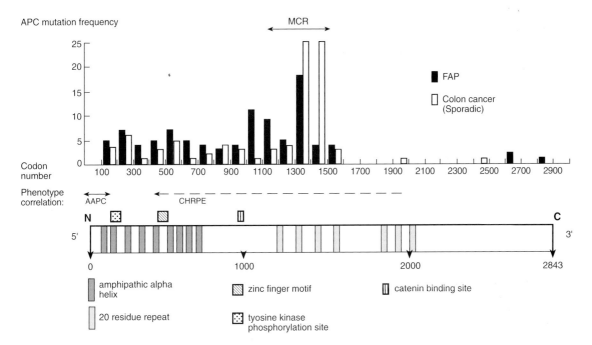

Fig. 4.9 Schematic representation of the mutation frequency and protein structure of *APC*. The height of the bars in the graph represents the number of mutations detected at that codon number: note the clustering of somatic mutations within a relatively small region, around the middle of the protein termed the 'mutation cluster region'. Some genotype–phenotype correlations are shown by the dashed arrows. The site of germ line mutations in FAP appears to correlate with the number of polyps, if these occur before codon 160 or so. This pattern is referred to as an attenuated form, or AAPC, because such pedigrees demonstrate a milder phenotype (usually less than a thousand polyps). CHRPE (see Table 4.2) does not appear to occur unless the mutation is present in or after exon 9.

Some important structural motifs are represented, although their functional relevance has yet to be established. The first 55 amino acids appear to be sufficient for protein homo-dimerization Also of specific interest is the catenin binding site. Catenins are known to be associated with epithelial cadherin molecules which are important for cellular adhesion. Therefore, it may be that *APC* mutations somehow indirectly disrupt cellular adhesion, or, alternatively, mutant *APC* may, in certain circumstances, incorrectly signal downstream pathways involved in the regulation of growth inhibition through contact with other cells.

quent in LFS. Segregation analysis suggested that the observed cancer distribution was best described by an autosomal dominant mode of inheritance and that a tumour suppressor gene was likely to be implicated. This has been confirmed recently by demonstrating that inactivating mutations of the *p53* gene (for 53-kilodalton protein) are associated with a variety of sarcomas, leukaemia, lung and breast cancers (Malkin *et al*. 1990). Thus, kindreds with germ line mutations of the *p53* gene can now be screened closely from a young age for the development of tumours, as their risk is extremely high.

The p53 protein was originally independently identified in the late seventies, as it was shown to bind the large T antigen of the SV40 DNA virus in cells transformed by this virus. Serum antibodies to this protein were shown to be present in animal tumour models as well as in patients with breast cancer. Whereas the protein was shown to accumulate in the nucleus of transformed cell lines, it could not be demonstrated in normal cells. Techniques of classical genetics had identified the human coding sequence in 1985. However, it was only in the late 1980s, when it was demonstrated that altered or

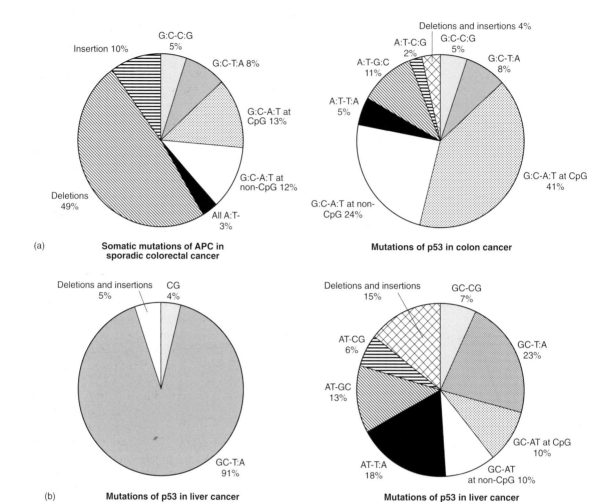

(a) **Somatic mutations of APC in sporadic colorectal cancer**

Mutations of p53 in colon cancer

(b) **Mutations of p53 in liver cancer :Area of high incidence**

Mutations of p53 in liver cancer :Area of low incidence

Fig. 4.10 (a) Representation of the distribution of the specific types of characterized *APC* and *p53* mutations in sporadic colorectal carcinoma. To appreciate the significance of the relatively random pattern of mutations, two charts of *p53* mutations in hepatocellular cancer (HCC), the commonest cancer world-wide, are shown alongside (b). In high incidence areas of HCC, where the aetiological associations are strong, due to the hepatitis B virus and aflatoxin (a peanut mould), there is a striking preponderance of guanine (G) to thymine (T) (and so correspondingly cytosine (C) to adenine (A)) transversions. Similarly, more than 40 per cent of *p53* mutations in lung cancer are GC to TA mutations, largely associated with cigarette smoking. In direct contrast, in low incidence areas, the types of mutations are fairly evenly distributed. The *APC* and *p53* charts in sporadic colorectal tumours are similar, in that *no* obvious bias to a specific class of mutations is seen. This suggests that mutations in these genes in colorectal carcinoma are *unlikely* to be caused by specific environmental (or in this case, dietary) mutagens as these often tend to cause a particular type of mutation. Cytosine to thymine transitions are the commonest type of spontaneous mutations in eukaryotic genomes, owing to the relative ease of methylation of cytosine followed by spontaneous deamination. CpG denotes a dinucleotide, where this type of deamination frequently occurs.

mutant forms were increased in human cancers, that its importance became clearer. By a combination of allele loss studies after the gene had been mapped to 17p13, and mutation analysis in colorectal tumours, it was shown to be a human oncogene behaving essentially like a tumour suppressor.

p53 currently has the distinction of being the most commonly mutated gene in cancers arising from a wide spectrum of tissues. Hence it is not surprising to learn that it has been implicated in the control of the cell cycle, as both a positive and negative regulator of transcription, and appears to be pivotal in deciding the fate of a cell in response to DNA damage. Indeed, it may coordinate genes that regulate genomic stability, and has been called 'the guardian of the genome' as its normal function appears necessary to decide whether, following certain forms of DNA damage, a cell should progress through the cell cycle or undergo active programmed cell death. Mutations which render *p53* dysfunctional may therefore allow cells to continue to propagate when they should otherwise undergo apoptosis. This has major implications regarding the way we treat cancers, as evidenced from clinical and experimental data showing an increased resistance (and poorer survival) to both chemotherapy and radiotherapy, in many tumours with *p53* mutations.

The paradox remains as to why the spectrum of tumours in the LFS does not encompass some common solid tumours, such as colon and small-cell lung cancer, whereas over a half of such sporadic tumours have *p53* mutations. The explanation may lie in the relative importance of *p53* in different tissues, especially with respect to the level of effective expression. It is thus noteworthy that sarcomas mostly have non-functional *p53* mutations whereas carcinomas have almost exclusively mis-sense point mutations.

It appears that *p53* has the characteristics of both a dominant oncogene, as demonstrated originally with its mutant forms, and as a recessive tumour suppressor gene in its normal (or wild-type) form, as it can curtail growth when transfected into transformed murine and human cells with mutant endogenous *p53*. It therefore appears that loss of the wild-type function may not be a prerequisite to abnormal regulation of cell growth, but that the presence of a mutant protein is in itself sufficient. This is termed a 'dominant negative' effect, in contrast to the requirement of recessiveness at a cellular level of classical tumour suppressor genes. However, mice that are homozygous for inactivating mutations (so that p53 protein expression is undetectable), appear to be developmentally viable but develop a spectrum of tumours at a young age, whereas heterozygotes develop tumours relatively late. This implies that one normal copy of *p53* can, to some extent, mitigate tumour formation and that gene dosage (haploinsufficiency) may be critical.

p53 mutations are detectable in over thirty tumour types and over 80 per cent of these are mis-sense mutations, usually in the hydrophobic mid-region of the protein which binds DNA. There is consequently a significant body of data that allows us some insight into its genetic epidemiology. A good example is in hepatocellular carcinoma (HCC), one of the most prevalent tumours on a world-wide basis. It has long been known that exposure to hepatitis B virus and to a peanut mould toxin, aflatoxin B_1, are synergistic risk factors for the development of HCC in certain geographical locations. In fact, in such areas, over three-quarters of the *p53* mutations are specific to codon 249 of the gene, and, strikingly, are invariably G to T transversions leading to a serine substitution at residue 249. However, in low risk areas, the mutations in sporadic HCC are distributed throughout the gene without a predilection for any specific site or type. The specificity for the codon 249 transversion mutations is confirmed by mutagenesis studies *in vitro*, which show that this is the change most expected from the mutagenic effect of aflatoxin B_1 (Fig. 4.10(b)). Similarly, cigarette smoke, and its constituent carcinogens, causes an identical transversion and this can be seen both in lung, and head and neck cancers. Likewise, in about 30 per cent of squamous cell carcinomas, there are tandem mutations where a CC is replaced by a TT in *p53*. As it is known that ultraviolet (UV) radiation specifically induces pyrimidine dimers, if these were incorrectly repaired such a change would persist, implicating UV radiation as a contributing factor. In contrast, in colorectal tumours, *p53* mutations do not have the G to T-type of transversion, indicating, as in the case for *APC* mutations, that such mutagens are probably not relevant for this type of cancer (Fig. 4.10(a and b)). Hence, particular mutations and their distribution act as molecular dosimeters of environmental carcinogen exposure providing a molecular epidemiological assessment of human cancer risk. This gives us an insight into not only the biochemical mechanisms responsible for the genetic lesions, but also the gene function and, of more immediate importance, it may suggest preventive measures to reduce tumour incidence.

4.4.5 Breast and ovarian cancer

As the lifetime risk of developing breast cancer in the Western world is high, at about 1 in 12, the probability of having affected relatives with the disease purely by chance is also, correspondingly, relatively high. The significant feature in those pedigrees with a strong family history has been the relatively young age of onset, and in some cases the presence of bilateral disease. In a subset of families with a high incidence of breast cancer, there is also an increased, though highly variable, incidence of ovarian cancer. Additionally, there are other syndromes associated with breast cancer such as Li–Fraumeni syndrome (discussed in the preceding section) and ataxia telangiectasia. In some families with familial colon cancer (see HNPCC, Section 4.5.2), there is an increased incidence of ovarian but not breast cancer. In all these cases there is a young age of onset and the pattern of inheritance follows an autosomal dominant mode.

In 1990 it was reported that some, but not all, breast cancer pedigrees showed linkage to chromosome 17q and the susceptibility gene in this region was labelled *BRCA1* (Breast cancer 1). Hence there was clear evidence of genetic heterogeneity right from the outset, suggesting the presence of other unidentified loci. Subsequent studies suggest that *BRCA1* is responsible for the disease in about two-thirds of all breast cancer pedigrees, and in almost all these cases there is a family history of ovarian cancer. The lifetime penetrance of developing breast or ovarian cancer in females who carry these mutations is estimated at over 70 per cent.

Analysis of both breast and ovarian tumours in families linked to 17q show frequent loss of the wild-type allele when compared with normal tissue. This loss of heterozygosity, as with *APC*, is highly suggestive that *BRCA1* is a tumour suppressor gene. However, the presence of other potential tumour suppressor genes on 17q (not linked specifically to breast cancer) confound this hypothesis somewhat.

BRCA1 was eventually cloned in 1994, by the analysis of expressed sequences within a region spanning 600 000 nucleotides (600 kb). It has turned out remarkably like the *APC* story in that the gene shares a similar size and complexity to *APC*, and has relatively little in the way of homology to other known proteins or motifs, making its functional analysis more difficult (see also Table 4.4a). The mutation-type pattern is also generally similar with the majority being either frameshift or nonsense, leading to a truncated protein product. However as yet, unlike *APC*, there is no evidence for a restricted mutation distribution throughout the gene and only weak evidence for a genotype–phenotype correlation with respect to an apparently higher incidence of occurrence of ovarian versus breast cancer, with mutations in the 5' half of the gene.

Demonstration of linkage at a second locus, termed *BRCA2* and positioned at 13q12–13, has recently been confirmed in some breast cancer families (see also Table 4.4b). Again, the pattern is of a highly penetrant, dominant gene with frequent allele loss. The relative proximity of the retinoblastoma gene to this locus again confounds the interpretation of this data. Interestingly, there is evidence that families with more than one case of male breast cancer, which is not surprisingly one hundred times rarer than female breast cancer, show linkage to *BRCA2* and rarely to *BRCA1*.

There is a genuine possibility that in the near future, mutation analysis of high risk individuals will be possible on a routine basis at a young age; the caveats being the management and interpretation of both a positive and negative result, respectively. In the former case, there is currently no optimal screening procedure for young women, leaving only the draconian measure of bilateral mastectomy as possibly secure. (There is no guarantee that residual epithelial cells will not be left behind after surgery, as often occurs currently with breast cancer surgery!) Conversely, the genetic heterogeneity, as well as the high risk of background or sporadic breast cancers, confounds the predictive value of a negative result.

4.4.6 The general extent of recessive genetic changes in tumours

There are an increasing number of examples of individually rare instances of clear-cut inherited susceptibilities to particular cancers. Each of these may, as in the case of retinoblastoma, p53, and APC, turn out to be of fundamental interest in providing clues to the genetic changes in non-familial cancers, even though the overall contribution to the incidence of cancer from these rare inherited susceptibilities is very small. Some examples are shown in Tables

Table 4.4a Cloned tumour suppressor genes and their involvement in known inherited cancer syndromes and sporadic tumours

Gene [Tumour suppressor unless stated]	Chromosomal location	Putative main function(s)	Familial syndromes/tumours (approximate heterozygote frequency per 10^5 population)	Known sporadic (or non-inherited) tumours with somatic mutations
p53	17p13.1	53 kDa transcription regulator (of G1 to S transition) cell fate after DNA damage	Li–Fraumeni syndrome Adrenocortical sarcomas, breast, leukaemia, brain *(2)*	Most commonly mutated gene; in up to 70% of tumours
RB1 Retinoblastoma	13q14	110 kDa transcription factor (regulation of G1 to S transition)	Retinoblastoma, osteosarcoma *(2)*	Retinoblastoma, osteosarcoma, lung, breast, prostate, and bladder
APC Adenomatous polyposis Coli	5q21	310 kDa cytoplasmic protein ? cell adhesion via β-catenin, (indirectly E-cadherin linked) ? microtubule stabilization	FAP, gastrointestinal carcinomas and desmoids (see also Table 4.2) *(8)*	Gastrointestinal tract (GIT) neoplasms including pancreas
WT1 Wilm's tumour	11p13	45 kDa transcription factor	Wilms' tumour: a specific childhood renal tumour *(<1)*	Only about 20% of sporadic Wilms' tumours are WT1 mutant
NF1 Neurofibromatosis type 1	17q11.2	280 kDa arasGAP GTPase (neurofibromin), a negative regulator of p21ras	Neurofibromas, sarcomas, glioma, and phaeochromocytoma (phaeo) *(29)*	Schwannomas
NF2 Neurofibromatosis type 2	22q12	66 kDa cytoskeletal membrane intercellular junction associated protein (merlin)	Neurofibromas, meningioma, and acoustic schwannoma *(3)*	Schwannoma and meningioma
VHL von Hippel–Lindau	3p25.5	34 kDa membrane protein ? function	Renal tumours, phaeo., and haemangioblastoma *(3)*	Sporadic renal tumours
BRCA1 Breast cancer 1	17q21	cytoplasmic protein with C-terminal zinc finger ? function; size ≈ 200 kDa	Breast, ovarian, ?prostate *(2)*	Possibly some ovarian, (but *not* breast tumours)
DCC Deleted in colorectal cancer	18q21.3-ter	153 kDa N-CAM (neural cell adhesion molecule)-like protein	Familial syndrome *not* clearly described	Colon tumours; in other GIT tumours total gene deletion has been described
MEN 2 Multiple endocrine neoplasia	10q11	RET protooncogene, receptor tyrosine kinase[1]	Phaeo. parathyroid and medullary thyroid tumours	

Hereditary non-polyposis colon cancer with the corresponding germ line mutations of the mismatch repair genes are not included here (see Table 4.6), as current evidence suggests that they may not be tumour suppressor genes in the classical sense.

[1] Only known example of an ocogene (as opposed to a tumour suppressor), whose mutations in the germ line place the host at risk of cancer. In tumours, expression of the DCC protein is low or absent.

Table 4.4b Mapped putative tumour suppressor genes in neoplasms and in familial syndromes

Gene symbol	Chromosomal location	Neoplasm(s) in familial cases
NB1	1p36	Neuroblastoma (no linkage studies yet, as familial cases are extremely rare)
MLM	9p21[1]	Melanoma
MEN 1	11q13	Multiple endocrine neoplasia; pituitary, pancreas, and parathyroid adenomas
BCNS	9q31	Basal cell naevus or Gorlin's syndrome, medulloblastoma, and skin tumours
RCC	3p14	Renal cell carcinoma
BRCA2	13q12–13	Familial breast cancer: probably also includes familial male breast cancer
BWS	11p15.5[2]	Beckwith–Widemann syndrome; Wilms' and other embryonal tumours

[1] Recently cloned, although some controversy remains as to the exact relevance of this gene; one report also suggests another possible locus on chromosome 1p.

[2] Not all BWS patients are linked to this locus.

4.4a and 4.4b. In addition, the use of RFLPs and the newer PCR-based CA repeat markers to search for allele losses in tumours has revealed examples of recessive changes in tumours that are not associated with a familial inherited susceptibility. The case of multiple endocrine neoplasia type 2A (MEN 2A) is interesting in this respect, since allele loss was shown for markers on chromosomes 1p and 22, while the gene for MEN 2A itself has been mapped to chromosome 10q11. However, loss of heterozygosity is rare at this locus, which has recently been identified as the ret protooncogene (which appears to be a receptor with tyrosine kinase activity). This makes it the first and only example, so far, of a classical oncogene which, if inherited as mutated, predisposes that family to a cancer susceptibility. It is likely though, that the sites of allele loss that are frequent in this syndrome are tumour suppressor genes, whose inactivation may be critical for tumour initiation or progression. Indeed, allele loss at 1p is common in many tumours, and there is a suggestion, using mouse models, that there is a strong phenotypic modifier for familial adenomatous polyposis within this region. There is already a wide range of suggested genetic changes in tumours, a number of which have been found in common tumours such as of the colon, breast, bladder, and lung. It seems clear that these recessive changes form an important counterpart to the dominantly acting oncogenes found initially through the study of the oncogenic viruses (see Chapters 9 and 10).

The general scheme, based on Knudson's model, that fits the data on retinoblastoma, FAP, and other tumours where recessive genetic defects have been uncovered, is illustrated in Fig. 4.11. The individual who is heterozygous for a defective gene carries a dominantly inherited predisposition to the cancer, which is only expressed after a further somatic change leading to recessive 'expression' at the cellular level in the cancer itself. The sporadic cases involving the same change, arise through two successive genetic events essentially knocking out the same gene function. A recessive mechanism could arise in a variety of ways, including genes that have inhibitory or negative controls over the production of growth factors (or their receptors) or important cell cycling control genes. Recessive mechanisms could also arise from positive control of differentiation, since blocking differentiation to achieve increased growth may be one of the mechanisms leading to tumour progression.

What is not clear to date, is whether being heterozygous for a defective tumour suppressor gene in some way compromises or deregulates the status of specific cells. For example, this might occur by marginally increasing cellular turnover or, alternatively, by increasing resistance to apoptosis, leading to an increased propensity to further somatic change even if this change were, as is likely, a random event. There are at least two mechanisms by which a defective gene in the presence of its normal counterpart might affect a cell. The first, or haplo-insufficiency (gene dosage) theory, would be through a straightforward reduction in the amount of protein transcribed by the defective gene, leading to an overall deficit. The second, could be through an inhibitory

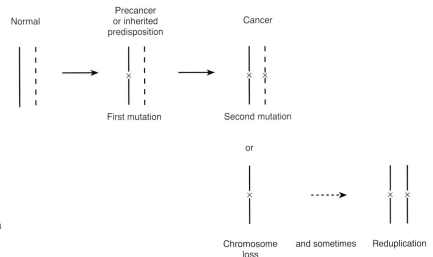

Fig. 4.11 Model for the two stages (or 'hits') involved in the recessive control of cancer.

effect of a transcribed but defective protein, on its normal counterpart, particularly if the proteins self-associate or homo-dimerize in some way. This is often termed a dominant–negative effect. There is evidence currently to support both these ideas with respect to specific circumstances.

4.4.7 Animal models of inherited cancer susceptibility

It has been known since the early 1950s, that tumours could be propagated vertically (i.e. from one generation to the next) in lymphoma or breast cancer-prone inbred mice strains. This was shown to be the result of infectious RNA tumour viruses, classic examples being the murine leukaemia (MuLV) and murine mammary tumour (MMTV) viruses. In this sense, the cancer susceptibility was not truly inherited but rather was through infection, even though this could occur as early as at fertilization. Many inbred mouse strains have also been classified with both varying degrees of spontaneous cancer-prone susceptibility and resistance to the development of cancer, with certain mutagens. Just as with humans, where genetic maps allow us to pinpoint susceptibility genes, in mice, the situation in many ways is even further advanced, as the progress in dense gene mapping has been relatively faster. Mouse breeding potentially allows for unlimited numbers of test candidates, over a relatively short time-span. Furthermore, on an evolutionary time-scale, human and mice genes are often over 80 per cent conserved (and even more, when functionally

important domains are assessed), providing us with a valid framework for mouse to human comparisons.

Recombinant DNA technology now also allows us to specifically design mice harbouring too many copies of a gene (transgenic mice), so that overexpression of that gene product will occur; or to create mice with prespecified mutations within a gene of interest through techniques of homologous recombination by specifically targeting that gene. The latter approach also allows us to engineer mutations that are nonsense or frameshift, so that the resulting product will either not be expressed or is present in a shortened or truncated (and therefore inactive) form. Such mice are often referred to as 'knockout' mice. This approach is an extremely powerful one in attempting to understand the relative role of a specific gene, and can allow a specific genetic defect to be correlated to a phenotypic level. Furthermore, crosses between engineered mice yield offspring from which one could potentially study the interaction of two or more abnormal genes, and so, for example, model the stepwise progression in human tumours.

There are currently several mouse models of three of the genes already discussed, *APC*, *p53*, and retinoblastoma (see Sections 4.4.2–4.4.4). The first of these will be discussed in more detail and the characteristics of some of the other models are listed in Table 4.5.

Through a mouse mutagenesis programme, a multiple intestinal neoplasia (Min), fully penetrant,

Table 4.5 Examples of mouse models of inherited cancer syndromes

Gene/inherited predisposition	Phenotype		
	Homozygotes	vs.	Heterozygotes
p53/Li–Fraumeni syndrome[1]	↑↑ predisposition to multiple neoplasms especially sarcomas—usually die by six months of age		↑ predisposition but less severe compared to homozygotes, as neoplasms develop at a later age (Females also show ↑ embryonic deaths)
RB1/Retinoblastoma	Embryonically lethal		Pituitary carcinoma
APC/familial adenomatous polyposis[2]	Embryonically lethal		Multiple intestinal polyps, predominantly of small intestine[3]
WT1/Wilms' tumour	Embryonically lethal		Do not develop Wilms' tumours
MSH2/HNPCC	Lymphomas at ≈ 2–4 months		Appear normal
PMS2/HNPCC	Lymphomas, sarcomas at ≈ 1 year; males infertile ?meiotic recombination defects		None obvious by 1 year

In 'knock-out' mice, the mouse homologue of the relevant human gene is replaced by a molecularly engineered equivalent but mutant DNA sequence, which is often designed to code for a truncated or non-functional protein to mimic the human disease state. This is usually done by the technique of homologous recombination in mouse embryonic stem cells, which, after transfection and appropriate selection, are inserted into a blastocyst, which forms a chimera. A proportion of these mice are then able to transmit the abnormal copy of the gene in their germ line.

[1] *P53* genetically engineered *transgenic* mice, that is mice that overexpress a heterologous mutant copy of *P53*, in addition to the normal background of two copies of mouse *P53*, have also been shown, in some cases, to have an increased propensity for tumour development, although the spectrum of neoplasms differs in various transgenic mice.

[2] The original model (or Min as described in the text) was fortuitously derived from a mutagenesis programme (i.e. not by homologous recombination). In some laboratory inbred strains the Min phenotype is surprisingly heavily suppressed. Subsequently, at least four knock-outs have been reported with the APC protein designed to truncate within different exons. These mice generally all show similar phenotypes to Min.

[3] Generally the polyps do not transform into carcinomas from the adenomas, although this has been reported for one of the later models with a C-terminal truncating mutation, it remains a rare event.

dominant phenotype was fortuitously selected. This was subsequently shown to cosegregate with the murine homologue of the *APC* gene (*mApc*) when a germ line nonsense mutation [codon 850: leu (T*T*G) → stop (T*A*G)] is present. This mutation is analogous to those found in human FAP kindreds and sporadic colorectal cancers. The murine and human coding sequences are 86 and 90 per cent identical at the nucleotide and amino acid levels, respectively, with conservation of important motifs. The homozygous state is embryonically lethal (during the second week), but heterozygous Min mice on a C57BL/6J background (a specific type of laboratory mouse inbred strain originally established in 1921), develop numerous, predominantly *small* intestinal adenomatous polyps within the first three months of life. Transformation to invasive carcinoma is rare, and metastases have not been observed. There is also an increased incidence of mammary tumours, which are not MMTV dependent. This was unexpected, as human FAP is not associated with breast cancer. However, there are

some extra-intestinal manifestations, such as desmoids, akin to the human disease. The Min mouse therefore provides a valuable model for the study of *APC* function, tumour biology, and approaches for preventing or treating polyps.

By crossing Min on to different inbred mouse strains, it was found that the intestinal polyposis could be almost completely suppressed. Using crosses between two different backgrounds and appropriately spaced genetic markers, a locus called MOM-1 (for modifier of Min) has been identified, which strongly modifies the Min phenotype. It is likely that when the human homologue of this locus is identified, currently mapping to a region in human chromosome 1p35–36, it will also have a substantial modifying effect on the phenotype of FAP patients. Interestingly, this region shows frequent chromosomal loss in a variety of human tumours, including colon cancer. This suggests that this modifying locus may be an important tumour suppressor gene. However, there is strong evidence that mouse strains that are also mutant (constitutionally null) for an enzyme called secretory phospholipase A2 (PLA2) are also highly sensitive to the effects of *APC* mutations. That is, mice that express normal levels of this protein are conferred strong protection against the normally deleterious effects of an *APC* mutation. Human secretory phospholipase A2 has been mapped to 1p35–36 but it is as yet unclear whether this gene has any modifying activity in FAP.

4.5 Systemic inherited susceptibilities

Part of the early evolutionary process must have been to ensure that cells are able to deal comfortably with hostile environments. This may be in many forms such as chemicals or toxins and ionizing radiation. When such agents can directly or indirectly damage DNA, there is the potential to affect genes that control cellular growth and so effect dysregulation. Even in prokaryotes, numerous sophisticated pathways are present that can prevent such damage. However, should DNA damage occur, there are many specific ways in which its fidelity is restored, dependent on the exact type of insult and consequent change that has occurred. If genes that are involved in DNA replication and repair are mutated, it is very likely (if the mutation is not lethal) that, subsequently, mutations of a specific type will accumulate. If such a change is in the germ line, then there may be an increased propensity to tumour formation at an earlier stage.

4.5.1 DNA repair deficiencies

The best known example of a systemic effect leading to an inherited susceptibility to cancer is the recessively inherited xeroderma pigmentosum (XP), which is cause by a deficiency in the ability to repair DNA. XP is rare, with an incidence of about 1 in 250 000, and is characterized by an extreme susceptibility to sunlight-induced abnormalities of the skin, frequently followed by malignant skin cancer. Cells from individuals with the disease are unusually sensitive to the sublethal effects of UV light, and, to a lesser extent, certain types of carcinogens, because they are defective in their ability to repair damaged DNA. Specifically, the UV-induced impairment is the abnormal joining of two adjacent bases in DNA leading to bulky dimer formation, which causes a distortion in the double helix. It is now

known that there are several different forms of the disease, probably all a result of mutations in different genes involved in the first step of the nucleotide excision–repair pathway of bulky dimers. There are at least seven such predisposing excision–repair cross-complementing genes cloned in humans and they appear to have either endonuclease- or helicase-type functions. It seems likely that the reason why XP individuals predominantly get malignant skin cancers is that this tissue is the most exposed to their susceptibility mutagen, normally UV radiation in sunlight. This exposure far exceeds that of internal organs from ingested mutagens, to which some XP individuals also appear to be sensitive. There are confirmed reports of XP patients with internal tumours.

The first DNA repair syndrome clearly identified with a molecular defect was Bloom's syndrome. This is also associated in some patients with a sensitivity to UV radiation, as well as an immunodeficiency. It has been shown that in at least one (possibly rare) form there is a defect in one of the DNA ligases, which is responsible for joining gaps between adjacent nucleotides in the DNA. There also appears to be a general decrease in the rate of chain elongation during the DNA synthesis phase, which may or may not be related. Several other diseases are also thought to be associated with DNA repair defects, giving rise to sensitivity to UV light or other carcinogens, and most of these are associated with a very significantly increased susceptibility to cancer. Notable among these disorders are ataxia telangiectasia, which is now also known to be a collection of diseases associated with different mutations in one single gene, and Fanconi's anaemia. These are all rare, recessively inherited syndromes, involving defects in some aspect of DNA repair leading to increased chromosomal breakage and rearrangements, multiple clinical abnormalities, often involving the neurological and immune systems, and an increased risk of developing cancer at a young age.

4.5.2 Mismatch repair and hereditary non-polyposis colonic cancer (HNPCC)

In addition to syndromes such as FAP and XP, which are dominantly and recessively inherited conditions, respectively, with a strong predisposition to cancer, there are other notable instances of 'cancer families' where there is a predisposition to several types of cancer but the inheritance is not necessarily clear-cut. This may be either because the pedigrees are small, but it is more likely to be becuase the penetrance of the cancers is relatively low or late, which can result in confusion with phenocopies, particularly if the background tumour incidence is relatively high. In 1966, Henry Lynch described two such families within which were, among other tumours, six instances of the ordinarily rare combination of primary colonic and endometrial carcinomas. In addition, as for the LFS, the cancers occurred at an early age. From this he proposed the existence of a disease complex called 'the cancer family syndrome' which was characterized by an increased occurrence of adenocarcinoma of the colon (principally of the right side in contrast to the usually more common left side), and endometrial and gastric carcinoma. From the patterns of inheritance, he suggested an autosomal dominant mode and further subdivided the syndrome into Lynch Syndrome I, which is used eponymously for site-specific (colon) cancer, and type II, which is colorectal carcinoma in association with other tumours. As opposed to colonic cancer in FAP, which arises on the background of an inherited predisposition to numerous polyps, familial cancers in the colon in the Lynch-type families are also called collectively HNPCC (hereditary non-polyposis colon cancer). This was specifically defined in pedigree terms as 'occurrence of early onset colonic cancer and/or other specific tumours in first degree relatives, spanning at least two generations'. Until recently the inheritance (thought initially to involve a tumour suppressor gene) of this disease has been an enigma to cancer geneticists. However, at least four genes have now been cloned within such families with a predisposition to colorectal carcinoma.

The unifying features among these genes is that they encode proteins that are involved in the repair of damaged DNA and, when mutated, appear to allow or 'generate' widespread genetic damage of a specific type, called replication slippage. It is known through studying gene-repair pathways in yeast and *Escherischia coli*, that a specific repair pathway exists called 'mismatch repair' because it appears to remove nucleotides that have paired up with the wrong partners in the DNA double helix, replacing them with the correct ones. In yeast and bacteria it had also been observed that mutations in such genes lead to specific types of genetic instability. Because short repeat sequences are particularly vulnerable to this type of damage, it is often observed as microsatellite instability (or genomic instability), normally as a high mutation rate at positions within CA repeats. Thus, a mutation in a gene in this pathway appears to give rise to an increase in mutation rate generally, as predicted.

The first clue to the nature of the mutation in the HNPCC families came from the observation that tumours from involved individuals had a uniformly high mutation rate for CA repeats, namely microsatellite instability. Then, because of the extraordinary conservation of function of the mismatch repair genes from *E. coli* through yeast to humans, it was shown that an *E. coli* human homologue mapped precisely to the location of one of the HNPCC genes on chromosome 2 (called *hMSH2*, for human mutator-S protein (in *E. coli*) homologue). It was an obvious further step therefore to screen this as a candidate gene and demonstrate that it was indeed mutated in the chromosome 2-linked cases of HNPCC. Three other genes in the mismatch repair pathway were then shown to correspond to other HNPCC families, with essentially indistinguishable phenotypes, but which mapped to different chromosomes (see Table 4.6).

Certainly, given the finiteness of the process of cancer progression, a mutation giving rise to an increase in the mutation rate may be advantageous, but, as in the theory underlying sexual evolutionary processes, the selective pressure for such a change (especially if it is recessive) must be secondary to mutations having a more direct effect on the independence and growth of potential cancer cells. Perhaps surprisingly, some sporadic tumours (i.e. not inherited) have also been shown to have mismatch repair mutations, and studies have confirmed that the tumour cell DNA can be 100 times more mutable compared with the normal counterparts. In sporadic colorectal tumours, less than 15 per cent appear to have mutations in the currently defined four mismatch gene repair pathways, although there is a suggestion that this percentage rises as the age of onset falls. It seems possible that in sporadic tumours these types of mutations play a similar role to those in *p53* in that the cells acquire, or are selected for, resistance to apoptosis.

4.5.3 Carcinogen metabolism

Inherited variations in the activity of enzymes that metabolize potential carcinogens are another source

Table 4.6 Cloned human mismatch repair genes and their homologues

Human genes	Mapping	*Sacchromyces cerevisiae* yeast	*Escherichia coli* prokaryotes
*h*MSH2	2p16	msh1-42	Mut S Initial mismatch recognition and methyl-directed DNA binding
*h*MLH 1	3p21–23	mlh1	Binds to Mut S-DNA complex
*h*PMS1[1]	2q31–33	pms1	Mut L (humans appear to have at least three homologues
*h*PMS2[1]	7p22	?	all probably involved in DNA binding)
?		?	Mut H Endonuclease
?		?	Mut U DNA helicase II
?		?	Dam Strand signal

In *Escherichia coli*, mutants that displayed a spontaneous marked increase in mutation rate helped elucidate the molecular systems responsible for the maintenance of genetic integrity in prokaryotes over 20 years ago. Biosynthetic mistakes are recognized and eliminated from the newly synthesized DNA strand by this system. In addition, it appears that in *E. coli*, some of these proteins also ensure the fidelity of genetic recombination by blocking cross-overs between sequences that have diverged genetically (see also Table 4.5). In humans, defects in mismatch repair cause replication errors (RER) in nucleotide repeat sequences, which is responsible for the microsatellite instability seen. Mutations in *h*MLH1 and *h*MSH2 appear to account for about 80 per cent of HNPCC. By contrast, it appears that the majority of sporadic colon cancers do *not* have RER positivity, although this may not be the case for the 2 per cent (or less) sporadic cases that occur in young patients under 35 years of age. One abnormal copy of each human gene appears sufficient to contribute to some degree of microsatellite instability, although the situation is not clear with *h*PMS2. Although HNPCC syndromes are inherited as autosomal dominant, the data as to whether a somatic 'second-hit' is absolutely necessary for tumour formation, are conflicting to date. Microsatellite instability has also been demonstrated in apparently phenotypically *normal* cells of patients with germ line mutations of PMS2 and *h*MLH1. This raises the important issue of the relevance of this type of instability in tumourigenesis.

[1] These genes have been mapped in sporadic cases only and no pedigrees carrying germ line mutations have yet been found.

of inherited systemic susceptibilities to cancer. Among the best known such enzymes are the mono-oxygenases, or cytochrome P450 enzymes (Wolf 1986). These enzymes are known to metabolize many substances from inert into reactive, or carcinogenic compounds. Thus, in the mouse there are differences between inbred strains in the level of the enzyme aryl hydrocarbon hydroxylase, which acts on certain hydrocarbons turning them into potent mutagens and carcinogens. These differences have been shown to be associated with differential effects of these hydrocarbons on the rate of tumour induction. Similar studies in humans were initially promising and suggested a single gene difference in susceptibility to induction of lung tumours by cigarette smoking, but these observations have not been confirmed. Inherited variations in various P450 enzyme activities are associated in humans with differential responses to a wide variety of drugs, termed pharmacogenetic variation. This is owing to the fact that the activity of the drugs is modified by these enzymes. One example studied involves differences in the ability to metabolize the drug debrisoquine. About 10 per cent of the population metabolize this drug slowly and so have severe side effects when given the drug at therapeutic doses. This reaction appears to be associated with a recessively inherited difference in the relevant hydroxylation enzyme, the susceptible individuals being homozygous for a less active form of the enzyme. A controlled study of cigarette smokers with and without lung cancer has shown a striking sixfold lower frequency of the slow metabolizers of debrisoquine among lung cancer cases (Ayesh *et al.* 1984). If confirmed, this would be a most important example of an inherited systemic susceptibility to the carcinogenic effects of an environmental agent, cigarette smoke, owing to differences in rates of carcinogen metabolism.

Most of the P450 enzymes have now been cloned. This means that it is now possible to study genetic variation in these enzymes at the DNA level and to test the association of slow and fast metabolism of debrisoquine with lung cancer by seeing whether detectable variation at the DNA level in the relevant enzyme, for example using RFLPs, associates with susceptibility to lung cancer among cigarette smokers. In the case of the debrisoquine sensitivity, the DNA-based studies have not yet confirmed the original pharmacological associations. These and other variations, such as in the glutathione-S-transferases and certain acetylases, may provide important clues to inherited susceptibilities to cancer through metabolism of carcinogens.

4.5.4 Immune response differences

A third major example of inherited systemic effects concerns immune response differences. The major human histocompatibility (HLA; human leucocyte antigen) system controls two main sets of cell surface determinants which are involved in interactions between lymphocytes and other cells in the control of the immune response. The system is highly polymorphic, that is, there are many differences between individuals with respect to the cell surface determinants. These differences make it necessary to match individuals for organ transplantation. HLA differences have also been shown to be associated with a variety of autoimmune- or immune-related disease, such as juvenile onset insulin-dependent diabetes mellitus, rheumatoid arthritis, and ankylosing spondylitis, most probably through inherited differences in specific immune responses. A number of associations between HLA and different cancers have been suggested, most notably with Hodgkin's disease, nasopharyngeal carcinoma (NPC) and Kaposi's sarcoma; in no case is the association as striking as that with the clear-cut autoimmune- or immune-related diseases. In the case of both NPC, associated with the Epstein–Barr virus, and Kaposi's sarcoma, also now known to be caused by a novel member of the herpesvirus family, an inherited immune response difference to the virus, or virally induced cellular determinants, is a plausible mechanism for an inherited difference in susceptibility to the cancer. Inherited immune response differences associated with HLA variation, as well as with variation in the other molecules of the immune system, notably antibodies and the T cell receptor, may be relevant in susceptibility to other virally induced human cancers. These include, for example, cervical and other cancers associated with the human papillomaviruses, the leukaemias associated with the various human T cell leukaemia viruses, and liver cancer associated with the hepatitis virus.

4.6 Types of family data and their interpretation

The simplest inherited susceptibilities are those, such as retinoblastoma, polyposis coli, Li–Fraumeni, the DNA repair deficiencies, and other inherited systemic susceptibilities, that follow a clear-cut Mendelian pattern of inheritance. In such cases, the nature of the genetic control is not in question,

and the challenge is to identify the specific genes involved and interpret their functions at the molecular and, subsequently, cellular level. There are, however, many examples of inherited susceptibilities that are not so easy to interpret. For example, the associations of debrisoquine slow metabolizers or HLA variants and particular cancers were not identified through family studies, but by looking at the distribution of a particular genetic difference in patients with a given sort of cancer compared with controls.

The classical approach to assessing a potential inherited contribution to a disease, in the absence of clear-cut Mendelian segregation, is to establish to what extent there is an increased incidence of the disease among the relatives of affected individuals. Often this involves, specifically, the study of twins, contrasting identical with non-identical twins. If there is a major inherited component, then the disease incidence among co-identical twins, that is the concordance, should be greater than that among co-non-identical twins. This is because the former share all their genes, while the latter on average share only half their genes, just as any brothers or sisters do. Studying twins brought up in the same household tends to average out the effects of environment. Twin studies tend to show a slightly increased concordance of cancer among identical as compared to non-identical twins, but the effect is marginal and the data very hard to obtain. More generally, studies on the incidence of particular forms of cancer among relatives of patients compared with that in the general population have often indicated an approximately two- to fourfold increase in incidence among relatives, especially for breast and childhood cancers. It is, however, very difficult to interpret these relatively modest increases as necessarily caused by genetic factors, since relatives also tend to share a common environment and this clearly could have a similar effect on incidence among relatives as do genetic factors. Thus, while such studies may suggest a limited genetic contribution to overall inherited susceptibility to certain cancers, they do not provide clear-cut answers and offer little or no prospect for further investigation.

Another approach to the problem of sorting out inherited susceptibilities, especially for the comparatively common cancers such as breast and colon cancer for which it is clear that the majority of cases do not show an obvious inherited component, is to ask whether there is, nevertheless, a subset of cases that tend to cluster in families. This would indicate a minority of cases associated with a clearly inherited susceptibility. Occasional very striking examples of clusters of cancers within a single family have often been described, and an example is shown in Fig. 4.12. The difficulty with this approach is in assessing whether the familial clustering is really significant. Obviously for a relatively common cancer, some cases will cluster in families simply by chance, and appropriate statistical methods must be used to distinguish these from familial clustering owing to Mendelian segregation of a gene associated with an increased susceptibility. Statistical models for the expected distribution of different genetic types can be fitted to such families, but such models rarely provide a clear-cut answer to the interpretation of familial clusters.

The study of familial clustering as a basis for identifying inherited susceptibilities is also subject to another major difficulty. This is the fact, easily demonstrated, that even if a disease does not show any obvious familial clustering, it may nevertheless have a major genetic component. Suppose, for example, there exists a dominant gene that increases the chance of getting a particular form of cancer by a factor of 10 say, from one in a thousand to one in a hundred. If the gene is rare, then in most families where it occurs it will only occur once in one of the parents. Then, for example, only in $(1/100)^2 = 1/10\,000$ of such families with two offspring will both of them have the cancer, and the chance of a sib of an affected sib being affected is only $1/200$. Even if the gene gives rise to a 10 per cent chance of getting the cancer, only 1 per cent of families with two children with the gene present once in either parent will have pairs of affected sibs. Nevertheless, even when the gene frequency is as low as 0.05 per cent, it could still be contributing as much as 50 per cent to the total incidence of the particular form of cancer with

which it is associated. Here, one would have a situation where a particular gene was responsible for 50 per cent of the incidence of one form of cancer, and yet because only 10 per cent of the people with the gene get the cancer, there would be very few examples of familial clustering. However, in those families where pairs of sibs are affected, most pairs will both carry the relevant susceptibility gene. It is this that provides the clue to the objective study of such inherited susceptibilities, because if an inherited Mendelian marker difference can be found for a gene that is reasonably close to the one actually causing the inherited cancer susceptibility, then this marker will also tend to be associated with pairs of affected sibs. In other words, if one finds a genetic marker whose distribution among affected pairs of sibs is distorted compared with Mendelian segregation, then this marker must be linked to a gene causing an inherited susceptibility.

This principle can be illustrated using as an example, the association between HLA and Hodgkin's disease. A weak association between certain HLA markers and Hodgkin's disease was first observed in 1967. This was subsequently confirmed by many other studies, but its significance is only a result of the fact that the association was studied so extensively. The maximum relative risk, a simple measure of the relative increase in the frequency of a particular HLA determinant among people with Hodgkin's disease compared with controls, was only about 1.3–1.6 compared, for example, with relative risks of close to 100 or more for the association of HLA type B27 with ankylosing spondylitis. Now, although the vast majority of cases of Hodgkin's disease are sporadic, a small proportion, perhaps up to 3 per cent of cases, occur in families with two or more affected individuals. Within such families, HLA typing can establish whether the affected pairs of sibs with Hodgkin's disease are

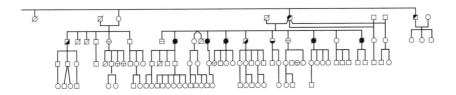

Fig. 4.12 Pedigree of a family with multiple cases of cancer (S. Cartwright and J. G. Bodmer, personal communication). Circles, females; ◔, carcinoma cervix; ◑, carcinoma liver; ●, carcinoma breast; ◑, carcinoma stomach; ⊖, cervical dysplasia; ⊕, ovarian cysts. Squares, males; ◪, carcinoma bronchus; ◪, skin basal cell carcinoma; ⊟, papilloma bladder. A diagonal slash through the symbol represents death of the individual.

HLA identical (namely have inherited the same HLA chromosome complement from each parent), share only one HLA chromosome but not the other, or have neither chromosome in common. The expected frequency of these three situations on the assumption of Mendelian segregation, and in the absence of any association within the families between HLA and Hodgkin's disease, is 1:2:1. Overall, among 32 sib pairs studied in this way, 16 were found to be HLA identical, 11 shared one HLA chromosome, and 5 none, a highly significant departure from the expected Mendelian 1:2:1, or 8:16:8, ratio. The data thus clearly show an association between the HLA segregation in the families and Hodgkin's disease. This is exactly as expected if there is a gene in, or close to, the HLA region which confers susceptibility to Hodgkin's disease. Thus, in the case of Hodgkin's disease, the family data provide the most convincing evidence for an association with the HLA system. This approach can clearly be generalized to any situation where there is more than one member of a family with Hodgkin's disease. The question asked is whether the HLA distribution is distorted among the individuals with Hodgkin's disease, compared with what could be expected from the normal pattern of Mendelian segregation. Interestingly, it has also now been shown that for Hodgkin's disease, there is a significantly increased risk to identical twins both being affected compared with non-identical twins.

The HLA system was originally chosen for study in the case of Hodgkin's disease because of the association between the mouse H2 system (the equivalent to HLA) and certain types of virally induced murine leukaemias. For most examples of familial clustering of cancer, there is no such clue as to which genetic marker should be studied. In this case all that one can advocate is a systematic search for a genetic marker that is distorted in its segregation among individuals with cancer within a family. While this may seem a haphazard approach, the range of genetic markers available for such studies is now vastly increased using recombinant DNA techniques as described in Section 4.3, and so such systematic surveys are a realistic possibility. Through them, it should be possible to identify, for any significant familial clustering of an inherited cancer susceptibility, one or more genetic markers sufficiently close to the gene actually causing the susceptibility. Such a gene would be detected by a distortion in its expected Mendelian segregation among the individuals in the family who have cancer. In our view, this is now the only satisfactory way of establishing an inherited susceptibility other than finding the gene, which itself gives rise to that inherited susceptibility.

This is the general principle that underlies the analysis of the association between HLA and Hodgkin's disease discussed above. Clearly, the ability to detect a distortion in the marker distribution among individuals with cancer in families will be a function of how close the marker happens to be to the susceptibility gene. In practice, even a recombination fraction of 10 per cent would readily allow the detection of a segregation distortion. It can be calculated that approximately 250 markers regularly spaced at a 10 per cent recombination fraction interval are needed to cover the complete human chromosome set. This, therefore, in principle, would be the maximum number of markers needed to be tested on a set of families, in order to find one or more sufficiently close to the gene actually causing an inherited susceptibility for it to be identified.

4.7 Conclusions and future prospects

Although inherited susceptibility to cancer may contribute no more than 20 per cent of overall cancer incidence in a direct sense, this is nevertheless both an important contribution in its own right and can help to provide major clues to the fundamental underlying causes of cancer, and to approaches for its prevention and treatment. Tissue-specific inherited changes can provide clues to genetic changes taking place during tumour progression in non-inherited cancers. Inherited susceptibilities connected with systemic effects, such as deficiencies in DNA repair, carcinogen metabolism, and immune response, provide major clues to potentially controllable environmental factors that cause cancer. In all cases, the ultimate challenge is to identify the particular genetic differences and their functional basis.

The use of DNA polymorphisms to find markers linked to cancer susceptibility genes in principle provides an avenue to the eventual identification of novel genes. The more closely the marker is associated within families with the cancer, the more likely it is to be near to the responsible gene and the easier it will be, therefore, eventually to isolate the gene itself, as has become almost routine with the availability of dense genetic maps and the advent of automated DNA screening technology. Indeed, the rate of progress in recombinant DNA technology has allowed the identification of many cancer susceptibility genes, leaving knowledge regarding their functions as the challenge for the immediate future. The analysis of retinoblastoma remains, however, the model example in this context.

As already emphasized, the genes for the P450 enzymes and other enzymes involved in carcinogen metabolism can now be studied using the DNA-based techniques for their association with inherited cancer susceptibilities. Sooner or later, all the genes for the DNA repair deficiency syndromes will be identified. Then, the question of whether there is an increased risk of cancer associated with an individual who carries just one copy of a defective DNA repair gene, that is one of the many in the repair gene complement, will become amenable to analysis using modern techniques.

A genetic marker that is closely linked to an inherited susceptibility may have considerable practical value even if it does not immediately lead to the identification of the specific genetic function involved in the susceptibility. First of all, such a marker may help to recognize heterogeneity in the predisposition, since different subsets of susceptibilities may show different patterns of linkage to different genetic markers. Secondly, within families, the linked marker defines a high risk group, the identification of which may be very valuable. For example, individuals identified as being at high risk may be treated prophylactically, as is now the case for polyposis coli. Such individuals may also be useful for studies of the physiology of the difference between high and low risk groups, which should help to identify the underlying functional basis for a particular inherited susceptibility. It may also be possible to do case–control studies comparing high and low risk groups within families, in order to identify factors that may interact with a genetic predisposition.

Recombinant DNA technology leads to identification of the genetic steps, one at a time, that take a cell from the normal to the cancerous state. Already, for example, in the case of colorectal cancer, relevant genetic changes have been identified at specific regions on chromosomes 5, 12, 17, 18, and probably also 1. Many of these genetic changes can already be identified using archival material stored in the form of paraffin blocks from tumour biopsies. With the further development and refinement of DNA-based

techniques and approaches to growing out samples of cells from tumours and their surrounding tissues, it will become possible to identify all the genetic steps and their sequence during tumour progression, as well as their functional significance. This genetic profile must be the ultimate classification of a tumour, through which one must hope to find new approaches either to prevention or to early detection and to treatment. Already, there is evidence for the presence of *p53* mutations within certain tumours correlating not only to a poorer prognosis, but also to a relative resistance to both chemotherapy and radiotherapy.

Sooner or later, through the collaborative efforts of the Human Genome Project, we shall have essentially the whole DNA sequence of the human genes and some definition of all the basic functional units. When this situation is reached, having found a linked marker for a particular inherited susceptibility, it may be possible simply to look up the genes with relevant functions that are in its neighbourhood, and through that, focus on the actual genetic difference responsible for the inherited susceptibility. There can be no doubt that the application of recombinant DNA techniques, coupled with epidemiological and genetic studies, will in due course unravel the full genetic contribution to the initiation and progression of cancers both at the germ line and somatic cell levels. Simultaneously, much will be learnt about normal cellular growth and development.

In summary, major advances in the next few years are likely to encompass a further understanding of the function of important genes already cloned and their interaction in cellular pathways. Animal models engineered with specific mutations are likely to further facilitate this knowledge. This should stimulate new ideas in therapeutic approaches, including drug design, to treatment. Advances in mutation screening and analysis in susceptibility genes should allow effective prophylactic and preventive practice and, possibly of even greater significance, the building of epidemiological molecular databases which may pin-point or provide clues to specific environmental hazards. Automation will make feasible the identification of genes with lower penetrance or with modifying effects on the 'major' susceptibility genes, and this will help us to improve genetic profiling and ultimately provide a fuller understanding of the biological basis of sporadic tumours.

References and further reading

General

Ayesh, R., Idle, J. R., Ritchie, J. C., Crothers, M. J., and Hetzel, M. R. (1984). Metabolic oxidation phenotypes as markers for susceptibility to lung cancer. *Nature,* **312**, 169–70. The paper on the association between debrisoquine metabolism and lung cancer owing to cigarette smoking.

Bodmer, W. F. (ed.) (1982). Inheritance of susceptibility to cancer in man. *Cancer Surveys,* **1**, 1–186. Contains a range of articles covering many of the topics surveyed in this chapter.

Fearon, E. R. and Vogelstein, B. (1990). A genetic model for colorectal tumorigenesis. *Cell,* **61**, 759–67. A review of the evidence supporting the stepwise hypothesis of adenoma to carcinoma in colon cancer

Fialkow, P. J. (1972). Use of genetic markers to study cellular origin and development of tumors in human females. *Advances in Cancer Research,* **15**, 191–226.

Franks, L. M. (ed.) (1988). Somatic cell genetics and cancer. *Cancer Surveys,* **7**, 225–371. A series of papers on genetic aspects of cancer as revealed by somatic cell genetic techniques.

Harnden, D., Morten, J., and Featherstone, T. (1984). Dominant susceptibility to cancer in man. *Advances in Cancer Research,* **141**, 185–245. A review of certain aspects of inherited susceptibility to cancer.

Knudson, A. G. (1986). Genetics of human cancers: review. *Annual Reviews of Genetics,* **20**, 231–51. A previous statement of Knudson's ideas.

Knudson, A. G. (1993). Antioncogenes and human cancers: review. *Proceedings of the National Academy of Sciences, USA,* **90**, 10914–21. An update of Knudson's ideas.

Lockhart-Mummery, (1925). Cancer and heredity. *Lancet,* **1**, 427–9.

McKusick, V. (1992). *Mendelian genetics in man,* (9th edn). Johns Hopkins University Press, Baltimore. The standard reference catalogue for inherited human diseases, including cancer.

Mulvihill, J. J., Miller, R. W., and Fraumeni, J. F., jun. (ed.) (1977). *The genetics of human cancer.* Raven Press, New York. An earlier collection of papers on cancer genetics which is still a very useful survey.

Omenn, G. S. and Gelboin, H. V. (ed.) (1984). *Genetic variability in response to chemical exposures,* The Banbury Report 16. Cold Spring Harbor Laboratory, Cold Spring Harbor, New York. A useful collection of papers on a whole variety of aspects of inherited differences in drug metabolism and their relationship to cancer incidence.

Willis, A. E., Weksberg, R., Tomlinson, S., and Lindahl, T. (1987). Structural alterations of DNA ligase I in Bloom syndrome. *Proceedings of the National Academy of Sciences, USA,* **84**, 8016–20.

Wolf, C.R. (1986). Cytochrome P 450: polymorphic multigene families involved in carcinogen activation. *Trends in Genetics,* **2**, 209–14. A review of the P450 enzyme systems.–

Familial adenomatous polyposis

Bodmer, W. F., Bailey, C. J., Bodmer, J., Bussey, H. J., Ellis, A., Gorman, P., *et al.* (1987). Localization of the gene for familial adenomatous polyposis is on chromosome 5. *Nature,* **328**, 614–16.

Dietrich, W. F., Lander, E. S., Smith, J. S., Moser, A. R., Gould, K. A., Luongo, C., *et al.* (1993). Genetic identification of Mom-1, a major modifier locus affecting Min-induced intestinal neoplasia in the mouse. *Cell,* **75**, 631–9. This paper demonstrates the power of modern mouse mapping techniques.

Groden, J., Thliveris, A., Samowitz, W., Carlson, M., Gelbert, L., Albertsen, H., *et al.* (1991). Identification and characterization of the familial adenomatous polyposis coli gene. *Cell,* **66**, 589–600. One of the two simultaneous papers describing the cloning of *APC.*

Kinzler, K. W., Nilbert, M. C., Su, L. K., Vogelstein, B., Bryan, T. M., Levy, D. B., *et al.* (1991). Identification of FAP locus genes from chromosome 5q21. *Science,* **253**, 661–5. One of the two simultaneous papers describing the cloning of *APC.*

Leppert, M., Dobbs, M., Scambler, P., O'Connell, P., Nakamura, Y., Stauffer, D., *et al.* (1987). The gene for familial polyposis coli maps to the long arm of chromosome 5. *Science*, **238**, 1411–13.

Solomon, E., Voss, R., Hall, V., Bodmer, W. F., Jass, J.R., Jeffreys, A. J., *et al.* (1987). Chromosome 5 allele loss in colorectal carcinomas. *Nature*, **328**, 616–19. This paper and that by Bodmer *et al.* (1987) describe the localization of the familial adenomatous polyposis gene and the demonstration of its likely role as a recessive genetic change in a relatively high proportion of sporadic colorectal cancers.

Spirio, L., Olschwang, S., Groden, J., Robertson, M., Samowitz, W., Joslyn, G., *et al.* (1993). Alleles of the APC gene: an attenuated form of familial polyposis. *Cell*, **75**, 951–7. This paper describes a genotypephenotype correlation in FAP.

Su, L. K., Kinzler, K. W., Vogelstein, B., Preisinger, A. C., Moser, A. R., Luongo, C., *et al.* (1992). Multiple intestinal neoplasia caused by a mutation in the murine homologue of the APC gene. *Science*, **256**, 668–70. This paper describes the murine model of FAP.

Retinoblastoma and p53

Cavanee, W. K., Dryja T., Phillips R., Benedict W., Godbout R., Gallie. *et al.* (1983). Expression of recessive alleles by chromosomal mechanisms in retinoblastoma. *Nature*, **305**, 779–84.

Hollstein, M., Sidransky, D., Vogelstein, B., and Harris, C. C. (1991). P53 mutations in human cancers. *Science*, **253**, 49–53.

Huang, H. J., Lee, J. K., Shew, J. Y., Chen, P. L., Bookstein, R., Friedmann, T, *et al.* (1988). Suppression of the neoplastic phenotype by replacement of the RB gene in human cancer cells. *Science*, **242**, 1563–6.

Lee E. Y., To H., Shew J., Brookstein R., Scully P., and Lee W. (1988). Inactivation of the retinoblastoma susceptibility gene in human breast cancers. *Science*, **241**, 218–21.

Malkin D., Li F., Strong L., Fraumeni J., Nelson C., Kim D., Kassel J., *et al.* (1990). Germ line p53 mutations in a familial syndrome of breast cancer, sarcomas and other neoplasms. *Science*, **250**, 1233–8

Whyte, P., Buchkovich, K. J., Horowitz, J. M., Friend, S. H., Raybuck, M., Weinberg, R. A., and Harlow, E. (1988). Association between an oncogene and an anti-oncogene: the adenovirus E1A proteins bind to the retinoblastoma gene product. *Nature*, **334**, 124–9. Describes the likely function of the retinoblastoma gene product and provides references to its initial identification.

HNPCC and mismatch repair

Bronner, C. E., Baker, S. M., Morrison, P. T., Warren, G., Smith, L. G., Lescoe, M. K., *et al.*(1994). Mutation in the DNA mismatch repair gene homologue *h*MLH1 is associated with hereditary non-polyposis colon cancer. *Nature*, **368**, 258–61.

Fishel, R., Lescoe, M. K., Rao, M. R., Copeland, N. G., Jenkins, N. A., Garber, J., *et al.* (1993). The human mutator gene homologue MSH2 and its association with hereditary nonpolyposis colon cancer. *Cell*, **75**, 1027–38.

Ionov, Y., Peinado, M. A., Malkhosyan, S., Shibata, D., and Perucho, M. (1993). Ubiquitous somatic mutations in simple repeated sequences reveal a new mechanism for colonic carcinogenesis. *Nature*, **363**, 558–61.

Lindblom, A., Tannergard, P., Werelius, B., and Nordenskjold, M. (1993). Genetic mapping of a second locus predisposing to hereditary non-polyposis colon cancer. *Nature Genetics*, **5**, 279–82.

Peltomaki, P., Aaltonen, L. A., Sistonen, P., Pylkkanen, L., Mecklin, J. P., Jarvinen, H., *et al.* (1993). Genetic mapping of a locus predisposing to human colorectal cancer. *Science*, **260**, 810–12.

Shibata, D., Peinado, M. A., Ionov, Y., Malkhosyan, S., and Perucho, M. (1994). Genomic instability in repeated sequences is an early somatic event in colorectal tumorigenesis that persists after transformation. *Nature Genetics*, **6**, 273–81.

Breast and ovarian cancer

Miki, Y., Swensen, J., Shattuck-Eidens, D., Futreal, P. A., Harshman, K., Tavtigian, S., *et al.* (1994). A strong candidate for the breast and ovarian cancer susceptibility gene. *Science*, **266**, 66–71. This paper describes the cloning of *BRCA1*, and the associated following paper the identification of mutations within the families.

Structure of DNA and its relationship to carcinogenesis

BEVERLY E. GRIFFIN

5.1 Introduction

Cells (and the intracellular substances secreted by them) make up the structural elements of the body. Within the nucleus of the cell resides its genetic information in the form of the polymeric material, deoxyribonucleic acid, or DNA. The integrity of this DNA is essential for the proper functioning of cells, their interactions, and, following naturally from this, the health of the whole organism. There are a few well-documented exceptions to DNA as the repository of genetic information. Some viruses carry their genetic information in ribonucleic acids, or RNA (see Chapter 8). Among these are viruses, designated *retroviruses*, that warrant serious consideration in any discussion about the genesis of cancer in avian and mammalian species. They code for an enzyme that converts their genomic RNA into DNA, which provides the origin of the term 'retro' or backward flow of information. Controversial suggestions have recently been put forward regarding the nature of the genetic agent in diseases such as scrapie in sheep and kuru in humans, where no infectious DNA or RNA has been identified and chemical or enzymatic reagents, which might be expected to destroy both, fail to abolish infectivity! It has been suggested by one school of scientists that the genetic information may indeed reside within protein molecules (so-called 'prions'), and models for protein replication have been put forward. However, at present this suggestion remains speculative and unconvincing.

The introduction to this chapter in the previous edition divided the study of DNA into 'seven ages'.

First was the age of the medical investigator, with the discovery by Miescher and colleagues in Germany over a century ago of a material in pus cells designated by them as 'nuclein'. Their finding alerted the scientific world to the existence of a hitherto unknown, and possibly important, cellular component. The second age, that of the chemist, was necessary to provide the definition of the component parts of DNA (and RNA), their chemical nature, and how they are linked to make up the polymeric species. Following this comes the age of the geneticist and the discovery that DNAs contain the genetic information essential for the continuity of most organisms. In the fourth age the molecular biologist defined the mechanisms by which DNA could pass on its genetic information. From this group of scientists came the concept of the linear relationship whereby DNA specifies the structure of RNA, which in turn specifies proteins (the so called 'central dogma' of molecular biology) and the concept of a triplet genetic code. The virologist provided much of the material and experimental designs for testing hypotheses proposed by molecular biologists and for identifying regulatory mechanisms that control gene expression, both quantitatively and qualitatively. The sixth age of DNA, that of the present, continues to belong to the biotechnologists and genetic engineers who turn academic exercises into practical reality, manipulating genes and their expression at will in the cause of medical or commercial progress and providing tools for probing the details of the biology of normal and abnormal cells. There are even firm plans for sequencing the human genome. At this junction it may be hoped that the history of DNA will not end like the famous Shakespearean diatribe on the 'seven ages of man' and in 'second childishness and mere oblivion, sans teeth, sans eyes, sans taste, sans everything'. This seems highly unlikely, and one can predict optimistically that the 'seventh age of DNA' will complete the circle, returning to the cell and the cell biologist, who will draw on all the knowledge acquired over the last 100 or so years (as outlined briefly in the discussion that follows) to unravel the intricate interactions, balances, and counterbalances in the normal cell and contrast them with lesions that give rise to the malignant cell.

We now know that each specific character in an organism is coded by a gene, a unit of genetic information, which produces its effect by specifying the production of a particular protein. The genes consist of long strands of DNA arranged in a very specific order. The DNA exists in close association with a group of small basic proteins known as histones, also arranged in an ordered manner with the protein molecules acting as wedges that have the correct shape to form the strands into coils. The structural unit is a nucleosome (Fig. 5.1) which is made up of a short length of DNA (about 200 nucleotide pairs— associated with a protein core of histones. The nucleosomes are attached to each other by a short piece of linker DNA (about 60 base pairs) like strings of beads, which are themselves organized into coils or supercoils by associated non-histone proteins. Individual nucleosomes are too small to be genes (the average gene is thought to be about 1000 nucleotides), and act as packing devices. Recently it has proved possible to crystallize nucleosomes and thus precisely determine their three-dimensional structure. When genes are inactive, the DNA and protein molecules are closely packed. When the genes are active, that is, being transcribed, the protein DNA complex opens up into a different, more accessible structure to allow the process of gene expression to take place. Alterations in cell behaviour may be brought about by changes in the structure of the DNA, i.e., mutation, or by perturbations in the mechanisms that control gene expression. Although we now have a great deal of information on changes in DNA structure and their relationships to neoplastic development (to be discussed later in this chapter), our knowledge of control of gene expression is much more limited. There is convincing evidence that methylation of DNA, particularly at CpG base pairs is one method

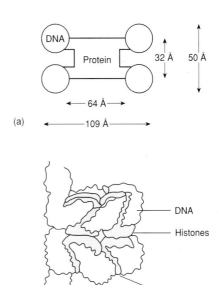

Fig. 5.1 Diagram showing substructures of a nucleosome. DNA strands in the nucleosome surround a core of histones and are continuous with linker strands of DNA above and below: (a) cross-section along axis; (b) from the side (from Richards *et al.* 1977).

by which control is exerted, in that such sites are often found to be transcriptionally inactive. Recent evidence suggests that methylation may enhance DNA coiling or induce curvatures in coils, provoking physical distortions that markedly alter transcription. Research in this area and into the relationship between mutation and gene expression should ultimately lead us to an understanding of cancer and of its control.

5.2 Components of DNA

DNA is composed of three relatively simple chemical species, namely, heterocyclic (nitrogenous) bases of which four are normally used, a five carbon atom sugar (deoxyribose), and phosphoric acid. The bases themselves are of two types, one a six-membered ring species designated a 'pyrimidine', and the other a fused five- and six-membered ring species designated a 'purine'. By convention, pyrimidines as classes are abbreviated as Y, purines as R, and the rings are numbered as shown in Fig. 5.2. In spite of their apparent simplicity, purines and pyrimidines

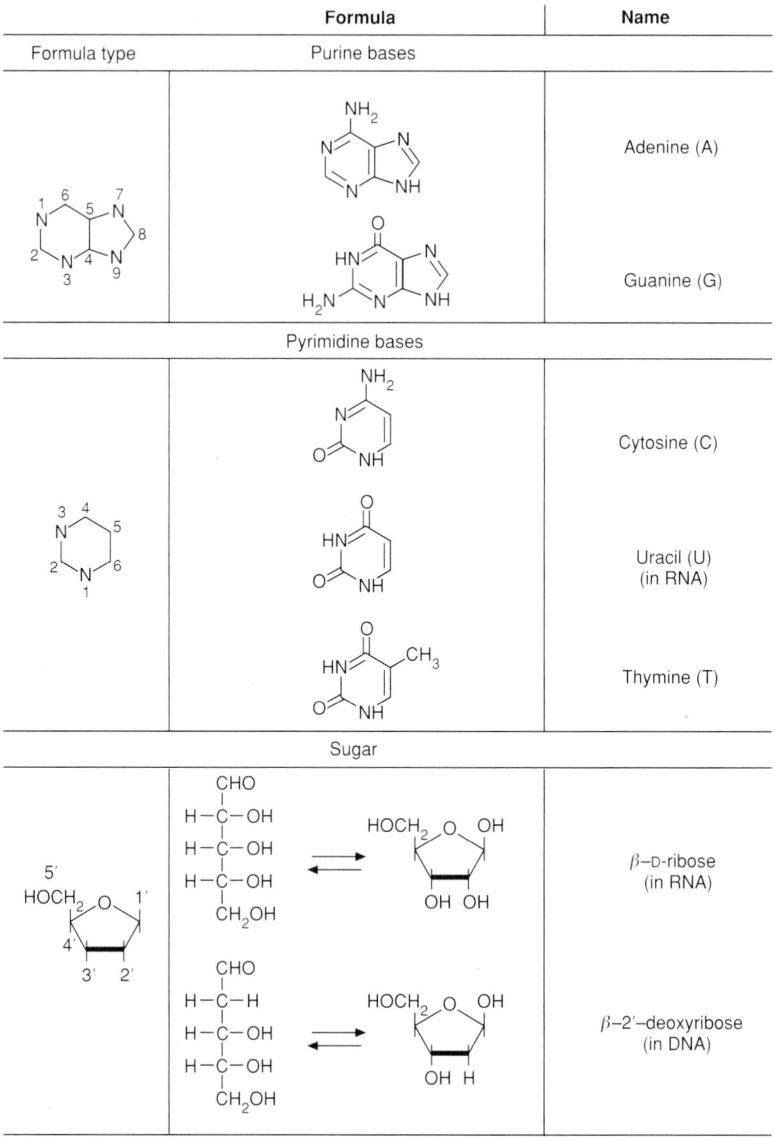

Fig. 5.2 Structures, numbering systems, and abbreviations of the heterocyclic (nitrogenous) bases, and five-carbon sugar moieties that are found in DNA and RNA. The numbering system currently in use for the six-membered pyrimidine ring is to be regretted, since the original system wherein the corresponding rings in both purines and pyrimidines were numbered alike is a simpler system. Further, the latter was used in the classical hydrolytic studies of Chargaff, where he showed that, regardless of the system used for isolation of DNA or its overall base content, there was a conserved correspondence between the ratios of A:T and G:C. That is, the 'oxy' function in the 6-position of one purine was matched by a 6-amino function in the pyrimidine, and vice versa. Chargaff's work provided the basis for the well-known Watson Crick hypothesis of complementary structures in a double-stranded DNA and ultimately to the 'double helix' model of DNA. The pentose sugar numbers carry a 'prime' designation when this moiety is linked to the bases, to distinguish them from numbers given to the latter.

have the capacity for determining many of the physical and biological properties of individual DNAs. Thus, it is important to understand their chemistry. The structures of the two pyrimidine residues, cytosine (C) and thymine (T) that exist in DNA are shown in Fig. 5.2. Theoretically, both these species can exist in a number of tautomeric forms although the isomer shown in Fig. 5.3 is that normally found in DNA. None the less, it is relevant to consider the other forms, as illustrated for cytosine, since pyrimidines trapped in one of these alternatives (as for examples by alkylation) can lead to mutations in

DNA. The various species result from a simple form of keto–enol (or imino–amino) tautomerism, that is, the interconversion between a double bonded oxygen atom ($=O$) and its singly bonded hydroxyl ($-OH$) counterpart which occurs by shift of a pair of electrons and hydrogen moiety, or, alternatively, by a comparable mechanism between an $=NH$ and $-NH_2$, moiety.

Similarly, in the case of the two purines that make up DNA, guanine (G) and adenine (A), various tautomeric forms exist, but for native DNA those shown in Fig. 5.2 persist. In other words, for both

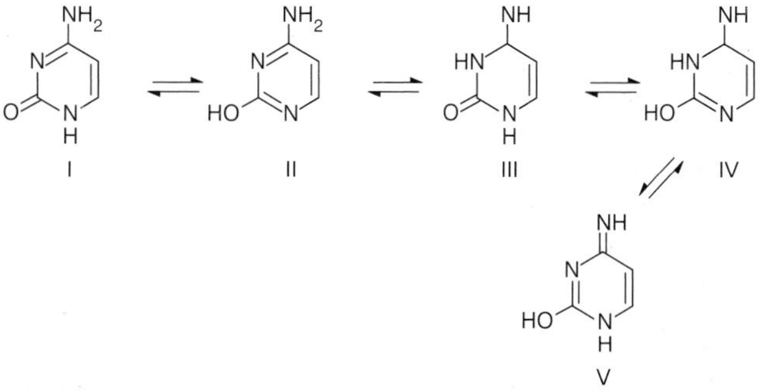

Fig. 5.3 An example of tautomerism, illustarted by the tautomeric forms of the pyrimidine base, cytosine. Form I is that commonly found in DNA, but forms III and V are also theoretically capable of existing under suitable conditions. Similar tautomeric forms can exist for the other bases that make up DNA (or RNA) and can often be 'trapped' as such by mutagenic and carcinogenic reagents, thus perturbing the structure.

pyrimidines and purines in DNA under normal circumstances the exocyclic oxygen atoms exist in the keto ($=$O) form, whereas the exocyclic nitrogens exist in an amino ($-$NH$_2$) form. This tautomeric preference in DNA can be altered, for example, by radical changes in pH or chemical modification, events frequently accompanied by important changes both in the physical and biological properties of the DNA.

Three of these heterocyclic bases, C, G, and A, also make up the building blocks of RNA. The fourth residue in DNA, thymine (T), is replaced in RNA, for reasons that are not wholly understood, by a similar molecule designated uracil (U) which lacks a methyl group at position 5. Similarly, in the DNA of many plants, 5-methylcytosine (5-MeC) is frequently found in place of cytosine (C), again for reasons that are yet to be defined but may be related to the maintenance of fidelity of DNA. This base also occurs infrequently in mammalian DNA. The role of modified or altered bases in DNA and RNA is clearly of great functional significance and may be important in control of gene expression in a cell. This is an area that is being explored.

In small RNA species called transfer (t) RNAs, which are important in protein synthesis, many unusual modified bases are found, as shown for one such tRNA in Fig. 5.4. The relative absence of 'unusual' bases in DNA may reflect the fact that error-free replication is vital to the maintenance of any specifics, and modifications could increase the likelihood of error (mutation).

In DNA (and RNA), the heterocyclic bases are covalently bound to the pentose sugar moiety, 2 deoxyribose (or ribose), through an N-glycosidic bond. This link traps the carbohydrate in one of its tautomeric forms, that of a β-D-deoxyribose, see Fig. 5.2. (In RNA, the corresponding sugar moiety is β-D-ribose.) The combination of a heterocyclic

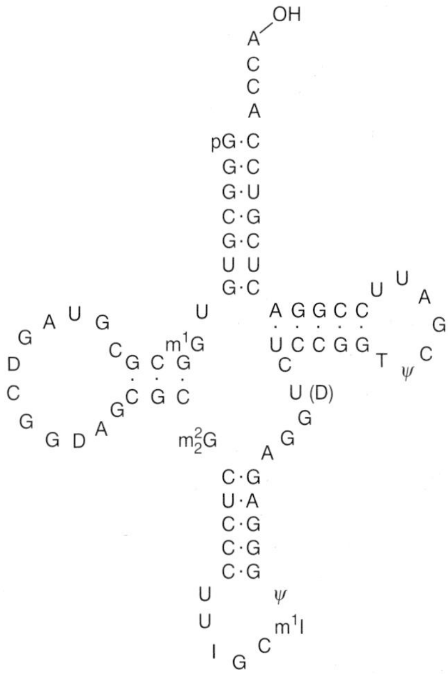

Fig. 5.4 The structure of one of the small transfer (t) RNAs, alanine tRNA, important in protein synthesis, showing some of the so-called 'minor bases' common to this kind of RNA, but not known to be ubiquitous in DNA or other RNA. Transfer RNAs carry amino acids to the sites of protein synthesis on ribosomes. It can be seen that more than 10 per cent of this particular molecule is composed of bases such as methylated guanines (m^{1}G, m$_2^2$G) or inosine (I) which are not normal components of nucleic acids. Similar types of modifications are found in other tRNAs and ribosome RNAs. (ψ is pseudouracil.)

base linked to the sugar is called a *nucleoside* or *deoxynucleoside*, as shown in Fig. 5.5 (see also Table 5.1).

The third component of DNA, phosphoric acid, is covalently linked to the pentose sugars by a phos-

Table 5.1 Standard nomenclature

Base	(deoxy)Nucleoside	Abbreviation	(deoxy)Nucleotide
Cytosine	(deoxy)Cytidine	C	(deoxy)Cytidylic acid
Thymine	Thymidine	T	Thymidylic acid
(Uracil)	(Uridine)	(U)	(Uridylic acid)
Guanine	(deoxy)Guanosine	G	(deoxy)Guanylic acid
Adenine	(deoxy)Adenosine	A	(deoxy)Adenylic acid

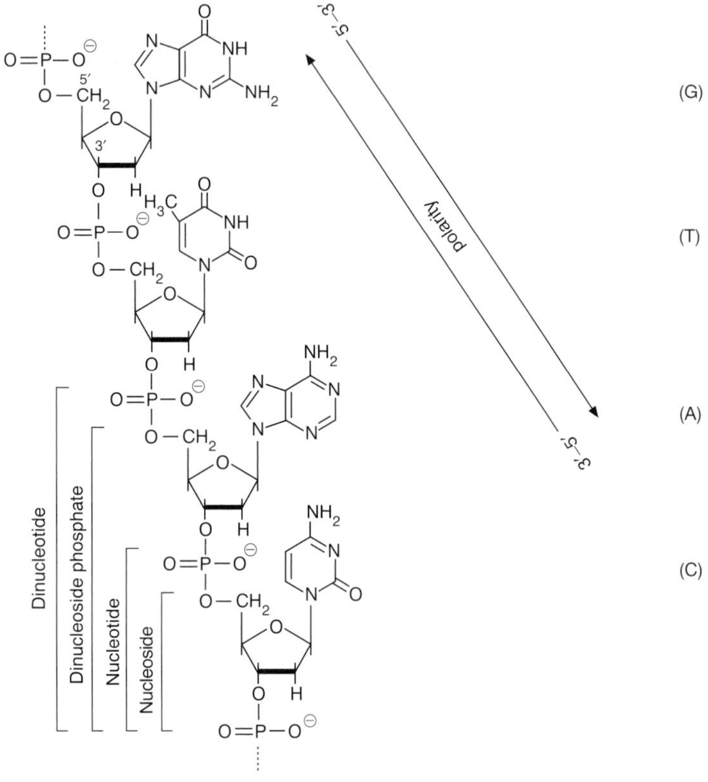

Fig. 5.5 Schematic representation of a tetranucleotide, GTAC, which illustartes the chemical linkages found in DNA, the terminology used to describe individual chemical entities, and the concept of polarity, important in any consideration of the double-stranded nature of DNA. The polarity must also be known before the structure of a polypeptide (protein) can be predicted from a DNA sequence.

phate ester bond to produce, initially, a *nucleotide*. Nucleotides, *per se*, especially in the cases where the sugar component is ribose, have many functions in cells. For example, they further combine with other molecules of phosphoric acid to produce compounds (such as adenosine triphosphate) that act as energy sources in many biochemical reactions. They also combine with other organic molecules to produce coenzymes, or they cyclize to produce signalling molecules important in regulating cellular functions.

A nucleotide, linked to another nucleoside through a phosphodiester bond, produces in an initial reaction a dinucleoside phosphate, which on

phosphorylation gives a *dinucleotide*, part of the backbone of either DNA or RNA (see Fig. 5.5). The determination of the nature of the links involved in generating these species was one of the important contributions of the chemists in this field, since it provided the basis for our present understanding of the structure of DNA. It was found that the $5'$ position of the deoxyribose in one nucleotide was covalently bound to the $3'$ position of another by diester bonds with phosphoric acid (for numbering of the sugar, see Fig. 5.2). This linkage determines the polarity, sequence, and structure of the chain of molecules that compose nucleic acids, whether they be DNA or RNA (Fig. 5.5). It is interesting at this stage to note that for many years the macromolecular nature of DNA went unrecognized. Since only four major bases were evident from the hydrolysis of DNA, the compound was assumed to be a tetranucleotide and, as such, obviously lacked the capacity to be the genetic entity required even by the simplest of cells.

5.3 The genetic material

The DNA of most cells is double stranded. In the case of many viruses, it is also circular. A polymer composed of nucleotide components with a 5′-3′ polarity binds to another (complementary) polymer with a 3′–5′ polarity to create the double-stranded DNA (Figs 5.5 and 5.6). The recognition of the nature of the bonds that link one strand of a double-stranded DNA with its partner, and the fact that these bonds are very specific, provided the basis for the explanation of the mechanism by which

DNA alone could encode genetic information. The groundwork for this important discovery came from analysis of the components released when DNA from a variety of sources was subjected to chemical hydrolysis. These experiments showed that although the base compositions, that is, the percentages of the various pyrimidines and purines, could vary enormously between species, a common relationship between bases was maintained such that the ratio of G:C or A:T always gave a figure that was about 1.0. These data, together with X-ray crystallographic evidence that showed the regularity of the structures of DNA, led not only to the very important suggestion of the nature of the base pairing between strands of DNA and its specificity, but recognition by Crick and Watson of how this could explain the key biological role of DNA. A model of the 'double helix' that arose from these combined studies is shown schematically in Fig. 5.6, wherein a C residue on one strand of DNA, wherever it occurs, is always 'paired' with a G residue on the opposite strand,

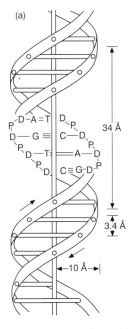

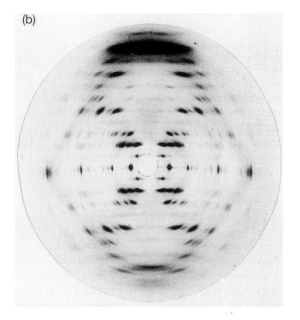

Fig. 5.6 (a) Schematic representation of the B form of double-stranded DNA, together with its dimensions as derived from X-ray crystallographic analyses, and (b) its corresponding X-ray diffraction pattern (courtesy of Dr A. G. W. Leslie). Complementary bases (A and T, G and C) in opposing strands are held together by hydrogen bonds, as shown (see Fig. 5.7). This structure produces grooves of two different sizes in

DNA, designated 'major' and 'minor', which can act as sites of entry to DNA by chemicals, enzymes, etc. (D represents the deoxyribose moiety, P phosphate, and A, G, T, C the respective heterocyclic bases). The remarkable accuracy of the model of DNA has now been confirmed at the atomic level using a technique called scanning tunnelling microscopy (Driscoll *et al.* 1990).

(a)

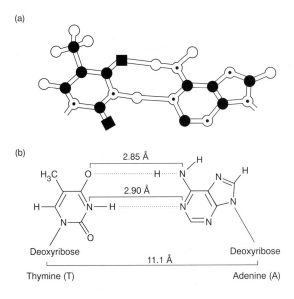

(b)

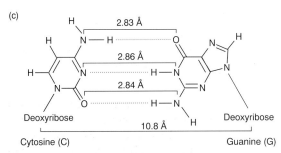

Thymine (T)   Adenine (A)

(c)

Cytosine (C)   Guanine (G)

Fig. 5.7 (a) A schematic representation of the links between the pyrimidine, thymine, and its purine complement, adenine. (b) and (c) The hydrogen bonds formed between the base pairs T/A and C/G, respectively, and the distances found between the base links in double-stranded DNA. In general, the strength of a hydrogen bond is proportional to its distance. Here it is seen that not only are there three such bonds in the C/G partnership, but also that they are generally shorter. The energy required to separate these complementary bases is thus greater than that required for T/A base pairs. Hydrogen bonds determine the specificity that exists in DNA and can be considered the 'watchdogs' of fidelity during DNA replication, or transcription of RNA.

likewise A with T (Fig. 5.7). The order in which the bases appear prescribes the genetic information. It is relevant to note that the bonds that link heterocyclic bases to sugars, and the latter to phosphates, are all covalent and as such very strong, requiring considerable energy to break. On the other hand, the so-called 'hydrogen bonds' (H bonds) that link one base residue to another to form double-stranded DNA are, by their nature, very weak bonds (less than 3 kcal of energy is generally sufficient to cleave a hydrogen bond compared with more than 10 times this for the weakest covalent bond). The strength of the attachment between strands of DNA is thus in large part a consequence of the fact that many such H bonds are involved in the interaction between strands of DNA.

Of great relevance biologically is the fact that when, during mitosis, the strands of DNA separate and each single strand is then copied to reproduce double-stranded DNA, the specificity of base pairing ensures that a faithful, albeit complementary, replica of the coded DNA is made and the fidelity of the gene for future generations is maintained. If mistakes occur, however, as they do from time to time, normal cells have a variety of important functions that recognize individual errors and make the necessary repairs.

Following on the discovery of the mode by which fidelity of genetic information can be maintained was the elucidation of the mechanism by which the sequences of bases on any particular region of a strand of DNA could specify the sequence of amino acids in a corresponding protein, that is, how the genetic information is actually encoded within the DNA. The colinear relationship between DNA, RNA, and proteins is such that (except in the case of retroviruses) a gene containing an 'antisense' version of information maintained in DNA, is faithfully copied into a complementary 'sense' version of a species of RNA known as messengers (or mRNAs) Using the specific base pairing discussed above (that is, for example, CAT in DNA would specify AUG in mRNA), RNA messenger, using blocks of trinucleotide sequences as its code, in turn specifies the amino acids and their order in a protein. But why a 'triplet' code? There are only 20 essential amino acids and four distinct nucleotides, so a doublet code would be inadequate, whereas a triplet could specify 64 amino acids (more than enough). The precise nature of the code, as worked out with mixtures of synthetic oligonucleotides, is shown in Table 5.2. Certain amino acids, for example, methionine (MET), are only encoded (specified) by one particular triplet (in this case AUG). In other cases, the coding is 'degenerate' and more than one triplet can specify a given amino acid. For example, proline (Pro) is encoded with two C residues and a third base which can be either C, U, A, or G. This degeneracy, together with the three

Table 5.2 The genetic code

	U	C	A	G	
U	PHE	SER	TYR	CYS	U
	PHE	SER	TYR	CYS	C
	LEU	SER	STOP	STOP	A
	LEU	SER	STOP	TRP	G
C	LEU	PRO	HIS	ARG	U
	LEU	PRO	HIS	ARG	C
	LEU	PRO	GLN	ARG	A
	LEU	PRO	GLN	ARG	G
				ARG	
A	ILE	THR	ASN	SER	U
	ILE	THR	ASN	SER	C
	ILE	THR	LYS	ARG	A
	MET	THR	LYS	ARG	G
G	VAL	ALA	ASP	GLY	U
	VAL	ALA	ASP	GLY	C
	VAL	ALA	GLU	GLY	A
	VAL	ALA	GLU	GLY	G

The first letter of the triplet is in the left hand vertical column, the second in the horizontal axis, and the third in the right hand vertical column.

triplets (UAG, UGA, and UAA) that specify the termination of translation of a nucleotide triplet into an amino acid, is such that all 64 potential triplet codons play some role in the specification of protein structures. Although the frequency of usage of individual codons appears to be species specific, all are used. The universality of this code has only been challenged fairly recently with the discovery that triplets that normally specify translational 'stops' are used as coding sequences in some species, such as certain mitochondrial DNA. The exceptions would appear to be rare however.

Mitochondria are important organelles that provide the bulk of the ATP (adenosine triphosphate) for eukaryotic cells and contain enzymes that catalyse many cellular reactions. It is generally speculated that this energy-converting organelle has been derived from a more primitive body, such as a virus, and has evolved together with its host, developing a symbiotic relationship with it. (The nearest equivalent to mitochondria in other species are the chloroplasts of plants.) Aside from its novel genetic code, mitochondrial DNA (16.5 kilobases in size) is also unique in being transmitted exclusively by maternal inheritance. The mitochondrial genome codes for at least 13 different proteins and it has

long been suspected, but remains unproved, that defects in mitochondrial genes may be important in the genesis of at least some forms of cancer. On the other hand, the clinically and biochemically heterogeneous mitochondrial myopathies and encephalopathies—inborn errors of metabolism—are beginning to be better defined. In several recent reports, deletions or mutations (evidenced by restriction enzyme polymorphisms) in mitochondrial DNA have been specifically associated with human disease, in particular with the Kearns–Sayre syndrome and Leber's hereditary optic neuropathy. It remains to be seen whether there is a strong association with cancers, but as aberrant growth is a marker for these pathologies and mitochondria provide cellular energy, with the newer molecular methods available for research into genetically inherited diseases, it would seem to be a fertile area for further exploration.

Space-filling models of DNA usually represent it in its most stable (B) form. The dimensions of B DNA (Fig. 5.6) are derived from X-ray diffraction studies. (Similar studies suggest RNA exists in a less compact, or A form, type of helix.) As far as is known, B DNA structurally represents most of the DNA in a cell, and almost certainly that which is 'coding' (specifying proteins). However, for reasons yet to be resolved, much of the DNA in a mammalian cell would appear to be non-coding and has even been referred to as irrelevant (or 'junk') DNA. Biologically, this is a difficult concept to accept with regard to highly conserved, and conservative, organisms. It seems more probable that such DNA, although not directly related to coding, has a function yet to be recognized. In this regard, it is interesting that experimental data suggest that certain specific DNA sequences, such as regular repeats of purines and pyrimidines, may specify alternative structural forms of DNA, which in turn might play roles in regulation of gene expression or other cellular functions which might be modulated by DNA, as well as in intracellular DNA recombination.

The crystal structure of a hexadecanucleotide (C–G–C–G–C–G–T–T–T–T–C–G–C–G–C–G) shows this molecule to adopt a 'hairpin' configuration with the four T residues forming a loop; hairpin structures have been postulated to be important in DNA replication. Recently it has also been shown that certain guanine-rich sequences in DNA can self-associate under physiological salt concentrations to form parallel four-stranded complexes (Sen and Gilbert 1988). It has been postulated that such sequences, which occur in immunoglobulin switch regions, gene promoters, and chromosomal telomeres, may bring together the four homologous chromatids (see Glossary) during meiosis. Moreover, if the hypothesis that guanine-rich regions might be involved in meiosis is correct, such sites could be crucial in forming the (postulated) structures required for pairing homologous chromosomes during this stage of cell division.

Before turning to other aspects of DNA, two further topics should be noted briefly. One concerns the remarkable solubility of this highly polymeric species. Since water solubility is not a common property of most highly polymerized materials, the explanation for the great solubility of DNA must lie in its capacity to form specific interactions with water. The phosphodiester bond generated by the interaction of phosphoric acid with hydroxyl groups of sugar residues in nucleosides creates not only the backbone for DNA, but also leaves a single acidic residue on the phosphate moiety that, at the normal pH of a cell, should be negatively charged (Fig. 5.5). *In vivo*, this charge is neutralized by cations, such as Mg^{2+}, to generate a macromolecular version of a 'salt', which is capable of interacting both electro-

statically or through hydrogen bonding with water. In support of this notion, DNA isolated from cells is neutral and contains many molecules of water of hydration. Moreover, once deprived of its water of hydration, DNA is remarkably difficult to redissolve.

The second point is that DNA in the nucleus of a cell is not 'naked'. Rather, it is found in association with histones and other proteins to produce a characteristic and fairly regular structure (Fig. 5.1). DNA in association with histones is known as 'chromatin'. Further organization of chromatin produces the highly ordered chromosomes whose structures are specific and unique within each individual organism. A number of proteins have now been discovered that bind to regulatory regions of DNA adjacent to genes and allow transcription of these genes (Santoro *et al.* 1988). It is interesting to note that the DNA of some viruses also appears to be organized as 'mini-chromosomes', which, none the less, have regions that do appear to be 'naked' and act as origins of DNA replication. Whether the same is true for higher organisms with regard to areas relevant to the initiation sites of DNA replication remains to be seen.

5.4 'Informational' DNA

It is becoming increasingly apparent that not all DNA is used in the strictly genetic sense to 'specify genes'. Moreover, even within genes, there are signals that determine the function of a particular region (domain) within a protein. For example, some DNA sequences specify structural motifs in proteins. One encodes a leucine at every seventh amino acid that allows the designated region in the protein to form an α-helix (Landschultz *et al.* 1988). The leucine side chains from one protein interdigitate with those of another protein, forming a 'leucine zipper' that holds the molecules together. This dimer in turn can interact with DNA to regulate gene expression. Metal binding sites are also important components of many regulatory proteins and sequences specifying these have been located in a number of DNAs. The best characterized of these is the 'zinc finger' motif (Klug and Rhodes 1987), which juxtaposes two cysteines, two histidines, two aromatic amino acid residues, and one leucine with the appropriate spacing to bind zinc (see Fig. 5.8). These domains in turn attach the regulatory protein to recognition sequences in the appropriate gene.

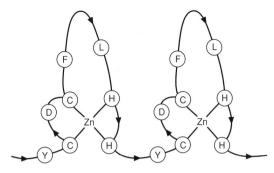

Fig. 5.8 A schematic folding arrangement for repeated zinc finger motifs in the *Xenopus* transcription factor IIIA (TF III A). Each domain is centred on a tetrahedral arrangement of Zn ligands. Ringed letters represent conserved amino acids; cysteine(C) and histidine (H) form bonds with zinc, and other amino acids, leucine(L), phenylalanine(F), tyrosine(Y), and aspartate (D), may form a structural core. This protein mini-domain allows interaction with DNA (adapted from Klug and Rhodes 1987).

Yet other motifs in DNA determine the subcellular localization of proteins, the best studied being the signals that specify nuclear or nucleolar localization and the sequence G–C–C–A–A–T which has been implicated both in eukaryotic transcription and in DNA replication.

Thus, little by little, the evidence is building up that allows patterns in DNA sequences to be recognized and the fine structure information in DNA to be understood. In the long run, such understanding should allow 'gene therapy' to become a realistic proposition.

5.5 DNA damage

As mentioned earlier, many of the agents that produce mutations in DNA do so by altering the tautomeric form of a base (Fig. 5.3) such that inaccuracies occur during DNA replication which may be reflected in the transcription of DNA into RNA. In many cases, these mutations may be 'silent' in that they occur in the 'wobble' allowed at the third base (degenerate) position of some of the triplet codons (Table 5.2). In other positions within a codon, mutations could lead to an alteration of amino acid structure, which, if protein function were not therefore impaired, might be allowed. In fact, such alterations can even lead to mutants with selective advantages over the 'wild-type' species.

Other alterations could be positively harmful and, if not repaired, ultimately lethal either to the cell, or in the case of cancer-causing lesions, if such there are, to the whole organism. In addition to mutations produced by exogenous agents, such as certain organic and inorganic chemicals, X-irradiation (see Chapters 6 and 7), etc., there is always a background level of mutation in a cell produced by the hydrolytic interaction of water itself with DNA. Such damage includes hydrolytic cleavage of the glycosidic bond resulting in depurination (Fig. 5.9) or depyrimidination, and ultimately in strand breaking, or deamination of exocyclic amino groups. For example, cytosine converted to uracil (an abnormal base in DNA) by deamination would produce a 'mismatch' during DNA replication which could ultimately lead to the concomitant alteration of the structure of a protein. It has been calculated that the rate of release of purines from double-stranded DNA occurs at a rate of about 10^4/day/10^{10} bases (in rat liver cells), whereas depyrimidination occurs with a slightly lower frequency (about 5×10^2/day/10^{10} bases). Deamination proceeds marginally more slowly than depyrimidination. Were normal cells not endowed with a variety of mechanisms to combat such lesions, it can be seen that water alone could

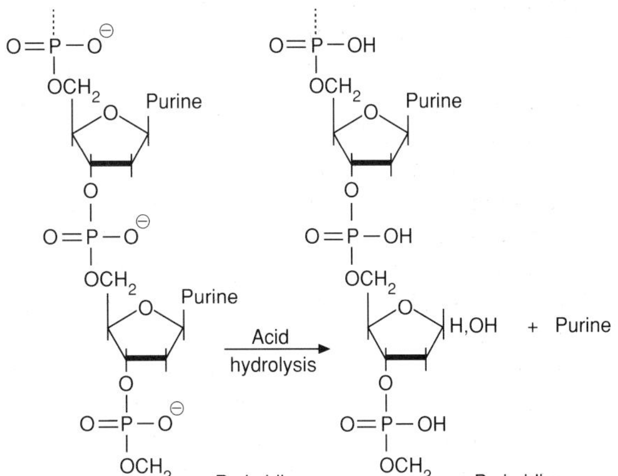

Fig. 5.9 A schematic representation of one of the well-characterized lesions of DNA, that of depurination. Loss of purine (or pyrimidine) base, if not repaired, can lead to DNA chain breaks.

pose a serious threat to the accurate survival of genetic information. Hydrolysis could also lead directly to phosphodiester bond cleavage, disrupting the DNA backbone itself. Although theoretically possible, this mode of damage is not thought to be of great physiological relevance, although the alkylation of a phosphodiester (to a phosphotriester) could create a more labile substrate for hydrolysis. The role of phosphotriesters in DNA damage of mammalian DNA is only beginning to be investigated, and its effect assessed.

Most cells have a limited capacity to correct lesions produced in DNA by exogenous or endogenous reagents. A variety of different repair processes have been identified, and some of them are well characterized, at least in bacteria. There is no compelling evidence to suggest that higher organisms do not have repair processes comparable in type and effect to those found in the better studied *Esherischia coli*. In normal individuals, these processes must effectively compete with the background levels of mutations in DNA. It is obvious, however, that in individuals deficient (or defective) in one or more of the repair processes, and probably in ageing populations in general, this delicate balance can be disturbed, with deleterious consequences. One of the most telling examples of this comes from studies on cells from patients with Bloom's syndrome (Willis and Lindahl 1987). Such individuals are known to have a greatly increased risk of developing cancer and have now been shown to be deficient in DNA ligase I, an enzyme likely to be involved in both DNA replication and repair. Ligase I can, for example, catalyse the joining of blunt-ended DNA fragments *in vitro*. A defect in ligase I could account for the increased sister chromatid exchanges (see Glossary) found in individuals suffering from Bloom's syndrome.

Many mutagens are also carcinogens (see Chapters 6 and 7). Some of the best studied agents that act on DNA are the simple alkylating agents, whose biological effect can be directly related to their site of action (Fig. 5.10). Some of the most damaging agents, which can be shown to induce tumour formation in animal models *in vivo*, are those that modify the oxygen moiety at the 6-position of guanine and lead to the creation of an unusual tautomeric form of this base in DNA. This modification alters two of the sites normally used in forming base pairs with cytosine, and can lead to a site-specific error during DNA replication.

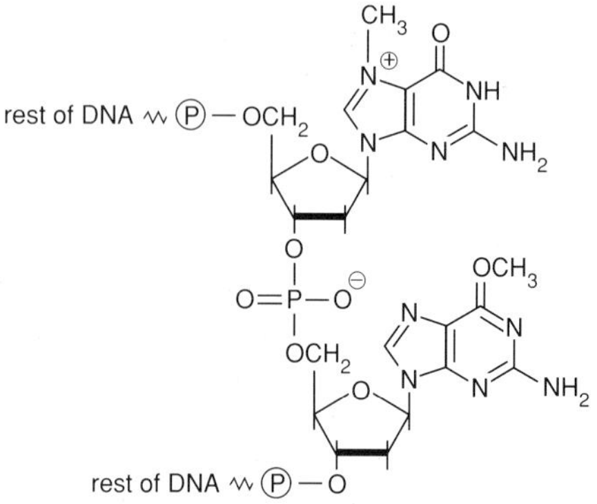

Fig. 5.10 Two of the well-characterized lesions produced at guanine sites in DNA by simple alkylating agents. Modification of the N-7 position (on the five-membered heterocyclic ring) generates a positively charged species, but is essentially 'silent' since it has no effect on base pairing in DNA. Conversely, methylation at the O-6 postion of the six-membered ring, if not repaired, is a dangerous lesion, being both mutagenic and carcinogenic.

Significant, and certainly of great biological importance for the individual, is the fact that by far the most reactive site to alkylating agents in DNA is, however, the N-7 position of guanine; lesions at this site within coding sequences should be essentially harmless since they have little effect on normal hydrogen bonding. None the less, it can be seen how the build-up of such lesions in DNA, by creating multiple positive charges, could be deleterious in other ways. Efficient repair pathways do exist to remove *N*-7-methylguanine from DNA.

It has been shown by a variety of methods that during evolution, transforming (or tumorigenic) retroviruses arose by incorporation of cellular DNA into the genome of weakly or non-transforming viruses. A most interesting finding is that, in some instances, the difference between a viral oncogene and its normal cellular counterpart is the presence of mutations in the former, which lead to simple amino acid alterations in the protein specified by the respective genes (see Chapter 9). One of the most promising aspects of the high technology that now attends the analysis of DNA is that it provides the tools for investigating alterations in potentially normal functions that accompany malignancies. Noteworthy in this regard is the identification of the chromosomal deletions that give rise to (or result from) retinoblastoma and other tumours (see

Chapters 4 and 10). It would be surprising if such changes were not fairly widespread.

5.6 DNA manipulation

The fact that mammalian DNA can be amplified by recombinant DNA technology and (potentially) expressed in both prokaryotic and eukaryotic systems makes many experiments possible that would hitherto not have been feasible. This should engender a sense of optimism, and even adventure, in those interested in exploring the cellular and molecular biology of cancer. It has, for example, already allowed *inter alia*, a sequence homology to be observed between some of the normal growth factors of cells and those of viral and cellular 'oncogenes', implying a function for the latter in uncontrolled cell growth (see Chapters 9 and 11). Many vector systems for generating recombinant DNAs that can be amplified by replication in bacterial systems, and even expressed in bacteria or mammalian cells, have been generated.

A detailed description of nucleic acid molecular biology used for this purpose is beyond the scope of this chapter; however, a brief account may be given here to explain some of the terminology and methods employed. The applications are discussed elsewhere in this book. Perhaps one of the most important tools comes from the discovery of enzymes known as restriction endonucleases in many bacteria. The restriction enzymes recognize specific sets of DNA sequences in double-stranded DNA and cut both strands of DNA at or near these sequences. In some instances, the enzymes cut through both strands at a single point generating blunt-ended molecules, whereas with others, the cuts are at precisely spaced points along the two strands and generate overlapping ('sticky' or overhanging) ends. Various other enzymes are available for filling in or cutting back at these ends. These techniques allow unrelated DNA molecules to be joined together (ligated); in particular this is of use for propagating sequences from eukaryotic organisms in prokaryotic hosts such as bacteria. For example, the entire genetic information (genome) of human chromosomes can be ligated to bacteriophage (bacterial virus) DNA, giving rise to a 'library' of human DNA from which homogeneous clones can be isolated, amplified, and manipulated further (e.g. for nucleotide sequence analysis, for mutagenesis experiments,

for gene expression studies, etc.). One of the most common techniques is to isolate a specific clone of interest and label it with a radioisotope so that it can be used as a probe to examine the gene in various DNA or RNA preparations (see Chapters 4 and 12). In the example cited in Chapter 12, human DNA was cut with a restriction enzyme, the fragments of DNA were separated by size by electrophoresis through a gel, and then were transferred to a filter. The filter was exposed (hybridized) to a radioisotopically labelled probe for an immunoglobulin locus and the specific binding (hybridization) was measured by exposure of the filter to X-ray film. In the specific example shown, the study examined whether the immunoglobulin locus had been rearranged, compared with the germ line sequences, during differentiation of B lymphocytes. Similar techniques have been applied to the study of cellular oncogenes (see Chapters 4, 9, and 11).

Such genetic manipulations are as yet in their infancy, and not wholly without pitfalls, as is beginning to be recognized. For example, genes expressed in heterologous systems may produce functions that are without activity in their normal hosts, possibly as a consequence of incorrect or incomplete protein modification which could result in aberrant folding or unusual instability. Further, gene functions expressed at abnormally high levels, even in homologous systems, can lead to unexpected effects, including cell death. 'Dose response' may prove a difficult problem to solve, at least in terms of defining underlying mechanisms of gene action within a cell. Another basic problem for biotechnology appears to be the expression of genes in the wrong cellular compartment following introduction of DNA into cells (transfection). The critical problems for gene manipulation now appear to be not how to 'clone' and express a particular part of DNA, or even a particular gene, but how to introduce it into a cell and regulate its expression so as to obtain data *in vitro* that are meaningful in terms of *in vivo* responses.

Essentially, what is implicit in the above discussion is the fact that all the 'rules of the game' have not yet been determined, although great progress has been made. It is significant that the need for regulation of gene expression is now being widely recognized. With this in mind, vectors have been developed that allow control of DNA replication and many of them contain RNA polymerase promoters that can be additionally regulated by such external agents as temperature, hormones, or heavy metals.

One of the other basic problems in gene manipulation and expression arises from the fact that in mammalian cells mRNAs are often not colinear with respect to genomic DNA. Rather, they reflect the fact that enzymatic processes have occurred in the cytoplasm, subsequent to transcription, which have 'spliced' together non-adjacent regions of RNA to produce the functional messengers for proteins. For expression of such genes *in vitro*, the messenger itself must first be isolated and reverse transcribed into DNA, before the latter can be introduced into suitable vector systems and studied. This process is both tedious and frequently unsuccessful, particularly in the case of mRNAs that are present in low copy numbers in cells and/or are unstable. In attempts to circumvent this, interesting new classes of vectors, have been developed. These are hybrid DNAs with elements derived both from plasmid and viral sources, such that for expression they can be 'shuttled' between bacteria and mammalian cells (Cepko *et al.* 1984), and even packaged as retrovirus particles, thus allowing recovery of input material. Since the latter contain all the signals for retrovirus transcription, these vectors provide the capacity for correctly splicing, in an *in vitro* system, the input DNA. Thus the latter should be re-isolable as a reversibly transcribed copy of its message. These vectors have, however, a size constraint that may limit their usefulness for many mammalian genes.

Gene manipulation is the basis of a new approach to medicine designated 'gene therapy'. For example, if 'cancer genes' can be identified and defined, they should be subject to manipulations (for example, controlled, site-specific mutagenesis) that could render them inactive, and even possibly subjects for 'therapy' if corrected genes could be substituted for the aberrantly expressed ones. Such problems for the future deserve thought. An interesting alternative approach just beginning to be explored involves the use of complementary (antisense) sequences of mRNAs, which, upon being introduced into cells, should, at least theoretically, be capable of binding to the messenger and rendering it inactive. This potentially fruitful avenue is at present being widely examined with particular regard to the prevention of expression of aberrant genes, but the approach has proved successful in only a few specific cases to date.

5.7 Conclusion

An essentially historical approach to DNA has been presented here because it shows how many scientific disciplines have been, even indirectly, involved in taking us to a point where we can begin to approach the problem of human cancer in a non-empirical manner. At the moment it seems ironic, and paradoxical, that one of the few human cancers that has been firmly associated for over twenty-five years with a viral infection (e.g. Burkitt's lymphoma with Epstein–Barr virus), is still preferentially treated with massive doses of cyclophosphamide, an alkylating agent and potent carcinogen. (Indeed, cyclophosphamide is a drug of choice in the therapy of many human tumours.) The aim of understanding at a molecular level the pathological process defined broadly as 'cancer' is obviously to be able to control it. Ideally such containment should come about by a less empirical manner than that presented as an example above, where, although the disease is initially eradicated, the patient is left with many undesirable lesions and, in a large proportion of cases, the tumour reappears and, notably, is no longer susceptible to treatment.

At least one success story can be cited as arising from application of the scientific method, and that is the control of herpes simplex by the drug Acyclovir. Among others, patients immunosuppressed prior to and subsequent to transplant therapy become immediately susceptible to the effects of reactivation of herpesviruses. Once the existence of a thymidine kinase gene was identified in herpes simplex virus, specific antagonists of the kinase enzyme were sought. The drug, Acyclovir, a nucleoside analogue, was developed; it blocks a vital step in the enzyme pathway and thus counters the reactivation of herpes simplex viruses, and provides protection for the patient. If cancer(s) can be related to specific sequences of DNA, it should be possible, in a similar fashion, to search for their control.

References and further reading

Alberts, B., Bray, D., Lewis, J., Raff, M., Roberts, K., and Watson, J. D. (1994). *Molecular biology of the cell.* Garland Publishing, New York.

Bramhill, D. and Kornberg, A. (1988). A model for initiation at origins of DNA replication. *Cell,* **54**, 915–18.

Cepko, C., Roberts, B. E., and Mulligan, R. C. (1984). Construction and applications of a highly transmissible murine retrovirus shuttle vector, *Cell,* **37**, 1053–62.

Chattopadhyaya, R., Ikuta, S., Grzeskowick, K., and Dickerson, R. E. (1988). X-ray structure of a DNA hairpin molecule. *Nature,* **334**, 175–9.

Driscoll, R. J., Youngquist, M. G., and Baldeschwieler, J. D. (1990). Atomic-scale imaging of DNA using scanning tunnelling microscopy. *Nature,* **346**, 294–6.

Glover, D. M. (ed.) (1985). *DNA cloning. A practical approach.* IRL Press, Oxford.

Gluzman, Y. (ed.) (1982). *Eukaryotic viral vectors.* Cold Spring Harbor Laboratory, Cold Spring Harbor, New York.

Klug, A. and Rhodes, D. (1987). 'Zinc fingers': a novel protein motif for nucleic acid recognition. *Trends in Biochemical Sciences,* **12**, 464–9.

Landschultz, W. H., Johnson, P. F., and McKnight, S. L. (1988). The leucine zipper: a hypothetical structure common to a new class of DNA binding proteins. *Science,* **240**, 1759–64.

Laskey, R. A. (1987). The cell nucleus. *British Medical Journal,* **295**, 1121–3.

Lindahl, T. (1979). DNA glycosylases, endonucleases for apurinic/apyrimidinic sites, and base excision-repair. *Progress in Nucleic Acid Research and Molecular Biology,* **22**, 135–92.

Messer, W. and Noyer-Weidner, M. (1988). Timing and targeting: the biological functions of dam methylation in *E. coli. Cell,* **54**, 735–7.

Radman, M. and Wagner, R. (1988). The high fidelity of DNA duplication. *Scientific American,* August, pp. 24–30.

Richards, B., Pardon, J., Lilley, D., Cotter, R., and Wooley, J. (1977). The substructure of nucleosomes. *Cell Biology International Reports,* **1**, 107–15.

Santoro, C., Mermod, N., Andrews, P. C., and Tjian, R. (1988). A family of human CCAAT-box-binding proteins active in transcription and DNA replication. *Nature,* **334**, 218–34.

Sen, D. and Gilbert, W. (1988). Formation of parallel four-stranded complexes by guanine-rich motifs in DNA and its implications for meiosis. Nature, **24**, 364–6.

Singer, B. and Grunberger, D. (1983). *Molecular biology of mutagens and carcinogens.* Plenum Press, New York.

Siomi, H., Shida, H., Nam, S. H., Nosaka, T., Maki, M., and Hatanaka, M. (1988). Sequence requirements for nucleolar localization of human T cell leukaemia type I px protein which regulates viral RNA processing. *Cell,* **55**, 197–209.

Willis, A. E. and Lindahl, T. (1987). DNA ligase I deficiency in Bloom's syndrome. *Nature,* **325**, 355–7.

Wolffe, A. (1995). *Chromatin: structure and function* (Second edition). Academic Press, London.

6

Chemical carcinogenesis

RAYMOND TENNANT, CAROLINE WIGLEY, AND ALLAN BALMAIN

6.1 The role of chemical carcinogens and mutation in human cancer

As outlined in Chapter 1 and considered in detail in this and subsequent chapters (see Chapters 7, 8, and 9), carcinogenesis is a multistage process. The first step is known as initiation and is followed by one or more promoting events. These stages in the stepwise process of carcinogenesis have been detected in man and in animals and can now be analysed, as illustrated later. Each stage may be influenced by different factors. From epidemiological data and animal studies, and most recently from molecular analysis of tumours, there is little doubt that chemical agents are involved at some stage, although there are many other contributing factors. Many potentially carcinogenic agents are present in our diet and environment. There is convincing evidence that the site of action of most of these agents is the genetic material in cells; many known and suspect chemical carcinogens cause mutations. Even so, it is not entirely clear whether a change in DNA sequence is needed. We include in our definition of mutation gross DNA changes such as rearrangements and should bear in mind that heritable changes in gene expression, while not mutational events at the sequence level, might have similar effects on the cell phenotype.

Occupational exposure has provided categorical associations and clear evidence for induction of cancers in humans by over 70 chemicals or agents. Presumptive evidence of carcinogenicity exists for about 35 other chemicals or industrial processes. There is uncertainty or conflicting evidence for many other chemicals, but for most of the estimated over 13 million chemicals listed by Chemical Abstract Services, there are no clear data for judging their carcinogenic potential. Thus, knowledge about the properties of known carcinogens, and an understanding of the mechanisms by which they induce cancer, are critical for identifying potential carcinogens.

As with reproductive, immunological, behavioural, neurological, or teratological effects induced by chemicals, the induction of cancer often involves the same toxicological principles of exposure, pharmacokinetics, tissue distribution, metabolism, and cell injury. The nature of the interactions between chemicals and animal tissues gives information for predicting potential carcinogenic hazards. Accumulated data are available that provide information on structure-activity relationships for many classes of chemicals. These permit prediction of the carcinogenic potential of a chemical based upon critical structural 'alerts' or substructural determinants (see Section 6.7.2). Similarly, studies in genetic toxicology have developed biological assay systems *in vitro* and *in vivo* that provide additional information regarding the relationship between events at the subcellular level and carcinogenesis.

6.2 Epidemiological evidence

As discussed in Chapter 3 epidemiological methods have led to the identification of many carcinogens by analysing variations in the frequency of cancers in different human populations and seeking relationships to causal factors. A few examples illustrate the situation. The classic example was described in 1775 by Percival Pott who noted that chimney sweeps had a high incidence of cancer of the scrotal skin attributed, quite correctly, to chronic contact with soot—a mixture of chemicals including polycyclic hydrocarbons which were later shown to be carcinogenic in animals. Earlier, clinical observations by John Hill in 1759 provided the first association between inhaling tobacco snuff and oronasal cancer.

Many important epidemiological findings have been based upon clinical observations and these methods account for the recognition of most of the human carcinogens that have been classified by the International Agency for Research on Cancer (IARC). These are listed in Table 6.1. In some cases they represent groups of chemicals or industrial processes where the actual carcinogen or carcinogens could not be defined but where epidemiological evidence was sufficient to suggest a causal relationship. β-Naphthylamine and other aromatic amines have been linked to bladder cancer in workers in the dye industry, whereas industrial exposure to nickel and some chromates has been strongly implicated in the causation of cancers of the respiratory system. There are also naturally occurring carcinogens that may be present in the diet. A good example is a substance present in bracken fern which may cause tumours in the alimentary tract in animals and possibly in humans in areas where fern hearts (fiddles) are eaten as a delicacy. Other intestinal carcinogens may be formed in the gut by the action of intestinal microorganisms or substances in the diet or in the bile. Better known, but less well defined, is the chemical carcinogen(s) in tobacco smoke associated with lung cancer (see Chapter 3). Some of the chemicals included in the list such as vinyl chloride, 4-amino biphenyl, bis(-chloromethyl)ether, and others were first recognized as carcinogens through studies in animals and later verified by epidemiological data.

There are limits to the power of clinical observation and epidemiology to identify potential cancer causes unless a high prevalence of a specific type of tumour can be clearly associated with a given risk factor. The remarkable achievements of clinical observation and epidemiology in the eradication of infectious diseases were possible, in large part, to the fact that causal associations could be made between risk factors, such as bacteria or viruses, and specific diseases because methods existed for isolating the suspected agent and for demonstrating that the isolated agent could induce a similar disease state in experimental animals. With cancers induced by a chemical or environmental agent, it is not always possible to identify the precise agent because of the long latent period between exposure and onset of disease. Also, even appropriate experimental methods may not always demonstrate an aetiological association. For example, although many clinical and epidemiological studies show a strong correlation between lung cancer and smoking, the actual carcinogen has not yet been identified. One of the problems is the fact that most cancers develop late in life and may occur long after exposure to the aetiological agent(s). Since a number of factors such as age, race, sex, duration of exposure, genetic make up, life style, etc., are involved in the induction of the most common cancers, it is more difficult to identify their relative importance.

We now know that almost all chemicals implicated by epidemiologists as human carcinogens can cause cellular mutations in the conventional sense, i.e. localized base changes in DNA, but there are a few exceptions. Asbestos causes cancer of the pleural cavity (see Chapter 3) but is not mutagenic in classical mutagenesis test systems, e.g. the Ames test (see Section 6.7.2). However, it has been shown to induce gross chromosomal changes such as non-disjunctions in mammalian cells, probably because of binding to the spindle apparatus during mitosis. The resulting gene imbalance may be an important step in the generation of aneuploidy which is fre-

Table 6.1 Chemicals with proven carcinogenic activity in humans

Chemical (or industrial process)[1]	Main type of exposure[2]	Main route of exposure[3]	Target organ(s) in humans[4]	Target organ(s) in mice[4]	Mutagenicity (sal/rodent bone marrow aberrations or MN)[5]
Aflatoxins	Environmental, occupational	Ingestion, inhalation	Liver	Liver, lung	+/+
Aluminium production	Occupational	Inhalation	Lung, bladder	na[6]	na[4]
4-Aminobiphenyl	Occupational	Inhalation, ingestion, skin contact	Bladder	Liver, bladder	+/+
Analgesic mixtures containing phenacetin	Medicinal	Ingestion	Urinary tract	Urinary tract	+/+
Arsenic compounds	Occupational, medicinal, environmental	Inhalation, ingestion, skin contact	Skin, lung, liver, bladder, kidney, colon	Lung[7]	−/+
Asbestos	Occupational, environmental	Inhalation, ingestion	Lung, gastrointestinal tract	Peritoneum	−/na
Auramine manufacture	Occupational	Inhalation, ingestion, skin contact	Bladder	Liver	+/−[4]
Azathioprine	Medicinal	Injection, ingestion	Haemopoietic system, skin, liver	Haemopoietic system	+/+
Benzene	Occupational	Inhalation, skin contact	Haemopoietic system	Haemopoietic system, lung	−/+
Benzidine	Occupational	Inhalation, skin contact, ingestion	Bladder	Liver	+/+
Betel quid with tobacco	Cultural	Oral	Oral cavity, larynx	Skin	+/+
N,N-*bis*(2-chloroethyl)-2-naphthylamine (Chlornaphazine)	Medicinal	Ingestion	Bladder	Lung	+/+
Bis(chloromethyl)ether and chloromethyl methyl ether	Occupational	Inhalation	Lung	Skin, lung	+/na[4]
Boot and shoe manufacture and repair	Occupational	Inhalation	Nasal cavity, bladder	na	na[4]
1-(2-Chloroethyl)-3-(4-methylcyclohexyl)-1-nitrosourea (Methyl-CCNU)	Medicinal	Injection	Haemopoietic system	Haemopoietic system[7]	+[8]/+[9]
Chlorambucil	Medicinal	Ingestion	Haemopoietic system	Lung, haemopoietic system, ovary	+/+

				Muscular system	
Chromium compounds (hexavalent)	Occupational	Inhalation	Lung	Lung	+/+
Coal (gasification, tar pitches, tars)	Occupational, medicinal	Inhalation, skin contact	Skin (scrotum), lung, bladder	Skin, lung	+/na
Coke production	Occupational	Inhalation	Skin (scrotum), lung, bladder	na	+/na[4]
Cyclophosphamide	Medicinal	Ingestion, injection	Bladder, haemopoietic system	Bladder	+/+
Diethylstilboestrol (DES)	Medicinal	Ingestion (acts transplacentally)	Uterus, vagina (in offspring)	Uterus, vagina, cervix, ovary, mammary	−/+
Erionite	Environmental, occupational	Inhalation	Lung	Lung	na
Furniture and cabinet making	Occupational	Inhalation	Nasal cavity	na	+/na[4]
Haematite mining (radon)	Occupational	Inhalation	Lung	Lung[7]	na[4]
Iron and steel founding	Occupational	Inhalation	Lung	na	na[4]
Isopropyl oils	Occupational	Inhalation	Nasal cavity, larynx	na	na[4]
Magenta, manufacture of	Occupational	Skin contact	Bladder	na	+/na[4]
Melphalan	Medicinal	Ingestion, injection	Haemopoietic system	Haemopoietic system, lung	+/+
8-Methoxypsoralen + UV	Medicinal	Skin contact	Skin	Skin	+/na
Mineral oils, untreated and mildly treated	Occupational	Skin contact	Skin (scrotum)	Skin	+/na
MOPP (and other combined therapies)	Medicinal	Injection, ingestion	Haemopoietic system	na	+/+
Mustard gas	Occupational	Inhalation	Lung, larynx	Lung	+/na
Myleran	Medicinal	Ingestion	Haemopoietic system	Haemopoietic system, thymus, ovary	+/+
2-Naphthylamine	Occupational	Inhalation, skin contact, ingestion	Bladder	Liver	+/+
Nickel (nickel-refining industries)	Occupational	Inhalation	Nasal cavity, lung, larynx[7]	Muscular system, lung	−/na
Oestrogens (steroidal)	Medicinal	Ingestion	Uterus, mammary gland	Mammary gland, uterus, pituitary gland, vagina, cervix	na

Table 6.1 Chemicals with proven carcinogenic activity in humans (contd.)

Chemical (or industrial process)[1]	Main type of exposure[2]	Main route of exposure[3]	Target organ(s) in humans[4]	Target organ(s) in mice[4]	Mutagenicity (sal/ rodent bone-marrow aberrations or MN)[5]
Oral contraceptives (Combined)	Medicinal	Ingestion	Liver	Pituitary gland, mammary gland	na
Soots, tars, and oils	Occupational, environmental	Inhalation, skin contact	Lung, skin (scrotum)	Skin	+/na
Talc-containing asbestiform fibres	Occupational	Inhalation	Lung	None[10]	−/−
The rubber industry	Occupational	Inhalation, skin contact	Haemopoietic system, bladder	na	na[4]
Tobacco products, smoke, smokeless	Recreational	Inhalation, oral	Lung, oral cavity, bladder	Lung, skin	+/+
Treosulphan	Medicinal	Ingestion	Haemopoietic system	na	+/+
Vinyl chloride	Occupational	Inhalation, skin contact	Liver, brain, lung, haemopoietic system	Mammary, lung, Zymbal gland, skin, liver	+/+

[1] The precise chemical(s) responsible may not be known.

[2] The main types of exposure mentioned are those by which the association has been demonstrated; other exposures may occur.

[3] The main routes of exposure given may not be the only ones by which such effects could occur.

[4] IARC Monographs, Suppl. 7, 1987.

[5] Shelby, M. D. and Zeiger, E. (1990). Activity of human carcinogens in the Salmonella and rodent bone-marrow cytogenetics tests. *Mutation Research*, **234**, 257–61, 1990.

[6] na—Either the results were unavailable to the IARC Working Group; the test was inadequate; or the assay was not done.

[7] There is indicative evidence for these organs.

[8] *JNCI* **65**, 149 (1980).

[9] *Mutation Research*, **286**, 101 (1993).

[10] National Toxicology Program, Technical Report 421.

Adapted from Tomatis et al. (1978). *Cancer Research*, **38**, 877–85.

quently observed during tumour progression. Diethylstilboestrol, a synthetic steroid hormone, was given in the past to prevent miscarriages in pregnant women; later it was found to cause vaginal tumours in female offspring at puberty by a mechanism that does not seem to involve DNA mutation in the strict sense. The role of mutations in tumour production is discussed in Chapter 4 and chromosome changes are considered in Chapter 10.

There are some instances where there may be an increased tissue susceptibility to the tumour-inducing activity of carcinogens. In some rare conditions, an inherited trait predisposes affected members of a family to develop a particular cancer (see Chapter 4). This led Knudson and others, as has already been mentioned, to propose that the first event in carcinogenesis involved DNA mutation and that this mutation could, in rare instances, be transmitted in the germ cell line from parent to offspring. As a rule, this first or initiating mutation occurs after birth, in a target somatic cell. One heritable cancer-predisposing condition, xeroderma pigmentosum (XP), is one of the best understood of a group of conditions where something is known about the defect. Individuals with XP suffer from a deficiency in their ability to repair DNA damaged by UV light in particular; this is demonstrated in cell cultures prepared from small biopsies of a patient's skin. The skin exposed to sunlight in XP patients is at risk of developing cancer, providing a very strong argument linking DNA damage (and, by implication, its faulty repair or lack of repair), mutation, and cancer.

6.3 Evidence from animal studies

Considerable support for the evidence from epidemiological studies came when, early this century, Japanese workers showed for the first time that a number of potent hydrocarbon carcinogens cause cancer when applied to the skin of rabbits. Subsequently, many other suspected chemicals were shown to be carcinogenic by similar techniques. Nowadays, most drugs, food additives, etc., are tested on laboratory animals, usually rodents, for general toxicity and long-term carcinogenicity (see Section 6.7.1). Very many substances have now been shown to be tumour producing in experimental animals. Some produce tumours at the site of application, e.g. on the skin. Others may produce tumours at the site of absorption, e.g. the foresto-

mach if given by mouth, or at the site of the breakdown (metabolism), e.g. in the liver, or in the excretory organ, e.g. kidneys or bladder (see Table 6.1). In some instances, a carcinogen may not produce tumours or may do so in an entirely unexpected organ. For example, the carcinogens dimethylbenz-(a)anthracene and nitrosomethylurea, when given by mouth, cause breast cancer in female rats, but have to be given at a particular time in the development of the breast during puberty. There seems to be a critical sensitive period, which depends on the hormonal status of the cells (see Chapter 14). If nitrosomethylurea is given at an earlier stage to a pregnant animal it acts transplacentally to produce tumours of the nervous system in the offspring. Interestingly, tumours arising in these two tissues are specifically associated with activation of different protooncogenes, e.g. Harvey *ras* (Ha-*ras*) in mammary carcinomas and *neu* in Schwannomas of the nervous system. Similar complex factors may operate in other tissues also, so that exposure to a carcinogen is necessary, but not sufficient, for cancer induction in these cases. Intensive long-term administration by several different routes is essential if possible toxic and carcinogenic effects are to be excluded by animal screening tests. This is considered in more detail later (see Section 6.7.1)

6.4 Molecular evidence

If cancer can be caused, partly or wholly, by chemical carcinogens inducing mutations in DNA, the powerful techniques of modern molecular biology can be used to detect differences between the DNA of normal and tumour tissue from a single individual cancer. The cellular oncogenes (c-*oncs*) are one group of genes for which comparisons of DNA sequences have shown mutations in human tumours (see Chapters 9 and 10). Members of the *ras* oncogene family, in particular, have been shown to be mutated, usually around codon 12 or 61, leading to the production of proteins with specific amino acid substitutions at these positions. Examples of these mutations have been found in a proportion of virtually all human tumour types, including carcinomas of the bladder, colon, pancreas, and skin, and also sarcomas, lymphomas, and leukaemias. We know that these highly specific mutations must affect the function of the c-*onc* because the mutant gene, but not its normal homologue, can dramatically alter the phenotype of cells in culture that have been transfected with the tumour DNA (see Chapter 9). Different oncogenes tend to be activated preferentially in different tissues after carcinogen treatment. This may be related to the observation that carcinogen interaction with DNA is non-random throughout the genome and may depend on the degree of condensation of the chromatin, or on the extent of DNA methylation at particular loci. This will, of course, vary with the differentiated phenotype of the target cell and may explain why a particular oncogene is activated more often in one type of tumour than in another. Since many of the oncogene protein products that have been identified are linked with the process of growth factor responses, either as analogues of a factor itself, a receptor, or part of the intracellular signalling mechanism (see Chapter 11), it is likely that a mutated oncogene product would show altered interactions with other molecules in the finely tuned system that regulates the growth of the cell.

Agents other than chemicals can cause mutations. Irradiation is known to damage human DNA (see Chapter 7), and some viruses may also be mutagens when they integrate into host cell DNA (see Chapter 8). We must turn to experimentally induced cancer in animals to find direct evidence that chemical carcinogens can cause mutations such as those in c-*onc* genes that have been linked to cancer causation in humans (see Chapter 9). One of the first examples of this came from the induction of breast tumours in female rats by nitrosomethylurea, a DNA alkylating carcinogen. All nine tumours in one experimental series contained an 'activated' *ras* gene (Ha-*ras*-1), and one of the genes that was isolated and analysed in detail showed that the same amino acid codon (at position 12 of the protein) was mutated as in the human cancers of unknown causation mentioned earlier. Evidence that the carcinogen causes the mutation directly, through interaction with DNA (see Section 6.5.2), is also provided by sequence analysis of the mutations. The change in nucleotide sequence observed is precisely that predicted from the known reaction between the particular carcinogen and a specific DNA base. For example, nitrosomethylurea methylates the O-6 position of guanosine residues and this adduct is known to mispair with thymidine during DNA replication (see Chapter 5). Thus, the observed G:C to A:T transition at position 12 of the protein is generated. A wide spectrum of different *ras* mutations is found in tumours of the breast, skin, and liver which are induced by carcinogens with different DNA-binding properties. In many, but not all, cases, the specific mutations observed can be correlated with the particular base involved in adduct formation.

Convincing as this might seem, many questions remain to be answered: only a minority of human tumours contain mutant oncogenes of the sort we have just described, whereas in other cases (e.g. colon or pancreatic carcinomas) the frequency is as high as 40–95 per cent. Moreover, one member of the *ras* family appears to be the preferred 'target gene' in each case. For example, Kirsten-*ras* (Ki-*ras*) is the most frequently mutated gene in colon or pancreatic tumours, whereas Ha-*ras* or neuro-blastoma-*ras* (N-*ras*) are more often mutated in bladder tumours and leukaemias, respectively. The reasons for this apparent specificity, which is also observed in animal model systems, are unclear but may be related to the route of exposure or tissue-specific metabolism of certain carcinogens. The evidence that the mutant genes are causal in the development of the cancers that contain them is persuasive; the tumours are usually clonal in origin and the mutation is present in every cell, suggesting that the first cell in which the molecular change occurred had a selective advantage. In some cases, *ras* mutations may be an early event or even the initiating event in tumour formation, whereas in others there is evidence that mutations occur during tumour progression.

A great deal of attention has been devoted to *ras* mutations simply because this was the first human oncogene to be described in some detail. There is therefore a natural tendency to 'search where there is light', but the impression should not be given that these are the only genes involved. Many human and animal tumours have apparently normal *ras* genes, indicating that such mutations are not necessary for tumours to develop. Other genes must be involved in generating the complex cancer phenotype. Some of these may be alternative protooncogenes which can be activated in a positive sense by mutation, but there is strong evidence that recessive mutations can also play an important role. Wilms' tumour of the kidney (see Chapter 10) and retinoblastoma (see Chapters 4 and 10) are rare childhood cancers associated with the loss or inactivation of genes on chromosomes 11 and 13 respectively, particularly involving the so-called tumour suppressor genes (see Chapters 4, 9, and 10). There is increasing evidence that loss of these tumour suppressor genes is also implicated in the generation of the more common human cancers which have no clear hereditary pattern (see Chapter 4). Since, in principle, it is easier to inactivate a gene functionally by mutation or deletion than to activate a protooncogene in a specific way, the tumour suppressor genes may constitute important targets for carcinogenic chemicals at some stage of tumorigenesis.

6.5 Experimental approaches to the study of carcinogenesis by chemicals

6.5.1 The biology of cancer induction in animals: precancer and multistage models

Studies on the experimental induction of cancer by chemicals in laboratory animals introduced several new concepts, particularly the multistage theory (Fig. 6.1). Carcinogens fall into two groups, complete and incomplete. The former can produce tumours on their own, whereas the latter cannot and require subsequent exposure of the treated (initiated) cells to promoting agents, which are not carcinogenic in themselves. Promoting agents can also lead to the development of tumours when applied to tissue previously treated with a subthreshold dose of a complete carcinogen, which would not in itself produce tumours. Polycyclic aromatic hydrocarbons and the nitrosamines are complete carcinogens and can act as initiators and promoters. The complexity of the situation is illustrated by urethane, an incomplete carcinogen when applied to the mouse skin but a complete carcinogen in the lung. Promoting agents are less well defined but seem to be specific for particular tissues. One group, the phorbol esters extracted from some plants, act as tumour promoters in skin. Other classes of promoting agents have been identified more recently, such as the teleocidin and aplysiatoxin classes. These were first identified from fungal and algal sources, respectively. Aplysiatoxins were found to be responsible for outbreaks of a condition known as 'swimmer's itch' in waters off the Japanese coast. Sporadic algal blooms produced a highly irritating substance in the water which caused dermatitis. An important finding is that most promoting agents appear to act in a way similar to the phorbol ester class, binding to the same specific receptor molecule, protein kinase C (PKC), and activating the same intracellular signalling mechanism (see Section 6.5.2). There are other

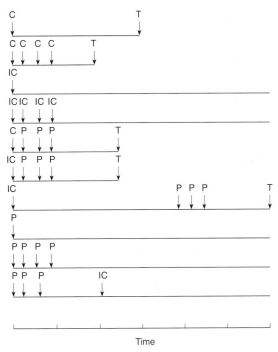

Fig.6.1 Initiation and promotion in carcinogenesis. Schematic representation of various schedules of treatment of mouse skin with a complete or incomplete carcinogen and tumour promoter. Different combinations and sequences in time are shown horizontally. Tumours result after different latent periods only from schedules where 'T' is indicated. C, carcinogen; P, promoter; T, tumour; IC, incomplete carcinogen.

classes of tumour promoters that do not directly interact with or activate PKC, but the non-phorbol-like chemicals are less well characterized.

Many promoting agents appear to act, at least in part, through their ability to cause irritation and inflammation. Many also interfere with intercellular communication through gap junctions between cells. This has led to theories that involve the response of initiated cells to the 'normalizing' influences of surrounding unaffected cells, as a critical component of promoter function. There is experimental evidence for this in studies on cellular transformation in tissue culture, but this has not yet been confirmed *in vivo* in studies on the effects of tumour promoters on gap-junctional communication between skin cells. In culture at least, isolated cells show tumour-like characteristics after carcinogen treatment at a much higher frequency than cells in dense cultures.

It is likely that the effects of promoters are multiple and that different cell types will respond differently to the same agents. This is currently an active area of research.

During experimental carcinogenesis in various tissues, macroscopic and microscopic changes in the affected tissues, which precede the appearance of tumours, have been defined (see Chapter 1) as altered discrete focal areas within the carcinogen-treated region. These focal areas of abnormal tissue are intermediate in character between normal and malignant. In time, further changes occur in these foci culminating in the development of overt cancer. The cells in the precursor foci have an increased risk of cancer development compared with normal tissue, i.e. they are precancerous. The process will be illustrated by describing three experimental animal systems for inducing cancer of epithelial tissues in skin, liver, and large bowel (colon and rectum). In the colon system, in particular, there are similarities to tissue changes in humans that, from epidemiological evidence, are considered to be precancerous. This suggests that the experimental animal models are a valid way of studying the disease and may provide clues to possible means of medical intervention.

Carcinogenesis in mouse skin is the classic model system in which two stages in the process of cancer development, initiation and promotion, were first described. A single application of a subthreshold dose of a chemical carcinogen is applied to the shaved dorsal skin and this results in the initiation of an unknown number of cells which, if they are left without further treatment, will persist for a very long time without showing any apparent changes. If a second class of chemical agent, a tumour promoter, is subsequently applied to the same area at any time, even a year later, and the treatment is repeated regularly, benign tumours (papillomas) appear. They are believed to arise from some of the initiated cells in the carcinogen-treated skin. A small proportion of these papillomas may develop into fully malignant tumours with or without further applications of promoter. The two classes of chemical agents used appear to have different mechanisms of action (see Fig. 6.1).

Initiating agents and complete carcinogens are almost always DNA damaging (genotoxic) and it seems very likely that the initiating event involves some form of carcinogen–DNA interaction and subsequent damage (see Section 6.5.3). Initiated cells persist in the tissue long after the initiating agent has disappeared and the lesion produced is both stable and heritable, i.e. it has the characteristics of a mutation. Conversely, most promoting agents are not mutagenic, although in some cases they may modify gene expression. It is now thought that promotion itself consists of several steps, and that promoting agents too may be either complete, and able to perform all functions, or incomplete, and active at only one or a few stages. A third term, progression, is usually reserved for the process by which cells of a benign or malignant tumour acquire more and more aberrant characteristics—the bad to worse principle of tumour evolution.

Similar sequences of events occur in other tissues. Cancer of the liver can be induced by chemical carcinogens fed to rats. For example, aflatoxin B_1, a mould product which may contaminate certain foods in the tropics, is one of the most potent liver carcinogens known. In all probability it contributes to the high incidence of human liver cancer in the tropics; it seems to act in combination with hepatitis B infection (see Chapter 8). One of the earliest effects of chronic aflatoxin B_1 treatment is the appearance of nodules of hyperplastic, probably precancerous, liver cells. These nodules have a range of enzyme abnormalities distinguishing them from surrounding normal tissue. Iron is lost from the precancerous nodules but glycogen stores increase. In the liver, there seems to be an absolute requirement for cell proliferation before nodules can be induced. Aflatoxin is toxic and kills many liver cells. The tissue then regenerates to restore the lost mass. [The powers of regeneration in the liver are remarkable; in rats three-quarters of the organ can be removed surgically (partial hepatectomy) and regenerative proliferation will restore the original tissue mass within weeks.] Partial hepatectomy can, in fact, act as a promoting stimulus in rat liver carcinogenesis, and tumours arise in the regenerated liver after an initiating, prehepatectomy treatment with a carcinogen. Neither chemical promotion nor surgical treatment alone is sufficient for cancer induction in the adult animal. Interestingly, in young weanling rats, where the liver is growing rapidly during normal development, there is no need for a proliferative stimulus and an initiating dose of carcinogen alone will induce cancer. Indeed, stimulation of cell division appears to be a necessary component of the promotion stages of carcinogenesis in most, if not all, tissues, but it is not usually sufficient in itself. Some types of hyperplastic stimuli are more effective than others. Promotion is obviously a complex process which is only recently becoming better understood, particularly with the development of cell culture model systems for studying this aspect of carcinogenesis (see Section 6.7.2).

Cancer in the colon induced by dimethylhydrazine in rats or mice shows well-defined precancerous stages. A sequence of pathological changes (Fig. 6.2) can be observed before overt carcinomas develop, and the type and amount of altered colon epithelium depends on carcinogen dosage as well as length of treatment. Submucosal glands become abnormal (dysplastic), and benign polyps (adenomas) arise with increasing incidence with both dosage and time. Histologically, carcinomas can be shown to develop directly from polyps and, more rarely, from abnormal glands, indicating that these are precancerous stages in colon carcinogenesis. This is precisely the conclusion reached by pathologists from observations on human colon cancer. In families with familial polyposis coli (see Chapter 4), affected members develop multiple polyps of the colon and rectum at an early age and at least one polyp will almost certainly become carcinomatous within about 10 years. Usually, the entire colon is removed surgically before this time. This offers the pathologist a unique opportunity to study the precancerous lesions, which in other circumstances would escape clinical detection. Most pathologists agree that, in polyposis patients, focal areas of carcinoma develop almost invariably from pre-existing polyps (or more rarely from microscopic glandular abnormalities) and that the polyps represent a precancerous stage. The adenomas themselves can be classified according to their potential for malignant change. Size (above 1 cm^2) and the presence of a particular histological pattern (villous) is accompanied by a statistically increased chance of cancer developing from a particular polyp. Thus there may be additional, more advanced precancerous stages in the multistage sequence, but these are

less well defined (see Fig. 6.2). It is thought that precancerous polyps may also occur in the general population but are few in number and arise sporadically later in life, preceding the cancer by a similar 10- or 15-year interval. The animal carcinogenesis model of colon cancer is thus especially suitable for the study of factors (including dietary components) suspected, from epidemiological studies, of being involved in the adenoma (or polyp) to carcinoma progression sequence. For instance, bile acids and their derivatives may have promoter-like activity (see earlier); this has already been shown in animal experiments. In addition, a few laboratories are beginning to make use of cell culture techniques to investigate precancerous cells from polyps *in vitro* (see Section 6.5.5).

6.5.2 Mechanisms of carcinogen activation and action

One of the most critical determinants of chemical carcinogenesis is the manner in which a chemical is metabolized, activated, or detoxified by exposed individuals. Each chemical class is potentially subject to a different metabolic pathway and a variety of enzymes may be involved in the fate of a single chemical. A predominant gene family involved in the metabolism of many chemicals is the cytochrome P450 enzymes. They constitute a supergene family since they are highly polymorphic genes for which many variants exist between species and between individuals, and the expression of which can be tissue specific. This polymorphism is believed to account for individual variation in response to a variety of known drugs and chemicals. These enzymes, which number in the hundreds, have been codified into families to reflect sequence homology. In addition to gene polymorphisms, there can also be wide variations in the basal level of expression between individuals or species and in the inducibility of individual P450 enzymes. Since tobacco

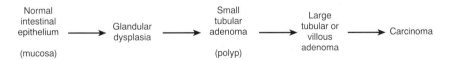

Fig. 6.2 Flow diagram showing the presumptive precancerous stages between normal and malignant tissue, identifiable histologically in human colorectal epithelium. Note: arrows indicate the direction of increasing potential for malignant change, not that cells necessarily pass through all of the precancerous stages between normal and malignant tissue.

smoke is composed of polyaromatic hydrocarbon and *N*-nitrosamines, which are substrates for P450 enzymes, individual susceptibility has been related to their expression. Certain phenotypes, such as the capacity to hydroxylate the drug debrisoquine, have been associated with lung cancer susceptibility. There are many other enzymes that may also be important in susceptibility to carcinogens, including flavin mono-oxygenase, transferases, prostaglandin synthetases, and others, but generally they have not been characterized for a role in chemical carcinogenesis as extensively as the P450 enzymes.

Until the late 1960s, some of the most potent carcinogens, the polycyclic aromatic hydrocarbons, were unable to mutate cells in culture. We now know that this is because many carcinogens need to be metabolized by cellular enzymes to a reactive derivative before they can be effective, and the test cells used were deficient in one or more metabolic functions and were unable to activate the chemical. Similarly, these (and most other) chemicals must be metabolized to electrophilic derivatives before they become carcinogenic. In animals, metabolism usually happens in the target cells from which the cancer will develop; most reactive metabolites have short half-lives in solution in body fluids. Occasionally, activation may occur in the liver. The capacity for metabolism is genetically determined and may be species specific. For instance, the guinea pig lacks a critical enzyme for the activation of acetylaminofluorene (AAF) to its active metabolite, *N*-hydroxy-AAF, and is thus resistant to its carcinogenic effects. There are also differences between tissues in the extent of metabolic activation of a particular chemical and in the relative extents of deactivation (or detoxification) and activation to the ultimate carcinogenic derivative.

6.5.3 DNA repair

What then happens to DNA that has been modified by alkylation or by the formation of nucleic acid adducts with large bulky hydrocarbon molecules? Are there mechanisms by which a cell detects and repairs such lesions so that its DNA sequence of bases is faithfully restored? The primary consequence of the metabolism of chemicals to electrophilic intermediates is the covalent adduction of these forms to DNA. If cells are in the process of DNA replication and the adduct cannot be removed before the affected sequence is replicated, a muta-

tion is induced. This is the prototypical 'tumour initiation' event if it occurs in a protooncogene or other gene that is involved in the pathway by which a specific cancer develops. There are also potentially important consequences if carcinogens adduct RNA or specific proteins, but such effects are probably secondary to the adduction to DNA which can induce heritable change if the mutation is not lethal.

The presence of adducts can be used as markers of exposure. Of the available methods, the use of ^{32}P-postlabelling has found wide application. DNA from exposed individuals is enzymatically digested to nucleotides, and incubated with ^{32}P-ATP and polynucleotide kinase, separated chromatographically, and quantitated. This and other methods have been utilized to detect tobacco-specific *N*-nitrosamine, polyaromatic hydrocarbon, and other adducts in a variety of human tissues.

The processes by which adducts and other DNA lesions are detected and repaired have been established in prokaryotic systems, and enzymes involved in recognizing, excising, and repairing the carcinogen-induced damage have been identified. Much less is known about mammalian cells, but it seems certain that inefficient or faulty (error-prone) repair of DNA is important in some types of cancer.

The most compelling evidence for a role for DNA repair mechanisms in chemical and environmental carcinogenesis has been derived from the study of heritable cancer-predisposing syndromes. Among the best studied is the induction of skin cancers in individuals with the xeroderma pigmentosum (XP) syndrome. Individuals carrying this mutation have a defect in the capacity to repair UV-induced DNA damage. Exposure of normal skin to a high level of UV radiation in sunlight results in the induction of lesions in the DNA of basal epidermal cells, the predominant form of which is dimerization of pyrimidine bases (e.g. TT). This defect appears to be responsible for the high sensitivity of XP patients to UV-induced skin cancers. This defect does not appear to account for the general sensitivity of Caucasians (particularly those of Anglo-Saxon descent) to UV-induced non-melanoma skin cancer. While some repair deficiencies or errors may occur in the repair process, it is also likely that the cancers may arise as a consequence of unrepaired lesions that result from excessive exposure to sunlight.

Other heritable, cancer-prone syndromes that may involve defects in DNA repair mechanisms include ataxia telangiectasia (AT), Fanconi's anaemia, and Bloom's syndrome, which have high incidences of chromosome breakage. Each of these syndromes is associated with specific cancer susceptibility or the development of cancers at specific sites that may arise as a consequence of the genetic defect itself or as a consequence of increased susceptibility to some environmental agents (e.g. X-rays). A heritable cancer-predisposing syndrome, hereditary non-polyposis colon cancer (HNPCC), has provided evidence for a role for DNA mismatch repair genes. The defect is recognized as a dinucleotide repeat instability that gives rise to mis-sense mutations resulting in apparent predisposition to several types of cancers.

In summary, most carcinogens need to be activated metabolically to be converted to the ultimate carcinogen that binds to DNA, modifying accessible DNA bases in a precise way throughout the genome, depending on the dose and extent of metabolic activation. It is likely that small errors in repairing this damage or, on a larger scale, complete chromosome breakage, perhaps owing to lesions on both DNA strands in the same vicinity, are important. Thus, mutations at the DNA sequence level, or those involving gross changes such as large deletions, translocations, and mechanisms leading to a functionally homozygous state at particular loci (see Chapter 10), are strongly implicated in the mechanism of carcinogen action.

6.5.4 Transgenic mice

In the past decade it has become possible to introduce new genes or genes that are differently regulated, or to ablate entirely the function of specific genes in the germ line of mice. These mice, and now other transgenic animals, are created by injection of the cloned gene into pronuclei of fertilized ova which are then implanted into a foster mother made pseudopregnant by mating with a vasectomized male. The ablation or 'knock-out' of genes is achieved by homologous recombination in embryonic stem cells between a gene carrying a mutation and the normal endogenous gene. The stem cells are then implanted into a foster mother. The consequence of integration of the transgene is that all cells in the individual and its progeny carry the gene. By this technique it is possible to delete specific genes, alter the expression of a gene, insert it in an ectopic location, insert mutated genes or

additional copies of normal genes, and finally to analyse the consequences.

Transgenic models have particular applicability in the identification of genes that play specific roles in developmental processes and in studying the role of specific genes in carcinogenesis. Since the mice are isogenic to the control animals in all but the transgene, it is also possible to analyse chemical–gene interactions. In most cases, introduction of a transgenic oncogene produces an animal model that is genetically initiated and which exists in a preneoplastic state. In many cases, the oncogene has been linked to transcriptional promoters capable of directing expression to specific tissues. Studies using a variety of oncogenes linked to various tissue-specific promoters are providing new insights into the processes of carcinogenesis.

A transgenic model that has been very informative is a mouse strain in which the *p53* tumour suppressor gene (see Chapter 9) has been knocked out ($p53^{-/-}$). In the nullizygous state (i.e. both alleles inactive), the animals develop cancers relatively early in life, particularly lymphomas. These cancers arise in normal mice but do so later in life. The *p53* gene plays a very broad role at molecular and cellular levels in controlling cell proliferation (see Chapter 9). When *p53* function is lost, the errors, whatever their nature, can be expressed more readily. It is interesting to note that tumours develop in the *p53*$^{-/-}$ mice in a tissue-specific manner indicating that there is some genetic tissue basis; that is, that they are non-random. Further study of the genetic basis of these tumours may help to identify the types of processes controlled by the *p53* gene.

The hemizygous mice (i.e. *p53*$^{+/-}$) have a relatively low incidence of spontaneous cancers during the first six months of life, but develop lymphomas and soft-tissue sarcomas at a later stage, most of which have lost the wild-type allele of the *p53* gene. These mice are also more sensitive to the effects of mutagenic carcinogens than mice with the normal ($p53^{+/+}$) genotype. The *p53*$^{+/-}$ mice have not shown high sensitivity to non-mutagenic carcinogens. These hemizygous mice can also be used to define genes that cooperate in neoplastic processes. For example, Balmain and co-workers have shown that the incidence of benign skin tumours carrying H-*ras* mutations induced by chemical initiation is unaffected in hemizygous mice in comparison with wild-type litter mates. However, progression to malignancy is greatly accelerated in the *p53*-deficient animals, suggesting that this gene operates primarily at the late progression stage of carcinogenesis. The role of *p53* in tumour development is, however, very complex and is still the subject of intense study. Cross-breeding of *p53*-deficient mice with animals carrying *ras* oncogenes as transgenes in some cases leads to increased tumour progression, but in others there is either no difference or the tumours completely fail to develop in the absence of wild-type *p53*. The latter results suggest that some aspects of *p53* function may be beneficial or necessary for the development of certain classes of tumour.

Many other transgenic mice with protooncogenes, oncogenes, growth factor or receptor genes, viral genes, etc. have been created utilizing a variety of promoter constructs. There are also increasing numbers of mice with ablated genes being created and more will soon become available. Another valuable model is one that utilizes genes derived from *E. coli* which can be vectored by λ phage. Both *lacI* and *lacZ* genes have been utilized to create a mouse line for chemical mutagenesis studies. It is possible to measure tissue- and cell-specific mutagenesis by packaging genomic DNA in phage particles that are plated on to susceptible *E. coli* under conditions that select for or identify mutant colonies. These lines hold the promise of providing a mutation assay that overcomes some of the limitations of the Ames *Salmonella* mutagenesis assay (see Section 6.7.2) by providing for endogenous distribution and metabolism of the chemicals.

6.5.5 Cellular transformation *in vitro*

Transformation is a term used for changes seen in tissue culture whereby more or less normal cells become altered to resemble cancer cells. This can happen spontaneously as a rare event whose frequency depends on a variety of factors and on the species. Cells from some rodents, e.g. mouse, transform spontaneously in culture whereas human and avian cells rarely (if ever) do. Physical agents (see Chapter 7), chemicals, and viruses (see Chapter 8) can transform cells *in vitro*. In many cases where the cell transformation system is well defined, near-normal, diploid cells can be converted with reasonable efficiency into cells that can grow into invasive tumours if they are put back into a suitable animal host. The converted or transformed cells in culture are then said to be tumorigenic, and the process by

which they became so can be studied as a model for carcinogenesis *in vivo* (spontaneous or induced).

Many different culture systems for studying transformation have used mesenchymal or 'fibroblast' cells (see Chapter 1) which rarely give rise to malignant tumours spontaneously in humans or laboratory animals. They probably do not provide a very good model system for studying the relationship between cell differentiation and neoplasia, but they are easy to grow and manipulate in culture and they have certainly provided us with ways of studying some fundamental aspects of carcinogenesis. For instance, the system devised by Heidelberger and his group used a clone of mouse embryo fibroblast cells called C3H/10T$_{1/2}$ (Reznikoff *et al.* 1973). One parameter of transformation that correlates well with tumorigenicity in this cell system (as it does in many others, but not invariably) is the appearance of a property known as anchorage-independent growth (AIG). Most normal cells need to be anchored to and spread on a solid substrate before they can divide and form a colony or clone from a single cell. Some cancer cells are able to grow and form colonies when suspended in a semi-solid medium such as soft (0.33 per cent) agar in tissue culture medium. If untransformed C3H/10T$_{1/2}$ cells are treated with a chemical carcinogen, a small proportion of the cells will grow in soft agar and these cells are also usually tumorigenic. The frequency of transformation to this phenotype can be measured after correction for the proportion that survived the carcinogen-induced toxicity. The efficiency with which certain carcinogens transform cells to AIG has been used by some scientists as a rapid screening test for chemicals that might cause cancer (see Section 6.7.2), but it is not as reproducible as other tests and is not widely used. There are many other changes that can be induced in cell culture by carcinogens and for which there is evidence of a link with the cancer cell phenotype. Changes in components of the filamentous cytoskeleton of cells is one such example. Since none of these markers of transformation in culture is invariably associated with cancer cells, their role in carcinogenesis remains an area of active investigation and dispute (see Chapter 1).

As mentioned earlier, some aspects of carcinogenesis cannot be studied in simple fibroblast cell systems; namely, those concerned with differentiation and tissue homeostasis (the balance between cell renewal by division and cell death in a defined population)—a key abnormality in cancer. Some aspects of these properties can be investigated in specialized systems such as in differentiated epithelial cell cultures. Methods have been established for growing some of these more fastidious cell types from rodent and human tissues. It has been shown conclusively that chemical carcinogens, such as the hydrocarbons benzo(*a*)pyrene and dimethylbenzanthracene, can induce transformation and eventually tumorigenic potential in epithelial cells treated with the carcinogen in primary culture, i.e. cells grown directly from animal tissues. Various types of rodent cells have been used, including skin keratinocytes, salivary gland duct cells, epithelium from the respiratory system, and urinary bladder cells. All of these epithelial systems demonstrate one feature particularly clearly: transformation, like carcinogenesis, is a multistage process. There is a relatively long period of time between treating normal cells with a chemical, sometimes just for a single short exposure, and the eventual emergence of cells that will grow as tumours in an appropriate animal host. During this long latent period, more or less discrete precancerous stages occur wherein the cells appear altered in a characteristic way but are not yet capable of forming tumours in an animal. Some of these intermediate stages are probably equivalent to the precancerous stages in carcinogenesis observed *in vivo* (see Section 6.5.1), but a comparison of the molecular changes *in vivo* and *in vitro* will be necessary to determine whether the sequence of events is the same. Among the properties that frequently alter during the precancerous stages in transformation are chromosome number (which usually increases, and often nearly doubles, the normal complement), loss of dependence on growth-stimulating factors in serum (see Chapter 11), increased ability to grow clonally from single cells (clonogenicity) or at a reduced cell density, and the acquisition of a prolonged or indefinite life span in culture (immortality—an escape from senescence). We know very little about the factors that govern progression through these precancerous stages. Further studies will investigate the effects of tumour promoters, identified from animal experiments, and other known modifiers of gene expression which do not conform to the carcinogen/mutagen category of initiating agents.

6.5.6 Precancerous cells *in vitro*

Human cells of all types and, in particular, normal epithelial cells which give rise to the common human cancers, are extremely resistant to transformation by chemicals in culture. The reasons for this are poorly understood. It is now possible to culture epithelial cells directly from some tissues that are already precancerous. The early stages of transformation in these cells, especially the stage(s) leading to immortality and the capacity for indefinite propagation *in vitro*, may have already taken place. We can now study such cells and try to identify the factors that lead to the development of more malignant cell properties, or, conversely, those that induce reversion to a more normal state. This approach is most useful where the precancerous tissue is readily available, usually through surgical procedures. In patients with familial polyposis coli, diseased tissue is removed surgically. Polyps from these surgical specimens have been cultured successfully and immortal cell lines have been derived from about one specimen in five which survived the initial preparation procedure and remained uncontaminated by intestinal microorganisms. The uterine cervix, oral tissues, oesophagus, and trachea also provide suitable precancerous tissue from biopsies, but work using these tissues is in its early stages.

6.6 The role of tumour promotion in human cancer

6.6.1 Epidemiological evidence

While most of the known human chemical carcinogens (Table 6.1) and those that cause cancer in experimental animals are positive in screening tests designed to detect mutagenic activity (see Section 6.7), some do not fall into this category. It has been known for some time that there are many components with biological activity in cigarette smoke and that not all of these have the hallmarks of classical mutagenic/carcinogenic chemicals. We now believe that some constituents act to promote the development of cancers from cells of the respiratory epithelium that harbour covert mutations, perhaps in oncogenes. Such promoters (see Fig. 6.1 and Section 6.5.1) must be applied regularly over a long period of time to achieve the eventual completion of the carcinogenic process. This may partly explain the striking relationship between lung cancer incidence and duration of smoking (see Chapter 3).

Other agents whose probable role in carcinogenesis is to promote rather than initiate tumour development include those contained in, or influenced by, the diet. High dietary fat has been linked epidemiologically with increased bowel cancer risk. This may be a reflection of consequent high levels of bile acids, some of which have been shown to promote colorectal cancer in experimental animal models. Hormones can also act as growth-promoting factors, which may in some circumstances create an environment in which initiated cells have a selective advantage. Obviously, the situation is complex and much experimental work needs to be done to correlate cancer risk statistics in human populations with identification of the causative agents and analysis of their modes of action.

6.6.2 Mechanisms of tumour promotion

Evidence for the role of some chemicals as promoters of tumour development comes from data on experimental animal model systems. Some of these systems are described in the preceding section. The generally applicable conclusion is that activation of an oncogene by mutation, which can be seen as an initiating event, does not in itself lead to cancer development. Promoting influences, such as the activity of hormones on a hormone-dependent tissue, the mammary gland at puberty for instance, are necessary for complete carcinogenesis. An activated oncogene may be linked experimentally to DNA sequences which, under hormonal control, promote expression of the gene, when introduced into early embryos (to produce transgenic animals) (Stewart *et al.* 1984). Tumours develop, as predicted, predominantly in the tissues that respond to the hormonal stimulation. Presumably this is a result of activated oncogene expression under hormonal control. However, the situation is more complex than this, since expression of the activated oncogene can be detected in a wider range of hormone-dependent tissues than those that give rise to tumours. This indicates that the hormone, in addition to stimulating expression of the oncogene, has other effects on the target tissue which promote tumour formation.

The primary cellular target for some tumour promoters is thought to be an intracellular kinase known as protein kinase C (PKC). The endogenous mechanism of PKC activation is by binding diacylglycerol, which is in turn generated by growth factor-stimulated turnover of membrane-bound phosphatidyl inositol (see Chapter 11). Some tumour promoters are chemically similar to diacyl-

glycerol, and can consequently bind directly to PKC causing its 'translocation' (receptor translocation) to the cell membrane and the activation of pathways leading to DNA synthesis and cell division. This picture, however, represents a vast oversimplification of the true situation. Several members of the PKC family exist and it is not known which of these is critical for tumour promotion. In addition, some promoting agents that do not resemble phorbol esters do not bind PKC, and conversely, other agents which bind PKC are either inactive as tumour promoters or, paradoxically, can inhibit promotion. It is therefore unlikely that the mechanism of promoter action involves only this pathway.

Although tumour promoters do not bind to DNA and are non-mutagenic in bacterial test systems (see Section 6.7.2), there is now evidence that promoters nevertheless have effects at the DNA level. The phorbol ester promoters have clastogenic effects on some mammalian cells, i.e. they cause single strand breaks in DNA. This probably involves the generation of 'active oxygen' species within the cells which are known to cause such breaks. Indeed, some chemicals that induce active oxygen molecules can act as tumour promoters; for example, benzoyl peroxide. One possible explanation of this phenomenon is that the non-specific DNA damage caused by these agents induces a regenerative response which accounts for their tumour-promoting ability, but this is far from being understood at the moment.

Other documented effects of tumour promoters are the induction of gross chromosomal changes in epidermal cells, both *in vivo* and *in vitro*. While these events may lead to changes in the function of critical genes, alterations in controlling elements, or development of homozygosity at certain chromosomal loci, there is as yet no evidence that such changes are critical for the selection of initiated cells rather than a result of the toxic effects of the promoting agents used.

6.7 Screening for carcinogens

6.7.1 Animal carcinogenicity tests

The importance of testing any substance for its carcinogenicity is obvious although none of the methods in current use is completely satisfactory. Laboratory rodents are now the most widely used species as they have life spans that are short enough to develop tumours that involve long latent periods (as a proportion of the life span) or delayed responses and they can be inbred and maintained easily. The pathology and incidence of spontaneously occurring tumours is well defined and can be compared to tumours produced after chemical exposure. Most known human carcinogens and many other chemicals will produce tumours in experimental animals under appropriate, although sometimes very artificial, conditions. In fact, it is required by law that any new chemical introduced for use in or by humans (such as medicines, cosmetics, food additives, weed and pest killers, agricultural fertilizers, household cleansing products, to give a few examples) must be tested in laboratory animals for their long-term effects. This is enormously costly in time and expenditure so it is vital that tests should be carefully planned and informative. This requires a knowledge of the way in which chemicals are metabolized (see Section 6.5.2) and excreted in different species and whether these characteristics are appropriate to the human situation. For instance, the guinea pig would be inappropriate for testing AAF since it lacks the enzyme necessary to convert this chemical to its active, carcinogenic form. In practice, most tests are done on rats and mice, male and female, which are exposed for a long period, often one to two years, to the maximum tolerated dose. The route of administration usually depends on the likely mode of human exposure, by inhalation, in the diet or drinking water, or through skin contact. After the necessary length of time, animals still surviving are examined for tumours which can be confirmed as malignant by a pathologist.

The US Public Health Service has compiled the results of various chemical carcinogenesis studies in animals but there are problems. Over 800 chemicals have been studied by various methods, using variable doses of chemicals of sometimes uncertain purity, variable numbers of animals, and different routes of administration and periods of exposure. Thus, while an extensive database exists, much of the information is not useful because it is not possible to make direct comparisons between studies because of the wide range of variables encountered.

Today, rats and mice continue today to be the primary species used for carcinogen bioassays. The experimental procedures have been highly standardized under the aegis of the US National Toxicology Program. While a high degree of standardization can impose limitations on studies with certain chemicals, there is much to be gained in the reduction of variables. In the conventional bioassay protocol, mice and rats of both sexes are treated with incremental doses of chemical for two years, followed by a complete post-mortem evaluation. Except for a relatively few well-known and well-studied chemicals that are highly carcinogenic, most chemicals are carcinogenic to rodents only after prolonged exposures (> 60 per cent of the animal's life span). As shown in Table 6.1, there is a high concordance between the known human carcinogens and the induction of tumours in rodents. However, the known human carcinogens constitute only a small portion of the 800 chemicals studied in rodent bioassays. Thus, there is often uncertainty about whether all results in bioassays should be extrapolated to humans. Since the induction of tumours varies as a function of dose, duration or route of exposure, and genetic background or gender of rodents, multiple variables can influence bioassay results. However, this model represents the best available system with which to identify potential human carcinogens prospectively.

The process of determining whether the results of rodent bioassays represent direct human health hazards enters the discipline of risk assessment in which efforts are made to extrapolate quantitatively a potential human risk based upon the chemical dose and frequency of tumours induced by a given chemical. Data provided by the rodent bioassays may serve as the primary source of information for government regulatory actions. No other methods have yet emerged to supplant the rodent bioassay, although extensive efforts are underway to develop *in vitro* and other shorter term *in vivo* techniques. The primary justification for continued dependence upon rodent bioassays is the high correlation between the tumorigenicity in rodents of the majority of organic chemicals that have been defined as known human carcinogens (Table 6.1). Evidence of mutagenicity by a chemical provides strong corroborative evidence of carcinogenicity, as the majority of the chemicals that are known human carcinogens are also mutagenic. Among the chemicals that produce carcinogenic responses in both rats and mice, there is a very high proportion that are also mutagenic *in vitro* or capable of inducing chromosomal damage in whole animals, so mutagenic activity provides a strong risk factor of probable human carcinogenicity when combined with the ability of the chemical to induce tumours in both mice and rats.

As discussed earlier, human cancers are thought to take many years to evolve after the initiating event in a susceptible target cell. This can range from about 10 years up to almost the total lifetime of an individual. This fact alone poses a very real problem for the experimenter who wants to confirm the safety of a potentially useful chemical. Animal studies still form the main acceptable evidence for food and drug safety authorities throughout the world, and yet they are very time consuming and expensive. As an example, to test one compound thoroughly for carcinogenic activity in two species (rats and mice) costs approximately £500 000 at 1989 prices and takes up to three years.

As it became apparent that most compounds with proven carcinogenic activity were genotoxic, a number of more rapid tests were developed as first-order screens for large numbers of chemicals at between 1 and 10 per cent of the cost of animal experiments, depending on the type and number of rapid tests used.

6.7.2 Rapid screening: *in vitro* tests for carcinogens and mutagens

Rapid developments in understanding the structure and function of DNA and progress in microbial genetics have provided new insights and tools for identifying genetic damage caused by chemicals. Recognition that the mutagenic effects of radiation could be linked to induction of cancers stimulated efforts to identify the mutagenic potential of chemicals. In addition, there was great concern that both radiation and chemicals, if they could produce demonstrable somatic genetic effects, could also have important effects on the germ line to create heritable mutations that would be passed from generation to generation. Thus, the field of genetic toxicology emerged in response to concerns over the widespread dissemination of potentially hazardous environmental chemicals.

A large number of different tests have been put forward over the last few years as potentially useful indicators of carcinogenic activity. After a series of comparative trials, the authorities in most countries have reached agreement on the type of evidence that would be acceptable. This requires a compound to have been tested in assays measuring mutation (both in bacteria and in mammalian cells in culture) and for their ability to cause chromosome breakage both *in vivo* (in the animal) and in cell cultures. The

results of a battery of about four rapid screening tests selected from within these categories should, if the results are unequivocal, provide information on the potential carcinogenicity of a chemical which would be accepted by safety authorities in lieu of long-term animal data.

There are several problems in evaluating the usefulness of such rapid screening tests and in extrapolating from mutagenesis assays *in vitro* to carcinogenicity in animals and thence to the potential human cancer risk incurred by exposure to a suspect chemical. It is wise to assume that any chemical that is capable of causing mutation is a potential carcinogen. However, the expression of carcinogenic potential varies markedly between species, even between those that are as close (in evolutionary terms) as rats and mice. Regulatory authorities are continually updating and revising test protocols to minimize the chance of undue exposure to carcinogens.

The most well known and widely publicized rapid test for chemical carcinogens takes the name of its originator, Bruce Ames (Ames *et al.* 1975). This test assesses the mutagenicity of chemicals, with or without metabolism, by activating enzymes (from a crude subcellular fraction, S9, of rat liver, a rich source of membrane-bound enzyme activity including the mixed function oxidases, MFO) in a range of specially selected strains of *Salmonella* bacteria. These bacterial strains have each been constructed in the laboratory to detect mutations of a specific kind. For instance, one strain is able to indicate a particular nucleic acid substitution which alters one base pair to another in bacterial DNA after exposure to a DNA-damaging agent. Another strain detects chemicals able to cause frameshift mutations (whereby addition or deletion of one or more nucleic acids other than a multiple of three causes the whole reading frame of the triplet code to be thrown out of phase), when the encoded protein is drastically altered. The bacteria used as test strains are themselves mutants and are unable to make a particular amino acid essential for their growth, such as histidine. The test then detects whether a particular chemical can cause the specific base pair substitution or frameshift mutation needed to revert the mutant bacteria to their wild-type capacity for synthesizing the essential amino acid. This is done because the investigator can most easily score the number of bacterial colonies that do grow on an incomplete nutrient agar substrate (one which does not supply the particular amino acid). Most carcinogenic chemicals induce a wide range of mutations which may kill the bacteria, so it is important to test a chemical at a dose giving an acceptable level of toxicity that can be measured separately under non-selective conditions. Obviously a positive result is one in which a chemical induces a significant increase in reverted (auxotrophic) bacteria capable of forming colonies on a selective (deficient) nutrient agar substrate where the unaffected bacteria cannot grow (see Fig. 6.3).

The Ames test is probably one of the least expensive and most rapid tests available (taking only a couple of days) to detect a property, namely mutation, common to most human carcinogens. However, there are some drawbacks to the test which mean that the results obtained with it should be considered suggestive rather than conclusive evidence for or against the carcinogenicity of a suspect chemical compound. First, the complete spectrum of enzymes involved in metabolizing a variety of carcinogens is not present in the particular liver microsome fraction (S9) component of the assay mixture. This means that although mutagenic derivatives of a chemical may be generated by the microsomal enzymes, they may not be the ones produced by an intact cell or in the body, and so present a different picture of the chemical's potency. It is even possible that a false positive or negative result might be obtained for similar reasons. In practice, the Ames test, using a battery of four *Salmonella* strains each designed to detect a particular type of mutation, has achieved greater than 90 per cent accuracy in predicting both carcinogens and non-carcinogens in 'blind' trials. However, the relative potency of the chemicals was predicted less accurately in quantitative comparisons between different classes of chemicals.

Because mammalian cell DNA is more complex than bacterial DNA, mutation tests in mammalian cells *in vitro* must also be performed, even though they are rather more complicated to do and take longer to produce results. The mutations most commonly used are deficiencies owing to DNA sequence modification in either hypoxanthine phosphoribosyl transferase (HPRT) or thymidine kinase (TK), enzymes involved in nucleic acid synthesis (see Fig. 6.4), or to a mutation that reduces the capacity of the drug ouabain to bind at the cell surface and block membrane transport. The most commonly used mutation is HPRT deficiency (HPRT) because,

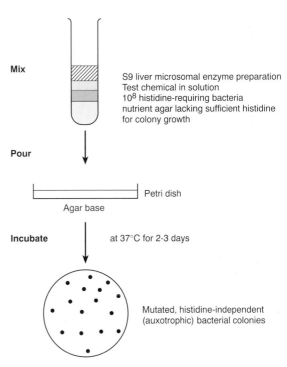

Fig. 6.3 Diagram showing the basic Ames test procedure for detecting mutagenicity of chemicals in bacteria. A panel of similar tests is generally used, each designed to detect different chemical activities and types of mutation in order to predict carcinogenic potential.

although recessive, it can be induced at relatively high frequency owing to its location on the X chromosome, i.e. inactivation of the single gene copy in male cells is sufficient for expression of the mutant phenotype. The assay procedure involves treating suitable mammalian cells (often Chinese hamster fibroblasts) with a suspect chemical, with or without activation by the S9 rat liver cell enzyme fraction. The treated cell population is assessed: (i) for its ability to grow from single cells to form clones as a measure of the degree of toxicity of the chemical (reduction in clone formation compared with untreated cells), and (ii) for the number of mutations in a given number of cells cultured in the presence of the drugs 6-thioguanine or 8-azaguanine. Unaffected cells take up the selective drug, incorporate it into nucleic acid, and are thus killed. Mutated cells fail to do so because they lack HPRT of the salvage pathway and cannot utilize base analogue drugs. They depend solely on the alternative biosynthetic pathway and are spared. They grow to form

Fig. 6.4 Diagram showing the biochemical pathways utilized in the synthesis of nucleic acids. The biosynthetic (*de novo*) pathway can be blocked by aminopterin and the alternative salvage pathway can be abolished by mutation in hypoxanthine phosphoribosyl transferase (HPRT) or thymidine kinase (TK) genes. This is detected by cellular resistance to the cytotoxic base analogue drugs 6-thioguanine (or 8-azaguanine) and bromodeoxyuridine, respectively. Mutation in a forward direction (HPRT or TK phenotypes) or reversion of mutants to wild-type (resistance to aminopterin) are increased in frequency by many chemical carcinogens.

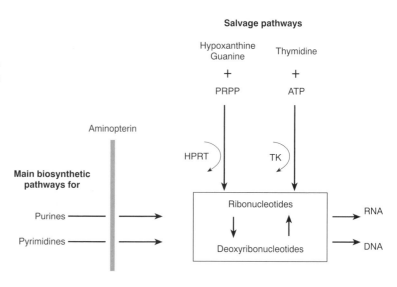

clones of mutant cells which can be stained and counted after one to two weeks, and their numbers expressed as a mutation frequency within the surviving fraction (after correction for toxicity of the suspect chemical). Relative to the control 'background' level of mutation in untreated cells, an elevated mutation frequency would indicate that the suspect chemical has potential carcinogenic activity.

Together with the development of the *Salmonella* mutagenesis assay system, important advances have also been made in the field of cytogenetics and *in vitro* mammalian cell culture. For example, improvements in the ability to capture large numbers of cells in metaphase through the use of the chemical colchicine or other techniques, and the development of banding methods (see Chapter 10), has permitted widespread application of cytogenetic studies in the search for chromosomal damage. Stable chromosome aberrations induced by radiation are used as biological dosimeters of exposure. This in turn encouraged the search for chemically induced chromosomal effects. At the same time the increasing ability to culture mammalian cells *in vitro* provided a resource that was valuable both to cytogeneticists and to cell biologists.

Chromosome mutations, e.g. aberrations such as chromatid breaks (see Chapter 10) caused by chemicals, are also good indicators of carcinogenic activity and this property forms the basis of the second pair of screening tests. The *in vivo* assay relies on the

living animal to activate the test chemical, if this is necessary, after it has been fed or injected, and metabolism may occur in the liver or in the target cells. In this test, target cells are usually from the bone marrow where blood cell precursors are dividing rapidly and are highly sensitive to DNA-damaging agents. At several times after injecting the chemical, samples of bone marrow cells are prepared for chromosome analysis (see Chapter 10). Chromosomes in the metaphase part of the cell cycle, just before cell division, are condensed and relatively easy to see. Many metaphase chromosome spreads are analysed and the average numbers of breaks, or discontinuities, in the chromatid arms of each chromosome are counted. Significant increases above the spontaneous background level indicate that the chemical may be carcinogenic. The same kind of analysis may be performed on cells in tissue culture, which can either be human blood lymphocytes in short-term culture or permanent cell lines of human or rodent origin. These are treated with the chemical *in vitro*, with or without the metabolizing S9 enzyme preparation, and chromosomes prepared at two or three times thereafter to find the peak of chromosome breaking activity; this may vary, but is generally at 24–48 hours.

Although the *Salmonella* mutagenesis assay identified many potential carcinogens, some carcinogens failed to induce mutations in the *Salmonella* assay. This stimulated efforts to use cytogenetic methods, mammalian cell transformation and mutation, or other assay methods to identify potential carcinogens that might be missed using the *Salmonella* assay system alone. This led to the emergence of many other methods to measure mutagenesis or induced DNA damage in cultured mammalian or *Drosophila melanogaster* cells. Successful application of these methods to a variety of chemicals was due, in large measure, to the recognition that most mutagens must undergo some form of metabolism in order to create the mutagenic intermediates. Tissue homogenates (S9 fractions) were used to accomplish this enzymatic conversion. The method is not without some limitations because the liver homogenates cannot accommodate species- or tissue-specific metabolism, nor the complex variety of enzymatic alterations that chemicals might undergo *in vivo*. Thus, there were known intrinsic limitations on the use of any *in vitro* system when attempting to match the results directly from these systems to effects that were observed in whole animals.

The recognition by Dr Leo Sachs and colleagues at the Weizmann Institute in Israel that cells from Syrian hamster embryos could be morphologically transformed by exposure to selected carcinogenic chemicals suggested that it might be possible to use mammalian cell systems to screen for chemicals that had carcinogenic potential. Subsequently, other cells were established in continuous culture, primarily from mouse embryos, that also appeared to be appropriate targets for morphological transformation. It was soon possible to produce clonal cultures that had the ability to grow autonomously and produce tumours when injected into recipient animals (see Section 6.7.1).

Many other assay systems were proposed as *in vitro* methods of identifying potential carcinogens and by 1980 over a hundred systems had been described. The task of determining the extent to which systems properly predict the carcinogenic potential of chemicals in animals and humans has been termed *validation*. This determines parameters such as *sensitivity* (the proportion of known carcinogens that are detected in the assay) and *specificity* (the proportion of known non-carcinogens detected by the assay system, i.e. the proportion of false positive results that the assay might generate). International efforts were mounted to validate test systems, the most comprehensive of which was the Genetox Project conducted by the US Environmental Protection Agency. The project compiled the results that had been reported in the scientific literature on specific assays and specific chemicals. Scientific work groups evaluated the data to establish a consensus on the most acceptable data and methods and various cross-comparisons were made. Results of this extensive effort did not give definitive answers. The two major impediments to achieving objective evaluations were the absence of an adequate number of chemicals in common between the various assay systems and, most importantly, the absence of a significant number of non-carcinogens with which the specificity of the assays could be determined. Subsequently, the US National Toxicology Program conducted a detailed evaluation of 110 chemicals that included a high proportion of chemicals that had not demonstrated carcinogenic activity in two-year rodent bioassays. The chemicals were tested in assay systems measuring mutagenesis and chromosomal effects to determine the relative sensitivity and specificity of the assays and their ability to discriminate between rodent carcinogens and non-carcinogens. This effort demonstrated that the *Salmonella* mutagenesis assay produced the most reliable data in terms of sensitivity and the absence of false positive responses. However, none of the other assays complemented the *Salmonella* assay, thus indicating that these assay systems detected common properties of chemicals, i.e. interaction with DNA, as they were developed to do. However, some also detect toxic chemical properties that are unrelated to genetic toxicity and to carcinogenicity.

As *in vitro* systems utilize exogenous S9 liver homogenate fractions to activate the chemicals metabolically, there appeared to be some intrinsic limitations in the assays because about half of the carcinogens in the studies failed to demonstrate a consistent pattern of genetic toxicity. However, it is equally plausible that these chemicals exhibit their carcinogenic potential independently of their ability to interact directly with DNA. An extensive analysis of the structure of many chemicals by Dr John Ashby supports the concept that the majority of chemicals that are mutagenic to *Salmonella* possess specific structural 'alerts' for electrophilic potential consistent with their ability to mutagenize *Salmonella* and to react in other genetic toxicity assays. The group of carcinogens that was not mutagenic did not demonstrate any apparent structural features that were consistent with mutagenic potential. Thus, there are alternative mechanisms of carcinogenesis that do not involve direct interaction with cellular DNA. Theoretically, it should be possible to compensate for the limitations imposed by the use of *in vitro* metabolic activation systems by studying the genetic toxicity of chemicals in whole animals. To that end, over a hundred chemicals were evaluated for the ability to induce chromosome damage *in vivo*. However, even these assays do not significantly complement the *Salmonella* assay, thereby providing little additional evidence for non-mutagenic mechanisms of carcinogenesis. Figure 6.5 gives a diagram of chemical structures associated with electrophilic potential. These structures are incorporated into an artificial molecule in order to illustrate the various electrophilic groups which correlate with both mutagenic and carcinogenic potential. Analysis of the structure of chemicals that do not show electrophilic groups, but which are tumorigenic, has not resulted in the identification of structure-activity relationships that predict non-mutagenic carcinogens.

Thus, *in vitro* systems are valuable in the identification of mutagenic chemicals, and the association between mutagenic potential and the ability to induce tumours in rodents is very high. Among the human carcinogens shown in Table 6.1 and among the chemicals that induce cancers in both rats and mice, a very high percentage are mutagens. Thus, mutagenicity is a clear risk factor for carcinogenic potential, but the absence of a mutagenic effect in an *in vitro* or *in vivo* system does not necessarily indicate that the chemical lacks carcinogenic potential in rodent bioassays.

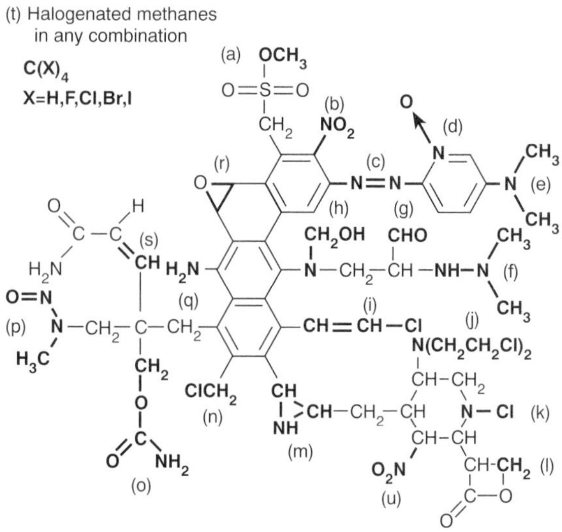

6.8 Prospects

6.8.1 Early diagnosis of precancerous conditions

With most precancerous lesions, there are no problems for the patient, who is probably unaware of their presence. In rare circumstances, a large adenoma of the bowel for instance may cause obstruction or bleed chronically and require surgery, but generally the lesions are asymptomatic. These situations are distinct from some other clinical conditions, such as ataxia telangiectasia and Down's syndrome, where obvious multiple abnormalities exist, including an increased risk of particular cancers to which the clinician will already be alerted.

Fig. 6.5 Modified version of the model compound upon which structural alerts to genotoxicity are based. The structure shown earlier in Ashby and Tennant (1988) has been supplemented with a centre of Michael reactivity (s). Halomonocarbons (t) have been added as a separate structure because their potential genotoxicity will probably not become evident when attached to a larger molecule. Thus, α,α-dichlorotoluene (PhCHCl$_2$) should not be considered as an active analogue of dichloromethane (CH$_2$Cl$_2$), just as aniline (PhNH$_2$) is not usefully considered as an analogue of ammonia (NH$_3$). The structural subunits are as follows: (a) alkyl esters of either phosphonic or sulphonic acids; (b) aromatic nitro groups; (c) aromatic azo groups, not *per se*, but by virtue of their possible reduction to an aromatic amine; (d) aromatic ring *N*-oxides; (3) aromatic mono- and di-alkylamino groups; (f) alkyl hydrazines; (g) alkyl aldehydes; (h) *N*-methylol derivatives; (i) monohaloalkenes; (j) a large family of N and S mustards (β-haloethyl); (k) *N*-chloramines (see below); (l) propiolactones and propiosultones; (m) aromatic and aliphatic aziridinyl derivatives; (n) both aromatic- and aliphati-substituted primary alkyl halides; (o) derivatives of urethane (carbamates); (p) alkyl *N*-nitrosamines; (q) aromatic amines, their *N*-hydroxy derivatives, and the derived esters; (r) aliphatic epoxides and aromatic oxides; (u) an aliphatic nitro group, as present in tetranitromethane (Tennant and Ashby 1991). Qualifications or refinements of these units are discussed in Ashby and Tennant (1988). The *N*-chloramine substructure (k) has not yet been associated with carcinogenicity, but potent genotoxic activity has been reported for it (discussed in Ashby and Tennant 1988).

The main clinical problems in cancer usually arise when metastasis occurs to distant parts of the body (see Chapter 2) so that local surgical excision or radiation therapy is no longer feasible. By definition, precancerous tissues of epithelial origin have not invaded the underlying stroma (see Chapter 1) although the individual cells may be highly abnormal in other respects. There can only be the possibility of metastasis once invasion has taken place. In some tissues, such as breast, this may take place when the cancer is very small, but cancer cells must at least have penetrated vessels in the stroma. Is there any way of detecting abnormal precancerous tissues before invasive properties are acquired? In some cases there may be. The haemoccult test used to detect cancer of the colon and rectum relies on the fact that many cancers ulcerate and bleed chronically and blood can be detected biochemically in the faeces. Thus a simple screening test can often help in diagnosing cancer in individuals with bowel problems, when malignancy is suspected. In fact, many precancerous adenomas of the large bowel, particularly the more advanced ones, will also be detected with this test, and can be removed surgically. In the near future, it should be possible to use a similar approach to detect more specific products of premalignant colon cells in faecal samples, either actively secreted into the bowel lumen or shed from dead cells. The problem is whether this type of test will be practical for the population as a whole, perhaps only for those over a certain age, or just for high risk individuals with a family history (see Chapter 4). Similar principles could, theoretically, apply to products of abnormal tissues released into other body fluids. Screening for cervical precancerous lesions using a smear from the cervix to look for abnormal cells is a well-known example of a different technique used to identify potential cancers before the risk of invasion and metastases arises (see Chapter 21). Apart from these examples, screening for overt cancer of various tissues and organs presents a great problem, with little chance at present of finding precancerous lesions by current insensitive and, for the most part, non-specific methods. It is in this area of clinical cancer research that much effort is needed, particularly where clinicians and scientists in the laboratory can combine efforts and devise sensitive diagnostic procedures. Monoclonal antibody technology will undoubtedly have a major influence in this area (see Chapters 17, 18, and 21).

6.8.2 Understanding and preventing tumour progression

Very little is known about the factors that govern the fate of precancerous lesions and determine whether or not a cancer develops and progresses. Some clues have come from epidemiological studies (see Chapter 3) but information is sparse. To take the example of cigarette smoking, where components of the smoke are thought to promote development of lung cancer in the later stages of carcinogenesis. This tumour progression phase can be retarded by stopping smoking however long ago the habit was established (see Chapter 3). In the case of liver cancer, hepatitis B virus infection and chronic hepatitis probably act as promoting influences, particularly in the Third World (see Chapter 8). It is likely that this occurs through the creation of tissue damage, which in turn stimulates regeneration, a situation which is known from animal experiments to allow expression of chemical carcinogen-induced genetic changes, culminating in cancer. Improved availability of preventive measures, particularly viral vaccines, would almost certainly reduce the overall incidence of this cancer. It may also be effective to modify the diet, or hormonal status, in individuals with precancerous lesions of particular tissues or in those in a high risk group for cancer development.

Much more needs to be done to identify potential promoting agents for the common cancers and thus the means for intervention in the process of tumour progression. It may be more practicable to arrest the development of the disease or slow its progress sufficiently for it to cease to be life threatening, than to prevent its initiation.

6.9 Summary

Numerous chemicals and environmental factors have been shown to cause cancer in humans and animal models. Most known human carcinogens are represented by chemicals or processes encountered in occupational exposure, drug therapy (particularly chemotherapy), and environmental exposures such as sunlight and tobacco use. The high concordance between the capacity of the known human carcinogens to induce cancer in rodents, and to demonstrate mutagenicity *in vitro* suggests that many other agents that are mutagenic and carcinogenic in rodents, but for which no clear clinical or epidemiological evidence exists, may also be human carcinogens. The most problematic agents are those that are not mutagenic and that show limited capacity to induce tumours in rodents. There are many important factors that can mitigate or enhance the effects of carcinogens that involve inherited susceptibility. With the multitude of genes that influence chemical metabolism and distribution, and DNA repair, and the many other factors within the life style such as diet, geography, social customs, etc., it is clear that the risk for environmental carcinogenesis is not equally distributed among all people. Important goals of current research efforts are to determine the various mechanisms by which known carcinogens act and to identify and define the function of specific genes that confer increased susceptibility, or which are the targets of environmental carcinogens.

References and further reading

Ames, B. N., McCann, J., and Yamasaki, E. (1975). Methods for detecting carcinogens and mutagens with the *Salmonella*/mammalian-microsome mutagenicity test. *Mutation Research*, **31**, 347–64.

Ashby, J. and Tennant, R. W. (1988). Chemical structure, *Salmonella* mutagenicity and extent of carcinogenicity as indicators of genotoxic carcinogenesis among 222 chemicals tested in rodents by the U.S. NCI/NTP. *Mutation Research*, **204**, 17–115.

Ashby, J. and Tennant, R. W. (1991). Definitive relationships among chemical structure, carcinogenicity and mutagenicity for 301 chemicals tested by the U.S. National Toxicology Program. *Mutation Research*, **257**, 229–306.

Balmain, A. and Brown, K. (1988). Oncogene activation in chemical carcinogenesis. *Advances in Cancer Research*, **51**, 147–82.

Barrett, J. C. and Preston, G. (1994). Apoptosis and cellular senescence. In *The molecular basis of apoptosis in disease*, pp. 253–81. Cold Spring Harbor Laboratory Press, New York.

DeCosse, J. J. (1983). Precancer. *Cancer Surveys*, **2**, 347–518.

Farber, E. (1986). Some general principles emerging in the pathogenesis of hepatocellular carcinoma. *Cancer Surveys*, **5**, 695–718.

Franks, L. M. and Wigley, C. B. (ed.) (1979). *Neoplastic transformation in differentiated epithelial cell systems in vitro*. Academic Press, Orlando.

Freeman, A. E. (1980). Induction of mammalian cell transformation by chemical carcinogens: basic considerations. In *Mammalian cell transformation by chemical carcinogens* (ed. N. Mishra, V. Dunkel, and M. Mehlman), pp. 37–45. Senate Press, Princeton, New Jersey.

IARC Monographs. Suppl. 2 (1980). *Long term and short term screening assays for carcinogens: a critical appraisal*. IARC, Lyon.

Moolgavkar, S. H. and Knudson, A. G., jun. (1981). Mutation and cancer: a model for human carcinogenesis. *Journal of the National Cancer Institute*, **66**, 1037–52.

Reznikoff, C. A., Bertram, J. S., Brankow, D. W., and Heidelberger, C. (1973). Quantitative and qualitative studies of chemical transformation of cloned C3H mouse embryo cells sensitive to post-confluence inhibition of cell division. *Cancer Research*, **33**, 3239–49.

Rosenberg, M. P. (1993). Transgenic mouse models of cancer. In *The molecular basis of human cancer* (ed. B. Neel and R. Kumar), pp. 397–432. Futura Publishing Company, New York.

Shields, P. G. and Harris, C. C. (1993). *Principles of carcinogenesis: chemicals in cancer—principles and practice of oncology*, Vol. 1, (ed. V. T. DeVita, S. Hellman, and S. A. Rosenberg), pp. 200–12. J. B. Lippincott, Philadelphia.

Stewart, T. A., Pattengale, P. K., and Leder, P. (1984). Spontaneous mammary adenocarcinomas in transgenic mice that carry and express MTV/myc fusion genes. *Cell*, **38**, 627–37.

Tennant, R. W. and Ashby, J. (1991). Classification according to chemical structure, mutagenicity to *Salmonella* and level of carcinogenicity of a further 39 chemicals tested for carcinogenicity by the U.S. National Toxicology Program. *Mutation Research*, **257**, 209–27.

Willis, A. E., Weksberg, R., Tomlinson, S., and Lindahl, T. (1987). Structural alterations of DNA ligase 1 in Bloom's syndrome. *Proceedings of the National Academy of Sciences, USA*, **84**, 8016–20.

Yuspa, S. and Poiret, M. C. (1988). Chemical carcinogenesis: from animal models to molecular models in one decade. *Advances in Cancer Research*, **50**, 25–70.

7

Radiation carcinogenesis

G. E. ADAMS AND R. COX

7.1 Introduction

7.1.1 The problem

Although humans have always been exposed to natural background ionizing radiation, there is considerable doubt whether in the past such exposures have had any significant role to play in the aetiology of human cancer. Radiation carcinogenesis is a twentieth century problem, as indeed are the problems of carcinogenic risk from many other hazards to which society is exposed. Cancers induced by ionizing radiation are indistinguishable from most cancers arising from other causes and their occurrence can only be identified by a statistical analysis of excess incidence over the 'natural' incidence. However, rapid developments are taking place in the molecular genetics of cellular control mechanisms including the identification of mutant markers in growth control genes, e.g. *p53* (see Chapter 9). That, coupled with the increasing evidence that gross deletions are common in cytogenetic abnormalities caused by radiation suggests that specific markers of radiation-induced cancer will be identified in the not too distant future. At present, much of our information on human radiation carcinogenesis is derived, therefore, from epidemiological sources. Studies of occupational exposure of diagnostic radiologists, uranium miners, and workers in the nuclear industries, for example, have provided some infor-

mation. Much more, however, has come from analyses of cancer incidence in patients exposed to radiation for medical purposes, either for diagnosis or for treatment of non-malignant conditions.

Another major source of information has been the long-term follow-up of survivors of the atomic bombs dropped in 1945 on Nagasaki and Hiroshima. This Life Span Study has been in progress since 1950 and has achieved a remarkable level of precision, particularly in regard to the dosimetry. In many cases, the precise location of the individuals and the shielding effect of buildings and other structures is now known accurately.

Studies on radiation carcinogenesis in experimental animals have addressed problems such as the pathogenesis of the various cancers that have been identified, interspecies variation, the relationships between cancer induction and cell mutation and other cellular phenomena, dose relationships, and, most important of all, the validity or otherwise of animal experiments for assessing radiation risk in human populations. While such studies have provided much information on the biology of radiation carcinogenesis, estimates of radiation risk in humans still rest heavily on the data from epidemiological studies. As in other fields of carcinogenesis, knowledge of events at the cellular and molecular level is essential to an understanding of radiation carcinogenesis, a complex multistage process that extends from the very early physical, chemical, and cellular changes initiated by the absorption of radiation to the delayed effects that only appear many years later.

The energies of photon or particulate radiations emanating from radionuclides, X-ray sets, and particle accelerators are vastly in excess of those of the chemical bonds in biological molecules. Ionization, i.e. electron ejection from atoms with which the radiation interacts, is therefore the primary initial event. The time-scale over which energy is imparted to the atom is governed by the speed of the particle (usually at or near the velocity of light), the dimensions of the atom, and the extent of energy loss. A quantum of γ radiation, or an energetic α particle, will pass through a small molecule and deliver energy to it, in a time between 10^{-17} and 10^{-18} seconds. The subsequent physical, chemical, and biological processes that follow this event are only expressed as an induced cancer perhaps 30 years or more later. Thus the time-scales of the earliest physical and the latest biological effects of radiation can differ by as much as a factor of 10^{27}. Therefore, it is not surprising that the interpretation of radiation carcinogenesis in terms of the primary physical and molecular events is a complex undertaking.

7.1.2 The temporal stages of radiation action

It is convenient, though not rigorously precise, to classify the many processes of radiation action into four stages; namely, physical, chemical, cellular, and tissue effects (Table 7.1).

The physical stage Radiation deposits its energy in discrete packages. Their magnitude and spatial distribution depend on factors such as the energy of the radiation, the nature of the absorbing medium, and particularly the type of radiation. The 'densely ionizing' radiations (i.e. α-particles, protons, and neutrons) lose energy over a much shorter distance than do the 'weakly ionizing' X- and γ-rays. The biological effectiveness of the particulate radiations in cell killing, mutagenicity, cell transformation, and carcinogenic potential are substantially greater than the weakly ionizing or low 'LET' radiations (LET or 'linear energy transfer' is a measure of the rate at which energy is imparted to the absorbing medium per unit distance of track length). The physical descriptions of the tracks of ionizing radiation passing through a cell differ considerably between X- or γ-rays (low 'LET') and particulate radiation such as α-particles. Such tracks can be simulated from theoretical analysis using Monte Carlo calculations, and this has given much insight into the problem of energy distribution in irradiated cells. This is discussed later in the context of molecular mechanisms of radiation action.

Interaction of radiation with an atom ejects an electron, or electrons, in less than $\approx 10^{-16}$ s. The

Table 7.1 The temporal stages of radiation action

1.	*The physical stage*	
	10^{-18}–10^{-17} (s)	Fast particle traverses small atom or molecule
	10^{-16}	Ionization: $H_2O \rightarrow H_2O^+ + e^-$
	10^{-15}	Electronic excitation: $H_2O \rightarrow H_2O^*$
	10^{-13}	Molecular vibrations: dissociation
	10^{-12}	Rotational relaxation: $e^- \rightarrow e^-$ aq
2.	*Physicochemical and chemical stage*	
	10^{-10}–10^{-7} (s)	Reactions of e^- aq and other free radicals with solutes in radiation tracks and spurs
	10^{-7}	Homogeneous distribution of free radicals
	10^{-3}	Free radical reactions, largely complete
	Seconds, minutes, hours	Biochemical changes (enzyme reactions)
3.	*Cellular and tissue stage*	
	Hours	Cell division inhibited in microorganisms and mammalian cells; reproductive death
	Days	Damage to gastrointestinal tract (and central nervous system at high doses)
	Months	Haemopoietic death; acute damage to skin and other organs; late normal tissue morbidity
	Years	Carcinogenesis and expression of genetic damage in offspring

ejected electrons have energy greatly in excess of atomic ionization potentials and cause many more of the secondary ionizations responsible for the subsequent chemical changes that lead to biological damage. The secondary electrons lose energy by collision and eventually undergo dipole interaction. This involves electrostatic interaction between the negative charges of the secondary electrons and the slight positive charge associated with the hydrogen atoms in water. This polarization in water is a result of the higher electronegativity of the oxygen atom compared with that of hydrogen. The interaction in aqueous media is complete in about 10^{-12} s ('the dielectric relaxation time'). The trapped electron, or, as it is called, 'the hydrated electron' $[e^-(aq)]$, has, in many respects, the properties of many free radicals. It can diffuse considerable distances and can undergo rapid reaction with many diverse types of chemical structures including those present in most biological molecules. Its formation marks the transition to the chemical stage of radiation action.

The chemical stage The chemical stage of radiation action is concerned mainly with the formation and reaction of molecular fragments such as free radicals and excited molecules. Roughly speaking, radiation energy deposited in the cell is partitioned according to the relative proportions of the constituent atoms (at least for the low atomic number elements normally represented in biological tissue). This is known as 'the principle of equipartition of energy' and implies that about 80 per cent of the overall energy deposited in the cell by ionizing radiations initially occurs in the aqueous component. This is why so much attention in the past has been devoted to the study of the radiation chemistry of water and aqueous solutions.

The hydroxyl radical (OH), an oxidizing species of high reactivity, is formed very quickly from the ionized water molecule, H_2O^+, by interaction with neighbouring water molecules and by rapid dissociation of excited H_2O molecules. The reactive hydrogen atoms and hydrated electrons are the corresponding reducing equivalents so that, overall, water radiolysis is described by the simple equation

$$H_2O \rightarrow H[+e^-(aq)] + OH$$

Some of the radicals interact together to form molecular hydrogen and hydrogen peroxide. The remaining radicals diffuse away from the radiation track and react with other molecules in the environment.

There is much evidence that damage to biological molecules caused by free radicals contributes to loss or change of cellular function following irradiation. The problem that remains is to identify those reactions that are relevant to the observed cellular response to radiation. The time-scales for these reactions are very short and most will be complete in times much less than a millisecond. Others, however, will take longer.

The cellular stage Ultrastructural changes in cells can sometimes be observed a short time after irradiation. Local protrusions of the plasma membrane, for example, can be observed within minutes of exposure of cells to a relatively high dose of radiation. Within a few hours these changes are followed by membrane distension and later by invagination of the nuclear membrane. These effects are accompanied by changes in the permeability of the membrane and loss of essential enzymes. However, the more important effects (i.e. the loss of, or changes in, cellular function that occur at much lower radiation doses) can only be observed after longer periods. Loss of reproductive capacity is only evident when the cell fails to divide, and chromosomal changes or cellular mutations are observable only after sufficient cell divisions have taken place to allow the analyses of aberrant cells in the total population. Similarly, measurement of changes in the repair capacity of irradiated cells, a process that is normally complete within a few hours of irradiation, usually requires clonal analysis of irradiated populations. Nevertheless, the stages in the cell cycle when radiation damage is most critical are now known. Mammalian cells are usually most radiosensitive during mitosis and very early in the G_1 phase, and are usually at their most resistant in early S phase, although this is very dependent on radiation quality. Cellular sensitivity to low LET radiation is usually much more variable than it is to high LET radiation.

The tissue stage The response times of mammalian tissues to radiation exposure vary widely, as do their sensitivities. The observation that mammalian cells show maximum sensitivity to radiation during mitosis predicts firstly that the fertilized mammalian egg cell (zygote) would be highly sensitive to radiation, and secondly that, in the animal, the most radiation-sensitive tissues would be those that turn over rapidly. This is indeed the case. The rapidly dividing proliferating stem cells of the hae-mopoietic system and the intestinal epithelium are particularly sensitive and respond more quickly than do the moderately sensitive tissues such as lung and the basal layer of the skin. Cells that do not normally divide except after an appropriate sti-mulus, i.e. parenchymal cells of the liver and con-nective tissue, are less sensitive still, and cells that divide only during embryonic development are the least radiosensitive. The time of onset for normal tissue damage and mortality depends on the radia-tion dose. The nature, origin, and expression of ra-diation injury at the tissue level are classified according to the organ in which such injury occurs. The International Commission on Radiological Protection (ICRP) (ICRP 1977) made a clear dis-tinction between so-called stochastic and non-sto-chastic effects. The former are those where the probability of injury but *not* the severity, increases with radiation dose. Non-stochastic effects, how-ever, increase in severity with increasing dose and also usually show a threshold dose below which *no*

discernible damage occurs. Examples of non-sto-chastic effects resulting from injury to a substantial population of cells include induction of visual de-fects such as cataract formation, lung fibrosis, in-fertility, loss of function in the gastrointestinal tract, and suppression of stem cell production in the bone marrow.

Stochastic effects can result from injury to a single cell, or a small number of cells, and include induc-tion of some genetic abnormalities and, in particu-lar, cancer.

The essential features of stochastic and non-sto-chastic effects are illustrated in Fig. 7.1 (taken from ICRP 1984).

7.2 Radiation and human cancer

7.2.1 Radiation dose and radiation risk

Radiation dose to tissue is expressed in terms of absorbed energy per unit mass, the gray (Gy),

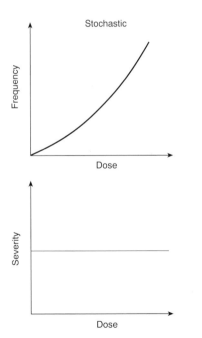

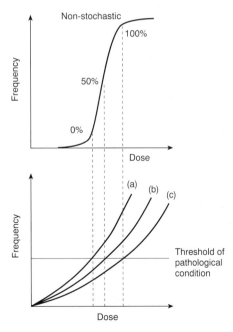

Fig. 7.1 Dose–effect curves illustrating stochastic and non-stochastic effects. The upper and lower plots on the left of the figure illustrate that the frequency of a stochastic effect increases with radiation dose, but not the severity. The upper and lower plots on the right of the figure show how the frequency and severity of a given radiation injury of a non-stochastic type

increase with radiation dose in a population of mixed susceptibilities (a, b, and c). The severity increases most rapidly with dose in the most sensitive group (curve a) and reaches a level of clinical detectability at a dose lower than those for the other two subgroups (curves b and c). Redrawn from ICRP (1984).

which is 1 joule/kg. The older unit, the rad, still in common use, is equivalent to 100 ergs absorbed per gram of tissue and is equal to 0.01 Gy. Carcinogenic potential depends upon absorbed dose and is greater per unit dose for high LET radiations than for low LET radiations. The latter type becomes less effective per Gy as the dose falls, which is not the case for high LET radiation. This means that, for example, neutrons that are five times more effective than gamma rays at a given dose may be relatively much more effective than gamma rays over a lower dose range. This dose dependence of relative biological efficiency (RBE) is a problem in assessing risk following exposure to a mixture of radiation qualities. This has been encountered in the analysis of the atomic bomb data from Japan.

Estimates of cancer risk may be made in various ways. *Additive* risk expresses the number of *excess* cases per unit of time per unit of dose in a given number of exposed individuals. The *multiplicative* or relative risk model expresses the ratio of the risk in the irradiated population to that in a non-irradiated control group. Additive risk has the advantage of specifying the number of individuals involved and is the approach favoured by UNSCEAR (United Nations Scientific Committee on the Effects of Atomic Radiations) in the absolute risk model. For example, a risk of 10^{-4} implies one excess cancer over a given period, in a population of 10 000 individuals, each of whom has received an average dose of 1 Gy.

The magnitude of the risk to the population at large from environmental radiation remains a topic of constant enquiry. It has been calculated that for an 'average' individual exposure of say 25 millisieverts per year, risk of any single gene mutation would appear to be 1 in 20 000. This takes no account of variations in individual radiation sensitivities, cancer proneness, or other genetically based mechanisms of radiation damage in sensitive groups in the population. Without doubt, the *overall* risk from the normal levels of environmental radiation to the population at large is very low. Nevertheless, the search for higher risk subgroups remains important.

7.2.2 Radiation epidemiology

Numerous long-term studies are in progress on human populations that have been exposed to radiation. These studies ask questions about overall cancer incidence, excess of individual cancers, latency periods, and, where possible, doseresponse relationships in groups of individuals exposed to radiation arising from occupation, the environment, and diagnostic or therapeutic medical procedures (BEIR 1980, 1988; UNSCEAR 1988, 1993, 1994).

Occupational exposure Excess lung cancers have been observed in underground workers including uranium miners, fluorspar miners in Newfoundland, and some Swedish zinc and iron ore miners. The cancers are owing to α-particle radiation from inhaled radon gas emanating from radium present in the ores. Risk estimates are complicated by the long average latency period of 20 years, difficulties of assessing dose, and the evidence that heavy cigarette smoking substantially increases the risk.

Painters of luminous watch dials have been exposed to radiation through ingestion (by brush licking) of substantial quantities of radium-226 and radium-228. These isotopes concentrate in the bone matrix and emit short-range α-particles. Results from a large US study have revealed 62 bone sarcomas and 32 carcinomas of the mastoid and paranasal sinuses in a total of about 2000 female dial painters. No more than one case would have been expected.

Environmental exposure Exposures to natural sources of radiation are very low. It has been estimated, for example, that by the age of 65 the average US citizen has accumulated the equivalent of only 0.12 Gy from all natural sources and 0.04 Gy from man-made sources. However, concern is increasing in several countries, including the UK, that there is a small, but significant risk to health arising from exposure inside dwellings to the radioactive gas radon. This element has three naturally occurring isotopes, radon-219, radon-220, and radon-222 of which only the last two are of radiological consequence. Of these, radon-222 is the more important because of its longer half-life (3.824 days). Radon-222 is formed in the uranium-238 decay series and is environmentally important because it decays (by α-particle emission) to form products or 'daughters' that are themselves radioactive. Radiation doses to the individual arise predominantly from irradiation of lung epithelium by α-particles from the decay products. Radon generated in rock, soil, and building materials, used for example as infill, diffuses readily and can attain relatively high levels, particularly in poorly ventilated rooms. Radon decay products form small ion clusters with water molecules or react chemically with vapours present in air. These decay products can become attached to aerosol particles and ultimately enter the body by inhalation.

A recent survey has estimated that in the UK the total average annual effective dose-equivalent from radon is about half of the radiation dose received from natural sources. This is misleading, however, since there is much regional and individual variation in domestic exposure to radon. In some cases, annual doses may be 1–2 orders of magnitude higher than the average and it is estimated that about 20 000 dwellings in the UK, mostly in the south-west of the country, require action to reduce radon levels indoors. The calculation of excess lung cancer risk to the population arising from exposure to radon is fraught with uncertainty because of the assumptions involved. However, one calculation using current risk estimates (O'Riordan 1988) indicates that about 1500 persons may die annually from lung cancer associated with exposure to radon and its decay products. To put this in context, however, this figure is somewhat less than 4 per cent of the total annual death rate from lung cancer in the UK and about one-quarter of the death rate from domestic accidents.

The possibility has been raised that inhaled radon may contribute to the incidence of leukaemia. While there is no direct evidence for this, Henshaw and colleagues (Richardson *et al.* 1991) have pointed out that the solubility of radon daughters in fat cells in bone marrow is much higher than would be anticipated. Calculations suggest that such levels could be important in inducing radiation damage in bone marrow stem cells *in situ*.

Although the *average* individual dose from man-made sources of environmental exposure is very low, substantial exposure has occurred in some select groups of individuals. For example, exposure to short- and long-lived radioisotopes of iodine in the fallout from atmospheric weapons testing is responsible for excess thyroid cancer found in a small group of 240 female Marshall Islanders. Estimates of thyroid doses vary between 0.15 and 15 Gy.

The main source of data in the field of exposure to man-made environmental radiation is the Life Span Study on survivors from the atomic bombs dropped on Japan. This study has followed about 80 000 survivors who were briefly exposed to the radiation. Cancer incidence in this population is compared

with that in 26 500 age-matched, non-irradiated controls. A total of 180 excess cancer deaths occurred over the period 1950–74, corresponding to an increase over control of about 5 per cent, although this figure is misleading since a large proportion of the irradiated population received low doses relative to the remainder. First, excess cancer has occurred mainly in the groups receiving a whole body dose of 1 Gy or greater and, secondly, the excess will undoubtedly increase after total lifetime follow-up. A further four-year follow-up has shown that the *total* cancer mortality from all causes has increased by 24 per cent. Figure 7.2 shows the *relative* risk of cancer mortality for various sites over the period 1950–78. The excess leukaemia prominent over the first twenty-year period is obviously still present although analysis has shown that it is no longer significant over the last four-year period. Conversely, there is now evidence of increased rates for cancer of the stomach, lung, breast, and urinary tract, and, for the first time, excess risk of colonic cancer and multiple myeloma. These data clearly illustrate the remarkably long latent periods in some types of radiation-induced cancers. Final risk estimates will have to await the entire postirradiation life span. Calculation of risks is also complicated by factors such as age at irradiation, sex, variation in dose-response relationships for different cancers, and differ-

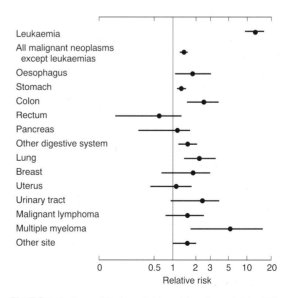

Fig. 7.2 Life Span Study: relative risk of mortality (90 per cent confidence intervals) for specific types of cancer (1950–78) (Kato and Schull 1982).

ences between incidence and mortality, which may be influenced over a protracted period by improvements in therapy.

There is considerable debate in the UK over reports of increased incidence of childhood leukaemia in the vicinity of some nuclear installations. In particular, small but statistically significant excesses of leukaemia have been identified in the populations living near the two nuclear reprocessing plants at Sellafield in Cumbria and Dounreay in the north of Scotland. The question as to whether or not these leukaemia clusters arise from man-made sources of radiation, or even radiation at all, is too complex to be discussed in detail here. However, some brief comment can be made. In consideration of the Sellafield cluster, Gardner and colleagues proposed in 1987 that the cluster could be a result of preconceptual irradiation of the fathers who worked at the Sellafield plant (Gardner *et al*. 1990). It is possible to calculate, from an estimate of the dose received, the magnitude of the risk factors that would have to apply in order for the cluster to be attributed to parental irradiation. Such risk factors would have to be about 2 per cent per Gy for a lifetime dose to about 20 per cent per Gy for a six-month dose. These are several orders of magnitude higher than those determined for non-malignant genetic abnormalities arising from parental irradiation.

UNSCEAR has calculated that the *total* genetic risk for all loci in F_1 and F_2 humans following parental irradiation is only about 0.3 per cent per Gy. However, some support for the Gardner hypothesis has been provided by studies of cancer induction in the offspring of mice irradiated preconceptually.

However, Doll and colleagues (1994) have examined the Sellafield cluster in the light of knowledge of radiation genetics, any possible heritability of childhood leukaemia, and the records of children of the irradiated atomic bomb survivors. They have concluded that, while a real cluster of leukaemia in young people has occurred near Sellafield, radiation is *not* responsible and other explanations must be sought.

Background levels of radiation in the environment rose substantially in the early sixties owing to fallout from nuclear weapons testing. At their peak, these levels were greatly in excess of the measured background levels in the vicinity of the reprocessing plants. It is argued (Darby and Doll 1987) that if the leukaemia clusters *were* attributable to these discharges then the relatively much larger doses from

nuclear fallout received by the general population during the weapons testing period should have caused a material increase some years later in the risk of childhood leukaemia elsewhere in the country. Analysis of temporal fluctuations of childhood leukaemia incidence in the UK as a whole and in Scandinavia showed no convincing evidence of an increase in incidence attributable to fallout let alone any increase comparable with that found around Dounreay. There are, however, some reservations and uncertainties concerning the estimate of radiation dose arising from ingestion of radionuclides from reprocessing waste, particularly if such nuclides become disproportionately concentrated in relevant tissues.

Cook-Mozaffari *et al*. (1989) have considered the distribution of cancer mortality in England and Wales. Estimates were made of relative risk associated with social class, rural status, population size, health authority region, and, in particular, proximity to one of 15 nuclear installations. The results confirm that there is an excess mortality from leukaemia, particularly lymphoid leukaemia, in the 0–24 age group in districts with some of the population resident within 10 miles of a nuclear installation, during 1969–78. The excess risk of persons under 25 years is small but statistically significant for all leukaemias (relative risk, RR = 1.5, $P = 0.01$), lymphoid leukaemia (RR = 1.21, $P = 0.01$), and Hodgkin's disease (RR = 1.24, $P = 0.05$). There is also, however, a significant deficiency of mortality from lymphoid leukaemia for persons aged 25–64 years (RR = 1.24, $P = 0.05$). Analysis provided no positive evidence that the increase in leukaemia is a result of environmental pollution from the installations.

A hypothesis in which an infective agent, unrelated to radiation, is considered to be involved in the aetiology of leukaemia, has been investigated by Kinlen (1988, 1995). The nuclear reprocessing plants at Dounreay and Sellafield were built in unusually isolated places where, it is postulated, herd immunity to widespread viral infections tended to be lower than average. The hypothesis is based on the premise that influxes of populations into previously isolated areas lead to epidemics of certain infections and that leukaemia is a rare response to some viral infections. Sellafield and Dounreay were identified as extreme examples of such communities. The town of Glenrothes in the rural district of Fife in Scotland was identified as a unique test of the hypothesis. Glenrothes, which is not near any nuclear installation, underwent a rapid expansion during the fifties and sixties. The community remained relatively isolated until the opening of a major road bridge in 1964. For the period 1951–67, there is a significant excess of leukaemia deaths below age 25 (10 observed and 3.6 expected). This excess is mainly accounted for by deaths at ages below 5 in the relevant period 1954–9. No excess was found for the period 1968–85. It is concluded that at least some of the excess leukaemia cases near the nuclear installation at Dounreay and Sellafield could be attributed to an infective agent mechanism since these locations represent even more extreme degrees of isolation combined with population influx.

Chernobyl In April 1986, a major nuclear accident occurred in a reactor in a nuclear installation in the Ukraine. Following the explosion, a huge cloud containing much radioactive debris drifted over a large area of northern Europe. The level of contamination in some parts of Belarus, Ukraine and the (now) Russian Federation was substantial. Careful examination has been made of any increase in childhood cancer in the years following the accident and a recent report (Stsjazhko *et al.* 1995) has described a substantial increase in thyroid cancer in children. The magnitude of the increase is very dependent on geographical region but, as an example, the *annual* rate of thyroid cancer for Belarus in children aged under 15 at diagnosis is 30.6 per million for the years 1991–4, compared with 0.3 for the period 1981–5. It has been estimated that for the population that continued to live in the region and to consume locally produced milk for the three months following the accident, the major dose to the thyroid arose from iodine-131 which is concentrated in the thyroid. Possible other consequences of the contamination from Chernobyl in regions and countries affected will be the subject of investigation for many years to come.

Medical exposure The evidence for cancer induction by radiation used for various medical treatments for non-malignant conditions is too substantial to review here, but a few general points can be made. Excess thyroid cancers have been observed in children and young adults treated with X-rays for enlarged tonsils, enlarged thymus, and nasopharyngeal disorders, and ringworm of the scalp. There is equivocal evidence of excess cancer in patients treated for hyperthyroidism with iodine-131, probably because the epithelial cells are killed by the high local doses of radiation.

Excess cases of leukaemia and cancers of the uterus, kidney, and bladder have occurred in women treated with pelvic irradiation for non-malignant gynaecological disorders. For example, leukaemia incidence in one group of patients had a two- to threefold increase over that expected. Excess breast cancer has also been reported in women who received fairly high doses of X-rays for treatment of mastitis during the period 1940–55, or during fluoroscopic examinations.

Two large current epidemiological studies are particularly significant. During the period 1935–57, in excess of 14 000 patients with ankylosing spondylitis were given a course of X-rays to ameliorate pain associated with the disease. Follow-up of earlier studies by Doll and colleagues (Weiss *et al.* 1994) have shown that cancer mortality was significantly greater than expected from the national rates for England and Wales with a relative risk of 1.30. Increased rates were found for leukaemia, non-Hodgkin's lymphoma, multiple myeloma and cancers of the oesophagus, colon, pancreas, lung, bones, connective and soft tissue, prostate, bladder and kidney. Relative risk decreased with time after irradiation, for all cancers, following an initial increase. While the increase in relative risk for lung cancers had completely disappeared 35 years after first treatment, it is noteworthy that it was still significantly high for other cancers although at a lower level than in earlier periods.

There is much concern over the risks arising from the ingestion of radionuclides such as radium and plutonium. These isotopes, which concentrate in the bones, decay by emission of energetic, short-range a-particles which can irradiate various regions of the bone matrix. Relevant to this are the results of studies on patients who were given multiple intravenous injections of radium-224 over a period of months to treat tuberculosis and ankylosing spondylitis. This isotope is short-lived (half-life of 3.6 days) and therefore decays while still on bone surfaces. In one study involving 681 adults and 218 juveniles (0–20 years) 18 and 35 cases of bone sarcoma, respectively, were reported, where an incidence rate of only 0.2 would have been expected (Gössner *et al.* 1985). Five cases of leukaemia have been reported in the higher age group but none occurred in the younger group. Two cases would have been expected in a normal population of comparable size, age, distribution, and follow-up time. It is pointed out, however, that the excess cases may not have been caused by the radiation in view of the possible leukaemogenic effect of the pain-killing drugs taken by spondylitic patients during the relevant period.

The induction of acute myeloid leukaemia (AML) has also been observed in experimental animals treated with such radionuclides. Deposition of the isotope on bone surfaces can lead to heavy irradiation of the marrow. Figure 7.3 is a neutron autoradiograph of plutonium-239 in trabecular bone and marrow of the mouse lumbar vertebrae. A thin section of bone is mounted on plastic sheet and placed in a nuclear reactor. Neutron-induced fission fragments of the plutonium and other fragments damage the plastic. After etching of the plastic, the fission fragment tracks show as black lines. Irradiation of the bone marrow is clearly evident.

7.2.3 Dose response relationships

The epidemiological data on radiation-induced leukaemia generally, its relatively short latency period, and the substantial evidence available from experimental laboratory studies, combine to make leukaemia the most suitable model for studying doseresponse relationships. Such information is essential for an understanding of the molecular and cellular aspects of radiation carcinogenesis as well as the calculation of risk for radiological protection purposes.

Figure 7.4 compares the dose response for mortality from all forms of leukaemia as observed in the ankylosing spondylitis study with that for induction

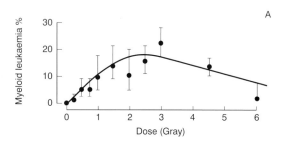

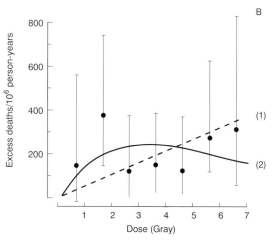

Fig. 7.4 Comparison of dose–response data for induction of myeloid leukaemia in male CBA/H mice after brief exposures to 250 kVp X-rays (a) (Mole *et al.* 1983) with excess mortality rate from leukaemia (as a function of mean bone marrow dose) in irradiated spondolytic patients (b) (Smith and Doll 1982). Line 1, linear dose–response relationship; line 2, linear dose–response relationship with cell-killing component included.

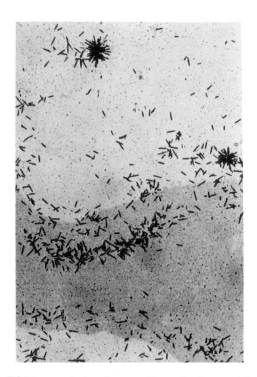

Fig. 7.3 Neutron-induced autoradiograph of α-particle tracks from plutonium-239 in mouse bone (see text).

of acute myeloid leukaemia in male CBA/H mice. The more precise experimental data clearly show an initial rise with increasing dose followed by a decrease at even higher doses. The human data are consistent with this type of response, as indeed are data for several other radiation-induced human and animal tumours. The overall response curve is influenced by two factors. The probability of a malignant transformation at the *cellular* level rises with increasing dose. However, when the dose is sufficient to sterilize (kill or prevent cell division) some cells, the number that survive, and are therefore capable of transformation, *falls* with increasing dose. The counterbalancing of these two effects results in the overall dose response for cancer induction.

Various empirical expressions have been used in attempts to describe the overall doseresponse relationships for human cancer induction although the lack of accurate data on radiation dosage is often a problem. For the experimental AML data in CBA/H mice, the curve fits the expression $P = \alpha D^2 e^{-\lambda D}$ reasonably well where P is the probability of induction, D is the radiation dose, and α and λ are constants. Knowledge of the response relationship for inactivation of the cells at risk would permit derivation of the response relationship for neoplastic transformation.

7.3 Cellular and molecular processes

7.3.1 Cell inactivation

A radiation dose of about 1 Gy leads to about 2×10^5 ionizations within the mammalian cell, of which approximately 1 per cent occur in the genomic material. A primary consequence is breakage of DNA strands. Of the 1000 or so strand breaks that occur, almost all disappear within a few hours, either by spontaneous rejoining, or by enzyme-mediated repair (see Chapter 5). Some breaks remain, possibly as aligned double-strand breaks, and these are the major cause of loss of viability of some cells. Nevertheless, at this dose, some 40 per cent of the irradiated cells retain the capacity for growth despite the large amount of chemical damage sustained by the cells. Much of the initial chemical damage caused by the radiation is therefore of no consequence to the fate of the cell. Only a very small part of the damage, caused perhaps by the fairly rare

local deposition of a large amount of energy near critical molecular sites, is important.

Useful information has been obtained from studies of the relative cytotoxic, mutagenic, and transforming abilities of radiations of different LET. Figure 7.5 shows typical dose–response 'survival' curves for cells in tissue culture irradiated with either low LET X-rays or high LET α-particles. High LET radiations invariably are more effective and frequently show an exponential dose relationship (linear on the semi-log plot in Fig. 7.5). In contrast, low LET dose responses are curved when plotted similarly, although, in some instances, the initial curvature observed at lower doses is followed by an exponential response. The LET differences in response are owing to the very different spatial patterns of the initial atomic and molecular damage. There is a greater probability of double-strand break formation from a single α-particle track than there is from either a single X-ray track or from the alignment of two single-strand breaks arising from two X-ray tracks. Many physical models based on such processes have been proposed to account for the shapes of dose–response curves based on the 'accumulation' of damage or 'interaction' of sublesions. There are, however, alternative explanations.

The spatial patterns of energy deposition by low and high LET radiation are very different over the scale of cellular, subcellular, and macromolecular dimensions (Goodhead 1988). Monte Carlo

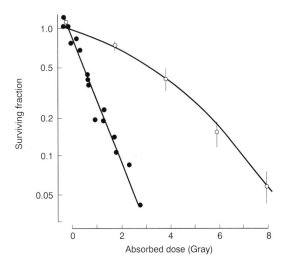

Fig. 7.5 Survival curves for V79 cells irradiated with low LET X-rays (○) and high LET α-particles (●) (from Thacker *et al.* 1982).

methods can be used to analyse and simulate radiation tracks passing through a cell. Figure 7.6 shows the results of such calculations for material irradiated with γ-rays or slow α-particles. For γ-rays, energy deposition occurs through the cell although there is much heterogeneity on a smaller scale. There are about 1000 tracks of energy deposition within the cell for a dose of 1 Gy. In contrast, energy deposition from α-particles occurs over a much smaller number of very narrow tracks. A dose of 1 Gy in this instance would correspond to only about four tracks. Even though numerous, the tracks from λ-rays are unlikely to deposit energy in given short lengths of chromatin. When energy deposition does occur, it will be in the form of individual ionizations or excitations arising in fairly isolated clusters. Although the likelihood of energy deposition from α-particles within a given section of chromatin is small, when it does occur, the amount of energy deposited is very much larger, with presumably greater consequences with regard to molecular damage in the region.

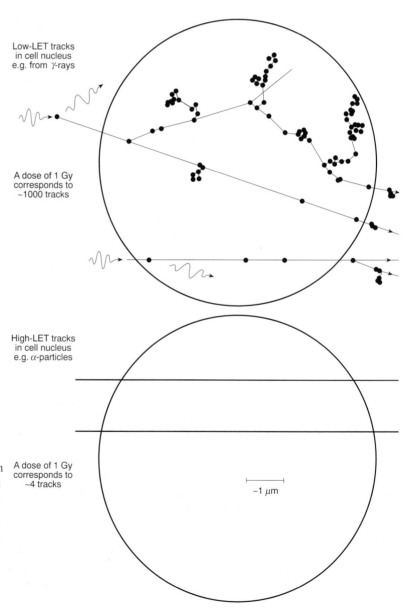

Low-LET tracks
in cell nucleus
e.g. from γ-rays

A dose of 1 Gy
corresponds to
~1000 tracks

High-LET tracks
in cell nucleus
e.g. α-particles

A dose of 1 Gy
corresponds to
~4 tracks

~1 μm

Fig. 7.6 Schematic representation of a cell nucleus irradiated with two electron tracks from γ-rays (low LET) or two α-particle tracks (high LET). A true scale diagram would require that the clusters of ionizations at the track ends be much more compact. From Goodhead (1988).

Cells irradiated at low dose rates or with intermittent radiation show reduced inactivation. The effect of such treatments on the shape of doseresponse curves has been explained on the basis of enzyme-mediated 'restoration' or 'repair' processes. There is direct evidence that single-strand breaks are much more readily repaired than double-strand breaks and therefore repair processes should be more efficient for low LET irradiation. The presence of a shoulder on low LET and survival curves is consistent with the existence of repair mechanisms which become inactivated, or more probably saturated, at higher doses.

7.3.2 Chromosome damage, cell mutation, and genetic instability

Chromosomal aberrations Radiation causes a variety of structural aberrations in mammalian chromosomes only some of which are lethal. Most of these aberrations appear to result from interactions between two or more lesions and can be conveniently grouped as exchanges (interchanges, intra-arm interchanges, and inter-arm intrachanges) and breaks or discontinuities. Not all such aberrations lead to cell death nor do those that are transmissible necessarily have detectable genetic consequences. The position of the cell in its cycle (or its status with regard to DNA duplication) leads to two types of aberration observed at metaphase (see Chapter 10). These are *chromosome type*, where both sister chromatids are involved in exchange for a given locus, and *chromatid type* where only one is affected. Radiation produces both types of aberration in contrast to most chemical chromosome-damaging agents, which cause only the latter type of aberration, as a rule.

Since cell sterilization and chromosome aberrations involve damage at the DNA level, one might expect some common types of behaviour in radiation dose–response relationships. The efficiency of aberration induction for low LET radiations falls at low dose rates and for intermittent, or fractionated, radiation. Figure 7.7 compares the efficiencies for the formation of asymmetrical interchanges (dicentric aberrations) in human lymphocytes irradiated with single doses of either γ-rays or fission neutrons. As for cell inactivation, the high LET neutrons are substantially more effective than the low LET γ-rays on an equidose basis.

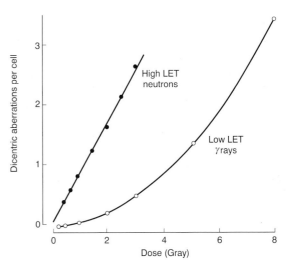

Fig. 7.7 The different effficiencies of high LET fission neutrons and low LET γ-rays in causing dicentric chromosome aberrations in human lymphocytes (combined data of Lloyd *et al.* 1975, 1976).

Single gene mutation and DNA repair The scale of the initial radiation chemical lesions and that of the chromosomal aberrations observed at the light microscope level are separated by several orders of magnitude. The considerable length of nuclear DNA associated with the nucleosomes is duplicated and packaged in a very precise configuration in 25-nm fibres which are themselves folded and coiled into the structure of the metaphase chromosome (see Chapter 5). The small-scale molecular changes that reveal themselves as major changes in chromosomal structure must involve considerable amplification. Further, it is likely that modification of some of the initial molecular changes will occur long before these chromosomal changes are observable. Studies at the single gene level provide a much higher degree of resolution.

Radiation-induced mutation in specific genes in target somatic cells is one plausible explanation for the initiation of cancer. It is useful therefore to consider briefly some of the molecular characteristics of mutations induced by radiation in somatic cells cultured *in vitro*. An end-point frequently used in radiation mutagenesis is the induction of thioguanine resistance in various mammalian cell lines. Resistance is a result of the induced reduction in activity of the enzyme hypoxanthine phosphoribosyl transferase (HPRT) whose normal function is to enable cells to incorporate purines from the growth medium (see Chapter 6). The coding gene is located on the X chromosome and therefore only one gene alteration may be required to show mutant behaviour. This allows elevation of mutation frequencies to be observed at fairly low radiation doses. Indirect evidence from various biochemical, cytogenetic, and immunological studies (Thacker 1986) has indicated that the majority of radiation-induced mutations at the HPRT locus are associated with deletions and/or rearrangement of DNA sequences within the HPRT region. In general terms, the evidence indicates that radiation-induced *point* mutation at this locus is either infrequent or masked by large rearrangements and deletions. This contrasts with mutation at HPRT by both ultraviolet (UV) light and chemicals, where point mutation appears to be the dominant mechanism. There are striking examples where irradiation of stem cell populations can lead to very large deletions which are *not* lethal to the cells in which the changes have taken place. Cattanach *et al.* (1993) have observed large, non-lethal chromosomal deletions in the offspring of mice following irradiation of parental spermatogonia. Remarkably, deletions of up to 10 per cent of an entire chromosome can be sustained without loss of fertility (see Table 7.2). One may speculate on the consequence of losses of large amounts of chromosomal material with respect to cancer induction. Deletions of such magnitude imply the loss of many genes in the affected chromosomes. There are many genes in the human genome controlling various mechanisms associated with cell progression, differentiation, apoptosis, and processes involved in cellular signalling pathways. It is clearly possible for a growth advantage to be given to an irradiated cell population by loss of function of one or more such genes occurring as a result of random radiation action. The probability, per unit dose, of such an event occurring would be clearly many times greater than that for a *specific locus* mutation where a direct

hit on a particular gene would be required. It is partly for this reason that there is rapidly increasing interest in radiation effects on genetic control mechanisms.

It is interesting that the efficiencies of radiation in causing cellular inactivation and mutation often appear to be quantitatively related. An example is shown in Fig. 7.8, again for mutation at the HPRT locus. The plot of mutation frequency corrected for cell lethality, against the logarithm of the fraction of the irradiated population that survives the radiation, is linear. This relationship is not affected by variations in the shapes of the individual radiation doseresponse curves for both mutation and cell kill between the different cell types. It is difficult to reconcile this behaviour in terms of two independent lesions leading either to cell death or to mutation. Thacker has argued that the repair process used by the cell in attempting to deal with the initial radiation damage is not entirely error free. If the probability of the repair system for *changing* the genetic material relative to that for *elimination* of the lesion in order to give non-mutant survivors is fixed, this would explain the constancy of the slope for the data in Fig. 7.7. To what extent such behaviour holds for high LET radiations has not been fully explored.

Ionizing radiation acts fairly non-specifically therefore to produce a very broad spectrum of types of molecular damage in DNA. The question as to which of these many different molecular lesions are biologically important remains largely unanswered. However, applications of gene transfer and recombinant DNA techniques to problems of mammalian cell radiosensitivity and DNA repair has

Table 7.2 Radiation-induced gross deletions produced by spermatogonial irradiation

Mutation	Chromosome	Deletion size (%)
Del(10)S1^{12}1H	10	10
Del(10)S1^{18}2H	10	3
Del(1)Sp^{1}3H	1	2

Data from Cattanach *et al.* (1993).

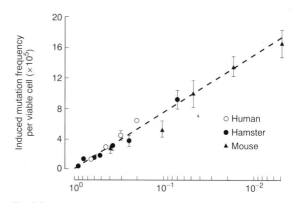

Fig. 7.8 Mutation survival relationships for the radiation induction of thioguanine-resistant mutants of cells from different species (from Thacker 1979).

yielded important information, particularly with regard to the role of DNA strand scissions in cellular radiosensitivity.

Studies on the autosomal recessive human genetic disorder, ataxia telangiectasia (AT) are particularly relevant to the role of DNA repair in oncogenesis. AT is a disease that is characterized mainly by neuromotor dysfunction, immunodeficiency, proneness to T cell neoplasia, and high radiosensitivity both *in vitro* and *in vivo*. Transfer of plasmid encoded genes containing inactivating DNA strand scissions into both normal human and AT cell lines has shown that AT cells exhibit greatly elevated *misrepair* of these scissions. This readily explains both the radiation sensitivity and apparent repair deficiency associated with the disorder (Cox *et al.* 1986). It is suggested that such *misrepair* might thereafter affect sequence-specific DNA recombination processes associated with maturation of the B cell immunoglobulin and T cell receptor systems and be implicated, therefore, in the immunodeficiency and the specific chromosomal rearrangements that characterize T cell neoplasia in AT. There is evidence in support of a close link between repair deficiency, enzyme (recombinase) function, and T cell neoplasia; firstly in that a chromosomal translocation (t7;14) observed in a T cell leukaemia in an AT patient involved aberrant recombination of the T cell receptor β gene and, secondly, reduced DNA topoisomerase II activity in AT cells.

Genetic instability It has generally been assumed, on the foundation of much evidence, that radiation-induced abnormalities observable in cells at the chromatid or chromosomal level that are non-lethal to the cell are *clonal* in nature. Such clonality implies that descendant cells can carry and express non-lethal abnormalities that are identical to those originally laid down in the ancestral irradiated cell. This is now being challenged. It is known, for example, that *delayed* cell death can occur and this has been attributed to the late expression of lethal mutations arising in the descendants of irradiated cells. Also, considerable clonal heterogeneity with regard to cell viability has been reported. Of particular interest is the finding that descendants of irradiated stem cells can show random *de novo* abnormalities in descendant cells that were not present in the irradiated ancestral cell. These have been observed both at the chromosomal level and through gene mutations. Transmissible genomic instability at the chromosomal level has been observed in primary cultures of both murine and human bone marrow stem cells (Kadhim *et al.* 1992, 1994). The instability is manifested by both chromatid and chromosomal random changes in cells in descendant clones.

It is perhaps significant that these changes in bone marrow stem cell cultures have been observed following irradiation by α-particles but so far, not by X- or γ-radiation. The spatial distribution of intracellular energy deposition along the track of an energetic α-particle is vastly different from that associated with transmission of X- or γ-radiation. The clustering of damage caused by an α-particle can be considerable even for the passage of a *single* α-particle through the genomic material of a cell. This transmissible instability has been observed under conditions where the probability of more than one α-particle track passing through a cell nucleus is very low indeed.

7.3.3 Radiation transformation and oncogenesis

There are clear dose–response interrelationships for radiation-induced cell inactivation, chromosomal rearrangements, and mutagenesis. One may ask: are such interrelationships of value in understanding mechanisms of radiation carcinogenesis?

There is now much research directed towards developing cellular systems *in vitro* that can be used to describe events associated with oncogenic transformation induced by radiation (see Hall 1988). In some established cell lines, neoplastic transformation can be induced by various agents, including some chemicals and radiation. Such transformed cells can induce tumours when reimplanted into the animal from which they were originally derived, or when transplanted into immunologically compatible hosts. Transformed cells *in vitro* usually display characteristics such as loss of anchorage dependence *in vitro*, loss of contact inhibition, and changes at the DNA level.

Radiation transformation *in vitro* was first observed by Borek and Sachs in 1966 using short-term cultures of Syrian hamster embryo cells. Transformation is indicated by the appearance of 'piled up' colonies on the culture plates. The C3H/10T$_{1/2}$ cell line (see Chapter 6) is also used frequently for radiation transformation studies. These fibroblast-like cells show normal contact inhibition when grown in confluent monolayer, but radiation treatment causes morphological changes. Colonies appear that overgrow the confluent layer and cells from these colonies can give rise to fibrosarcomas after inoculation into the appropriate animal host. Transformation efficiency can be expressed as a frequency per irradiated cell or per surviving cell. A disadvantage of this system is that the cells are less stable than the cells of the short-term hamster embryo cell system and spontaneous transformation may occur. Studies with this and other transforming systems show decreased transformation efficiency with decreasing radiation LET. This is in line with the trends for cell lethality and chromosomal aberration described earlier. Dose–response curves for γ-irradiated $10T_{1/2}$ cells show the 'bell-shaped' curves sometimes observed in experimental and human carcinogenesis (see Section 7.2.2 and Fig. 7.4). This is illustrated by the transformation data in Fig. 7.9 for $10T_{1/2}$ cells exposed to γ-radiation. Correction of the bottom curve, which is expressed as transformants per exposed cell, to take account of those cells that do not survive the treatment, gives the dose–response curve for the remaining cells that are at risk.

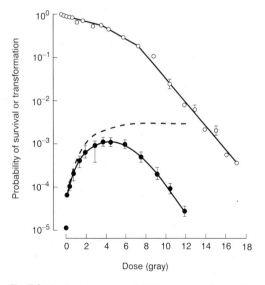

Fig. 7.9 Radiation survival (○) and transformation (●) data for $10T_{1/2}$ cells exposed to cobalt-60 γ-rays (1 Gy/min) (from Elkind *et al.* 1983). Transformation frequency corrected for cell loss due to inactivation is represented by – – – –.

7.3.4 Molecular studies in radiation oncogenesis

Although studies on DNA repair and mutagenesis provide valuable information on processes that may underlie the initiation of oncogenesis, the principal approach to the problem now centres largely on direct molecular analysis of somatic cells carrying lesions that may be associated with the neoplastic phenotype.

In the $10T_{1/2}$ cell line, utilization of DNA-mediated gene transfer techniques has shown that the transformed phenotype in $10T_{1/2}$ cells can be transferred to murine NIH/3T3 cells (Borek *et al.* 1987) (see Chapter 9). The identity of the specifically oncogenic DNA sequences in $10T_{1/2}$ cells remains to be established.

A major problem in the study of radiation oncogenesis at the cellular and molecular level remains the limited available cell lines. Mostly these are immortalized rodent fibroblast lines and the relevance of single cell responses to the more complex 'whole organ' responses that influence oncogenesis *in vivo* is a problem that is not just confined to radiation research. Nevertheless, these problems are recognized and much effort is currently devoted to the development of better model systems *in vitro*.

Radiation can activate oncogenic viruses under some circumstances. The so-called radiation leukaemia virus (RadLV) is a member of a class of retroviruses (see Chapter 8) first isolated as a leukaemogenic activity in cell-free extracts from radiation-induced thymic lymphomas in mice. Fractionated whole-body X-irradiation can produce up to 100 per cent lymphoma incidence in C57BL/Ka mice. These tumours express the virus in the primary tumour and in serial syngeneic transplants. Injection of cell-free extracts intrathymically gives rise to identical tumours in the same strain of mouse. The induction of myeloid leukaemia in RFM/Vn mice following irradiation is also associated with virus infection.

Ras oncogene activation occurs in some murine thymic lymphomas induced by radiation. Whilst some degree of codon specificity has been reported to be associated with Ki-*ras* activation, it is still not possible to relate these events directly to the initiation of neoplasia. It is feasible that they are associated with some late event in neoplastic development (virus and oncogene activation are discussed in detail in Chapters 8 and 9).

The problem of the interpretation of specific molecular changes in overt neoplasms is compounded in radiation oncogenesis because radiation is so generally non-specific in its capabilities for damaging DNA, notwithstanding the existence of radiation fragile sites (see below). Radiation causes many types of chemical damage in DNA of which only a few may be relevant to oncogenesis. An alternative approach to the problem of initiation of radiation oncogenesis lies in the search for chromosomal markers in preneoplastic cells. In essence, if such neoplasia-specific chromosomal effects exist, it may be possible to track these back in animal systems to the immediate postirradiation phase in the target organ.

Trisomy of chromosome (ch) 15 is known to occur in a high proportion of spontaneous and induced murine thymic lymphomas and there is evidence for duplication of a specific region of ch15 containing the *myc* and *put-1* oncogenes. Trisomy 15 may be detected also in thymocytes from irradiated mice 12–18 weeks after exposure. In some animals, however, a translocation marker (tl; 5) is observed at earlier times. It is suggested that this translocation is an early event in lymphomagenesis, whereas trisomy 15 may only contribute to neoplastic progression (McMorrow *et al.* 1988).

Fragile sites It has often been assumed that radiation-induced breaks in the genomic material of the cell are mostly random. However, there is increasing evidence that the cytogenetic abnormalities caused by radiation often involve particular breakpoints. A case in point is the occurrence of cytogenetic abnormalities on chromosome 2 (ch2) in CBA mice with radiation-induced acute myeloid leukaemia (see Section 7.2.3). Bouffler *et al.* (1993) have investigated a particularly common breakpoint on this chromosome occurring in the bone marrow from both irradiated normal mice and leukaemic mice. They have isolated and characterized two telomere-like sequences which are associated with ch2 breakpoints. In particular, one sequence has 2–3 telomere repeat units at either end of an inverted head-to-head structure. The frequency of hybridization of this clone to ch2 bands, as shown by fluorescence *in situ* hybridization techniques (see Chapter 10), was found to correlate well with the frequency of radiation-induced breakpoints in each band. This association with telomere-like structures suggests the existence of preferential sites for radia-

tion-induced deletions and rearrangements that may be important in sensitivity to radiation-induced cancer.

7.3.5 Radiation and the cellular stress response

In a rapidly expanding field there are numerous examples of various chemical and physical agents that are toxic to cells at high doses, and elicit protective responses at low doses. These so-called 'shock' or 'stress' responses are evident in primary organisms, mammalian cells in culture, and, in some cases, at the level of organized tissue. Stress responses are usually transient in nature and often involve the onset of resistance to higher doses of the same agent, or, in some instances, resistance to other agents. Other manifestations of the stress response at the cellular and subcellular level, include enhanced DNA replication, induction of mitogenesis, the up-regulation of some genes controlling protein synthesis, the onset of protein phosphorylation and other effects involved in mechanisms of signal transduction in cells, and, particularly, changes in expression of various genes controlling cell growth, proliferation, and differentiation.

Stress agents include physical agents such as heat, UV light, and ionizing radiation. Chemical and biochemical stress agents include hypoxia and hyperoxia, some cytotoxic drugs, glucose deprivation, cytokines, and tumour promoters. The fact that such widely differing agents elicit the stress response suggests that the stress response may be part of an evolutionary cellular defence mechanism in that agents that threaten the proliferative or functional integrity of a cell may increase the expression of mechanisms that are normally involved in such processes. It is in this regard that such stress responses may be a factor in enhancing the risk of cellular transformation.

There are many homologies in effects of stress-inducing agents. Table 7.3 gives examples indicating common stress responses induced by a wide variety of different agents. Some examples of stress responses specifically induced by ionizing radiation are listed in Table 7.4.

The literature includes various accounts of activation by low radiation doses of key effector molecules in signal transduction mechanisms within cells, including some protein kinases. Protein kinase C (PKC) and mitogen-activated protein kinase (MAP

Table 7.3 Homologies in cellular stress responses

Effect	Agent
Enhanced expression of heat shock protein hsp70	Heat, hypoxia, reoxygenation after hypoxia, UV
Enhanced expression of haemoxygenase	UV(A), heat, hypoxia, H_2O_2
Up-regulation of protein kinase C enzymes	Heat, X- and γ-radiation, hypoxia, UV(A)
Glucose-regulated proteins	Glucose deprivation, hypoxia
Mitogenesis	H_2O_2, t-butylhydroperoxide, UV, ionizing radiation, hypoxia
Drug resistance	Drugs, hypoxia, γ-radiation
Increased metastatic potential	UV, TPA, γ-radiation, hypoxia, glucose deprivation, acidosis

Table 7.4 The radiation stress response

Low doses of ionizing radiation induce:

Temporary radiation resistance

Enhanced expression of numerous proteins

Up-regulation of some protein kinases involved in cellular signal transduction

Increase in metastatic potential in B16 melanoma cells

Enhanced expression of a cell adhesion molecule ($\alpha_{IIb}\beta_3$)

Changes in regulation of cell cycle control

kinase) are protein-serine/threonine kinases which are important regulators of diverse cellular processes, including metabolism, proliferation, and differentiation (see Chapter 11). Expression of both kinases is enhanced by low doses of radiation. In addition to changes observed at the transcription level (Woloschak *et al.* 1990), changes in PKC have been observed in the phosphorylation status of one of the isozymes, PKC-α. Such changes were observed directly using Western blot techniques employing monoclonal antibodies that are ·specific to the phosphorylated amino acids (serine and threonine) within the protein but are non-reactive against the unphosphorylated protein. The increased induction of phosphorylation of PKC occurs mainly in the nuclear fraction within the cell. Unlike the PKC activator and tumour promoter activator (TPA), radiation stress does not induce any translocation from the cytosol to the membrane. However, like TPA, radiation *does* induce a complete redistribution of MAP kinase from the cytosol to the nucleus.

Notwithstanding the evidence that low doses of radiation can induce resistance to the lethal effects of radiation, the stimulating effect of such low doses of radiation on genetic mechanisms involved in cell control and progression suggests the involvement of stress responses in radiation carcinogenesis. One example of a possible link between induced resistance and cancer induction is the effect of radiation on transgenic mice carrying mutant alleles of the *p53* 'antioncogene' (see Chapter 9). Lee and Bernstein (1993) have observed that mice transgenic for *p53* mutants show increased radioresistance of various haemopoietic cell lineages. Other experiments have shown that whole-body irradiation of transgenic *p53* mutant mice produces a very high frequency of tumours compared with control mice carrying normal *p53* (Kemp *et al.* 1994).

There is evidence that radiation can up-regulate expression of at least one cell adhesion molecule (see Chapter 2). Onada and colleagues (1992) have observed, using a lung colony model in mice, that B16 melanoma cells irradiated *in vitro* with γ-rays in the range 0.25–2.5 Gy, give rise to increased seeding of tumour colonies in the lung when injected into syngeneic hosts. Radiation doses in this range significantly increased cell adhesion to fibronectin. Consistent with this was the finding that irradiated cells showed a large increase in the $\alpha_{IIb}\beta_3$ integrin receptor. The enhanced expression of this cell adhesion molecule receptor was transient, and returned to normal within 2–4 hours following irradiation. There is clearly scope for more studies of this kind now that monoclonal antibodies for a variety of cell adhesion molecules are becoming available.

7.3.6 Some free radical aspects of radiation carcinogenesis

Radiation carcinogenesis is a multistage process conveniently divided into *initiation* and *promotion* phases. Free radical processes are involved in both. The initial intracellular chemical damage caused by radiation must be mainly free radical in nature since the local energy deposition is greatly in excess of the normal bond energies of all the affected molecules. Many radiation chemical studies on DNA systems *in vitro* have led to a fairly complete knowledge of the various types, structures, and reactions of DNA free radicals produced by radiation action. The fundamental problem that remains to be solved, a problem common to the molecular action of other types of carcinogens, is the identification of the *specific* types of free radical chemical damage critical to the onset of the multistage process of carcinogenesis.

Radioprotectors It has long been established that various types of molecules containing the reactive sulphydryl group, –SH, influence radiation response. The effects include protection against: (i) cell lethality and mutagenesis *in vitro*, (ii) acute radiation morbidity *in vivo*, and (iii) late effects including radiation-induced life shortening. There is much evidence that these protective effects are a direct result of the relative weakness of the sulphur–hydrogen bond in the sulphydryl compounds. Free radicals produced either by the radiation or in subsequent chemical reactions can be 'restored' or 'repaired' by transfer of a hydrogen atom from the sulphydryl group of the protector. Such processes have been observed directly in various radiation chemical model systems using fast response pulse radiolysis techniques, i.e.

$$X^{\cdot} + RSH \quad \rightarrow \quad XH + RS^{\cdot}$$
$$\text{(free radical)} \qquad \text{(protector)}$$

Sulphydryl compounds can also inhibit radiation-induced carcinogenesis. The effect is complicated, however, by the protective effect of these agents against cell lethality and life shortening. The reduction in the number of potential tumour cells and the shortening of the time in which late tumours can be expressed influences their radiation-induced incidence. Protection against both these effects can lead to an apparent *increase* in incidence and this has been observed for some tumours. However, there is more consistency in the data for radiation-induced thymic lymphomas. Figure 7.10 shows the protective effect of a mixture of radioprotective compounds (most containing sulphydryl groups) on the incidence of thymic lymphomas in irradiated C57 mice.

Superoxide dismutase Evidence that free radicals are involved in the promotional phases of radiation carcinogenesis comes from studies with the enzyme superoxide dismutase (SOD). This enzyme is a powerful catalyst for the removal of the superoxide radical anion (O_2^-) ultimately formed in many cellular electron transfer processes. It has been proposed that this radical (or one of its reaction products, the hydroxyl radical) is highly damaging to the cell and that SOD has evolved as a natural cellular defence mechanism against free radical injury.

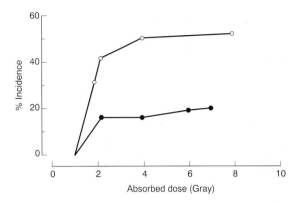

Fig. 7.10 Incidence of thymic lymphoma in C57BL male mice irradiated with 650 R X-rays ($\bigcirc$). Protective effect of a mixture of radioprotective agents ($\bullet$) (from Fry 1983).

There is evidence that this enzyme inhibits radiation transformation in the $10T_{1/2}$ and in the hamster embryo systems, but, interestingly, does not need to be present at the time of irradiation. It does require, however, *prolonged* postirradiation exposure. The hypothesis that free radicals are involved in the promotional phase of radiation carcinogenesis is supported by transformation experiments using chemical promoters and SOD. The phorbol ester tumour promoter TPA, for example, substantially increases radiation-induced cell transformation but the effect is completely eliminated by treatment of the cells with SOD. The mechanisms of inhibition of free radical processes involved in tumour promotion are obscure but a plausible explanation may lie in the ability of SOD to inhibit free radicals involved in lipid peroxidation in cellular membranes.

7.3.7 Interaction of radiation and chemical carcinogens

Of particular concern in the field of radiological protection and the assessment of risk is the question of possible interaction between radiation and environmental carcinogens. Many experimental *in vivo* studies have been carried out to assess interactions between radiation and chemical carcinogens. Overall, the evidence is equivocal. A complicating factor is the life-shortening effect of radiation which may mask any interactive influence of a chemical carcinogen. Nevertheless, there are experimental data indicating positive interactions, particularly after fetal exposure. The carcinogen ethylnitro-sourea (ENU) can act transplacentally in inducing various tumours in the offspring of mice treated with the chemical before birth. Leukaemia incidence is greater after both ENU and X-irradiation than with each agent alone. Interestingly, the incidence of radiation-induced ovarian tumours is also increased by exposure to ENU even though no such tumours were observed when ENU was administered without radiation. While such studies may highlight possible additional risks associated with combined exposure to radiation and chemical carcinogens, progress in understanding the mechanisms of such interactions must ultimately derive from the cellular and molecular approach.

Notwithstanding their limitations, the *quantitative* cellular transformation systems currently available have provided some information. For a general discussion see Nygaard and Simic (1983) and Cerutti *et al.* (1987). Radiation transformation *in vitro* can be potentiated by various chemical agents including some drugs used in cancer chemotherapy, tumour promoters such as TPA, thyroid hormone extracts, and particularly, pyrolysates of protein foods such as Try-P-2 (3-amino-1-methyl-5*H*-pyrido-4,3-*b*-indol). The transforming efficiency of 1.5 Gy of X-irradiation in hamster embryo cells, for example, is increased 20-fold by the addition to the medium of only 0.5 µg/ml Trp-P-2.

Information on the potentiating effects (and indeed inhibiting effects) of various other chemical agents on radiation-induced cellular transformation is steadily accumulating. The major problems in applying such information to the problems of human radiation carcinogenesis are the limitations of the *quantitative* transformation assay systems currently available. Established rodent cell lines of fibroblastic origin may not be appropriate models for investigating human radiation carcinogenesis since human tumours arise mainly from epithelial cells. Transformed human epithelial cells can behave quite differently from transformed cells of rodent origin. Nevertheless the rapid accumulation of knowledge on the various stages involved in the transition of a normal primary cell to a frankly malignant phenotype will eventually lead to the establishment of an assay system that is sufficiently quantitative for studies in radiation carcinogenesis. When that point is reached, there will be a much firmer basis for assessing radiation risk in the human population.

References and further reading

BEIR (1980). National Academy of Sciences. National Research Council. Committee on the Biological Effects of Ionizing Radiations. *The effects on populations of exposure to low levels of ionizing radiation: 1980.* National Academy Press, Washington, D.C.

BEIR (1988). National Academy of Sciences. National Research Council. Committee on the Biological Effects of Ionizing Radiations. *Health risks of radon and other internally deposited alpha-emitters*, BEIR IV. National Academy Press, Washington, D.C.

Black, D. (1984). Report of independent advisory group. *Investigation of the possible increased incidence of Cancer in West Cumbria.* HMSO, London.

Borek, C. and Sachs, L. (1966). In vitro cell transformation by X-irradiation. *Nature*, **210**, 276.

Borek, C., Ong, A., and Mason, H. (1987). Distinctive transforming genes in X-ray transformed mammalian cells. *Proceedings of the National Academy of Sciences, USA*, **84**, 794–8.

Bouffler, S., Silver, A., Papworth, D., Coates, J., and Cox, R. (1993). Murine radiation myeloid leukaemogenesis: relationship between interstitial telomere-like sequences and chromosome-2 fragile sites. *Genes Chromosomes and Cancer*, **6**, 98–106.

Cattanach, B. M., Burtenshaw, M. D., Rasberry, B., and Evans, E. P. (1993). Large deletions and other gross forms of chromosome imbalance compatible with viability and fertility in the mouse. *Nature Genetics*, **3**, 56–61.

Cerutti, P. A., Nygaard, O. F., and Simic, M. G. (ed.) (1987) *Anti-carcinogenesis and radiation protection.* Plenum Press, New York.

Cook-Mozaffari, P. J., Darby, S. C., Doll, R., Forman, D., Hermon, C., Pike, M. C., and

Vincent, T. (1989). Geographical variation in mortality from leukaemia and other cancers in England and Wales in relation to proximity to nuclear installation, 1969–78. *British Journal of Cancer*, **59**, 476–85.

Cox, R., Debenham, P. G., Masson, W. K., and Webb, M. B. T. (1986). Ataxia telangiectasia: a human mutation giving high frequency misrepair of DNA double strand scissions. *Molecular Biology and Medicine*, **3**, 229–44.

Darby, S. and Doll, R. (1987). Fallout, radiation doses near Dounreay, and childhood leukaemia. *British Medical Journal*, **294**, 603–7.

Doll, R., Evans, H. J., and Darby, S. C. (1994). Paternal exposure not to blame. *Nature*, **367**, 678–80.

Elkind, M. M., Han, A., Hill, C. K., and Buonaguro, F. (1983). Repair mechanisms in radiation-induced cell transformation. In *Proceedings of the 7th international congress of radiation research* (ed. J. J. Broerse, G. W. Barendsen, H. B. Kal, and A. J. van der Kogel), pp. 33–42. Martinus Nijhoff, Amsterdam.

Fry, R. J. M. (1983). Radiation carcinogenesis: radioprotectors and photosensitizers. In *Radioprotectors and anticarcinogens* (ed. O. F. Nygaard and M. G. Simic), pp. 417–36. Academic Press, New York.

Gardner, M. J., Snee, M. P., Hall, A. J., Powells, C. A., Downes, S., and Terrell, D. (1990). Results of case-control study of leukaemia and lymphoma among young people near Sellafield nuclear plant in West Cumbria. *British Medical Journal*, **300**, 423–9.

Goodhead, D. T. (1988). Spatial and temporal distribution of energy. *Health Physics*, **55**, 231–40.

Gössner, W., Gerber, G. B., Hagen, U., and Luz, A. (ed.) (1985). *The radiobiology of radium and thorotrast*. Urban and Schwarzenberg, Munich.

Gray, L. H. (1965). Radiation biology and cancer. In *Proceedings of the XVIII annual symposium on fundamental cancer research*, pp. 7–25. Williams and Wilkins, Baltimore.

Hall, E. J. (1988). *Radiobiology for the radiologist*, (3rd edn). J. B. Lippincott, Philadelphia.

Hasan, N. M., Parker, P. J., and Adams, G.E. (1996). Induction and phosphorylation of protein kinase C-α and MAP-kinase by hypoxia and by radiation in V79 cells. *Radiation Research*, **145**, 128–33.

ICRP (International Commission on Radiological Protection) (1977). Recommendations of the International Commission on Radiological Protection, ICRP No. 26. *Annals of the ICRP*, Vol.1, No. 3. Pergamon Press, Oxford.

ICRP (International Commission on Radiological Protection) (1984). Non-stochastic effects of ionizing radiation, ICRP No. 241. *Annals of the ICRP*, Vol. 14, No. 3. Pergamon Press, Oxford.

Kadhim, M. A., MacDonald, D. A., Goodhead, D. T., Lorimore, S. A., Marsden, S. J., and Wright, E. J. (1992). Transmission of chromosomal instability after plutonium α-particle irradiation. *Nature*, **355**, 738–40.

Kadhim, M. A., Lorimore, S. A., Hepburn, M. D., Goodhead, D. T., Buckle, V. J., and Wright, E. J. (1994). α-particle induced chromosomal instability in human bone marrow cells. *Lancet*, **344**, 987–8.

Kato, H. and Schull, W. J. (1982). Studies of the mortality of A-bomb survivors. 7. Mortality, 1950–78, Part 1, Cancer mortality. *Radiation Research*, **90**, 395–432.

Kemp, C. J., Wheldon, T., and Balmain, A. (1994). p53-deficient mice are extremely susceptible to radiation-induced tumorigenesis. *Nature Genetics*, **8**, 66–9.

Kinlen, L. (1988). Evidence for an infective cause of childhood leukaemia. Comparison of a Scottish new town with nuclear reprocessing sites in Britain. *Lancet*, **i**, 1323–6.

Kinlen, L. J. (1995). Epidemiological evidence for an infective basis in childhood leukaemia. *British Journal of Cancer*, **71**, 1–5.

Lee, J. M. and Bernstein, A. (1993). p53 mutations increase resistance to ionizing radiation. *Proceedings of the National Academy of Sciences, USA*, **90**, 5742–6.

Lloyd, D. C., Purrott, R. J., Dolphin, G. W., Bolton, D., Edwards, A. A., and Corp, M. J. (1975). The relationship between chromosome aberrations and low LET radiation dose to human lymphocytes. *International Journal of Radiation Biology*, **28**, 75–90.

Lloyd, D. C., Purrott, R. J., Dolphin, G. W., and Edwards, A. A. (1976). Chromosome aberrations induced in human lymphocytes by neutron irradiation. *International Journal of Radiation Biology*, **29**, 169–82.

McMorrow, L. E., Newcomb, E. W., and Pellicer, A. (1988). Identification of a specific marker chromosome early in tumour development in g-irradiated C57BL/6J mice. *Leukaemia*, **2**, 115–19.

Mole, R. H., Papworth, D. G., and Corp, M. J. (1983). The dose-response for X-ray induction of myeloid leukemia in male CBA/H mice. *British Journal of Cancer*, **47**, 285–91.

Nygaard, O. F. and Simic, M. G. (ed.) (1983). *Radioprotectors and anticarcinogens*. Academic Press, New York. (Collected papers.)

Onada, J. M., Piechocki, M. P., and Honn, K. V. (1992). Radiation-induced increase in expression of the $\alpha_{IIb}\beta_3$ integrin in melanoma cells: effects on metastatic potential. *Radiation Research*, **130**, 281–8.

O'Riordan, M. C. (1988). *Notes on radon risks in homes*, Radiological Protection Bulletin No. 89, February 1988. National Radiological Protection Board, Chilton, UK.

Richardson, R. B., Eatough, J. P., and Henshaw, D. L. (1991). Dose to red bone marrow from natural radon and thoron exposure. *British Journal of Radiology*, **64**, 608–24.

Silver, A. R. J., Breckon, G., Masson, W. K., Malowany, D., and Cox, R. (1987). Studies on radiation myeloid leukaemogenesis in the mouse. In *Radiation research*, Vol. 2 (ed. E. M. Fielden, J. F. Fowler, J. H. Hendry and D. Scott), pp. 494–500. Taylor and Francis, London.

Smith, P. G. and Doll, R. (1982). Mortality among patients with ankylosing spondylitis after a single treatment course with X-rays. *British Medical Journal*, **284**, 449–60.

Stsjazhko, V. A., Tsyb, A. F., Tronko, N. D., Souchkevitch, G., and Baverstock, K. F. (1995). Childhood thyroid cancer since accident at Chernobyl. *British Medical Journal*, **310**, 801.

Thacker, J. (1979). The involvement of repair processes in radiation-induced mutation of cultured mammalian cells. In *Radiation research proceedings of the 6th international congress of radiation research* (ed. S. Okada), pp. 612–20. Japanese Association for Radiation Research, Tokyo.

Thacker, J. (1986). The use of recombinant DNA techniques to study radiation-induced damage, repair and genetic change in mammalian cells. *International Journal of Radiation Biology*, **50**, 1–30.

Thacker, J., Stretch, A., and Goodhead, D. T. (1982). The mutagenicity of α particles from plutonium-238. *Radiation Research*, **92**, 343–52.

UNSCEAR (United Nations Scientific Committee on Effects of Atomic Radiation) (1988). *Sources, effects and risks of ionizing radiations*. 1988 Report to the General Assembly, UN, New York.

UNSCEAR (United Nations Scientific Committee on Effects of Atomic Radiation) (1993). *Sources and effects of ionizing radiation*. 1993 Report to the General Assembly, UN, New York.

UNSCEAR (United Nations Scientific Committee on Effects of Atomic Radiation) (1994). *Sources and effects of ionizing radiations*. 1994 Report to the General Assembly, UN, New York.

Weiss, H. A., Darby, S. C. and Doll, R. (1994) Cancer mortality following X-ray treatment for ankylosing spondylitis. *Int. J. Cancer*, **59**, 327–38.

Woloschak, G. E., Chang-Liu, C. M., and Shearin-Jones, P. (1990). Regulation of PKC by ionizing radiation. *Cancer Research*, **50**, 3963–7.

8

Viruses and cancer

JOHN WYKE

8.1 Introduction

Different forms of human cancer show marked geographical variations in incidence that mainly reflect social rather than genetic differences in the populations at risk. This suggests that variable environmental factors are responsible for a great deal of cancer (Chapter 3). These environmental risk factors comprise three categories: (i) physical agents (such as X-rays or UV light, see Chapter 7), (ii) chemical agents (either directly carcinogenic or converted to carcinogens in the body, see Chapter 6), and (iii) infectious agents. Of the infectious agents, fungi, parasitic animals, and, most notably, bacteria, have all been considered as potential carcinogens, but it is viruses that have received the most attention as risk factors in neoplasia of vertebrates. This has been justified for two major reasons. Firstly, viruses are important causes of cancer in certain animals and they are being implicated increasingly in human neoplasia. Secondly, the laboratory study of tumour viruses has led to important insights into the mechanisms of carcinogenesis. These, however, are accolades conferred only with the benefit of hindsight and before we consider our present knowledge of virus-associated cancer in more detail it is worth surveying the development of the subject.

8.2 The history of tumour virology

8.2.1 Pioneer days

The first viruses were discovered towards the end of the nineteenth century as very small infectious agents, pathogenic for both plants and animals, that passed through filters capable of retaining the smallest bacteria. It was not long before comparable filterable agents were found to cause tumours in animals. The first of these, discovered by Ellermann and Bang in 1908, induced erythroblastosis (erythroid leukaemia) in chickens. Rous in 1911 and Fujinami and Inamoto in 1914 then showed that viruses could induce sarcomas in fowls. These findings created relatively little interest in the scientific community at large, perhaps because the diseases of chickens were thought to have little relevance for those of man, and for 30 years the study of chicken tumour viruses was an esoteric pursuit.

None the less, this period saw advances in other fields that would later become very significant. Selective breeding of laboratory mice produced some with high incidences of various cancers. This enabled Bittner, in 1936, to show that the high incidence of mammary carcinomas in some strains was due to transmission of a filterable virus. In the same decade, Rous, Shope, and others produced interesting studies on the virus-induced papillomas and carcinomas of rabbits, and work with chicken viruses gathered momentum. The next major advance occurred in 1951 when Gross discovered the first mouse leukaemia virus. This early postwar finding was not the beginning of a new era in tumour virology but the end of an old one. By the beginning of the 1960s our views on tumour viruses were changing rapidly. The momentum behind this change had several sources, the main ones being our growing understanding of both viruses and neoplastic growth and the development of techniques to advance this understanding by studies in tissue culture.

8.2.2 The nature of viruses

Viruses vary enormously in structure and complexity but they all share certain features that distinguish them from other forms of life. They do not have a cellular organization that is propagated by division of the whole entity, but can multiply only by replication of their genetic material (genome) (Collier and Timbury 1990). The genome comprises either RNA or DNA and the proteins it encodes usually serve in genome replication or as structural components that protect the genome and facilitate its spread from host to host. Depending on the complexity of the virus, host functions may or may not be required to aid genome replication and transcription, but all viruses require host ribosomal functions for translation of their messenger RNA and thus they are all obligatory intracellular parasites. This enforced intimacy with their host can take many forms, ranging from cytolytic viruses that overwhelm host functions, replicate rapidly, and kill the cell, to latent forms that seldom express their own functions and whose genome is replicated, in concert with that of the cell, by the host's own machinery. As we shall discuss later, this close sym-

biosis is also the reason why some viruses can cause cancer.

Some important human diseases are caused by viruses, providing incentives to develop laboratory systems for detecting, growing, and quantifying viruses, notably the use of tissue cultures to examine virus cytopathic effects (CPE). An important development was a virus assay, based on CPE, in which virus spread was limited and localized plaques of dead cells were thus produced on a layer of tissue culture cells. When similar assays were tried during the 1950s with certain tumour viruses, it was found that, instead of plaques of CPE, the viruses induced focal areas of piled up and morphologically altered cells (Fig. 8.1). Such behaviour was not entirely unexpected, for in the late 1930s it was shown that chicken sarcoma viruses could produce comparable changes in organ explants and on the chorioallantoic membrane of eggs. This tissue culture cell 'transformation' by tumour viruses provided a ready means to examine and quantify the effects of tumour viruses on cells, and it proved a great impetus to further research.

8.2.3 Cell transformation: 'tumours' *in vitro*

The full significance of the discovery that some (but by no means all) tumour viruses can transform cells *in vitro* can be appreciated by considering concepts then current on the nature of cancer. The availability of inbred laboratory animals, which facilitated the identification of some tumour viruses, also permitted experiments on the transplantation of tumours, and it was possible to show that with some tumours a single transplanted cell could cause a tumour in a previously normal animal. This focused attention on cancer as a disease of the single cell, a concept that accorded with a clonal origin of many cancers. Transplantation studies also demonstrated the stable heritability of the tumour phenotype and this, together with the knowledge that many carcinogens were also mutagens, emphasized the possibility that the initiating defect in cancer may often be a mutation in the genome of a somatic cell. The problem with this concept was demonstrating its validity. Every cell in a complex vertebrate contains tens of thousands of genes, so identifying the one or few that are altered in cancer appeared a hopeless task.

Cell transformation by tumour viruses seemed to offer a way round this impasse. The speed and efficiency of this event suggested to workers in the

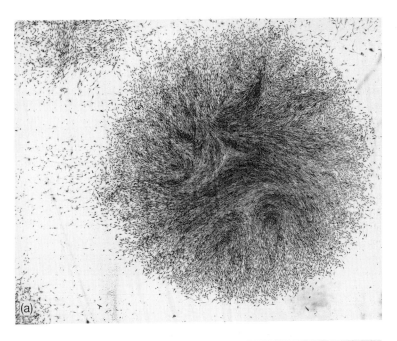

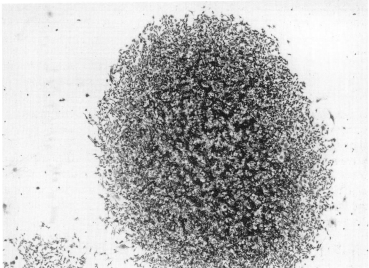

Fig. 8.1 Cell transformation by tumour viruses. (a) Shows a colony of uninfected cells of the Syrian hamster cell line BHK21/C13. The colony is flat and the cells are aligned in parallel array. In (b) a colony of the same cell line is shown after transformation with the small DNA virus, polyomavirus. The cells are piled up and disorientated.

1960s that it resulted directly from the functioning of a virus gene. Thus, to find a gene whose activity led to cancer one had only to sift through the genome of a virus rather than that of a cell. Since some tumour viruses contained only enough nucleic acid to encode three or four genes, this simplified the quest over 10 000-fold, bringing its potential achievement within the ambit of the techniques then available. This reasoning encouraged many researchers to investigate the genetics and biochemistry of virus-induced cell transformation and not

only has this led to the discovery of a number of tumour-inducing genes in viruses, but studies on the nature of these genes have had enormous conceptual implications for the whole of basic cancer research (see Sections 8.7.3, 8.7.4, and Chapters 3 and 9). It should be remembered, however, that these important advances had an element of serendipity in them for, as we shall discuss below, there are ways in which a virus might induce cancer that do not result directly from the action of one of its genes inside the tumour cell.

8.2.4 Modern concepts and questions

Tumour virology still concerns itself with two broad questions: the role of viruses in clinical neoplasia and the use of viruses in probing the mechanisms of carcinogenesis (Weiss *et al.* 1984; Wyke and Weiss 1984; zur Hausen 1991; Minson *et al.* 1994). We now know enough about viral genomes and host cell functions to understand how these two topics relate to one another in specific diseases (see Section 8.7). We also appreciate better the role of viruses as one component in what may be a multifactorial disease process, and this concept is taken into account when examining viruses as risk factors in human and animal cancer (see Section 8.3). Both these considerations are underpinned by the concept that cancer results from alterations in the presence, structure, or activity of certain genes in the cell, both oncogenes and tumour suppressor genes (see Chapter 9). Tumour viruses, by affecting these genes, played crucial roles in their discovery and viruses continue to be valuable in investigating their function.

8.3 Implicating viruses in experimental and natural cancers

How do we decide that an infectious agent is responsible for causing a given disease? The classic criteria were embodied in Koch's postulates of 1876 which stated that: (i) the agent should be found in all cases of the disease, its location corresponding with the observed lesions; (ii) the agent should be capable of isolation from the lesions and growth in pure culture outside the body; and (iii) the culture, when inoculated back into an animal, should produce the identical disease.

It is apparent that many pathogenic bacteria, let alone viruses, do not fulfil Koch's postulates but, when satisfied, these criteria provide convincing proof of causality. Many viruses have been shown to cause tumours in laboratory and domestic animals in this way, with the proviso that 'culture outside the body' has, perforce, been done on living cells, not inert media. Any doubts this raises about purity of the organism could, in theory, now be answered by molecular cloning of viral genomes in bacteria.

In contrast to the ease with which viruses have been implicated in animal tumours, their role in human disease has been extremely difficult to investigate. A major problem, of course, is the impossibility of ethically fulfilling Koch's third postulate; other animals can be used to test the oncogenicity of human viruses but the results they yield can be misleading. Attempts have been made to modify Koch's postulates by including evidence for the presence of viral genomes or proteins in the tumours (when infectious virus cannot be found) and by asking whether the person with a tumour shows a specific immune response against the candidate virus. However, even if positive, these tests only show that a virus is associated with a tumour, not that it is a cause. Good evidence for causality would, of course, be provided if elimination of virus infection (for instance by immunization) also eliminated the incidence of the tumour, but such evidence has not yet been provided for any major virus-associated human neoplasm.

A further problem in implicating viruses in human neoplasia is the complexity of the disease in humans. Many virus-induced tumours in animals occur in a high proportion of the infected population, often at a relatively early stage of the animal's short life span and, in the case of laboratory animals, selective breeding has enhanced these features. The virus is clearly a major risk factor in the disease. Human populations, in contrast, are usually outbred and the disease usually occurs towards the end of a long life span with a pattern of incidence that suggests a multifactorial causation (see Chapters 1 and 3). Indeed, the role of a virus in human neoplasia is often first hinted at by epidemiological data, the same data also showing that only a minority of the infected population develop tumours. Virus infection is thus usually one of a complex of interrelated risk factors that operate at different stages of development of a tumour, as shown in Fig. 8.2 (Wyke and Weiss 1984). This figure depicts three main groups of risk factors: those relating to virus infection, those concerning the cellular alterations involved in neoplasia, and those affecting the host response to both viruses and tumour cells. Let us consider how they may operate at three arbitrary stages in the evolution of a virus-associated neoplasm.

8.4 Risk factors predisposing to virus-associated neoplasia

The risk factors are shown diagrammatically in Fig. 8.2. In stage 1 a virus must infect the host and,

Risk factors in viral carcinogenesis

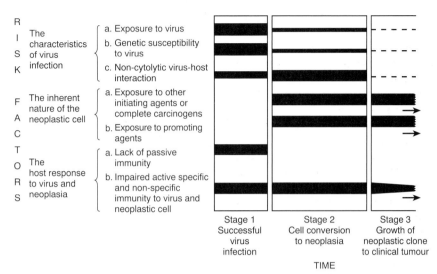

Fig. 8.2 Diagram of the relationship between the arbitrary stages of virus-associated neoplasia, the component features of the neoplastic process, and the risk factors that influence each of these features. Only the stages of neoplasia have a clear temporal relationship to one another, as shown on the abscissa. The breaks in the time-axis indicate that these stages vary in length and they are not shown to scale (in general stage 1 is likely to be relatively short and stage 2 is usually the longest period). The risk factors affecting either of the three features characterizing virus-associated neoplasia are shown on the ordinate and, as shown by the bars, they may operate at different, and often more than one, stages of the disease process. The thickness of the bars indicates the relative importance of each risk factor at each stage of neoplasia, broken lines indicating periods at which the risk factors are of uncertain significance.

depending on the mechanism by which it instigates neoplasia (see Section 8.7), infection must lead to persistence of virus genetic material in the host or to some stable virus-induced alteration in certain cells. Infection-related risk factors important at this stage are exposure to the virus (dose of virus and route of infection) and whether or not the host cells are susceptible to virus penetration and growth. The acquired resistance of the host, either by passive or active immunity (see Chapter 16), is also crucial, as in any other virus infection.

The requirements for stages 2 and 3 distinguish the pathogenesis of virus-associated neoplasia from that of acute cytolytic virus diseases. In stage 2, the conversion of an infected cell to neoplastic growth, the important characteristic of virus infection is the need to establish a non-cytolytic virus-cell association, since, obviously, only live cells can form tumours (an exception to this requirement may be those instances where the mechanism of virus onco-genesis is indirect, see Section 8.7.1). Some tumour-associated viruses, such as the retroviruses and hepatitis B virus, can replicate without causing massive cell death, while herpesviruses can persist in latent, inactive forms in living cells. Other tumour viruses, however, can only convert a cell to neoplasia if full replication of the virus is blocked, either because the host cell is unusual or the virus has some defect. In either case, the infection that leads to neoplasia is unusual and may not be apparent in other ways, yet another factor making it difficult to link virus infection to neoplasia.

The host cell is not necessarily a passive bystander in the lottery of whether or not a virus achieves infection without CPE. Many cells respond to infection with a variety of viruses by undergoing apoptosis, a multistep programmed cell death (see Chapter 9) which may consequently curtail the progress of viral infection (Vaux *et al.* 1994; Thompson 1995). The features of infection that induce an apoptotic response probably differ from virus to virus but a number of viruses counter this response by encoding proteins that inhibit apoptosis at various stages of the process. Apoptosis inhibition is a characteristic of many non-oncogenic viruses that achieve persistent infections but it may have particular significance for viruses that induce tumours. This is because apoptosis is also a cellular defence that eliminates cells with genomic damage. Cells that are resistant to apoptosis, by virtue of the viral genes that they express, are more likely to survive genomic damage that will predispose to subsequent neoplasia. Examples of this are given in Section 8.7.4.

Further complicating factors important at stage 2 are the requirements for (i) additional carcinogens or promoting agents (see Chapter 6); or (ii) the action of agents that affect host immune responses. In many virus-associated tumours of humans, such additional factors seem as, or more, important than virus infection itself.

Stage 3 in this sequence is the multiplication and progression of a neoplastic cell to form a clinical tumour. Infection-related risk factors are probably of little importance to this late stage in tumour evolution, although if expression of the virus persists it may serve as an antigenic target for host immune responses. Cocarcinogens, on the other hand, may remain important as tumour progression occurs (see Chapter 6). Impairment of the host immune response is also likely to remain important. There is, in fact, a pervasive connection between host immune deficiency and the development of virus-associated tumours, particularly in humans, which may be summarized as follows.

1. Immune mechanisms, such as T cell-mediated cytotoxicity, natural killer cell activity, and interferon, can reduce the growth of virus-induced tumours in laboratory animals (see Chapters 16 and 20).

2. Immune impairment is seen in many virus-induced tumours in animals. In some instances, as with agents that infect T cells, like Marek's disease virus and feline leukaemia virus, virus infection itself is immunosuppressive. In other cases a cocarcinogen has this effect, an example being the role of bracken fern in papillomavirus-associated alimentary carcinomas of cattle.

3. Human patients receiving immunosuppressive therapy show an increased incidence of a limited range of tumours, many of which are tumours in which virus infection has also been implicated. Indeed, so striking is this overlap that it has been suggested that viruses may play a role in all tumours whose incidence is increased in immune deficient individuals. However, in only one type of therapy-induced tumour has virus been directly implicated so far: the immunoblastic 'lymphomas' associated with Epstein Barr virus (EBV) (see Chapter 12).

4. Finally, immune impairment seems a risk factor in the natural history of a number of virus-associated human neoplasms. Notable among these are tumours linked to infection with the human T cell leukaemia virus (a retrovirus), certain papillomaviruses, hepatitis B virus, and the herpesvirus, Epstein Barr virus.

8.4.1 Searching for new viruses

This discussion points to a recurring triplet motif in naturally occurring viral cancers in animals and humans: (i) chronic viral infection, (ii) immune impairment, and (iii) cocarcinogens. These factors must be considered when asking where and how to implicate viruses in neoplasia.

The most promising tumours to examine are those whose incidence shows a clustering that can be either familial, geographic, or social/occupational, implying genetic or environmental factors, both of which can point to viruses, as can an increased prevalence in immunosuppressed individuals. Once candidate tumours have been identified, whole individuals and tumours should be examined for evidence of virus infection. Virus isolation may require *in vitro* culture of tumour cells, employing various stratagems to unmask latent viruses, including a search for appropriate cell types in which to propagate virus.

Isolation of a candidate virus will provide tools for a more detailed study of its association with the tumour but, failing isolation, a great deal may be learned by comparison with known tumour viruses, screening tumour cells for molecular evidence of virus infection, and examining hosts for seroepidemiological clues. If evidence is found for infection with a virus common in the population, then the features of the infection peculiar to the tumour-bearing hosts should be sought. Is the infection unusually persistent? Is the serological response abnormal? Is the virus in the tumour defective? Are unusual viral antigens expressed? Even when a virus cannot be identified, a specific tumour antigen may be an important clue to a viral aetiology.

In humans, epidemiological evidence is crucial (see Chapter 3), since it is impossible to test a causal role for the virus by animal inoculation. Case–control studies will further associate the virus with the tumour, and laboratory studies will indicate the features of high and low risk groups. Retrospective and, ideally, prospective studies of high risk groups should establish the temporal relationship between virus infection, other risk factors, and tumour development, so providing a basis to tackle the management of the tumour.

8.5 Important tumour viruses of animals and humans

The oncogenic viruses are a very diverse group. They include members of all the major families of DNA viruses that infect vertebrates, with the exception of the very small parvoviruses. On the other hand only one family of RNA viruses, the retroviruses, has generally accepted oncogenic members, although hepatitis C virus (an RNA virus resembling flaviviruses) has been implicated as a risk factor in human liver cancer. The tumour viruses vary greatly in the complexity of their genomes, in the types of neoplasms they induce, and in the requirement for cofactors in tumorigenesis. What do they have in common?

One almost universal feature is the importance of a DNA stage in the replication of the viral genome. The retroviruses are unique among viruses whose free infectious forms contain RNA, in that this genome is copied soon after infection into double-stranded DNA by an RNA-dependent DNA polymerase enzyme carried in the virus particle. Moreover, this DNA 'provirus' is then inserted ('integrated') by a covalent linkage into the host cell DNA (Weiss *et al.* 1984). Such integrations seem to be another frequent, but not invariant, hallmark of tumour viruses: whole or partial viral genomes are very often detected in tumour cell chromosomes. It is not clear why integration occurs so commonly since it is obligatory in only one of the mechanisms by which tumour viruses cause neoplasia (see Section 8.7.5). However, it may serve mainly to ensure a stable association between viral and host genomes during the lengthy development of a neoplastic cell lineage. In this context it is interesting that a number of poxviruses can induce cellular proliferation and, since some encode anti-apoptotic factors and proteins related to growth factors (see Chapters 11 and 20), this growth may be truly neoplastic, yet none of them induces stable progressing tumours. Could this be because they complete their life cycles in the cytoplasm of the cell and do not enter the nucleus?

Various groups of tumour viruses are shown in Tables 8.1, 8.2, and 8.3. These lists are representative and not comprehensive and for a fuller account the texts listed in Further reading should be consulted. Entries in the tables have been chosen because of (i) their historical or research interest; (ii) an intrinsically interesting pathogenesis; (iii) their importance as pathogens of humans and domestic animals; or (iv) their inclusion elsewhere in this chapter.

8.5.1 Retroviruses (Table 8.1)

This is a family of small viruses with RNA genomes of 5–10 000 nucleotides. Most tumorigenic members are in the oncovirus subfamily and, of the genera in this subfamily, by far the most important is the Type C virus genus.

The retroviruses of chickens were the first tumour viruses to be discovered and, together with comparable viruses of mice, they have played a crucial role in the history of tumour virology. They are still important in our attempts to understand the molecular basis of neoplasia (see Section 8.7.3 and Chapter 9), but only one group of avian retroviruses, the causal agents of fowl leukosis, is of commercial importance.

Two other important retrovirus pathogens of domestic animals are feline leukaemia virus and bovine leukosis virus (Onions and Jarrett 1987). The latter is of commercial importance in many parts of the world where it causes the most common malignancy in cattle. Leukaemia and lymphosarcoma are also the most frequent tumours of domestic cats but they account for only a fraction of the deaths attributable to feline leukaemia virus, which, together with feline immunodeficiency retroviruses, also causes anaemia, immunosuppression, and related diseases, making it now the most frequent non-traumatic cause of death among cats in developed countries.

The diseases caused by these cattle and cat retroviruses provide interesting parallels for a disease complex in humans associated with infection by a retrovirus group called human T cell leukaemia virus (HTLV). With all three agents the prevalence

Table 8.1 Some ocogenic retroviruses of animals and humans

Virus classification[1]	Viruses	Associated tumours	Other risk factors[2]
Oncovirus subfamily, Type B genus	Mouse mammary tumour virus	Mammary adenocarcinoma	Pregnancy (altered hormone levels), genetic susceptibility affecting endogenous virus production
Oncovirus subfamily, Type C genus	Avian sarcoma–leukosis virus complex	Various sarcomas, some carcinomas, lymphomas, and leukaemias	Genetic susceptibility affecting virus penetration, replication, and spread
	Avian reticuloendotheliosis virus complex	Lymphomas and leukaemias	
	Mouse leukaemia and sarcoma viruses	Various sarcomas, lymphomas, and leukaemias, some carcinomas	Genetic susceptibility affecting virus penetration, replication, and spread
	Feline leukaemia virus	Leukaemia, lymphosarcoma (mainly T cell)	Possible genetic susceptibility, concurrent infections
	Bovine leukosis virus	Lymphosarcoma, leukaemia (B cell)	Genetic susceptibility to development of lymphocytosis
	Primate leukaemia and sarcoma viruses	Fibrosarcoma, myeloid leukaemia	
	Human T cell leukaemia lymphoma viruses	Adult T cell leukaemia/lymphoma	
Oncovirus subfamily, Type D genus	Mason–Pfizer monkey virus	Fibrosarcomas	
Lentivirus subfamily	Human immunodeficiency viruses	Kaposi's sarcoma, B lymphoma	Concurrent infections with HTLV-1, human herpesvirus 6, Epstein–Barr virus, Kaposi's sarcoma herpesvirus
	Feline immunodeficiency viruses	B lymphomas	Feline leukaemia virus

[1] Classification is based upon virus particle structure and limited biological criteria. Evolutionary relationships being revealed by genetic comparisons may not accord with this taxonomy.

[2] Where known or suspected. The absence of listed risk factors does not imply that such factors are unimportant.

of infection in the population is greater than the incidence of neoplasia. Indeed, in the case of HTLV the associated tumour, adult T cell leukaemia/lymphoma, is rare and, even in areas where HTLV infection is widespread, only about 1 in 80 of the infected population develop the malignancy (presumably, unidentified cofactors are important in oncogenesis). Nevertheless, as with feline leukaemia virus, HTLV may induce diseases other than neoplasia. Two strains, HTLV-1, and -2, are associated with T cell malignancies while a third virus, identical to or closely related to HTLV-1, is strongly implicated in tropical spastic paraparesis, a chronic degenerative disease of nervous tissue.

An even more important group of human retroviruses, human immunodeficiency viruses (HIV), together with an almost identical simian agent (SIV), are grouped in the lentiviruses, a subfamily they share with feline immunodeficiency virus, equine infectious anaemia virus, visna virus of sheep, and others. Like many lentiviruses, HIV causes degenerative diseases of the immune and nervous systems, the most frequent manifestation being a T cell deficiency leading to acquired immunodeficiency syndrome (AIDS). HIV earns a place in this chapter because AIDS patients frequently develop otherwise rare mesenchymal tumours, such as Kaposi's sarcoma, which may affect connective tissues in many parts of the body (Weller 1994).

8.5.2 Small DNA viruses (Table 8.2)

The most important human oncogenic viruses are in this group (zur Hausen 1991). It is estimated that 200 million people, mainly in Third World countries, are chronically infected with hepatitis B virus and are at risk of developing cirrhosis (fibrosis of the liver) and primary liver cancer, a tumour that causes

Table 8.2 Some oncogenic small DNA viruses of animals and humans

Virus family	Virus	Genome size[1]	Host of origin	Associated tumours	Other risk factors[2]
Hepadnavirus	Hepatitis B group	3 kb	Human, apes, rodents, ducks	Liver cancer	In humans: alcohol, smoking, fungal toxins, other viruses
Papovavirus	Polyoma	5 kb	Mouse	Various carcinomas and sarcomas	
	SV40	5 kb	Monkey	Sarcomas (in rodents)	
	BK and JC	5 kb	Human	None in humans; neural tumours in rodents and monkeys	
	Papilloma	7–8 kb	Human	Genital, laryngeal, and skin warts Anogenital carcinoma	Smoking, herpes simplex viruses, immune suppression
				Laryngeal carcinoma Skin carcinoma	X-irradiation, smoking Sunlight, genetic disorders possibly affecting immunity
			Cattle	Genital, alimentary, and skin warts, may progress to alimentary carcinoma	Carcinogens and immune suppressants in bracken fern
				Skin carcinoma	Sunlight, genetic predisposition (lack of pigmentation)
			Other mammals	Papillomas, may progress to carcinomas	Experimentally, carcinogens such as methylcholanthrene

[1] In kilobases (kb); one kilobase is 1000 base pairs of nucleic acid.

[2] Where known or suspected. The absence of listed risk factors does not imply that such factors are unimportant.

about 500 000 fatalities per annum. However, even at this level it is clear that only a minority of those infected with the virus develop the tumour, and other risk factors, which may vary from area to area, must be important. Postulated factors include smoking, superinfection with another virus (the Delta agent), and consumption of alcohol or food contaminated with aflatoxin B, derived from the fungus *Aspergillus flavus*. Very similar viruses cause liver tumours in rodents and these should provide a good model for studying this important human disease.

One genus of the papovavirus family contains two important tools of the molecular biologist, polyoma and SV40, and two agents closely related to these that commonly infect humans, BK and JC virus. These latter have not been associated with any human tumour but they are frequently detected in immunosuppressed individuals, they transform cells in tissue culture, and they can induce tumours in rodents, so they are clearly still viewed with suspicion.

The papillomaviruses, in contrast, have long been known to cause tumours in many animals—benign warts (papillomas). However, it is now clear that these lesions can become malignant, but they have a natural history that may be very complicated. For instance, molecular biology techniques have revealed over 60 different papillomaviruses that infect humans alone, and those types commonly associated with benign growths may not be the same as the types found in malignant lesions (the most important of which is carcinoma of the uterine cervix). Moreover, the progression from benign to malignant growth can depend on several other predisposing factors (see Table 8.2) making it difficult to implicate a virus by epidemiological data alone. One example gives a flavour of this complexity. The very rare human disease epidermodysplasia verruciformis shows some familial clustering (suggesting a genetic component) and usually arises in young patients with congenitally defective cell-mediated immunity. It is characterized by disseminated skin warts of two main types from which can be isolated many different papillomaviruses. Carcinomas may later develop from one type of wart associated with a subset of these papillomavirus types. The carcinomas arise mainly in areas exposed to sun-

Table 8.3 Some oncogenic large DNA viruses of animals and humans

Virus family	Genome size[1]	Virus	Host of origin	Associated tumours	Other risk factors[2]
Adenovirus	30–50 kb	Types 2, 5, 12	Human	None in humans; sarcomas in hamsters	
Herpesvirus	130–250 kb	Frog herpesvirus	Frog	Adenocarcinomas	Ambient temperature
		Marek's disease	Fowl	Neurolymphomatosis (T cell)	Genetic predisposition of unknown basis
		H. ateles and *H. saimiri*	Monkey	Lymphoma, leukaemia (T cell)	
		Kaposi's sarcoma-associated herpesvirus/human herpesvirus 8	Human	Kaposi's sarcoma	Human immunodefiency virus infection
		Epstein–Barr virus	Human	Burkitt's lymphoma Immunoblastic lymphoma Hodgkin's disease Sinonasal non-Hodgkin's lymphomas	Malaria Immune deficiency
				Nasopharyngeal carcinoma	Salted fish in infancy, histocompatibility antigen phenotype
				Lymphoepithelioma-like carconomas (?)	
		H. simplex types 1 and 2	Human	Cervical neoplasia (?)	Papillomaviruses, smoking
		Cytomegalovirus	Human	Cervical neoplasia (?)	Immune deficiency, histocompability antigen genotype
Poxvirus		Various	Mammals	Epidermal or fibromatous hyperplasia—no progressive tumours	

[1] In kilobases (kb); one kilobase is 1000 base pairs of nucleic acid.

[2] Where known or suspected. The absence of listed risk factors does not imply that such factors are unimportant.

light. Thus specific papillomaviruses, immune deficiency, and a cocarcinogen (in this case UV light) all combine in the disease process. Factors of these three classes also operate in the genesis of alimentary carcinomas in cattle, emphasizing the triad of virus, cocarcinogen, and immune impairment as a common motif in many tumours.

8.5.3 Large DNA viruses (Table 8.3)

The adenoviruses cause mild non-neoplastic diseases in humans but the same strains can cause tumours in hamsters and, as a consequence, they have been studied intensively. There is no evidence that they play a role in human cancer, but these studies have been enormously fruitful for those interested in the basic molecular mechanisms of gene expression and regulation.

The herpesviruses are more significant pathogens. Marek's disease virus causes a commercially important disease of chickens characterized by a T cell proliferation that infiltrates nervous tissue (hence the description, neurolymphomatosis). Other herpesvirus types have been linked with human neoplasia. For two of these, the herpes simplex viruses and cytomegalovirus, the evidence that they play a causal role in certain cancers (Table 8.3) is intriguing but not conclusive (Macnab 1987). However, the recently identified human herpesvirus 8 is now widely accepted as a causative agent for Kaposi's sarcoma, hence its original name of Kaposi's sarcoma-associated herpesvirus (IARC Monographs,

1997). For other lymphotropic herpesviruses the causal link is also persuasive and, although some of these agents have only recently been described, EBV has long received considerable attention and is now considered a human carcinogen (IARC Monographs, 1997). Not only does EBV cause the non-neoplastic infectious mononucleosis (glandular fever), a disease particularly common in young adults, but it is also a major risk factor in nasopharyngeal carcinoma, a common malignancy in some heavily populated parts of the world such as southern China. Once more, however, we see the familiar pattern: infection is far more widespread than the incidence of the tumour, and other factors are clearly important. This is even more evident in the case of Burkitt's lymphoma, a B cell tumour of children in West Africa and New Guinea linked jointly to EBV infection and endemic malaria. A large proportion of children in these areas have experienced both known risk factors, yet only a small minority develop the tumour. What else is required for tumorigenesis? Specific chromosomal rearrangements seem to be an important prerequisite, but what favours such events and what are their biological consequences? These are discussed further in Chapters 9 and 10 but the answer can be given here—we do not know.

8.6 Prophylaxis and therapy of virus-associated neoplasia

Although we are clearly ignorant of many aspects of the pathogenesis of virus-associated tumours, the knowledge that a virus is implicated can be used in attempts to manage the disease at any of the three arbitrary stages of virus-associated neoplasia described above and in Fig. 8.2. In general these measures are more effective in veterinary medicine (where the health of the herd can override the survival of the individual) than in human practice.

8.6.1 Preventing virus infection

The level of oncogenic viruses in the hosts' environment can be reduced by hygiene and husbandry techniques, and by detecting and, if necessary, eliminating carriers. The latter approach has been used in managing diseases caused by the avian, feline, and bovine retroviruses and it has some limited applications in humans, for instance in detecting agents like

hepatitis B virus and HIV in donor blood intended for transfusion.

Increased genetic resistance to infection can be bred into domestic animals, an approach successful in developing chicken strains relatively resistant to both avian leukosis and Marek's disease.

However, in most cases acquired immunity to infection is the only option. Vaccines made from ground-up wart tissue have long been used as a prophylactic and, indeed, therapeutic measure against papillomas in animals, but the first successful commercial vaccines against a neoplasm were produced against Marek's disease and are a great boon to the poultry industry. A useful, but far from ideal, vaccine now exists against feline leukaemia but, in contrast to veterinary problems, proposals to produce vaccines against human oncogenic viruses have long been controversial, for several reasons: (i) in many instances the role of the virus in the tumour is uncertain; (ii) tumour production may be a rare outcome of infection by a widespread and not very pathogenic virus; and (iii) since tumours may result from an aberrant virus cell interaction, a classic vaccine, based on inactivated or attenuated virus, may itself pose a health risk. This last objection may be obviated by using purified immunogens produced by genetically manipulated portions of viral genomes or synthesized in the laboratory.

The first two considerations, however, suggest that the returns (in terms of improved health of the population) may not justify the outlay unless the virus causes significant disease in addition to its oncogenic potential (as is the case with HIV and hepatitis B virus), unless there are clearly defined, small, high risk populations, or unless the virus is the only clearly defined risk factor in the genesis of a common tumour (as with EBV-associated nasopharyngeal carcinoma).

These reservations, together with the problems of developing a safe and effective vaccine and delivering it to a susceptible population before they contract the virus, provide scope for other approaches. An alternative, popular with the pharmaceutical industry, is to limit infection, usually after it is clinically evident, with antiviral chemotherapy. This, too, poses problems inherent in the close symbiosis between viruses and their host cells, since drugs must be devised that are preferentially toxic for the virus. One approach focuses on processes essential to the virus and dispensable by the cell, such as reverse transcription by the retroviral RNA-dependent

DNA polymerase. Within these constraints, some widely used and moderately effective drugs have been developed against, for instance, herpesviruses and retroviruses.

8.6.2 Preventing cell conversion to neoplasia

The problems of tackling virus infection suggest that other potentially avoidable risk factors, which tend to operate at this stage, might provide easier targets for preventive measures. Such hopes, however, seem largely misplaced. In humans these risk factors include habits (notably smoking), dietary factors (which may be even harder to eliminate than smoking unless, like aflatoxin contamination, they are obviously undesirable), and other diseases. The most striking example of the latter is malaria, a risk factor in Burkitt's lymphoma in certain tropical areas but also a crushing disease problem in its own right in many parts of the world. Indeed, reducing or eliminating some of these risk factors would have benefits far beyond the reduction in cancer incidence, and this seems so evident that one doubts that the incentive of reducing cancer will work where other imperatives have so signally failed.

8.6.3 Tackling clinical neoplasia

Can a knowledge of tumour virology contribute to tumour diagnosis and therapy? So far such applications have been on a small scale but, in principle, a detailed understanding of the role of any given virus in cancer should aid diagnosis and prognosis by screening for characteristic viral genes or proteins, or a host response to them. It is harder to see how such knowledge could be applied to therapy, but there is the tantalizing example of interferon, a general antiviral agent produced by host cells after infection with many different viruses, which also has an antitumour effect in a few cases that is, as yet, poorly understood. There have also been instances of regression of virus-associated tumours in response either to viral antisera or to a 'vaccine' extracted from homogenized tumour. The latter effect, well known for papillomavirus infections, helps to justify attempts to produce vaccines against HPV-16 and HPV18, the two papillomaviruses most implicated in human cervical carcinoma. By the criteria mentioned in Section 8.6.1 above, venereally transmitted human papillomaviruses are not strong candidates for management by vaccination. Although there are high risk groups such as prostitutes, a very large proportion of the population in a sexually permissive society is at some risk of infection, which suggests the need for an extensive vaccination programme. Set against this is the fact that neoplasia is a relatively rare consequence of sexual promiscuity that might better be tackled by a screening programme allied to an education campaign (that would also help to reduce other venereal diseases). However, if vaccines against HPV can promote regression of cervical carcinoma, then they may play a greater role in its therapy than in its prevention.

Clearly, we will not advance much further with these considerations until we unravel the details of how a tumour virus subverts cell growth. Fortunately, as the next section describes, such understanding is beginning to take shape from the amorphous complexity of tumour virus behaviour.

8.7 The mechanisms of virus-induced neoplasia

We have already seen that workers in the 1960s set out to identify viral genes that directly converted normal cells to neoplastic growth. However, the many variations of intracellular parasitism exhibited by viruses could, in theory, permit neoplasia by a number of other mechanisms. Indeed, as we identify more tumour viruses so we are compelled to invoke an ever-widening spectrum of pathogenic mechanisms. In this section we will survey, with examples, these different modes of virus-induced neoplasia (Table 8.4).

The two major categories of the disease process are: (i) that in which the tumour cell ancestry must at some stage have been infected by the tumour-inducing virus; and (ii) that in which the tumour cell ancestry need not be infected by the virus. Neoplasia in the first category is a direct consequence of infection while in the second category it results indirectly, from infection of other cells (the terms intrinsic and extrinsic have also been used to describe these two mechanisms).

8.7.1 Indirect mechanisms: suppression and stimulation of cell proliferation

Most virus infections kill cells and if the cells of the host's immune system are targets for viral infection then immune deficiency, particularly an impairment of cell-mediated immunity, can result. The role of

Table 8.4 Mechanisms of virus-induced neoplasia

Pathogenic mechanism	Examples
Indirect	
1. Suppression of host immune system, impaired elimination of tumour cells	Avian reticuloendotheliosis viruses, feline leukaemia virus, HTLV-1, HIV-1, Marek's disease virus, cytomegalovirus
2. Stimulation of cell proliferation, increased 'targets' for other neoplastic changes	
(a) tissue regeneration after virus cytolysis	Probably hepatitis B and C viruses
(b) mitogenesis of immune competent or other cells	Possably some mouse leukaemia viruses, HTLV-1, HIV-1
Direct	
1. 'Hit and run': no crucial virus gene or structure whose persistence is essential Viral DNA or viral functions act transiently	Possibly some herpes viruses (including EBV), bovine papillomavirus
2. Crucial parts of viral genomes persist in tumour cells	
(a) virus carries a gene whose product directly or indirectly initiates and/or maintains neoplasia (oncogene)	
(i) oncogene descended from normal cell counterpart (*protooncogene*) in past evolution	Rous sarcoma virus, actue leukaemia viruses
(ii) oncogene directly transduced from protooncogene during virus infection	Feline leukaemia virus, avian leukosis virus
(iii) oncogene with no related normal cell counterpart	SV40, polyomavirus, papillomaviruses, adenoviruses, EBV, bovine leukosis virus, HTLV-1
(b) Insertional mutagenesis: virus DNA inserted in the host chromosome augments or destroys normal gene expression	Avian leukosis viruses, mouse leukaemia and mammary tumour viruses, woodchuck hepatitis virus and possibly some papillomaviruses

immune surveillance in cancer has been controversial (see Chapter 16) but, as we saw above, many virus-associated neoplasms occur in hosts with immune deficiency and it is possible that tumour cells arising in these hosts by unknown mechanisms are simply not eliminated. Viruses such as avian reticuloendotheliosis viruses, Marek's disease virus, feline leukaemia virus, HTLV, and cytomegaloviruses are known to have immune suppressive effects sometimes, but not always, associated with cytotoxicity. However, these agents also seem to have another, possibly direct, tumorigenic effect. One likely exception is HIV which does not appear to act directly in tumour causation. Its effect seems partly to be a result of immune impairment and a consequent inability to kill tumour cells arising by other mechanisms, and partly to other indirect mechanisms to be mentioned next.

Another possible consequence of virus infection is a reactive cell proliferation, the expansion of a cell population, increasing the chance of occurrence of a neoplastic change. In principle this proliferation can have several causes, one of which, regeneration of tissue damaged by virus cytolysis, has been invoked for liver carcinogenesis associated with hepatitis B

and C virus infections (Slagle *et al.* 1994). It is also possible that the frequently observed production of growth factors by virally transformed cells might stimulate hyperplasia of uninfected cells but the only good example of this plausible phenomenon is the induction of Kaposi's sarcoma in AIDS patients infected with HIV-1 and human herpesvirus 8 (Weller 1994). There is better evidence for chronic retroviral infection stimulating immune competent cells into proliferation. For example, in HTLV-1-associated B cell chronic lymphocytic leukaemia, the tumour cells are uninfected but recognize viral antigens (Mann *et al.* 1987). A similar mechanism also operates in HIV-1-associated B cell lymphomas, and variants have also been implicated in murine leukaemia virus-induced T cell lymphomas, although in this latter case the lymphoma cells are infected by the viruses, which additionally have a direct insertional mutagenesis component (see Section 8.7.5). Furthermore, virion constituents may mimic ligands for receptors on the surface of other cell types (see Chapters 9 and 11). If these receptors modulate normal cell growth and behaviour, chronic unscheduled binding of ligand analogues may lead to hyperplasia and then neoplasia.

This appears to happen with the viral envelope-derived oncogene of the mouse spleen focus-forming virus, which binds to the erythropoietin receptor, replacing the need for exogenous growth factors in erythroleukaemia. In a more complex example, mouse mammary tumour viruses (MMTV) encode polymorphic superantigens that stimulate developing and mature T cells, it being postulated that the latter release growth factors that drive proliferation of the MMTV-infected cells.

8.7.2 Direct mechanisms: the 'hit and run' hypothesis

It is conceivable that transient cell infection induces a heritable neoplastic change in the cell lineage and the infecting virus is then lost. In practice this mechanism is indistinguishable from the indirect modes described above. It can also resemble the direct mechanisms detailed below if specific viral functions are required only for the earliest steps of a multistage tumour evolution, as may occur with bovine papillomavirus and EBV. However, in other instances, notably herpes simplex virus and cytomegalovirus induced tumours, portions of the viral genome frequently persist. If neither the fragment of persisting virus, nor its location in the cell genome, show any discernible pattern, it is suspected that they represent the 'footprints' of an earlier 'hit and run' event whose significance cannot now be assessed (Macnab 1987). Since they are difficult to investigate, 'hit and run' and indirect mechanisms are usually only considered after failing to demonstrate tumour formation by one of the direct mechanisms described below.

8.7.3 Direct mechanisms: oncogenes with cellular ancestors

The viruses that most readily transform cells in culture (Fig. 8.1) and most rapidly induce tumours in animals are the chicken and mouse retroviruses that cause sarcomas and 'acute' (rapid) leukaemias, and the polyomavirus group of the papovaviruses. Using cell culture, mutants of these viruses with defects in transformation were obtained (Fig. 8.3) and analysis of these mutants defined transforming genes in the viruses. These genes, as predicted by the pioneer workers in this field, encode proteins necessary to initiate and/or maintain transformed cell growth, and they comprise two classes.

The retroviruses mostly contain transforming genes that play no part in virus replication and have, indeed, usually replaced portions of viral replicative genes in the virus genome (Weiss *et al.* 1984). These genes are related to sequences in normal host cells from which they are believed to have evolved after 'capture' of the cell gene by the virus in some ancestral infection. (Indeed, this evolution is apparently sometimes recapitulated when tumours are induced by certain chicken and cat leukaemia viruses.) These transforming genes were named viral oncogenes and the cellular counterparts became known as cellular oncogenes, or, since they presumably serve some crucial non-neoplastic function in the host, protooncogenes. These oncogenes, first brought to our attention by the retroviruses, encode aberrantly regulated components of the pathways that transmit signals from the cell exterior to nuclear and cytoplasmic responders, leading to altered cell growth and behaviour. Together with the tumour suppressor genes, which have generally countervailing effects, they are now central to studies on the molecular biology of cancer and are dealt with more fully in Chapters 9 and 10.

8.7.4 Direct mechanisms: oncogenes without cellular ancestors

The second class of transforming gene is exemplified by those in the DNA tumour viruses and in retroviruses such as bovine leukosis virus and HTLV-1. These genes are not derived from cellular ancestors but play a part in the virus life cycle and they induce neoplasia in a variety of ways.

One common mechanism is for a tumour virus protein to interact with a cellular tumour suppressor gene product, leading to the latter's inactivation or degradation (Vaux *et al.* 1994; Vousden 1994). Tumour suppressors comprise not only those genes whose loss contributes directly to the tumour cell phenotype, but also genes that protect the organism from the consequences of genomic damage and whose loss thus increases the chance of neoplasia developing (Chapter 4). Viral oncogenes interact with a number of members of this heterogeneous group.

The tumour suppressor protein pRB, which regulates the onset of cellular DNA synthesis, is functionally compromised by complexing with the T antigen of SV40 virus, the E7 protein of human papillomavirus (HPV), and the E1A protein of ade-

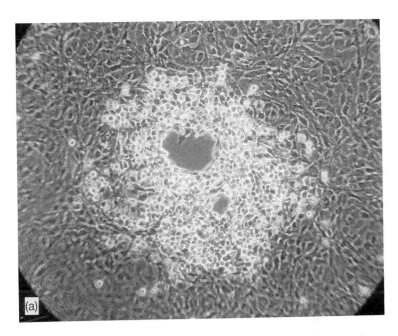

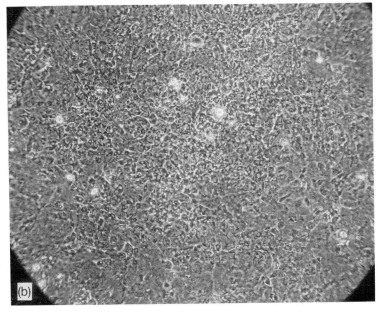

Fig. 8.3 Cell transformation by viruses with mutations in transforming genes. Some mutants of Rous sarcoma virus have 'temperature sensitive' defects in transformation. Infected cells grown at the 'permissive' temperature are transformed because the viral transforming gene functions normally. At the 'restrictive' temperature the gene is inactive and the infected cells are normal. (a) A focus of transformed cells on a chicken embryo cell monolayer induced by infection with a Rous sarcoma virus temperature-sensitive mutant and incubation at permissive temperature. The cells are rounded and detaching from the substrate, so that holes are appearing in the cell sheet. After photography the culture was incubated at restrictive temperature and four days later was photographed. (b) The cells are now flatter and more indistinct and the gaps in the cell sheet have been filled in. (×100 for both)

novirus. E1A protein has also been shown to induce apoptosis, suggesting that this is a host response to the aberrant DNA synthesis that results from pRB inactivation. In support of this view, the p53 protein, that elicits apoptosis in response to DNA damage (Lane 1994), is also inactivated by interaction with gene products of the same tumour viruses (SV40 T antigen, HPV E6 protein, and adenovirus E1B pro-

tein, respectively). Epstein–Barr virus also encodes anti-apoptotic functions, its BHRF1 protein having sequence and functional similarities to the cellular inhibitor of apoptosis, bcl-2, while its latency specific LMP-1 product up-regulates cellular bcl-2 activity. These viruses thus appear to encode the means to neutralize the apoptotic response that they themselves may induce.

Prevention of apoptosis is probably a significant feature of viral neoplasia but several tumour virus oncoproteins work in other ways. The function of the cellular protein ductin is compromised by binding to the bovine papillomavirus E5 protein (and homologous proteins in other papillomaviruses) or to the HTLV-1 p12 protein. Ductin, a component of intercellular gap junctions and intracellular proton pumps, can be regarded as a tumour suppressor, since loss of its function should affect both cell to cell communication and the down-regulation of responses to growth factors (Chapter 11). SV40 small T antigen apparently stimulates growth-promoting protein kinase signalling pathways by inactivating a protein phosphatase, an enzyme that can also be considered a tumour suppressor. The middle T antigen of polyomavirus also affects cell signalling but by a strategem that does not involve tumour suppressors, since it activates non-receptor protein tyrosine kinases that signal to growth-promoting pathways. Finally, bovine leukosis virus, HTLV-1, hepatitis B virus, and, probably, Epstein Barr virus all encode proteins that increase expression from their own genomes and, as a consequence, can trans-activate cellular genes, some of which are presumed to influence neoplasia.

In short, although this class of viral oncogenes has not directly identified cellular genes with a broader role in neoplasia it has indirectly revealed more complex, yet very important, features of the neoplastic process (summarized in Table 8.5).

8.7.5 Direct mechanisms: insertional mutagenesis

It appears, however, that many retroviruses without oncogenes induce neoplasia by a different means. The majority of retroviruses contain only the genes needed for their own replication, they cannot transform cells in tissue culture, they induce tumours after a long latency, and tumour induction results from a direct effect of the viral genome rather than from the action of a virus-coded protein.

Avian leukosis viruses (ALV) are retroviruses of this type and studies on the lymphomas they induce provided the following clues to this mode of pathogenesis. All or most of the cells in a lymphoma contain ALV proviruses integrated at the same site in the host DNA. There are two explanations for this: either the provirus is obliged to integrate at one location or the tumour is a clone, all its cells deriving from a single ancestor. The former possibility is eliminated by showing that ALV can insert itself at many sites in the normal cells of the host. It follows that, although many cells in the bird are infected, in only a very small minority of these cells does an event occur that promotes the clonal neoplastic growth of the cell. When lymphomas from different birds are compared, ALV proviruses are found integrated in the same region of the host DNA in over 90 per cent of them, although many of these proviruses are incomplete. The conclusion, that the site of provirus integration is vital to tumorigenesis, led to the postulate that the provirus acts as a mutagen whose insertion disrupts host gene expression in that

Table 8.5 Mode of action of viral oncogenes with no obvious cellular ancestor[1]

Virus	Inhibition of tumour suppression			Growth stimulation		
	pRb inhibition	p53 inhibition	Other anti-apoptotic effects	Ductin inhibition	Protein kinase stimulation	Transactivation
HTLV-1				p12		Tax
Hepatitis B virus		HBx (?)				HBx, Pre-S
Polyomavirus	Large T	Large T			Middle T	
SV40 virus	Large T	Large T			Small T	
Papillomavirus	E7	E6		E5 etc.		
Adenovirus	E1A	E1B				
Epstein–Barr virus	EBNA-5 (?)	EBNA-5 (?)	BHRF1 LMP-1			EBNA-1 (?)

[1] Viral oncogenes listed are those whose function has been identified. ? signifies that the biological role of an activity is uncertain. A gap means that an activity has not yet been convincingly ascribed to a virus gene product but does not mean that such an activity does not exist.

region (Weiss *et al.* 1984). You should note that this is the only one of these postulated pathogenic mechanisms in which virus DNA integration is obligatory.

This concept of 'insertional mutagenesis' has been supported by studies very similar to those described above on other virus-induced chicken tumours, on comparable tumours induced by some mouse leukaemia viruses, on adenocarcinomas caused by mouse mammary tumour virus, and on liver tumours caused by woodchuck hepatitis virus (Peters 1990). It has also been invoked to explain oncogenesis by hepatitis B virus and some papillomaviruses. How does the virus exert its mutagenic effect? Does it destroy host gene functions or stimulate them? Ablation of p53 function by proviral insertion has been found in Friend murine leukaemia virus-induced erythroleukaemias. However, in most cases host genes seem to be stimulated. Increased transcription of host DNA in the vicinity of an integrated provirus has often been detected, and this is generally ascribed to the action of elements in the provirus that increase transcription (such elements are required by the provirus to transcribe its own genes—see Chapter 9—and they are themselves subject to modulation by tissue-specific host cell factors, such that they are more efficient in some tissues than others). Moreover, in a number of instances it has been shown that the proviruses have integrated in the vicinity of, and increased transcription of, host protooncogenes. This further implicates such genes in neoplasia, and where a provirus has not integrated near a known protooncogene it is suspected that its integration site pin-points other genes that are important in tumorigenesis. We thus hope that new oncogenes will be identified in this 'guilt by association' process and this reasoning is pursued further in Chapters 9 and 10.

8.8 Conclusions

We have seen that viruses are important environmental carcinogens. In domestic animals they can be the predominant risk factors in some common and commercially important cancers. They are also implicated in about 15 per cent of human malignancies (zur Hausen 1991), although in humans the interplay between viruses and other risk factors may be very complex. Prophylactic procedures against infectious diseases have been used efficiently for over a century and it was hoped that similar approaches might prove successful in eliminating virus-associated cancer. However, the complexity of the disease process has frequently complicated such attempts and to improve management of these diseases we clearly need to understand more about the pathogenesis of virus-induced neoplasia.

Such basic studies have, in fact, already spurred advances in other directions. Genes in tumour viruses may directly mediate the neoplastic growth of the cells they infect, either as homologues of protooncogenes or as antagonists of tumour suppressor genes. Tumour virology has thus provided the first glimpses of genes that become altered in cancer cells, no matter what the precipitating cause of the disease may be. Much modern cancer research now aims to widen this window, to identify the full panoply of these oncogenes and tumour suppressor genes, to detect the functions of their products, and to determine how these functions affect normal and neoplastic cell growth and behaviour. The development of this work is reflected in the following chapters and we will leave it with one final thought. At various stages in its history, tumour virology has been dominated by the precepts and techniques of different scientific disciplines. Beginning with observations on whole animals, the field has become sequentially the preserve of the pathologist, the cell biologist, and the molecular geneticist. Now, with increasing emphasis on the products of oncogenes, the biochemist and protein chemist are coming to the fore. It is important that each of these disciplines realizes that it is looking at aspects of one biological question, and that it appreciates the accretion of understanding provided by its predecessors in the field. Only by such a breadth of view are we likely to close the circle and return to answer the questions that stimulated these studies—how do we prevent, diagnose, or treat malignant disease in the whole organism?

References and further reading

Collier, L. H. and Timbury, M. C. (ed.) (1990). *Topley and Wilson's principles of bacteriology, virology and immunity*, Vol. 4, *Virology*, (8th edn). Edward Arnold, London.

IARC *Monographs on the evaluation of carcinogenic risks to humans* (1997). Epstein-Barr virus and Kaposi's Sarcoma herpesvirus/Human Herpesvirus 8. **70**, IARC Press, Lyon.

Lane, D. P. (1994). Tumour suppressor genes and p53. In *Viruses and cancer* (ed. A. Minson, J. Neil, and M. McCrae), pp. 15–25. Cambridge University Press, Cambridge.

Macnab, J. C. M. (1987). Herpes simplex virus and human cytomegalovirus: their role in morphological transformation and genital cancer. *Journal of General Virology*, **68**, 2525–50. Tackles the difficult question of oncogenesis by herpesviruses that lack a specific oncogene.

Mann, D. L. De Santis, P., Mark, G., Pfeifer, A., Newman, M., Gibbs, N., Popovic, M., Sarngadharan, M. G., Gallo, R. C., Clark, J. and Blattner, W. (1987). HTLV-1-associated B-cell CLL: indirect role for retrovirus in leukemogenesis. *Science*, **236**, 1103–6. A primary source with useful references on indirect modes of neoplasia.

Minson, A., Neil, J., and McCrae, M. (ed.) (1994). *Viruses and cancer*. Cambridge University Press, Cambridge. Excellent and wide ranging reviews, several of which are quoted separately in this section.

Onions, D. E. and Jarrett, O. (ed.) (1987). Naturally occurring tumours in animals as a model for human disease. *Cancer Surveys*, **6**, 1–181.

Peters, G. (1990). Oncogenes at viral integration sites. *Cell Growth and Differentiation*, **1**, 503–10. A good short review.

Slagle, B. L., Becker, S. A., and Butel, J. S. (1994). Hepatitis viruses and liver cancer. In *Viruses and cancer* (ed. A. Minson, J. Neil, and M. McCrae), pp. 149–171. Cambridge University Press, Cambridge.

Thompson, C. B. (1995). Apoptosis in the pathogenesis and treatment of disease. *Science*, **267**, 1456–62.

Vaux, D. L., Haecker, G., and Strasser, A. (1994). An evolutionary perspective on apoptosis. *Cell*, **76**, 777–9. Two informative reviews on apoptosis.

Vousden, K. H. (1994). Cell transformation by human papillomaviruses. In *Viruses and cancer* (ed. A. Minson, J. Neil, and M. McCrae), pp. 27–46. Cambridge University Press, Cambridge.

Weiss, R. A., Teich, N., Varmus, H., and Coffin, J. (ed.) (1984). *The molecular biology of tumor viruses: RNA tumor viruses*, (2nd edn and Appendices). Cold Spring Harbor Laboratory, Cold Spring Harbor, New York.

Weller, I. V. D. (1994). HIV and predisposition to cancer. In *Viruses and cancer* (ed. A. Minson, J. Neil, and M. McCrae), pp. 293–306. Cambridge University Press, Cambridge.

Wyke, J. and Weiss, R. (ed.) (1984). Viruses in human and animal cancers. *Cancer Surveys*, **3**, 1–218.

Yoshida, M. and Seiki, M. (1987). Recent advances in the molecular biology of HTLV-1: *trans*-activation of viral and cellular genes. *Annual Review of Immunology*, **5**, 541–59.

zur Hausen, H. (1991). Viruses in human cancers. *Science*, **254**, 1167–73. More detail on the viruses important for human neoplasia.

9

Oncogenes and cancer

NATALIE M. TEICH

9.1 What is an oncogene?

The term oncogene has been used in several of the preceding chapters and will arise again in subsequent chapters. In this section, we shall try to amalgamate current knowledge and hypotheses of this fascinating subject from a more functional view. The generic name 'oncogene' was coined to delineate a gene capable of causing cancer. Obviously, this may be an oversimplified concept as the previous chapters have presented evidence that the genesis of a tumour is a complex issue involving multifactorial and/or multistep processes.

Some confusion may arise when reading this chapter and other chapters in the book regarding the nomenclature for genes. That is because there is no standardized format, particularly as some genes were discovered in mouse cells, others in humans, and still others in viruses, and different names were given to genes that eventually were known to be essentially the same. Genes described for human cells are usually written in upper case, italic type and their protein products in upper case roman type. Mouse genes are often given in lower

case italic type, their products as for those of human genes; those from *Drosophila* are italicized with the first letter capitalized if the gene is dominant. Specific oncogenes may be cited by a lower case first letter (c for cellular, v for viral), followed by a hyphen, and then the gene name in italic type. However, there may be further modifier terms. Hopefully, for the most part, we have maintained some degree of consistency.

9.1.1 First encounter: retroviruses

As discussed in Chapter 8, the family of RNA tumour viruses, Retroviridae, comprises a vast number of members from many animal species, with a wide range of pathogenic properties, including neoplastic and non-neoplastic diseases. The most common oncogenic viruses (such as long latency leukaemia viruses and the murine mammary tumour virus) contain genes for their replication only, and cause tumours by mechanisms grouped as insertional mutations, which may often take many months for clinical manifestation (see Chapter 8, Fig. 9.1, and below).

However, about 50 virus isolates have the interesting property of being able to induce tumours in infected animals after very short latency periods (generally days or weeks) and, furthermore, are often capable of causing morphological alterations in cells grown *in vitro* (transformation, see Chapter 8). Dissection of the genomes of these viruses showed that most of them had lost genetic information coding for their replicative genes (and hence were known as replication defective, albeit transformation competent, viruses). New genetic information was inserted in place of the deleted material (Fig. 9.1). By a variety of genetic techniques, this new set of sequences was shown to be responsible for the short latency and transformation-inducing capacities. Hence, the new sequences were designated as oncogenes, or *onc* genes. Nucleic acid sequencing and hybridization techniques revealed that the *onc* gene sequences of these 50 viruses were sometimes essentially identical and sometimes completely unrelated. Thus, approximately 30 different viral oncogenes (v-*onc* genes) were distinguished. Each of the separate v-*oncs* was given a different name, a three-letter word to define the virus from which it was isolated, which is italicized in type like other genes. This nomenclature is illustrated in Table 9.1.

The first important question to be asked was: where did the v-*onc* sequences come from? Again, nucleic acid hybridization studies were used to demonstrate unambiguously that the v-*onc* sequences were almost identical to sequences in the cellular DNA of the animal species from which the virus was isolated so that cellular DNA contains genes which when 'transplanted' (transduced) into retroviruses are cancer-causing genes. Moreover, it was shown that the *onc* sequences could be found in the DNA of every cell from virtually all higher vertebrate orders ('evolutionary conservation'). Thus, these sequences related to viral oncogenes are inherited from one generation to the next in the same way as one inherits genes for eye colour. It is clear, however, that these genes cannot be operating as cancer genes in cells (and indeed our own cells). How can we envisage this subtle but extremely important dichotomy? Firstly, one could imagine that the genes were never turned on (expressed) in animals. This is clearly not so, as messenger RNA (mRNA) molecules and also protein products of the genes can be found in different cell types, sometimes

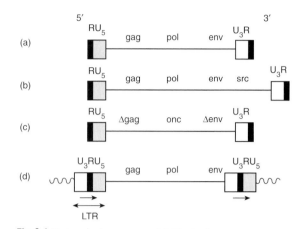

Fig. 9.1 Retroviral genomes. (a) Typical genome structure of a long latency leukaemia virus. The three replicative genes are shown: *gag*, the gene encoding the internal core structures; *pol*, encoding the RNA-dependent DNA polymerase enzyme known as reverse transcriptase; and *env*, encoding the envelope proteins inserted into the plasma membrane which becomes incorporated into mature virions. 5′ and 3′ denote the polarity of the molecule, as the RNA can serve directly as a mRNA molecule and be translated into protein (a positive strand genome). R denotes a short segment of RNA repeated at each end of the molecule. U_5 and U_3 denote non-coding, unique sequences at each end that contain the regulatory elements (the promoter and enhancer sequences) for viral transcription. (b) The structure of the Rous sarcoma virus of chickens, the only retrovirus that contains all replicative genes and, additionally, an oncogene (*src*). (c) Structure of the acutely leukaemogenic or transforming retroviruses. These genomes generally lack all or part of one or more of the replicative genes, thus rendering them defective for replication. The deleted sequences have been replaced by cellular sequences that confer the oncogenic potential (generically called *onc* genes). The extent of replicative gene deletion and location of the *onc* gene are distinct for each viral isolate. (d) Structure of the integrated virus (DNA provirus). The mode of replication of retroviruses generates duplicated ends known as long terminal repeat (LTR) structures in which the U_5 region is duplicated at the extreme 3′ end, and U_3 at the 5′ end. The LTRs are important for the integration of the provirus into chromosomal DNA and always generate a complete proviral DNA colinear with viral RNA. Another important feature is that the regulatory elements for viral transcription are now found also at the 3′ end of the molecule and thus can serve as promoters or enhancers for adjacent cell genes (denoted by the wavy lines).

Table 9.1 Retroviral oncogenes

onc	Retrovirus isolates[1]	v-*onc* origin[2]	v-*onc* protein[3]	Virus disease	v-*onc* product activity[4]	v-*onc* product location	Human chromosome
src	RSV	Chicken	pp60^{src}	Sarcoma	PK(tyr)	Inner side of plasma membrane	20q12–q13
	*r*ASV	Quail	pp60^{src}	Sarcoma	PK(tyr)	Inner side of plasma membrane	
fps	FuSV-ASV	Chicken	P130$^{gag-fps}$	Sarcoma	PK(tyr)	Plasma membrane	15q24–q25
	PRCII-ASV	Chicken	P105$^{gag-fps}$	Sarcoma	PK(tyr)	Plasma membrane	
	PRCIV-ASV	Chicken	P170$^{gag-fps}$	Sarcoma	PK(tyr)	Plasma membrane	
	UR1-ASV	Chicken	P150$^{gag-fps}$	Sarcoma	PK(tyr)	Plasma membrane	
	16L-ASV	Chicken	P142$^{gas-fps}$	Sarcoma	PK(tyr)	Plasma membrane	
fes	ST-FeSV	Cat	P85$^{gas-fes}$	Sarcoma	PK(tyr)	Plasma membrane	
	GA-FeSV	Cat	P110$^{gas-fes}$	Sarcoma	PK(tyr)	Plasma membrane	
	HZ1-FeSV	Cat	P100$^{gag-fes}$	Sarcoma	PK(tyr)	Plasma membrane	
yes	Y73-ASV	Chicken	P90$^{gas-yes}$	Sarcoma	PK(ytr)	Plasma membrane	18q21.3
	Esh-ASV	Chicken	P80$^{gas-yes}$	Sarcoma	PK(tyr)	Plasma membrane	
fgr	GR-FeSv	Cat	P70$^{gag-actin-fgr}$	Sarcoma	PK(tyr)	Cytoplasmic	1p36
ros	UR2-ASV	Chicken	P68$^{gas-ros}$	Sarcoma	PK(tyr)	Plasma membrane	6q22
abl	Ab-MLV	Mouse	P90–P160$^{gag-abl}$	Pre B cell leukaemia	PK(tyr)	Plasma membrane	9q34–qter
	HZ2-FeSv	Cat	P98$^{gag-abl}$	Sarcoma	PK(tyr)	Plasma membrane	
ski	Sk*n*-rASV	Chicken	P110$^{gag-ski-pol}$ P125$^{gag-ski-pol}$	Squamous carcinoma	?	Nucleus	1q12–qter
erbA	AEV-ES4	Chicken	P75$^{gag-erbA}$	?	Thyroid hormone receptor	Cytoplasm	(1): 17p11–q21
	AEV-R	Chicken	P75$^{gag-erbA}$			Cytoplasm	(2): 17
erbB	AEV-ES4	Chicken	gp65^{erbB}	Erythroblastosis and Sarcoma	Truncated EGF receptor PK(tyr)	Plasma membrane	7p13–p12
	AEV-R	Chicken	gp65^{erbB}				
	AEV-H	Chicken	gp65^{erbB}				
fms	SM-FeSV	Cat	gp180$^{gag-fms}$ gp140^{fms} gp120^{fms}	Sarcoma	PK(tyr) M-CSF receptor	Intermediate filaments, membranes	5q34
kit	HZ4-FeSv	Cat	P80$^{gag-kit}$	Sarcoma	*W* allele PK(tyr)	Plasma membrane	4q11–q21
sea	AEV-S13	Chicken	gP155$^{env-sea}$	Sarcoma, granulocytic leukaemia, and erythroblastosis	PK(tyr)	Plasma membrane	11q13
fos	FBJ-MSV	Mouse	pp55^{fos}	Osteosarcoma	DNA binding; complexes with *jun* (AP-1 transcription factor)	Nucleus	14q24.3
	FBR-MSV	Mouse	P75$^{gag-fos-fox}$	Osteosarcoma			
	NK24-ASV	Chicken	P100$^{gag-fos}$	Nephroblastoma			
mos	Mo-MSV	Mouse	P37$^{env-mos}$	Sarcoma	PK(ser, thr); oocyte maturation factor	Cytoplasm	8q11–q12
	Gz-MSV	Mouse	?	Sarcoma			
	MPV-MSV	Mouse	P34^{mos}	Sarcoma, erythroleukaemia, and myeloproliferation			

Table 9.1 Retroviral oncogenes (contd)

onc	Retrovirus isolates[1]	v-*onc* origin[2]	v-*onc* protein[3]	Virus disease	v-*onc* product activity[4]	v-*onc* product location	Human chromosome
sis	SSV	Monkey	P28$^{env-sis}$	Sarcoma	Truncated PDGF (B chain)	Membranes ? secreted	22q12.3–q13.1
	PI-FeSv	Cat	P76$^{gag-sis}$	Sarcoma			
	FT-FeSV	Cat	?	Sarcoma			
	TP2-FeSV	Cat	?	Sarcoma			
myc	MC29	Chicken	P110$^{gag-myc}$	Sarcoma, carcinoma and myelocytoma	DNA binding	Nucleus (P100 cytoplasmic)	8q24
	MH2	Chicken	P100$^{gag-mil-myc}$ P58^{myc}				
	CMII	Chicken	P90$^{gag-myc}$	Myelocytoma	Transcription factor		
	OK10	Chicken	P200$^{gag-pol-myc}$	Carcinoma			
	FeLV-*myc*	Cat	?	Granulocytic leukaemia			
crk	CT10-ASV	Chicken	p47$^{gag-crk}$	Sarcoma	Phospholipase C-related; regulator of PK(tyr) activity	Cytoplasmic	?
maf	AS42-ASV	Chicken	?	Sarcoma	?	Nucleus	?
cbl	CasNS-MSV	Mouse	P100$^{gag-cbl}$	Pre B leukaemia	Transcription activator	Nucleus	11q23.2-qter
jun	S17-ASV	Chicken	P65$^{gag-jun}$	Sarcoma	Complexes with *fos* (AP-1 transcription factor)	Nucleus	1p31–p32
myb	AMV-BAI/A	Chicken	p45^{myb}	Myeloblastosis	Transcription factor	Nucleus	6q22–q24
	AMV-E26	Chicken	P135$^{gag-ets-myb}$	Myeloblastosis and erythroblastosis			
rel	REV-T	Turkey	P64^{rel}	Reticulo-endotheliosis	Forms transcription factor with NF-KB	Nucleus	2p13–p12
raf	3611-MSV	Mouse	gP90$^{gag-raf}$ P75$^{gag-raf}$	Sarcoma	PK(ser, thr)	Cytoplasmic	(1): 3p25 (2): 4[5]
mil	MH2	Chicken	P100$^{gag-mil-myc}$	See above for *myc*			
Ha-*ras*	Ha-MSV	Rat	pp21^{ras}	Sarcoma and erythroleukaemia	GTP binding GTPase	Plasma membrane	(1):11p13 (2): X[5]
	RaSV	Rat	P29$^{gag-ras}$	? Sarcoma			
	BALB-MSV	Mouse	pp21^{ras}	Haemangiosarcoma			
Ki-*ras*	Ki-MSV	Rat	pp21^{ras}	Sarcoma and erythyroleukaemia	GTP binding GTPase	Plasma membrane	(1): 6p32-q13[5] (2): 12p12-pter
	NY-FeSV	Cat	?	Sarcoma			
ets	AMV-E26	Chicken	P135$^{gag-ets-myb}$	See above for *myb*	Transcription factor	Nucleus	(1): 11q23–q24 (2): 21q22

[1] RSV, Rous sarcoma virus; ASV, avian sarcoma virus; FeSV, feline sarcoma virus; FeLV, feline leukaemia virus; MLV, murine leukaemia virus; AEV, avian erythroblastosis virus; SSV, simian sarcoma virus; AMV, avian myeloblastosis virus; REV, reticuloendotheliosis virus; MSV, murine sarcoma virus. The other notations indicate specific viral strains.

[2] The origin denotes the species of animal from which the *onc* gene was transduced by a retrovirus. Note that in some cases the same *onc* gene has been transduced by retroviruses from different animals.

[3] The nomenclature has been standardized as follows: p, protein; pp, phosphoprotein; P, fusion protein between a retroviral replicative gene (*gag*, *pol*, or *env*; see fig. 9.1) and the *onc* sequence (note that this may influence the intracellular localization); gp or gP, glycoprotein. The numerals denote the molecular weight in kilodaltons, generally deduced from polyacrylamide gel electrophoresis.

[4] PK, protein kinase; tyr, tyrosine; ser, serine; thr, threonine; EGF, epidermal growth factor; PDGF, platelet derived growth factor; M-CSF, macrophage colony-stimulating factor. See text for further details.

[5] These genes lack introns and are probably not transcribed (pseudogenes).

expressed in particular stages of the cell division cycle. Secondly, one could speculate that *onc* gene products were overexpressed when under viral regulatory signals, i.e. in their viral form, compared with levels observed normally in cells. This possibility too has been ruled out for many of the cellular oncogene counterparts, but not for all. A third hypothesis is that the gene has cancer-inducing activity if expressed in the wrong place or at the wrong time. This theory is possible, there being no evidence at this time to rule it out definitively. A fourth alternative is that there are actual changes between the viral and cellular homologues. There is some evidence that such changes do occur, but again this does not apply to all oncogenes. Thus, a combination of all the qualitative and quantitative changes may be responsible for oncogenic activity. For clarity, the term protooncogene is used for the cellular species; sometimes, the cellular counterpart may also be called a c-*onc* gene, but this term has a connotation that the gene is an oncogene, and it is best to distinguish it instead as one with only a potential oncogenic activity.

Currently, there is very active and widespread research to sort out the properties and functions of v-*onc* genes and protooncogenes, both similarities and differences, in order to understand what may cause the potential carcinogenic activity to become an actual one. Many of the problems have been tackled initially with v-*onc* genes, which are more amenable to manipulation and dissection in the laboratory, and this will form the basis of the following sections.

The v-*onc* genes are useful for analysis of expression of the related protooncogenes in normal and tumour tissues. Messenger RNA preparations from different tissues, including embryonic tissues at different stages of development, were examined to look for both the level of expression and the size of the specific mRNAs (transcripts). (In general, the technique known as Northern hybridization was used, wherein mRNA molecules are fractionated by size during electrophoresis through agarose gels and then annealed to specific *onc* gene 'probes'.) The most consistent finding was that most of these genes are expressed at some stage in some tissue; that is, they are regulated genes and participate in the cell's normal differentiation programme. It also became evident that the cellular *onc* genes may be abnormally expressed in certain tumours owing to alterations in regulation, mutation, gene amplification, or chromosomal translocation (see also Chapter 10).

9.1.2 Second encounter: cellular oncogenes

While the RNA tumour viruses have given us a handle on nearly 30 oncogenes, there are probably at least 50 others that have been determined from studies on tumours. These have been found by three major approaches: (i) gene transfer; (ii) insertional mutagenesis mapping of virally induced tumours; and (iii) analysis of known chromosomal translocations or amplifications. This number is further increased by finding genes with sequence homology or biochemical (functional) homology to known oncogenes. While not necessarily true oncogenes (cancer inducing), the potential for oncogenicity is implied by analogy in these circumstances.

Gene transfer The primary method of gene transfer is often known by the name DNA transfection. The DNA is isolated from tumour cells and introduced into recipient cells. It may be added as a calcium phosphate precipitate to assist uptake, taken up following an electric shock (electroporation), or microinjected; the first is the most commonly used technique. The recipient cells are most usually the 'normal' immortalized mouse embryo fibroblast line, NIH/3T3. The NIH cells have several advantages in this system: (i) they are flat, contact-inhibited cells in monolayer culture; and (ii) their DNA can be distinguished in hybridization experiments from DNAs of other species (thus allowing identification of retained donor DNA). The first property is the most important as the general goal is to examine the transfected cultures for the appearance of morphologically altered (transformed) foci resulting from the expression of an introduced oncogene. This procedure is represented diagrammatically in Fig. 9.2. Although a lot of DNA is taken up by an individual cell, the majority of this material is degraded with time, and only a minority becomes stably incorporated into the cellular genome. To identify the gene responsible for the cell's transformed phenotype, transfection of DNA from the transformed cells is carried out a second and a third time; a procedure that eventually whittles down the amount of non-murine DNA carried over.

One of the surprises from such analyses was that cellular genes related to the already known *ras* genes of retroviruses were found to be responsible for the

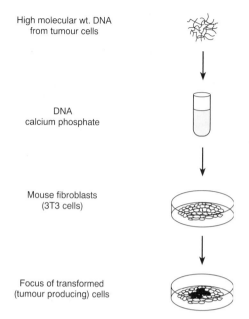

High molecular wt. DNA
from tumour cells

DNA
calcium phosphate

Mouse fibroblasts
(3T3 cells)

Focus of transformed
(tumour producing) cells

Fig. 9.2 DNA transfection. DNA isolated from tumour cells is introduced into recipient NIH/3T3 mouse cells. After several weeks, the monolayer is observed for foci of morphologically transformed cells. Repeated cycles of DNA transfection from transformed foci are generally performed. The transformed cells may be tested for tumorigenicity in nude mice. DNA from transfromed cells is also examined for retention and identification of donor cell sequences.

transformed phenotype in about 20 per cent of human tumours tested. This could be a result, at least in part, of the ability of NIH cells to respond morphologically to a given oncogene product, the need for the gene to be genetically dominant (e.g. lack of expression of an inhibitor gene in the NIH cell), and the need for the gene to be sufficient for the expression and maintenance of the transformed state. On second thoughts, perhaps it is not unusual to find that few genes other than *ras*-related genes have been identified as being 'activated' in tumours. This may be owing to the NIH cells being of the wrong lineage or species to respond to the effects of other genes. Or one may consider them to have a preneoplastic phenotype (see Chapter 6) as they already have the ability to grow continuously in culture; thus they may be more susceptible to genes whose effects are manifest during the later stages of tumour progression.

None the less, new oncogenes have been detected by this technique (Table 9.2).

Insertional mutagenesis Retroviruses lacking v-*onc* gene sequences carry only the genes required for replication; after infection, a DNA copy of their genome is synthesized and becomes integrated within the chromosomal DNA of the cell (the provirus, see Fig. 9.1). This event, by definition, is an insertional mutation and can have several consequences. The long terminal repeat (LTR) structures do not code for proteins but do contain the regulatory elements ('promoters' for initiation of transcription of mRNA molecules from the DNA, and 'enhancers' that may influence the levels of transcription of adjacent or distant genes) that permit transcription of the viral genes into mRNA molecules so that viral proteins are produced and incorporated into progeny virus particles. However, as shown in Fig. 9.1, the replication and insertion of a provirus leads to the generation of two LTRs; one may be used for the production of progeny virus whereas the other may be used for promotion of an adjacent cellular gene ('downstream promotion'). The first example of this phenomenon came from the examination of B cell tumours induced in chickens by avian leukaemia viruses (ALVs) lacking *onc* genes. Hybridization of LTR probes to tumour RNA revealed not only transcripts expected from the proviral genome but also some that contained an LTR but no viral sequences; the remaining sequences were derived from cellular genetic material. Further analysis showed that the cellular gene was in fact the counterpart of the *myc* gene already identified in several avian viruses (Table 9.1 and Fig. 9.3). The integration event resulted in the use of the LTR as a promoter for transcription of the cellular *myc* gene, leading to inexorable production of *myc* RNA and protein. Upon analysis of many of these B cell tumours, it was found that there was no specific integration of the ALV provirus at a unique site upstream of the *myc* gene; the integration sites in individual tumours were often several kilobases different from one another. ALV proviruses can integrate at a multitude of sites, even perhaps totally at random; however, the integrations near to *myc* presumably led to some selective advantage for the particular cell in proliferation, which might prime such cells for other neoplastic events to occur, or which might be oncogenic *per se*. Interestingly, the involvement of

Table 9.2 Non-retroviral oncogenes

Name	Tumour of origin	Method of detection	Human chromosome
hst/FGF4	Stomach tumour		11q13
N-myc[1]	Neuroblastoma	Amplification	2p23-p24
L-myc[1]	Lung carcinoma		1p32
neu[1,4]/ERBB2/ HER2	Mammary carcinoma		17
N-ras[1]	Neuroblastoma[2,3]	Transfection	1cen-p21
dbl	B cell lymphoma		
K-fgf (=hst)	Kaposi's sarcoma		11q13
mcf2	Mammary carcinoma		
mcf3	Mammary carcinoma		
met	Chemically transformed osteosarcoma cells		7p11-p14
neu	Neuroblastoma[4]		17
onc-D	Colon carcinoma		
ras related	Melanoma		
ret	T cell lymphoma		
Tlym-1, -2	T cell lymphoma		
trk	Colon carcinoma		
tx-1	Mammary carcinoma		
tx-2	Pre B cell leukaemia		
tx-3	Plasmacytoma		
tx-4	T cell lymphoma		
bcl-1	B cell leukaemia	Translocation[5]	11q13
bcl-2	B cell lymphoma		18q21
bcr	Chronic myelocytic leukaemia		22q11
tcl-1	T cell lymphoma		14q32
T$_k$NS-1	Plasmacytoma[6]		
int-1/Wnt-1	Mammary carcinoma	Insertional mutation[6]	12q14-pter
int-2/FGF3	Mammary carcinoma	(all rodent)	11q13
Mlvi-1, -2, -3	T cell lymphoma		
Pim-1	T cell lymphoma		
Pvt-2	Plasmacytoma		
RMO-int-1	T cell leukaemia		
fim-1, -3	Myeloid leukaemia		
evi-1, -2	Myeloid leukaemia		
Spi-1	Erythroid leukaemia		
fis-1	Myeloid and lymphoid leukaemia		

[1] Related to *onc* genes already known from retroviruses (see Table 9.1). The *neu* gene is related to the EGF receptor gene (*c-erbB*). Also called *c-erb2* or *HER2*.

[2] Also in rodent tumours.

myc promoter insertions has also been observed in murine T cell leukaemias induced by murine retroviruses, and in feline T cell leukaemias induced by feline retroviruses. Furthemore, the *erbB* oncogene (known as the counterpart of an oncogene isolated from avian erythroblastosis viruses, AEV) has also been activated by promoter insertion by other strains of ALV in situations where they induced erythroleukaemia instead of B cell leukaemia. In many of these instances, the integrated provirus is no longer intact, i.e. one of the LTRs, as well as coding sequences, may be lost, suggesting that the provirus itself is no longer required for maintenance of the neoplastic state (Fig. 9.3).

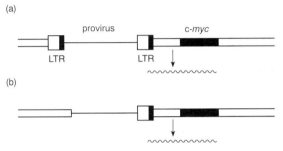

Fig. 9.3 Promoter insertion. In the example shown here, DNA from a B cell tumour (bursal lymphoma) of chicken induced by an avian leukaemia virus (ALV) has been examined for the site of provirus insertion. The provirus (shown as a single line bounded by LTRs) is located 'upstream' of the cellular gene known as *myc* and the viral LTR is being used as a promoter for the transcription of high levels of *myc* gene messenger RNA (mRNA), shown as a wavy line. For simplicity, the *myc* gene is shown as a contiguous element whereas it is actually composed of a 5′ untranslated exon and three coding exons separated by regions of non-coding sequences known as introns (the introns are also removed, 'spliced out', during the processing to mature mRNA molecules). (a) Provirus is intact. (b) Provirus shows deleted structure, lacking the 5′ LTR and some coding sequences.

[3] See also Table 9.5 for mutated N-*ras* genes in other human tumours.

[4] Rodent tumour.

[5] These genes represent breakpoint regions; no oncogenic potential has yet been demonstrated for any genes in this region.

[6] Targets of proviral insertion in rodent tumours. No oncogenic potential has yet been demonstrated for the activated gene *per se*.

A different phenomenon occurred when the integration sites for another retrovirus group, mouse mammary tumour viruses (MMTV, see Chapter 8) were mapped in a large number of tumours. As illustrated in Fig. 9.4, there were apparently clusters of regions where proviruses inserted. However, the LTRs in most cases could not be used to promote transcription of downstream genes. In the majority of tumours, it turned out that there were regions bounded by the provirus insertions and that this central region contained a gene that was activated in the tumour and silent in normal mammary tissue. The proviruses were oriented in a polarity that proscribed transcription of the central gene from the viral LTR, but presumably the enhancer element within the LTR was able to activate this cellular gene. In fact, (at least) two cellular genes may become expressed in this manner in different murine mammary carcinomas and have become known as the *int-1* and *int-2* loci (now known as *Wnt-1* and *FGF3*, respectively). Thus, a second mechanism of insertional mutagenesis has been identified. Integration sites in other tumours have delineated many more activated genes (Table 9.2). However, it must be stressed that many of these genes have not yet been shown to be oncogenes in a definitive test.

Chromosomal abnormalities Various chromosomal abnormalities have been detected in tumours by karyotype analysis of metaphase chromosomes; some abnormalities seem specific for a distinctive tumour type (see Chapters 4, 10, and 12). Because the *onc* genes mentioned above, whether originally identified in retroviruses or by gene transfer, all have cellular counterparts, each one can be mapped to a distinct region of a particular chromosome (see Tables 9.1 and 9.2 and Chapter 10). These two observations were linked in order to ask two questions. Firstly, did any of the known *onc* genes map in or near regions involved in abnormal tumour karyotypes? Secondly, could the abnormalities be used to discover new oncogenes?

The foreknowledge of promoter insertion of *myc* in ALV-induced B cell tumours quickly played a role. Burkitt's lymphoma is a B cell tumour of humans in which both Epstein-Barr virus and malaria are known cofactors (see Chapter 8). Additionally, it was previously known that tumour cells contained one of three chromosomal translocations (translocations refer to movements of genetic sequences from the normal chromosome site to another chromosome, see Chapter 10), involving part of the long arm of chromosome 8 becoming translocated to chromosome 14, 2, or 22 (the first occurring in approximately 90 per cent of tumours examined). The *myc* locus mapped to the long arm of chromosome 8 and it became obvious that it should be examined to determine whether it was translocated in these tumours. The simple answer was yes. Even more exciting was the finding that the *myc* locus translocated to regions containing different immunoglobulin loci (the heavy chain, k and λ light chains, respectively, on chromosomes 14, 2, and 22). Mechanistically, this meant that the *myc* locus could now be found adjacent to a highly transcribed gene (an important function of mature B cells being that of immunoglobulin production). The generation of the translocation also tended to have another effect; namely that the non-coding regulatory sequences of the *myc* gene were frequently

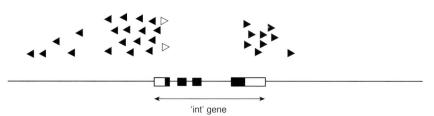

'int' gene

Fig. 9.4 Proviruses in mouse mammary tumour virus (MMTV)-induced breast tumours. The integration sites of MMTV proviruses in a large number of tumours have been mapped chromosomally. Each site is denoted by an arrowhead and the direction of the arrow shows the direction of transcription of the provirus (5′ to 3′). Note that the activated gene is in a central region (designated *int* for integration) around which the proviruses cluster and that the polarity of the provirus is in an orientation such that downstream promotion cannot occur. There are at least two well-characterized *int* loci, *int-1* and *int-2*; others may also exist.

'decapitated' from the gene, thus leaving it to the controls of its new chromosomal milieu. In most instances the altered *myc* allele was shown to be transcriptionally active while the non-altered one was silent. Moreover, the *myc* allele was sometimes located near the immunoglobulin enhancer element which could affect the level of *myc* transcription. Similar sorts of rearrangements also occur in immunoglobulin-producing tumours (plasmacytomas) of mice and rats.

Another particularly well-known translocation was the formation of the 'marker' Philadelphia chromosome in chronic myelocytic leukaemias (CML, see Chapters 10 and 12) which represents a translocation between chromosomes 9 and 22 (although other variants are known which may involve segments from three different chromosomes). The net result is that the *abl* locus (known from retroviruses) becomes transferred from chromosome 9 to sequences on chromosome 22. The *abl* gene is located rather a long distance away from the site of the breakpoint, the region being known as the breakpoint cluster region (*bcr*), and hence is presumably not dissociated from its upstream regulatory sequences, but transcription of the gene is abnormal in that the *abl* mRNA molecules are much greater in size than normal owing to the formation of *bcr–abl* transcripts.

Many other tumours contain recognizable translocations (see Chapter 10) and the translocation breakpoints of some of these have already been molecularly cloned. Although often listed as cellular oncogenes (e.g. some are included in Table 9.2), this remains a tenuous assignment until the sequences are shown experimentally to have neoplastic potential.

Another type of chromosomal abnormality seen in tumours is related to gene amplification and generally involves huge (100–1000 kilobases or more) DNA segments spanning many genes. The amplification may be observed microscopically as a homogeneously staining region (HSR) in which it occurs as a contiguous element in a chromosome, or as the formation of double minute (DM) chromosomes, which are additional tiny minichromosomes (although they lack centromeres and therefore may be lost, or segregate, during cell division). The availability of v-*onc* gene probes proved useful in demonstrating that HSRs and DMs observed in cell lines derived from various tumours contained *onc* gene amplifications (e.g. Ki-*ras* in a mouse adrenocortical

tumour cell line, *myc* in a human colon carcinoma line). Needless to say, these particular types of abnormalities require large degrees of gene amplification (large DNA segments repeated perhaps 50 or 100 times) to be detected by microscopic analysis of chromosomes. More sensitive techniques such as Southern blotting and hybridization (in which DNA is cut by endonucleases known as restriction enzymes, separated by size in gels, and transferred to nitrocellulose filters for hybridization to DNA probes) allow the detection of low levels of gene amplification, or indeed the disruption or rearrangement of a single gene (Table 9.3).

One particularly interesting finding is the N-*myc* amplification in neuroblastomas. This property is observed only in those tumours histologically defined as grades III and IV and thus may be a reflection of tumour progression towards a more advanced malignant state. Similarly, *myc* amplification in cell lines derived from small cell lung carcinomas is correlated with enhanced growth of the tumours when transplanted into nude mice.

None the less, it should be remembered that large segments of DNA are reiterated in these amplifications and the *onc* gene may be merely a passenger in this event. Thus, other genes in the amplified regions could have significant consequences.

Table 9.3 Ocogene amplification

Gene	Human tumour	Degree of amplification
c-*myc*	Promyelocytic leukaemia[1]	20
	Colon carcinoma	40
	Small cell lung carcinoma	5–30
N-*myc*	Neuroblastoma[1]	5–1000
	Retinoblastoma[1]	10–200
	Small cell lung carcinoma[1]	50
c-*abl*	Chronic granulocytic leukaemia	5–10
c-*myb*	Colon carcinoma	10
	Acute myeloid leukaemia[1]	5–10
c-*erbB*	Vulval carcinoma	30
c-Ki-*ras*-2	Lung carcinoma[1]	
	Colorectal carcinoma[1]	4–20
	Bladder carcinoma[1]	
N-*ras*	Mammary carcinoma	5–10

[1] Primary tumour material.

9.2 Identification of viral and cellular oncogene products

It is important to ascertain the physiological functions of oncogene products and to determine (or at least speculate) on how these products may lead to neoplastic changes within a cell. Such analyses include the subcellular localization of the gene product and deciphering biochemical functions associated with the expression of the product (see Table 9.1). To a large extent, these experiments rely on recombinant DNA technology (both *in vitro* and *in vivo*), specific antisera, and luck.

9.2.1 The tyrosine kinase family

src The Rous sarcoma virus (RSV) in chickens was one of the earliest retroviruses isolated and has turned out to be one of the most interesting from a genetic and biochemical standpoint. It is the only naturally occurring retrovirus with all replicative genes as well as an oncogene (see Fig. 9.1). The oncogene, v-*src*, was transduced from cellular DNA in such a way that the replicative genes of its presumptive parent virus (an avian leukaemia virus) remained intact, with the new sequences appearing appended to the viral *env* gene. Early genetic experiments showed that inactivation of the v-*src* gene by mutations or deletions left a long latency leukaemia virus that could no longer cause morphological transformation of cells in culture.

With recombinant DNA technology, it was possible to obtain molecular clones of proviral DNA and the v-*src* (and subsequently cellular *src*) gene was characterized down to its last nucleotide. Comparisons showed that the nucleotide sequences of the cellular and viral genes were essentially identical. Two major differences could be noted however: (i) the v-*src* gene lacks introns (sometime during the process of transduction this occurs with all oncogenes picked up by retroviruses wherein the introns are 'spliced' out); and (ii) the last (carboxy terminal) 12 coding amino acids of v-*src* were different from those of cellular *src* (which is also seven amino acids longer). Thus, transduction leads to splicing, truncation, and perhaps other sorts of recombinational events—a motif seen frequently in the derivation of the *onc*-containing retroviruses.

The next important breakthrough came with the development of an antiserum that reacted specifically with the *src* gene product, obtained from an animal bearing an RSV-induced tumour. The serum was used to show that the *src* gene product was located largely on the cytoplasmic side of the plasma membrane and was approximately 60 kDa in molecular weight. By metabolically labelling transformed cells with ^{32}P, it was shown that the protein was phosphorylated, and hence became known as $pp60^{v\text{-}src}$. The protein of the cellular gene also shared these properties and was called $pp60^{c\text{-}src}$. One of the most interesting discoveries from this study was that the protein was apparently responsible for its own phosphorylation (autophosphorylation) and also that it had the ability to phosphorylate the immunoglobulin (Ig) molecule in the antiserum that was used to identify it. Furthemore, both proteins were phosphorylated on tyrosine residues and thus the oncogene product was identified functionally as a tyrosine protein kinase. (Cellular enzymes that phosphorylated serine or threonine residues were known previously, but this was the first time that a tyrosine kinase was characterized.)

Several of the proteins phosphorylated by src are of interest. One is the protein vinculin, a component of the cytoskeleton network of mesenchymal cells, which is situated at areas of contact between cells or between a cell and a substrate (such as tissue culture dishes) known as focal adhesion plaques. The change in the phosphorylation pattern of vinculin could be responsible for some of the observable changes in transformed cells (rounding up, decreased adhesion to solid substrates, ruffling of the plasma membrane). Another interesting target is a protein known as p90 (so designated because it is 90 kDa in molecular weight) which with another protein (p50) serves to transport $pp60^{src}$ from its site of synthesis to the plasma membrane. While complexed with these two proteins, the *src* protein is neither phosphorylated nor does it exhibit kinase activity. The *src* product is also capable of phosphorylating lipids (i.e. it is a phospholipid kinase) such as phosphatidylinositol and diacylglycerol. These molecules are believed to function as 'second messengers' in response to growth factor stimulation, an important aspect of cell metabolism (see Chapter 11). Several enzymes of the glycolytic pathway are also targets for src kinase activity. Despite these identifiable changes, we are still a long way from demonstrating a direct link between these effects and the ultimate heritable change necessary for a cell to transform and develop into a neoplasm.

Guilt by association As further viral and cellular oncogenes were isolated, they were tested for a similar kinase function, and a number were found to be positive (Table 9.1). Nucleotide sequence data confirmed that there was a small region of sequence homology related to the shared biochemical activity.

Bearing in mind that a rather large class of genes were turning out to share this biochemical activity, oncogenes themselves were used as probes against genomic or cDNA libraries to pick up genes bearing sequence homology. As a number of these were isolated, it also became clear that the tyrosine kinases could be divided into two classes: (i) those that were membrane associated without clear transmembrane or extracellular domains (like *src*); and (ii) those that had apparent extracellular domains (like *erbB*) (Table 9.4). The latter class contained many members of the growth factor receptor category, with were of particular interest for studying proliferative stimuli.

There were two obvious questions at this stage. Do the cellular *onc* counterparts also display kinase activity? Could specific proteins in the cell be identified as target substrates? To the first question, the answer was generally yes, in that the *onc* proteins were capable of autophosphorylation, but often did not show any ability to phosphorylate Ig molecules. Answering the second question was more difficult. Levels of phosphotyrosine-containing

peptides in normal non-transformed cells are extremely low; thus, despite demonstrated kinase activity for c-*onc* gene products *in vitro*, their activity is virtually undetectable in cells. However, there is often a considerable elevation of phosphotyrosine in cells transformed with the kinase v-*onc* genes, suggesting that the v-*onc* products have greater activity. However, many different species of proteins seem to be affected rather than one or two specific target molecules. The demonstration of phosphotyrosine-containing peptides has been enhanced by the use of antibodies raised to recognize phosphotyrosine molecules, which are now readily available.

Lastly, one is interested in asking if any of these growth factor receptors can be turned into oncogenes by mutations similar to those of the viral counterparts [generally $5'$ (ligand binding) or $3'$ (catalytic) subunit truncation]. The insulin receptor (when truncated and inserted into a provirus) and the EGF receptor (when truncated in nature in tumours as the viral oncogene *erbB*) have proved to be true oncogenes; others remain to be tested.

kit The oncogene *kit*, first discovered in a cat sarcoma virus, is a transmembrane protein kinase like *fms* and *erbB* (see Table 9.4 and Chapter 11). What makes it stand out from the rest at this time is its apparent identity with the gene called *W* in mice. The initial relationship was hinted at by the finding that *kit* maps in the human genome at chromosome 4q11–q21, a region syntenic with mouse chromosome 5, where *W* maps. The *W* gene (or locus as it is called more familiarly) has been a gene of much interest since the 1950s because of its pleiotropic effects on the stem cells of at least three distinct lineages; in haemopoiesis (the animals suffer from severe macrocytic anaemia and mast cell defects), melanogenesis (the *W* stands for dominant white spotting which is an early discernible phenotype), and gametogenesis (the animals are infertile). Hence *kit* is also known as the receptor for stem cell factor. In some of the mutants of the *W* family one or another of these lineages may appear normal (e.g. the animals have normal red blood cells or are fertile), and the white spotting may occur to greater or lesser extents; these differences may represent the degree of penetrance of the gene or the extent of the mutant protein's kinase activity

Although the initial experiments only suggested that *W* and *kit* might be the same gene, more defi-

Table 9.4 Tyrosine protein kinases

Membrane-associated	Transmembrane
abl[1]	eph (eck, elk, erk . . .)
arg	erbB[1] (epidermal growth factor receptor)
fes[1]/fps[1]	erbB2/neu/HER2
fgr[1]	fms[1] (monocyte colony stimulating factor receptor)
fyn	Insulin receptor
mhck	Insulin-like growth factor type I receptor
lyk	kit[1] (W locus)
lyn/syn	mas
src[1]	met/HGFR
tkl	Platelet-derived growth factor receptor
tkr	ret
yes[1]	ros[1]
	sea[1]
	trk (A, B, C)

[1] First isolated as a retroviral oncogene.

nitive evidence of their identity was gained by: (i) the W^{19H} mutant which visibly lacks part of mouse chromosome 5 also lacks the *kit* gene; (ii) other *W* mutants have been shown to have point mutations in their *kit* gene sequence; and (iii) all *W* mutants lack functional (tyrosine kinase) expression of *kit* although *kit* RNA may still be present in tissue wherein *kit* is normally active (e.g. erythroid cell progenitors, mast cells, and testes). Interestingly, *kit* is also expressed at a high level in the brain, and is lacking in brain tissue of *W* mutant mice, although no noticeable defect in neurological function has yet been described! Taking these data further, there is interest in examining patients with two gene defects that map to this region of human chromosome 14q: those with the piebald trait (showing streaks of different hair colour and sometimes with mental retardation as well), and the haematological disorder known as Diamond-Blackfan syndrome.

The *W*/*kit* relationship is the first example of a germ line mutation in a mammalian protooncogene. However, its role in human cancer remains to be proven.

crk: an oncogene related to phospholipase C Another oncogene for which a biochemical function has been postulated is *crk* (for *CT*10 virus *regulator* of *kinase*) now known to have been transduced from chickens into two avian sarcoma viruses. Initial studies on the viral gene product showed that it did not have intrinsic tyrosine protein kinase activity like many other viral oncogenes, although cells transformed by the virus had elevated levels of intracellular phosphotyrosine proteins. When the putative amino acid sequence of *crk* was entered into a protein database, it was observed to have a sequence related to the enzyme phospholipase C, which plays a key role in signal transduction mechanisms, particularly in the activation of protein kinase C (see Chapter 11). These relationships suggest that the *crk* oncogene might function as a regulator of the endogenous non-receptor (membrane-associated) class of tyrosine protein kinases. Thus, once again an oncogene has been implicated as a potential disrupter of the cell receptor–growth factor recognition pathway.

9.2.2 The other kinases: *raf* and *mos*

Two other oncogenes, *raf* (also called *mil*) and *mos*, show kinase activity but in these instances serine and threonine are the substrate sites rather than tyrosine. Expression of *raf* (of which there are also several related genes) is fairly ubiquitous in mammalian tissues, and is involved in the kinase cascade of signal transduction (see Chapter 11). On the other hand, the oncogene *mos* was originally thought to be a pseudogene because the gene lacked introns and no expression could be detected in adult tissues. However, its expression was finally detected at very low level in testes and oocytes, and the pursuit was on for determining some physiological function in gametogenesis or early development. By far the most compelling evidence at this stage is its pattern of expression in the oocytes of the frog *Xenopus*. Although the cellular *mos* RNA is expressed from early oogenesis and persists through gastrulation, the protooncogene product, $pp39^{mos}$, rapidly appears following progesterone treatment (which stimulates maturation) and disappears extremely rapidly following fertilization. Investigations with *mos* RNA and monoclonal antibodies suggest that the *mos* protein is the key to holding the egg cell in metaphase arrest during meiosis and subsequently it becomes a relatively 'silent' gene. It is a little difficult to extrapolate from this scenario to the situation when the gene becomes oncogenic (as in the murine leukaemia virus transductions—Table 9.1—and in insertional mutagenesis in some rodent plasmacytomas) in which its role is as a proliferative signal rather than an antiproliferative one. Of course, it may be simply a question of its expression in the wrong cell type at the wrong time, or the altered gene product may phosphorylate different target substrates.

9.2.3 *ras* and GTPase activity

The *ras* oncogene was originally discovered in two murine retroviruses, known as Harvey and Kirsten murine sarcoma viruses (Ha-MSV and Ki-MSV). By nucleic acid hybridization, the oncogenes of the two viruses were non-homologous. This turned out to be owing to the degeneracy of the triplet code of DNA because the oncogene products from the two viruses were virtually identical, $p21^{ras}$. Moreover, it was found that both Ha-*ras* and Ki-*ras* were each found at two separate chromosomal loci, although in each case one locus appeared to be a pseudogene (a gene sequence lacking introns and thought to be untranscribed and thus not translated into protein, Table 9.1). Later, a gene showing homology to Ha-

ras and Ki-*ras* was detected in neuroblastoma DNA by transfection (see Table 9.2); this became known as N-*ras* and was mapped to yet another chromosome. These five different *ras* genes became known as the *ras* multigene family. By using conserved parts of the *ras* gene, a number of other *ras*-related genes have been detected in mammalian genomic DNA as well as in lower species, such as yeast; *rac* and *rho* genes are members of this extended family.

The viral p21^{ras} proteins were shown to have binding activity for guanosine triphosphate (GTP) and, in fact, enzymatically converted GTP to its di- and mono-phosphate forms. Thus, *ras* too is an enzyme, a GTPase. Comparisons of enzyme activity showed that p21^{v-ras} has less activity than p21^{c-ras}.

How did the change in activity come about? Nucleotide sequence analysis showed that in viral transductions (three separate isolates, the third being another capture of Ha-*ras*, see Table 9.1), the *ras* gene was intact, i.e. it was not truncated. But in each instance, there was one nucleotide change which in turn led to the substitution of a different amino acid compared to the cellular ras protein. The same event occurred in the neuroblastoma N-*ras* gene as well. These results, as well as those from other tumour transfections or site-specific mutagenesis *in vitro*, showed that changes in the ras protein at amino acid residues 12 or 13, or residues 59–61 almost invariably led to a change in the oncogenic potential (Table 9.5, see also Chapters 10, 11, and 12). The easiest explanation is that these changes lead to major alterations in the conformational (three-dimensional) state of the protein, thereby diminishing its activity.

Mutant *ras* sequences are the most frequently detectable alterations in some types of human tumours. In all cases tested to date, the single point mutations listed above are responsible for the changes in biological activity, keeping the protein in the active GTP form.

Another clue to *ras* function comes from studies on the yeast *Saccharomyces cerevisiae* which has two *ras* genes that stimulate adenylate cyclase. This finding led to the deduction that *ras* could be a regulator of adenylate cyclase similar to the known G-proteins that transmit signals from cell surface receptors ('second messages', see Chapter 11). Binding of GTP is necessary for activation of G-proteins and thus GTPase activity is a regulatory factor. The diminished GTPase activity of mutated ras proteins could lead to sustained effects on adenylate cyclase

Table 9.5 Mutated human *ras* genes

		Codon	
		12	61
c-Ha-*ras*-1[1]	Normal	gly	gln
	Bladder carcinoma	val	
	Lung carcinoma		leu
	Mammary carcinoma	asp	
c-Ki-*ras*-2[2]	Normal	gly	gln
	Lung carcinoma	arg	
	Lung carcinoma	cyc	
	Lung carcinoma	lys	
	Lung carcinoma		his
	Colon carcinoma	val	
	Bladder carcinoma	arg	
	Neuroblastoma	cys	
N-*ras*[3]	Normal	gly	gln
	Neuroblastoma		lys
	Teratocarcinoma	asp	
	Fibrosarcoma		lys
	Melanoma		lys
	Lung carcinoma		arg
	Leukaemia	asp	
	Rhabdomyosarcoma		his

[1] Mutated c-Ha-*ras*-1 also detected in a human melanoma.

[2] Mutated c-Ki-*ras*-2 also detected in human pancreatic carcinoma, gall bladder carcinoma, rhabdomyosarcoma, ovarian carcinoma, and acute lymphoblastic leukaemia.

[3] Mutated N-*ras* also detected in Burkitt's lymphoma, acute promyelocytic leukaemia, T cell leukaemia, acute myelocytic leukaemia, and chronic granulocytic leukaemia.

and the ensuing events in cell metabolism. The location of the ras protein on the cytoplasmic side of plasma membranes adds credibility to this hypothesis.

Another piece of evidence suggesting the involvement of ras proteins in signal transduction comes from studies using microinjection of anti-ras neutralizing antibodies into cells *in vitro*. The net result is a block to cell proliferation normally induced by a variety of mitogenic stimuli such as growth factors and activators of protein kinase C (see Chapter 11). Conversely, microinjection of ras protein into quiescent cells stimulates DNA synthesis. However, if such cells are treated so as to down-regulate protein kinase C, *ras* is unable to induce DNA synthesis. Interestingly, mutant ras protein-induced DNA synthesis also has an absolute requirement for insulin-like growth factor type I (IGF-1, see Chapter 11) whereas morphological transformation is independent of this factor. While the precise nature of the *ras* effector system remains unknown, a protein known as GAP (GTPase-activating protein) is implicated in the pathway by regulating the level of bound GTP (see Chapter 11).

9.2.4 Oncogenes with products related to growth factors

sis and platelet-derived growth factor activity The *sis* oncogene was originally found in a simian sarcoma virus and has a protein product, $p28^{sis}$, apparently found in the cytoplasm. The use of a computer database was the key to deciphering its physiological function. When the amino acid sequence of several tryptic peptide digests of the growth factor known as platelet-derived growth factor (PDGF) was entered into the database, it was immediately obvious that the amino acid sequence was highly homologous to that of the putative protein product of v-*sis*. Further experiments verified this observation, showing that v-*sis* represented a truncated form of the B chain of PDGF (see Chapter 11).

This observation was very exciting with regard to a central theme of tumours: continuous cell proliferation. Normally, PDGF is packaged in the subcellular blood components known as platelets, which are released by the disintegration of blood megakaryocytes. The release is generally triggered as a response to a wound and the local delivery of PDGF stimulates, for example, endothelial or epithelial cells around the wound to proliferate and fill in the gap. Once healing has begun, platelets are no longer released, thus decreasing local PDGF concentrations; the net result is that the cells become quiescent again. However, if PDGF were to be continuously produced, the cells would be constantly stimulated to divide. So the function of v-*sis* in virally induced tumours might be envisaged in one of two ways: (i) as an intracellular product that can still stimulate the specific PDGF receptor such that its 'signal' for cell division is transmitted to the cell nucleus (an autocrine mechanism); or (ii) as a secreted product interacting with specific PDGF receptors on its own, neighbouring (paracrine) or distant (exocrine) cells, thus stimulating cell growth.

Although PDGF (cellular *sis*) is overexpressed in at least one human osteosarcoma cell line, this does not seem to be a general feature of bone or other tumours so far examined.

int-2, hst, and K-fgf: genes related to basic fibroblast growth factor As mentioned above, the *int-2* gene was first identified as a target of proviral insertion in mouse mammary tumours. The effect of integration was the activation of this previously silent gene. In fact, when a variety of adult mouse tissues were examined, no *int-2* gene expression could be detected. Furthermore, when whole mouse embryos were surveyed, the only traces of expression were in early (6.5 day) embryos with a limited temporal and spatial distribution.

The amino acid sequence of the *int-2* gene product bears striking homology to the growth and angiogenic factor known as basic fibroblast growth factor (bFGF) which acts by stimulating the phosphorylation of the ribosomal 40S subunit (see also Chapter 11), and it is worth recalling at this stage that vascularization (angiogenesis) is required for development of a solid tumour (see Chapter 2).

Another gene, known as *hst*, was isolated from the amplified DNA of a human stomach tumour. Later, transfection techniques identified a gene from Kaposi's sarcoma (see also Chapter 8), called K-*fgf* owing to its relatedness to bFGF. Moreover, K-*fgf* and *hst* were found to be the same gene. An interesting finding arose once the *hst* gene was mapped chromosomally: it maps on chromosome 11q13 in humans within 35 kb of the *int-2* gene (similarly, the two genes are close together on mouse chromosome 7). Following the finding that *int-2* is amplified in about 10–20 per cent of human mammary carcinomas, it was also detected that *hst* was coamplified in many of the same tumours (including some of the murine tumours wherein *int-2* is expressed as a result of the integration of an MMTV provirus nearby). In contrast to the pattern found in mouse mammary tumours, however, *int-2* or *hst* mRNA has not yet been detected in any human tumour regardless of whether the genes are amplified. This result casts some doubt as to the significance of either of these genes in the mammary carcinogenic process. For this reason, there has been some interest in the *bcl*-1 gene (see Table 9.2), detected as a breakpoint of translocation in human leukaemias, which maps about 1000 kb away from *int-2* and *hst*, chromosomally. The fact that *bcl*-1 is generally not found to be within the amplified DNA segment (the 'amplicon') suggests that there may be another gene of major importance somewhere between the two genes.

There are at least seven members of the FGF family, including *int-2* also now known as *FGF3* and *hst* known as *FGF4*. Whether the other members of the family have oncogenic potential is as yet undetermined. Interestingly, there is also a multiplicity of FGF receptors with which the various FGFs may interact and hence there is a degree of complexity regarding which of the growth factor receptor combinations is most important in the normal development of any single tissue.

9.2.5 Oncogenes with products related to growth factor receptors

***erbB* and the epidermal growth factor receptor** The computer database was again fundamental in showing high levels of homology between the putative protein product of the v-*erbB* oncogene (from avian erythroblastosis viruses) and amino acid sequence derived from the receptor for the epidermal growth factor (EGF). As with v-*sis* and PDGF, the transduction of the cellular gene was a truncation event involving both the carboxyl- and amino-terminal coding portions of the gene. The v-*erbB* gene product is a faulty receptor; it lacks most of the external domain, including the binding site for ligand (EGF) and is also missing part of the intracytoplasmic domain (see Chapter 11). Interestingly, the EGF receptor is a protein that becomes modified by phosphorylation and possesses tyrosine kinase activity; both of these functional regions are retained in the v-*erbB* sequence. Going back to the central *sine qua non* of cell proliferation, we can suggest that these modifications to the EGF receptor protein may be sufficiently important to its conformational state so that a continuous proliferation signal may be generated in the absence of the appropriate ligand (which it cannot bind in any case).

Malfunction of the EGF receptor molecule also occurs in human tumours. For example, a truncated version is produced in a cell line derived from an epidermoid carcinoma of the vulva owing to gene amplification (and gene mutation presumably), as well as in several neurological tumours (for further discussion, see Chapter 11).

The oncogene *neu*, a transfectable gene from a carcinogen-induced rat neuroblastoma, is related, though non-identical, to *erbB* (see Chapter 11); it is generally called *erbB2* or *HER2*. Its ligand is as yet unknown.

***fms* and the macrophage colony-stimulating factor** The pattern of mimicry of a receptor is also observed with the oncogene v-*fms* (from a feline sarcoma virus). Studies on ligand and antibody binding provide evidence that v-*fms* has been derived from the receptor gene for macrophage colony-stimulating factor (M-CSF or CSF-1).

Others As mentioned above in detail, the protooncogene *kit* is a cell surface receptor for the interesting ligand known as 'steel' (or stem cell factor) from early mouse embryological studies. Likewise, the protooncogene *mas* is apparently the angiotensin receptor, and *sea* is a member of the insulin receptor family. Also, as discussed above, many of the tyrosine kinase oncogenes are cell surface proteins and are structurally related to known growth factor receptors. Hence it has been speculated that *abl* and *ros* may similarly represent growth factor receptors.

Lastly we must not forget that cytosolic or nuclear receptors, rather than cell surface proteins, exist for some of the hormones. One interesting example comes from the study of *erbA*, an oncogene originally detected in the avian erythroblastosis virus in which *erbB* was also first discovered (Table 9.1). It is now clear that *erbA* is the cellular thyroid hormone (triiodothyronine, T3) receptor.

9.2.6 Oncogenes with nuclear products

myc*, *myb*, *ets* and *ski Oncogene products located in the nucleus might be expected to have functions quite distinct from the oncoproteins mentioned above. One of the most facile hypotheses would be that these oncogenes might be involved in direct regulation of gene expression, perhaps serving as DNA-binding proteins to activate or inactivate transcription of a particular gene or set of genes. And indeed this has turned out to be the case, i.e. in many instances these oncogenes serve as transcription factors.

The *myc* oncogene, isolated from four separate avian sarcoma viruses, which induce sarcomas, carcinomas, and myeloid leukaemias, is perhaps the best characterized. One reason for heightened interest is its involvement in tumours caused by retroviruses lacking oncogenes, as well as its translocation and increased expression in tumours lacking retroviruses (e.g. Burkitt's lymphoma, see above). The *myc* gene is also a multigene family with the cellular *myc* homologue of v-*myc* and two distinct but related genes detected in neuroblastomas and retinoblastomas (N-*myc*) and small cell lung carcinomas (L-*myc*) (see Table 9.2).

The *myc* gene is expressed in many cell types suggesting that its normal function is in a pathway shared by most cells. There is often more *myc* product in cells actively proliferating, although levels are also high in the most mature macrophages whose differentiation programme is nearing the terminal phase. It has been speculated that increased levels of *myc* transcription in tumour cells (in situations where the regulation is governed by new promoter or enhancer elements) may represent deregulation of a negative feedback inhibition between the *myc* product and the *myc* gene, in situations where non-coding sequences have been removed or when the gene is amplified.

There has often been conflicting data as to the mechanism of action of the *myc* gene product. In this regard, it has now been shown that c-*myc* is effective in transcriptional repression as well as transcriptional activation and, perhaps also paradoxically, that it has a role in programmed cell death (apoptosis) as well as in processes of cell cycle progression. Particular interest has recently surrounded the distinct roles of two alternative translation products of the c-*myc* gene, c-Myc1 and c-Myc2. The intriguing observation that the ratio of c-Myc1 to c-Myc2 increases markedly upon cellular quiescence led to the discovery that c-Myc2 stimulates cell growth, whereas c-Myc1 appears to be growth suppressing.

A small protein, max, was originally identified through its interaction with *myc* family proteins and appears to be an obligatory partner for *myc* function. Myc–max heterodimers probably activate and max–max homodimers repress transcription of, as yet, unidentified target genes. Max has now been found to interact with at least two other proteins, mad and mxi1. Mad has been shown to abrogate the positive transcriptional activity of myc and to inhibit myc in cotransformation assays. This suggests that *mad* may antagonize *myc* function; it is rapidly induced upon differentiation, a time when *myc* is frequently down-regulated.

The *myb* gene, first detected in two avian myeloid leukaemia viruses, appears to be the best example of a cell cycle-dependent gene with levels highest during the G1 phase of growth. It is a DNA-binding transcription factor with a major role in haemopoietic cells.

Members of the *ets* family of transcriptional regulators play pivotal roles in physiological processes, such as embryonic development or immune response. The ets family proteins possess unique regulatory features because they bind DNA as monomers and their respective activities rely more on their ability to interact with other transcription factors than on their specific binding to a cognate DNA sequence.

Little is known about the *ski* oncogene detected in an avian carcinoma virus other than its size, chromosomal site, and nuclear location. It bears some homology to the helical domains in myosin, intermediate filaments, and lamins.

The *fos-jun* (and AP-1) connection The oncogene *fos* was originally discovered in 1982 to be the transforming region of the FBJ mouse osteosarcoma virus. Later it was also shown to be the oncogene of the FBR mouse osteosarcoma virus as well, and still later it was found in an avian virus (NK24) which gave rise to nephromas and fibrosarcomas with osteoid deposition *in vivo* (Table 9.1); these findings certainly imply a role for this gene in osteogenesis (formation of bone) although we now know several facts about *fos* that implicate its major role in tissues of nearly all types. The *fos* gene product is a nuclear phosphoprotein of 55 kDa. It is expressed constitutively in a few cell types, notably mature monocytes and cells of the placenta. However, in nearly all other cells, the *fos* gene becomes activated shortly after treatment with agents that induce differentiation (e.g. specific growth factors) or those that induce cell division (e.g. serum *in vitro*, PGDF, and the phorbol ester promoter, TPA). Increased levels of *fos* mRNA can be detected as early as 5 minutes following induction, making this one of the earliest nuclear events observed in response to mitogenic stimuli— a so-called 'immediate early' gene. However, the induction is only transient and diminishing levels of specific RNA are found by about 45 minutes after stimulation.

The oncogenic conversion in the retroviruses containing *fos* relies on the truncation of the 3′ end of the gene (coding and non-coding sequences) as well as the substitution of the gene's own promoter by the viral (or another strong) promoter. In the former situation, a motif (ATTTATTT...) in the 3′ noncoding region is removed; this motif is associated with relative mRNA instability, and hence the altered (viral) *fos* mRNA would have a longer half-life. In the latter situation, a region designated SRE (for serum response element) is no longer juxtaposed to the *fos* gene and hence the specificity of response to mitogenic elements of serum, for example, is lost. It is this short sequence, located about 300 bp upstream of the c-*fos* mRNA cap site, that mediates transcriptional activation of the gene. A 62-kDa binding protein (SRF, serum response factor) has been detected which binds to the SRE specifically.

Interestingly, even the earliest papers on *fos* mentioned its association with a cellular protein of 39 kDa (termed p39). The *p39* gene has since been recognized to be the cellular homologue of the viral oncogene *jun* first discovered in avian sarcoma virus S17 (see Table 9.1). The *jun* oncogene is highly related to a known mammalian transcriptional factor termed AP-1 (activation protein 1; it is also related to the yeast transcription factor known as GCN4). Hence the formation of the *fos–jun* complex can be seen to be involved in the regulation of transcription. Thus, a new motif for transformation might be the induction of transcriptional factors specific to different programmes of differentiation or cell division in various cell types. Since changes in gene expression following growth factor stimulation still occur in the presence of inhibitors of protein synthesis, the activity of transcription factors must be regulated at the post-translational level.

One other interesting feature of the *fos–jun* complex is the so-called 'leucine zipper'; regions of the proteins contain five leucine moieties at regular intervals separated by six residues forming a helix that would allow intercalation with similar regions on another protein bearing the same motif. Thus, the three-dimensional configuration of the two proteins allows for very specific binding between them, and to some extent accounts for their affinity to one another. This motif has since been found to occur in other nuclear protooncogenes (e.g. *myc* and its *max* and *mad* partners) as well as other possible transcription factors. Both fos and jun proteins form dimers, both homodimers and heterodimers, and it is the combination of which Fos (fos, fosB, FRA1 and FRA2) and which Jun (jun, junB, junD) proteins interact that specifies the transcriptional activity of the complex. The different heterodimers are known to be differentially regulated both in development and in adult tissues, and hence the particular dimer complex formed may be the determining fac-

tor in effecting a particular transcriptional activation pattern.

fos, like *myc*, may be involved in self regulation by virtue of its carboxyl amino acid sequences interacting with the 3′ non-coding regulatory sequences. How this effect modulates expression of other genes has yet to be discovered.

9.2.7 Other oncogenes

We have already seen that the cellular oncogenes may encode proteins that are growth factors, growth factor receptors, enzymes, transactivating DNA binding proteins, and other proteins involved in cell cycle regulation (Table 9.6). Each new oncogene is examined for these properties and oncogenes with other functions are being discovered. The major theme is that the normal gene counterparts are active, and presumably vital, to the functioning of cells, and abnormal properties may be attributed to mutation, truncation, amplification, or deregulation.

9.3 Tumour suppressor genes

9.3.1 Definition and conceptual views

The terms antioncogene and tumour suppressor gene are often used synonymously, although some investigators would use them in the negative or positive sense, respectively. Hence an antioncogene would be a gene whose repression, inactivation, loss, or dysfunction would lead to cell transformation or neoplastic conversion, whereas a tumour suppressor gene would be one whose activation, expression, or introduction would result in the suppression or inhibition of a tumorigenic phenotype. In addition, the term recessive oncogene has also been coined and previously used synonymously with tumour suppressor gene (given that oncogenes are thought to act in a dominant genetic fashion—or have a dominant rather than a recessive phenotype). None the less, tumour suppressor gene is now the preferred term.

The existence of tumour suppressor genes was suggested, in part, by the finding that, in somatic cell hybrids created *in vitro* by fusing a tumorigenic cell type with a non-tumorigenic one, the fused cell most often took on the characteristics of the non-tumorigenic parent. Furthermore, in interspecies hybrids (usually human × mouse hybrids from which the human chromosomes are selectively lost

Table 9.6 Functions of oncogenes

Growth factors	PDGFR/sis, int-2/FGF3, hst/FGF4, WNT1/WNT3
Tyrosine kinases	
Receptor-like tyrosine kinases	eph (eck, elk, erk, cek . . .), EGFR/erbB, fms, kit, ltk/tyk1, met, neu/HER2, ret, ros, sea, trkA,B,C
Non-receptor tyrosine kinases	abl, sck, fak, fes/fps, jak, tkf
Membrane-associated non-receptor tyrosine kinases	src, blk, fgr, fyn, hck, lck, lyn/syn, tkl, yes
Receptors lacking protein kinase activity	mas, mpl, α1β
Membrane-associated G proteins	Ha-ras, Ki-ras, N-ras, gsp, gip
Guanine nucleotide exchange proteins	SDC25
RHO/RAC binding proteins	bcr, dbl, ect2
Cytoplasmic protein serine kinases	bcr, clk, mos, pim1, raf/mil
Protein serine-, threonine-, and tyrosine kinase	sty
Cytoplasmic regulators	bcl-1, crk, nck
Transcription factors	bcl-2, ebl, erbA/THR, ets (elk), evi1, fos (fosB, FRA1, FRA2), gli-1, jun (junB, junD), myb (mbm2), myc, L-myc, N-myc, pax, rel, TAL1, ski, vav
Mitochondrial membrane factor	bcl-2
DNA mismatch repair genes	MLH1, MSH2
Unknown functions	akt, dlk, maf, mel, scc, tlm

in a random fashion with the continued passage of the cells in culture), the retention of human chromosome 11 (in the earliest experiments) is frequently associated with a normal morphological phenotype, whereas loss of this chromosome correlates with the neoplastic morphology. As a corollary to this, the introduction of a normal chromosome 11 into a tumorigenic cell led to a reversion of phenotype to normal morphological appearance; this situation is analogous to the retinoblastoma gene experiment discussed below.

The second situation that suggested the existence of tumour suppressor genes came from a variety of studies on familial cancers, in which a pattern of recessive inheritance requiring a two-hit phenomenon seemed to pertain (see Chapters 4 and 10).

In fact, tumour suppressor genes were first identified in inherited cancer syndromes, primarily through studies of rare cancers such as hereditary retinoblastoma and Wilms' tumour, and (of even further importance) were later shown to be involved in sporadic cancer as well. Recently, a second class of susceptibility genes, mismatch repair genes such as *MSH2* and *MLH1*, has been shown to be defective in hereditary non-polyposis colon cancers. Identification of these genes was facilitated by epidemiological studies of Mendelian patterns of can-

cers in families and advances in laboratory techniques to detect inherited mutations.

Over a dozen tumour suppressor genes have now been discovered (Table 9.7). Germ line mutation of tumour suppressor genes is associated with an inherited predisposition to a limited tumour spectrum, but somatic mutations in tumours are heterogeneous. The well-characterized tumour suppressor genes are involved in diverse functions including cell cycle regulation, check-point control, transcriptional repression, signal transduction modulation, and DNA repair—a pattern not too unlike the functions of classic oncogenes described above. The studies on tumour suppressor genes demonstrate that disturbance in cell proliferation, genetic stability, and cell death may all be part of a pattern that precedes tumorigenesis.

9.3.2 RB, retinoblastoma

One of the genetic highlights of the last decade is the identification of a gene involved in the formation of retinoblastomas. Retinoblastoma is a rare hereditary disease, occurring in 1 child in 20 000. In 40 per cent of cases, tumours are bilateral and more than one independently arising tumour may be present; these are the so-called familial tumours. Children with the

Table 9.7 Tumour suppressor genes

Gene	Chromosome	Neoplasms
APC	5q21–22	Familial adenomatosis polyposis
BCNS	9q31	Medulloblastoma
BRCA1	17q12–21	Breast and ovarian carcinoma
BRCA2	13q12–13	Breast carcinoma
CMAR/CAR	16q	Breast and prostate carcinoma
DCC	18q21	Colon carcinoma
INHA (α-inhibin)	2q33-qter	Gonadal tumours
MEN 1	11q13	Parathyroid, pancreatic and pituitary tumours
NF1	17q11.2	Neurofibromatosis type 1 (Neurofibroma)
NF2	22q12	Neurofibromatosis type 2 (Schwannoma, meningioma)
NM23	17q21.3	Neuroblastoma, colon carcinoma
p16/MLM/ MTS	9p21	Melanoma, pancreas adenocarcinoma, non-small cell lung carcinoma
p53	17p13.1	Breast, colon and lung carcinomas, osteosarcoma, astrocytoma, etc.
RB	13q14	Retinoblastoma, osteosarcoma, breast, bladder and lung carcinomas
VHL	3p25	von Hippel–Lindau syndrome (renal carcinoma, pheochromocytoma, hemangioblastoma)
WT1	11p12	Wilms' tumour

inherited mutant allele may later develop osteosarcomas but rarely get other tumours, even though all the cells in their bodies must bear the mutation. Hence, different cell types respond differently to germ line mutation of the retinoblastoma gene.

As expounded in Chapters 4 and 10, the inheritance of this tumour is often associated with the visible loss of part of chromosome 13 (specifically region 13q14). Sporadic cases occur and sometimes also exhibit obvious abnormalities of this chromosome. The pattern of inheritance suggests that the disease is caused by a two-hit phenomenon, as first postulated by Knudson: one of these changes occurs in the germ line and hence is genetic whereas the second presumably occurs early in life or perhaps during embryogenesis. Although one might argue that all tissues of the body are undergoing rapid and complex development during this period, it leads one to speculate that other tumours of the newborn might also arise from similar mechanisms (see discussions in Chapters 4 and 10).

In some instances where no visible deletion was apparent, when the DNA from tumours was compared to the DNA from the normal tissue of the same donor, the loss of heterozygosity (or a reduction to homozygosity) of loci near 13q14 (these changes are often detected by the use of restriction fragment length polymorphisms, RFLP) was often detected. Taken together, these findings suggested that absence or loss of a normal gene rather than the presence of an abnormal one was more likely to be the case here. The gene identified to this critical chromosomal region by Weinberg's laboratory in 1986 is called *RB1* and is found to be expressed in all cells and tissues tested with the exception of retinoblastomas—whereas normal retinal cells do express it. Thus, in the case of this tumour it would appear that absence of a gene product is a prerequisite for the development of the tumour.

What is known, so far, about the *RB1* gene and its product (generally known as RB, pRB, or p105)? The *RB1* gene is huge, about 200 kilobases in length, and has 27 exons coding for a protein of 105–110 kDa, called p105. The RB1 gene product is a ubiquitously expressed nuclear phosphoprotein that is hypophosphorylated through most of the 'resting' phase of the cell cycle. The state of phosphorylation is critical to its regulation of the G1 to S phase transition, and it is at this point in the cell cycle that it is thought to play its major role as a tumour suppressor.

The RB protein was found early in transformed cells as a complex with the nuclear proteins of several oncogenic viruses (e.g. the T antigens of SV40 and polyomaviruses, the E1A gene product of adenoviruses, and the E7 gene product of human papillomaviruses, HPV) in cells and tissues infected and transformed by these viruses (Table 9.8). Interestingly, SV40 large T antigen, adenovirus E1B, and HPV E6 bind p53, another cell cycle regulatory protein (see Section 9.3.3), suggesting that oncogenic DNA viruses have captured this mechanism to subvert cell replication machinery and to ensure that the enzymes for nucleotide synthesis are available for viral DNA replication. If the regions involved in RB binding are altered or mutated, binding of viral proteins is inhibited and their transforming activity is diminished.

Based on the absence of p105 RB in retinoblastoma tissues, it is logical to speculate that the amount (dosage) of the RB1 gene product might be important to its activity, whereby too little of

Table 9.8 RB and p53 protein binding partners

	RB	p53
Viral		
Adenovirus	E1A	E1B
Human papillomavirus	E7	E6
SV40	Large T antigen	Large T antigen
Cellular		
Transcription factors	E2F	SP1
		TBF (TATA binding protein)
	NF-IL6 (CCAAT binding factor)	CBF (CCAAT binding factor
Other	RBP-1 (RB binding protein)	hsp70 (heat shock protein 70)
	RBP-2 (RB binding protien)	mdm-2 (cellular oncogene)
		RPA (replication protein A)

the normal product (below the threshold value for function) would lead to expression of the oncogenic phenotype. It is also clear that the RB1 gene product, which is so ubiquitously expressed, must have a normal physiological function.

The primary role of RB is to regulate negatively the cellular G1 to S phase transition, and its growth inhibitory effects are exerted, at least in part, through the E2F family of transcription factors. E2F is a critical determinant of the G1–S phase transition during the cell cycle in mammalian cells, serving to activate the transcription of a group of genes that encode proteins necessary for DNA replication, such as dihydrofolate reductase, thymidylate synthase, DNA polymerase-a, ribonucleotide reductase, c-*myc*, N-*myc*, and *myb*. The expression of these genes is therefore inhibited by the binding of RB to E2F, which, in essence, sequesters the E2F and prevents its transcriptional function.

The RB–E2F complex becomes prevalent during G1, and phosphorylation of RB occurs close to the G1–S transition and releases it from E2F. Only hypophosphorylated RB binds to E2F; thus the state of phosphorylation becomes the critical factor in RB function, as phosphorylated RB releases E2F (Fig. 9.5). There are at least 10 sites on RB that are substrates for phosphorylation by the cyclin-dependent kinases (CDKs). Both cyclin E, which appears at the G1 restriction point, and cyclin A, which is newly synthesized at the beginning of the S phase, in conjunction with their CDK partners, can phosphorylate RB. A key component here could be CDK2 activity which is controlled by cyclin E. When CDK2 activity starts to increase rapidly in G1, owing to activation of a positive feedback loop, it reaches a critical level above which CDK inhibitors (CKIs) such as p21 WAF1 and p27 are no longer effective, and the cell then becomes independent of mitogenic and inhibitory signals and is committed to a new cell cycle.

Another cyclin-dependent control of RB is facilitated by cyclin D1 (also known as PRAD-1/

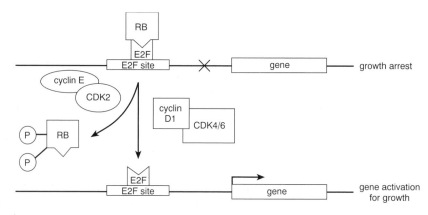

Fig. 9.5 RB–E2F interaction.

CCND1), a G1 cyclin that participates in the control of the cell cycle progression by interacting with RB. In some tumours, cyclin D1 is overexpressed and it is thought that this may lead to abrogation of the suppressive growth control of RB. The *CDKN2* gene, which encodes p16 (also known as INK 4 and MST1), inhibits CDK4–cyclin D1 phosphorylation of RB, preventing the G1–S transition. In turn, p16 expression is negatively regulated by functional RB protein, thus forming a feedback loop of regulation.

There are presumably a number of normal cell proteins that bind at the site where the viral oncoproteins bind; two such RB-binding proteins (RBP-1 and RBP-2) have been cloned. The binding of the viral proteins may then, in contrast, displace RB from its nuclear anchoring protein(s), causing it to be lost from the nucleus.

Hypophosphorylated p105 also associates with the ubiquitous transcription factor E1F; these complexes occur in G1 and function as transcription repressors in the presence of an RB-binding protein. One target of the complex is the promoter of the *CDC2* gene which is important for cell entry into the S phase.

RB1 is also involved in differentiation. The hypophosphorylated form of RB binds to NF-IL6, a member of the CCAAT/enhancer-binding protein (C/EBP) family of transcription factors. Interaction leads to enhanced binding activity of NF-IL6 to its cognate DNA sequences, thus leading to promoter transactivation by NF-IL6. These findings indicate a novel biochemical function of RB: it activates specific transcription factors important for differentiation (e.g. NF-IL6) and inactivates other transcription factors (e.g. E2F) that promote progression through the cell cycle. Such disparate mechanisms may help to explain the dual role of RB1 in cell differentiation and the cell division cycle.

RB1 can bind DNA itself in a non-sequence-specific manner, and has been shown to repress c-*fos* transcription and AP-1 transcriptional activity in cycling 3T3 cells. Furthermore, it can induce TGF-β1 gene expression in epithelial cells, in which TGF-β1 is a growth inhibiting factor, and repress its expression in fibroblasts, where TGF-β1 acts as a growth promoter.

There is also an RB1-related protein called p107 that binds the same viral proteins and also appears to have a role in cell cycle regulation. It has about 30 per cent sequence homology and binds similar transcription factors such as E2F. The transforming viral oncoproteins bind avidly to both p105 RB and p107.

Mutations In addition to retinoblastomas and osteosarcomas, mutations have been detected in a host of tumours including small cell lung (40 per cent), bladder (30 per cent), prostate (20 per cent), breast and cervical carcinomas, and some forms of leukaemia. In contrast to hereditary retinoblastomas, mutations in *RB1* in these other cancers are somatic rather than germ line.

Frameshift and chain termination mutations, deletions of entire exons, and point mutations are common. Many of these mutations affect domains between amino acids 393–572 and 646–772, which are involved in binding of viral oncoproteins (the same region as the E2F binding 'pocket' mentioned above).

Introduction of wild-type *RB1* genes into cells having inactivated *RB1* genes, or cells entirely lacking *RB1* genes (such as RB1$^{-/-}$ SAOS-2 human osteosarcoma cells) results in reversion to a more normal phenotype and loss of tumorigenicity in nude mice. Such reversal has been noted for a variety of retinoblastoma, osteosarcoma, and bladder and prostate carcinoma cell lines.

***RB1* knock-out mice** Knockout of genes is implemented by homologous recombination in mouse embryonic stem cells, followed by microinjection of the ES cells into blastocysts and implantation into foster mothers. *RB1* knock-out mice die before the 16th day of gestation. The major defects are massive neuronal cell death in the developing central nervous system and defective haemopoiesis, with a specific increase in the number of immature, nucleated erythrocytes. Heterozygous mice, in which only one *RB1* allele is knocked out, survive for up to 11 months; however, some of these animals then develop pituitary adenocarcinomas, although interestingly, none develop retinoblastomas. It appears that the remaining *RB1* allele is also lost in the pituitary tumours, fulfilling the two-hit mechanism for tumour development. Such data suggest that not all lineages rely exclusively on RB1 for control of cell proliferation and there are species differences in the target cells for neoplastic transformation after abrogation of RB1 function.

Summary *RB1* is a gene important in the control of cell cycling, regulated by its phosphorylation state. The growth inhibitory function of *RB1* can also be down-regulated by binding to viral oncoproteins, which bind to hypophosphorylated RB, or by mutations that alter the ability of RB protein to bind to its nuclear anchor protein(s). Thus, any of these three events—hyperphosphorylation, binding to oncoproteins, or mutations in the E2F binding 'pocket'—could have the same direct result: inability of RB to inhibit cell cycle progression. Normal cell cycle progression is mediated through normal mitogenic signals that turn on cyclins and CDKs that phosphorylate RB. Alterations to the cyclins, CDKs, and CKIs could lead to indirect mechanisms for affecting RB activity. The most general hypothesis for RB action as a cell cycle control gene, or tumour suppressor gene, is that RB binding to E2F prevents E2F from activating cell cycle progression genes and, conversely, phosphorylation of p105 allows the G1–S boundary to be passed.

9.3.2 *p53*

At this stage, we will survey the studies on a particularly important gene for tumorigenesis *p53* (also called *P53* and *TP53*). The gene was originally discovered because of finding its 53-kDa gene product in immunoprecipitates from cells transformed by SV40 virus as part of a complex with the viral large T antigen (see Table 9.8, and also Chapter 8). The p53 product can be detected in essentially all normal cells as well, although it is present at extremely low levels and appears to have a much shorter half-life, of only around 30 minutes, compared with p53 in transformed cells. Presumably, conformational differences in the mutant protein render it less susceptible to degradation, suggesting that the viral proteins stabilize p53 by formation of the complex. Further studies showed that p53 was present at above normal amounts in many different transformed and tumour cell lines not involving viruses. It is now known, in fact, that *p53* is the most frequently altered gene in cancers, occurring in approximately 70–75 per cent of all human tumours.

The very early studies suggested that *p53* could act as a dominant oncogene. However, comparisons at the DNA level of cloned *p53* from different tumour cell lines confirmed the presence of a mutated rather than the wild-type gene. Inactivation of *p53* is generally associated with the loss of the wild-type allele and the generation of a mutated, transforming one (dominant negative model) in a number of tumours (e.g. small cell lung carcinoma and mammary carcinomas in humans, leukaemias of mice and humans, etc.). Such data argue strongly for the role of *p53* as another tumour suppressor gene rather than as a dominant oncogene.

Many studies show a role for *p53* in cell cycle regulation. Firstly, introduction of wild-type *p53* into cells growing in culture usually blocks cell proliferation at the G1–S transition point in the cell cycle. Moreover, suppression of the neoplastic phenotype in culture and of tumorigenicity in nude mice is usually observed in such cells. Secondly, microinjection of cultured cells in G1 with anti-p53 antibodies inhibits DNA synthesis; however, during other phases of the cell cycle the cells proliferate normally, suggesting that p53 could be a requisite rate-limiting protein for progression through the cell cycle.

A role in metastasis is also hypothesized. A series of mouse leukaemias induced by the Abelson murine leukaemia virus (v-*abl*) became established as cell lines; all were tumorigenic *in vivo*, but only one failed to metastasize. This exception was a result of the integration of a helper murine leukaemia virus within the coding sequences of the *p53* gene, thus inactivating it. Upon introduction of an intact *p53* gene into these cells by transfection, the ability to metastasize was re-established.

The *p53* gene is located on chromosome 17p13 and has 10 coding exons. The 393 phosphoamino acid protein product contains five blocks of sequences highly conserved throughout evolution. The N-terminus contains the transactivating domain, whereas the C-terminus contains the nuclear localization signal, the DNA-binding domain, and sequences involved in protein–protein interactions.

Phosphorylation is an important regulator of p53 physiological activity, as was discussed above for many oncogenes and RB. There is a nuclear translocation domain near the CDK phosphorylation site on Serine-316, suggesting a cell cycle-dependent signal for nuclear translocation. The conformation of p53 is modulated by its phosphorylation state, and this alters its ability to bind to DNA, which occurs through tetramers. Mutant p53 cannot achieve the appropriate conformation and blocks wild-type p53 function by forming oligomers with it—hence the dominant negative effect.

The majority of p53 mutations are in the hydrophobic midregion of the protein, and binding to other cellular proteins and to DNA is disrupted by these mutations, indicating that the correct conformation is a crucial requirement for placing the functional domains in the right configuration.

Binding and transcription p53 can activate target genes by binding to specific DNA sequences located in their promoters. Binding to the relevant response elements in the promoters requires that p53 forms a tetramer, the formation of which may be inhibited by its binding to a mutant form of p53, to viral oncogene products, or to the product of a gene called MDM2 (see below). Many of these genes are associated with DNA replication, such as histone H3, DNA polymerase-α, and *myb*. Some other important genes include creatine kinase, growth arrest DNA damage inducible gene GADD45, MDM2, the cell cycle control gene CDC2, WT1 (see Section 9.3.3), and a gene called WAF1/Cip1 whose p21 product binds to cyclin-dependent kinases, inhibits their action, and arrests cells in midcycle. It also binds to the product of the replication A gene, RPA; both mutated and wild-type p53 can bind to RPA through its acidic activation domains and can inhibit its ability to bind to replication origins.

p53 negatively regulates a number of genes, including c-*fos*, c-*jun*, *hsp70*, *RB1*, interleukin-6, proliferating cell nuclear antigen (PCNA), and the multidrug resistance gene *MDR1*. On the other hand, p53 can also repress transcription from promoters that do not contain p53-binding sequences. There is evidence suggesting that one possible mechanism is by sequestering transcription factors, a situation very reminiscent of the model described above for RB1 and E2F. Furthermore, p53 can inhibit helicase activity and DNA replication.

One interesting interaction is with the gene known as MDM2, originally discovered because it was amplified on a double minute chromosome in transformed mouse cells (mouse *d*ouble *m*inute gene-2). This gene encodes a 90-kDa phosphoprotein that copurifies with p53. MDM2 can bind to and block p53-mediated transactivation. Overexpression of MDM2 in cells increases their tumorigenic potential and inhibits both the G1 arrest and apoptosis functions of the p53 tumour suppressor protein.

Overexpression can arise from amplification, as in 30 per cent of human bone and soft tissue sarcomas, and in about 10 per cent of malignant gliomas. Overexpression may also occur by increased gene transcription without amplification, e.g. in leukaemias and breast carcinoma cell lines. Interestingly, it has also been demonstrated that wild-type p53 can induce expression of MDM2, strongly suggesting that MDM2 is a biological target of p53. Thus, a tight regulatory feedback loop exists between both proteins.

To add further complexity to the plethora of functions attributed to p53, overexpression of wild-type p53 induces growth arrest at the G1 and G2M phases of the cell cycle, promotes differentiation and apoptosis in different situations, and may play a key role in the prevention of genetic instability induced by DNA damaging agents (see below).

Analysis of growth-arrested and -stimulated cells has shown that the localization of p53 varies during the cell cycle. Growth-stimulated cells contain p53 in the cytoplasm during G1 and in the nucleus during S phase; on progressing through the S phase, the p53 locates mostly to the cytoplasm. Experiments with a temperature-sensitive p53 mutant showed that, at the permissive temperature when cells are growth arrested, p53 was preferentially located in the nucleus, whereas in proliferating cells, at the restrictive temperature, p53 was mostly located in the cytoplasm.

Mutations High sequence homology for p53 exists between species, and it is in the conserved regions that one finds several hot spots for mutations in human cancers, strongly implicating these regions as important to its regulatory functions. Data suggest that transformation can be achieved with only amino acids 302–360 of murine wild-type p53; however, amino acids 22 and 23 located in the transactivation domain might also play a role in transformation.

Mutations of the *p53* gene have been reported for almost every type of human cancer, and they are particularly prevalent in colorectal tumours (up to 80 per cent), lung cancers (50 per cent), and breast cancer (40 per cent). Most of the mutations are missense point mutations in carcinomas, whereas in sarcomas, deletions, insertions, and rearrangements are more common and point mutations are rare.

Germ line mutations are observed in families with a high incidence of cancer. The Li–Fraumeni syndrome (see Chapter 4) is one such case; many members of these families have mis-sense and nonsense mutations in one *p53* allele and tend to get osteosarcomas, adrenocortical carcinomas, breast carcinomas, or brain cancers, often at an early age. Curiously, colon carcinoma is not prevalent in these families, even though *p53* mutations are often seen in colon cancer, suggesting that germ line mutations may make certain tissues more susceptible to further somatic mutations than others, or that some tissues have additional mechanisms for regulating cell proliferation that must be knocked out before *p53* mutations become important.

Thus, *p53* seems to manifest its effects through different phenotypes: (i) loss of function, in which a mis-sense mutation abrogates the ability of *p53* to block cell division or reverse a transformed phenotype; (ii) gain of function, as demonstrated by inducing a tumorigenic phenotype following the introduction of a mutant *p53* into cells lacking wild-type *p53*; and (iii) transdominant mutation observed when a mutant *p53* allele is introduced into cells bearing a wild-type allele, resulting in the formation of heteromeric proteins that override the normal inhibitory function of *p53* (dominant negative effect).

Overexpression is often an unfavourable prognostic indicator for several cancers, including breast, ovarian, endometrial, esophageal, lung and urinary bladder carcinomas as well as malignant melanomas.

Importantly, p53 accumulates in about 30 per cent of early dysplastic lung tissues, 70 per cent of lung carcinomas *in situ*, and 80 per cent of invasive tumours, indicating that abnormalities of p53 expression begin early in lung carcinogenesis. Such a finding may provide an extremely useful early diagnostic marker of this disease.

DNA damage and apoptosis As discussed below in Section 9.4.4, the 'anti-apoptosis' gene *bcl-2* can be down-regulated by means of a p53-dependent negative response element in the *bcl-2* gene. Interestingly, coexpression of the c-*myc* and *bcl-2* genes can overcome p53-induced apoptosis by altering the intracellular translocation of p53 to the nucleus. Not all types of apoptosis, however, are mediated by p53. For example, induction of apoptosis in thymocytes by gamma irradiation or the DNA-damaging drug etoposide is through a p53-dependent pathway, whereas that induced by glucocorticoids in thymocytes is not.

Apoptosis can be induced *in vitro*, for example, when spheroids of human lung cancer cells are transfected with a retroviral vector containing a wild-type *p53* gene. Whether such a method can be employed *in vivo* is still undetermined, but this implies that a therapeutic approach might be possible.

p53 enhances sensitivity to ionizing radiation and anticancer drugs. Thus the absence or mutation of p53 leads to an increase in cellular resistance to these agents, implying that cancer cells in patients can acquire resistance to chemotherapeutic agents or irradiation through mutation or loss of *p53*.

When DNA is damaged, there is increased synthesis of p53; p53 accumulates and stops DNA replication and cell division until DNA has time to be repaired. If this is not possible or the DNA repair mechanisms fail, p53 triggers a cell suicide response. Thus, in the case of massive damage to DNA in which repair is not possible, the cell dies. If p53 is mutated or lost, the cells continue to divide and replicate the damaged DNA, passing on mutations to daughter cells. Cells that do this are genetically less stable and accumulate further mutations and rearrangements, leading to the generation of an ever-increasing malignant state. Thus, loss of p53 causes cells to undergo a greater frequency of mutations and gene amplifications.

It is interesting to speculate that the MSH2 mismatch repair gene (see Section 9.4.3) may be a target for p53, a situation that would indicate a direct involvement of p53 in repair mechanisms. The final result—a decrease in radiosensitivity and chemosensitivity—is a bad prognosis for therapy.

In fibroblasts from patients with Li–Fraumeni syndrome, who already have an inherited *p53* mutation, they may lose the remaining wild-type *p53* allele; when they do, they have a greatly increased ability to amplify drug resistance genes (see Chapter 18).

Knock-out mice Mice homozygous for the null allele (i.e. no functional p53) develop normally, indicating that the gene is not necessary for the growth and differentiation of normal tissue. However, by about 6 months of age, these animals begin to develop a variety of neoplasms, including sarcomas, lung carcinomas, lymphomas, and embryonal carcinomas (quite reminiscent of the situation in humans). Thus, normal developing cells must have a redundancy of mechanisms to regulate cell proliferation, a conclusion similar to that reached for heterozygous *RB1* gene knock-out experiments described above. One hypothesis for the late development of tumours in the *p53* knock-out mice is that DNA damage begins to accumulate and p53 function is required to guard the genome from allowing DNA lesions to go unrepaired and passing mutations on to daughter cells.

9.3.4 *WT1*, Wilms' tumour 1

Wilms' tumour, or nephroblastoma, is an embryonal malignancy of the kidney with an incidence of approximately 1 in 10 000 live births. It occurs in both sporadic and familial forms, but only 1 per cent of Wilms' tumour patients have a positive family history. Like most tumours, it involves multiple genetic alterations affecting diverse genes. Early karyotype analyses showed major deletions on chromosome 11p13 to which the *WT1* Wilms' tumour suppressor gene 1 has now been localized. Other genes involved in these tumours have been identified: the *WT2* gene maps to 11p15 in the region of the Beckwith–Wiedemann locus, and the *WT3* locus localizes to chromosome 16q.

WT1 encodes a zinc finger-containing protein that shares homology with proteins in the early growth response gene family (see Chapter 11). Abundant *WT1* transcripts are found in the ovary, testis, uterus, and kidney, with lower levels in the heart and pancreas. Its pattern of expression suggests a critical role in normal mammalian urogenital development. WT1 can bind specific DNA targets within the promoters of many genes and both transcriptional repression and activation domains have been identified. On this basis, it is assumed that regulation of transcription is the basis of WT1 tumour suppressor activity. Interestingly, WT1 coimmunoprecipitates with a number of spliceosomal proteins, suggesting that it may also bind to RNA.

Germ line 'loss of function' mutations at the *WT1* suppressor locus are associated with a predisposition to tumours with mild genital system anomalies. In contrast, germ line mis-sense mutations within the DNA-binding domain often yield a more severe phenotype, known as the WAGR syndrome, which includes aniridia, genitourinary anomalies, and mental retardation.

WT1 represses transcription of several growth factors and growth factor receptors. Notably, WT1 can repress transcription of both the *bcl*-2 and c-*myc* promoters. As the *bcl*-2 and c-*myc* protooncogenes are essential for regulation of apoptosis and cell proliferation (see Section 9.4.4 below), the loss of functional WT1 may result in deregulation of the two genes, thus contributing to tumour formation. WT1 also suppresses synthesis of the epidermal growth factor receptor and induces apoptosis in *in vitro* systems; these mechanisms may contribute to its critical role in normal kidney development and to the immortalization of tumour cells with inactivated WT1 alleles.

9.3.5 Mammary carcinomas: *BRCA1* and *BRCA2*

In western Europe and the United States, approximately 1 in 12 women develop breast cancer. The aetiology of breast cancer involves a complex interplay of various factors, including genetic alterations. Because family history remains the strongest single predictor of breast cancer risk, attention has focused on the role of such genes in cancer-prone families. A small proportion, 5–10 per cent, of breast cancer cases, in particular those arising at a young age, are attributable to two highly penetrant, autosomal dominant susceptibility genes, *BRCA1* and *BRCA2*. *BRCA1* also confers higher risk of ovarian cancer and those with inherited alterations have up to a 94 per cent risk of developing breast and/or ovarian cancer by age 70. *BRCA2* confers a much higher risk of male breast cancer.

In 1994, the *BRCA1* gene, which is responsible for 45 per cent of hereditary early onset breast cancer, for the majority of coinheritance of breast and ovarian cancer, and for conferring increased risk also for colon and prostate cancer, was cloned. *BRCA1* is a large gene, located on human chromosome 17q21, and shows only limited homology to other known genes. It encodes a 190-kDa zinc finger protein of as yet unknown function. The BRCA1 gene product is a nuclear phosphoprotein in normal cells, including alveolar and ductal epithelial cells of the mammary gland. During pregnancy, there is a large increase in BRCA1 mRNA in mammary epithelial cells, suggesting that this increase parallels functional differentiation of the cells. Because high rates of breast cancer are associated with loss of BRCA1 expression, it is possible that this gene provides an important growth regulatory function in mammary epithelial cells. In the large majority of breast and ovarian cancer lines and samples of cells obtained from malignant effusions, however, BRCA1 localizes mainly in the cytoplasm rather than the nucleus. Absence of BRCA1 or aberrant subcellular location is also observed to a variable extent in histological sections of many non-familial breast cancer biopsies. These findings suggest that BRCA1 abnormalities may be involved in the pathogenesis of many sporadic breast cancers as well.

With the exception of some mis-sense mutations identified in the ring finger near the amino terminus of *BRCA1*, virtually all germ line mutations in the gene cause the novel BRCA1 protein to be prematurely truncated in length. Approximately 90 per cent of breast tumours in *BRCA1* families, 50 per cent of unselected breast tumours, and 65–80 per cent of unselected ovarian tumours have lost one allele of *BRCA1* by somatic deletion.

Another gene that confers an increased risk of breast cancer is the *BRCA2* gene, which maps to chromosome 13q12–q13 by linkage analysis. Mutations in *BRCA2* account for approximately 40 per cent of hereditary early onset breast cancer. Loss of heterozygosity is also observed in tumours of the prostate, ovary, cervix, colon, male breast, and ureter. Almost all breast tumours or tumour cell lines that show loss of *BRCA2*, also exhibit the simultaneous loss of *RB1* (at 13q14), thus suggesting that the genes may act in concert.

9.3.6 Others

The search for other tumour suppressor genes continues, stimulated by the knowledge that there are further chromosome segments carrying suppressors defined by cell hybrid experiments and defined karyotypic deletions associated with a variety of familial and sporadic cancers (see Chapters 4 and 10).

9.4 Interactions between oncogenes

At this stage, one should see an emerging pattern of the panoply of interactions between oncogenes and tumour suppressor genes. The following sections outline some of the ways in which these cooperative interactions were first deciphered.

9.4.1 Tripartite retroviruses

Perhaps one of the most unexpected results from studying v-*onc* genes was the discovery that a single virus genome often contained genetic information derived from two distinct cellular genes (often from two different chromosomes). The v-*src* gene of Rous sarcoma virus, as mentioned above, derives its carboxyl-terminal sequences from outside the cellular *src* gene; these sequences are apparently from about 1 kb downstream of the gene. The FBR strain of MSV, in addition to *fos*, contains sequences called *fox* from another location, which confer additional properties. Similarly, the AEV strain, ES4, differs from strain H; the former contains *erbA* and *erbB*, the latter *erbB* alone. Both strains cause erythroleukaemias but erythroid cells transformed in culture show differences in growth requirements and differentiation capacity depending on the specific virus strain. The GR strain of feline sarcoma virus shows fusion of part of an actin gene with the transforming *fgr* gene. Finally, two viruses have shown acquisition of sequences from two separate genes, each of which has oncogenic potential on its own: the avian myelocytomatosis virus, MH2, contains the oncogenes *myc* and *raf* (also called *mil*), and the E26 avian myeloblastosis virus contains *myb* and *ets*. The neoplastic potential of these viruses is expanded with regard to the types of tumours induced compared with viruses containing only one of the genes (see Table 9.1). In the case of v-*src* mentioned above, the unusual structure might have arisen by a large splicing event, but the others require more bizarre recombination. (However, it is still speculation whether transduction occurs at the DNA level between integrated provirus and adjacent cellular DNA, or at the RNA level between viral and cellular species, or by both mechanisms.)

9.4.2 Cooperative transformation

An old observation that primary rodent embryo fibroblasts, but not longer passaged or established cell lines, were generally refractory to morphological transformation by transforming viruses was the basis of a new assay for oncogene activity. For example, the dual expression of the genes encoding the nuclear (large T) antigen and the membrane-associated (middle T) antigen of polyomavirus (see Chapter 8) causes transformation, whereas neither alone has this capacity, although large T confers longevity ('immortalization' to continued cell growth). A similar relationship was found between unrelated oncogenes, e.g. the mutated alleles of Ha-*ras-1* (whether viral or cellular in origin) and *myc*. Eventually a pattern emerged of cooperation between a nuclear oncogene product and a cytoplasmic oncogene product (Table 9.9); the former also generally can immortalize non-established cells.

The discovery of cooperating oncogenes was particularly satisfactory given the multistage character of carcinogenesis, interweaving pathways of biochemical and physiological functions. But we have determined only the earliest step without generating clues to distinct targets or later cascades. Elucidation of the intermediate and final stages is necessary for both understanding and devising possible modes of intervention.

9.4.3 Multistep carcinogenesis: highways and byways

Colorectal cancers As discussed in Chapter 4, the aetiology of colorectal tumours has also recently

Table 9.9 Cooperating oncogenes[1]

Non-nuclear	Nuclear
Ha-*ras*-1[2]	v-*myc*
N-*ras*[2]	c-*myc*[3]
Polyoma middle T	Polyoma large T
Adenovirus E1b	Adenovirus E1a
	v-*myb*
	v-*fos*
	p53

[1] Manifestation of the transformed phenotype requires one oncogene from the nuclear group and one from the non-nuclear group.
[2] Mutated allele.
[3] Normal and rearranged forms when supplemented with a strong promoter.

been linked to the absence of a normal gene product. The story begins with the discovery of a mutant karyotype involving chromosome 5 in one patient who exhibited familial adenomatous polyposis (FAP, formerly the disease syndrome was known as polyposis coli) involving hundreds of tiny polyps in the large intestine and colon, some of which may convert to malignant papillomas with time, and in addition was mentally retarded (a circumstance that suggested that this person might have a larger genetic abnormality than people with FAP alone). By using probes from different region of chromosome 5, the defective region was discovered to be at 5q21. Taking these data a few steps farther, there were apparent rearrangements in this region in cells derived from polyps of FAP patients and in patients with colorectal cancer of a presumably non-familial (sporadic) origin. As colorectal tumours represent the second most common tumour in Western countries, it would seem that such tumour suppressor genes may exert a very important and frequent modality of carcinogenesis.

The adenomatous polyposis coli (*APC*) gene responsible for FAP was isolated in 1991, and germ line and somatic mutations of the *APC* gene have been identified (see Chapter 4). When the *APC* gene is the initial mutation, tumour development follows the 'loss of heterozygosity' (LOH) pathway (Fig. 9.6). Somatic mutations activating the Ki-*ras* oncogene and inactivating the MCC (mutated in colon carcinoma), DCC (deleted in colon carci-

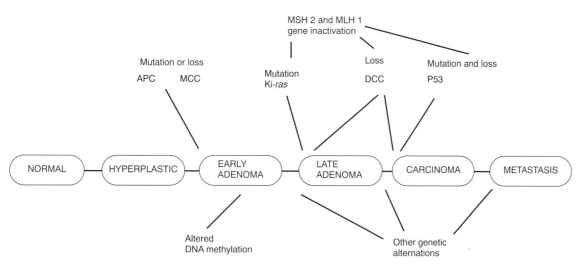

Fig. 9.6 Genesis of colon carcinoma.

noma), and p53 tumour suppressor genes accumulate in this pathway and mark the progression through polyp stages. However, another mechanism of tumour formation has recently been identified through the 'replication error' (RER) pathway when mismatch repair genes (such as MSH2 and MLH1) are altered (see Chapter 4). Germ line mutations inactivating one allele of these DNA mismatch repair genes may also be responsible for hereditary non-polyposis colorectal cancer (HNPCC) and seem to predispose affected individuals to a high frequency of early onset cancer. Thus the molecular mechanism of colorectal tumorigenesis now seems to be more complicated than was previously supposed: there is a convergence of mechanisms between familial and sporadic occurrence of these tumours as well as a divergence of mechanisms related to the genes initially involved.

Thyroid neoplasms Thyroid neoplasms represent another good model for studying the role of multiple mutations in epithelial cell multistep carcinogenesis because they comprise a broad spectrum of lesions with different degrees of malignancy. Medullary thyroid carcinoma (MTC) is a malignancy of the thyroid C-cells that comprises 5–10 per cent of all thyroid cancers. MTC occurs in both sporadic and familial forms, the latter making up 25 per cent of all MTCs and being comprised of three distinct syndromes: multiple endocrine neoplasia type 2A (MEN 2A), multiple endocrine neoplasia type 2B (MEN 2B), and familial medullary thyroid carcinoma, all of which have an autosomal dominant mode of inheritance.

Recent studies have established that the *ret* protooncogene is involved in the development of thyroid tumours, including medullary and papillary thyroid carcinomas. This oncogene was originally detected by transfection techniques using DNA from a T cell lymphoma. Germ line mutations of the *ret* protooncogene, a transmembrane receptor tyrosine kinase, were identified in MEN types 2A and 2B. MEN 2A point mutations involve cysteine residues in the extracellular domain that lead to disulphide-linked homodimerization of the ret protein on the cell surface, and subsequent activation of its intrinsic tyrosine kinase. On the other hand, a single point mutation in the tyrosine kinase domain was found in MEN 2B, as well as in 30–40 per cent of sporadic medullary carcinoma. This mutation

also resulted in activation of ret tyrosine kinase without the formation of its covalent homodimerization. Differences in the mechanisms of ret activation might account for the different phenotypes observed in MEN 2A and MEN 2B. In addition, somatic rearrangements of the *ret* protooncogene are frequently detected in papillary thyroid carcinoma, particularly from adult Europeans.

Interestingly, the same rearrangement was recently observed in approximately 60 per cent of papillary carcinomas of children from areas contaminated by the Chernobyl accident, suggesting that *ret* rearrangement can be induced as a direct consequence of radiation exposure.

As with familial adenomatosis polyposis, the use of genetic screening of individuals at risk of one of these syndromes has become integral to their clinical management. In those cases having a detectable mutation, surgical intervention is implemented, thus largely preventing aggressive metastasis of thyroid carcinoma, the main cause of death. Direct gene testing can also be used to demonstrate the lack of inheritance of a parental mutation in the *ret* protooncogene and thus obviates the need for the usual annual screening from age 5 years onwards.

The other main oncogenes involved in human thyroid carcinogenesis are *ras*, in the follicular tumour pathway, *trk* (nerve growth factor receptor) which is activated at high frequency in papillary thyroid carcinomas, and *p53*, particularly in the progression of either papillary or follicular adenoma to undifferentiated carcinoma. In experimental thyroid carcinogenesis, *ras* is again involved, with a correlation between the specific mutagenic agent used, the type of mutation, and the particular *ras* gene showing the mutation.

Further analysis suggests that two growth factor receptor genes are concerned with normal growth induced by thyroid-stimulating hormone (TSH); the TSH receptor and the IGF1 receptor may be involved in the progression of thyroid tumours of follicular pathology, whereas several tyrosine kinase receptors with unknown ligands or of uncertain physiological function are linked to papillary carcinoma. Thus, it seems likely that multiple oncogenes contribute to the genesis of thyroid tumours; however, one must always consider whether the mutations involved are causative of or consequences of the specificity of the tumour cells that predominate.

9.4.4 Apoptosis and *bcl-2*

The study of apoptosis is a rapidly growing field as its significance in terms of cancer is realized. Two gene families are of particular interest: the interleukin-1 beta-converting enzyme family of cysteine proteases and *bcl-2*. Both of these families are homologous to cell death genes in the earthworm *Caenorhabditis elegans*. Other genes with established roles in proliferation and differentiation control are also involved in apoptotic events: e.g. c-*myc* and *p53* which can invoke defective apoptosis, as discussed above.

The *bcl-2* protooncogene was originally detected as a common chromosomal translocation in non-Hodgkin's B cell lymphomas, arising from its location on chromosome 18 and juxtaposing it to the immunoglobulin heavy chain locus on chromosome 14, namely t(14;18)(q32;q21). This mechanism is similar to that of *myc* gene activation in Burkitt's lymphoma, discussed earlier (see Section 9.1.2), and the result is that there are abnormally high levels of expression resulting from placement of the gene under the influence of the highly expressed immunoglobulin heavy chain enhancer. The translocation occurs in about 85 per cent of follicular lymphomas, 20 per cent of diffuse large cell lymphomas, and 10 per cent of B cell chronic lymphocytic leukaemias (in this latter case, the translocation is to immunoglobulin light chain genes); the major breakpoint region is within the 3′ untranslated part of exon 3.

The gene does not fit the normal criteria for an oncogene, e.g. it does not transform or immortalize cells. However, the *bcl-2* gene holds a unique place in that its main action is to enhance lymphoid cell survival by inhibiting programmed cell death (apoptosis) rather than stimulating cell proliferation. Although the major group of epithelial cells expressing *bcl-2* protein are in proliferating zones, the survival advantage provided by *bcl-2* prolongs the life span, and allows proliferation, differentiation, and morphogenesis to proceed. Its expression in association with precancerous lesions suggests a role in the early stage of tumorigenesis. Thus, it may increase the likelihood of secondary genetic changes occurring which more directly effect tumorigenesis. It may also block *myc*-induced apoptosis in some systems, thus leading to cooperative transformation. However, not all mechanisms involved in induction of apoptosis can be prevented by *bcl-2*. For example, it can prevent apoptosis in embryonic neurones deprived of nerve growth factor (NGF) but not those dependent on other growth factors, or haemopoietic cells deprived of IL-3, IL-4, or GM-CSF but not those dependent on IL-2 or IL-6. This suggests that there are many contributing factors to the apoptotic pathway of a given cell type.

There are both positive and negative regulators of *bcl-2* function. A number of *bcl-2*-related genes have been identified, including *bcl*-X_S and *bcl*-X_L (and *bax*) which can render cells resistant to apoptosis and prevent *bcl-2* overexpression from preventing apoptosis, respectively.

Expression is associated with resistance to hormone therapy and recurrence in prostate carcinomas, whereas in lung and breast carcinomas, it is associated with a better prognosis. One hypothesis for the major mechanism of *bcl-2* action is that it stimulates an antioxidant pathway at sites of oxygen free radical generation. *bcl-2* can modulate the cytotoxicity of some anticancer agents by inhibiting the process of apoptosis; thus with better understanding of the functional and structural significance of proteinprotein interactions involving bcl-2, bax, and other members of the bcl-2 protein family, it may eventually be possible to develop novel pharmacological agents that improve tumour responses to currently available anticancer drugs.

9.5 Protooncogene expression in normal development and differentiation

Although molecular clones to probe for oncogene expression are available for many of the genes described above, it is a rather daunting task to examine many different tissues. In some cases, it is also difficult to obtain sufficient amounts of homogeneous cell populations and thus one is not always able to make direct comparisons between a neoplasm and its normal counterpart. This has left large gaps in our knowledge of oncogene expression during embryonic development, differentiation stages, or cell cycling (Table 9.10), although eventually this knowledge will be available.

One well exploited system is the examination of mouse embryos at different days of gestation. Genes such as *raf*, Ha-*ras*, Ki-*ras*, and *myc* are expressed throughout. The *abl* gene is highly expressed at day 10, corresponding to a period of fetal liver haemopoiesis, whereas *fos* peaks at later stages owing to

Table 9.10 Protooncogene expression

Gene	High expression[1]	Abnormal expression[2]
abl	Mid-gestation embryo, testes, spleen, thymus	Chronic myelocytic leukaemia
erbA	Mid to late gestation embryo	
erbB	Mid-gestation embryo	Squamous cell carcinomas, glioblastomas
fes	Bone marrow	Myeloid and lymphoid leukaemia
fms	Macrophage, placenta	Mammary and renal carcinoma
fos	Amnion, chorion, mature macrophages, growth factor stimulated cells	Choriocarcinoma
mos	Testis, oocytes	Plasmacytoma[3]
myb	Yolk sac, bone marrow, thymus	Myeloid and lymphoid leukaemia
myc	Ubiquitous	B cell lymphomas, promyelocytic leukaemia
raf	Ubiquitous	
ras	Ubiquitous	Numerous (see Table 9.3)
rel	Spleen	
ros	Kidney	
sis	Platelets	Osteosarcoma
ski	Cartilage, muscle, skin	
src	Spleen, macrophages, brain	Brain tumours
yes	Kidney	

[1] Most studies from experimental animals, principally mice.
[2] Human tumours or tumour cell lines.
[3] Rodent tumour only, gene activated by insertional mutagenesis (see Table 9.2).

high levels in the extraembryonic membranes, particularly the amnion, and *fms* expression is observed in the chorion. Other genes are not present at detectable levels. It is not facetious to speculate that protooncogenes are vital to embryogenesis and that we may eventually know their specific roles; however, we must not be surprised that often their functions and expression patterns in adult tissues are quite distinct from those seen in embryogenesis.

To study changes with regard to cell cycling and proliferation, several methods have been used. Most rely on selecting cells in the same phase of the cycle using a cell sorter that measures levels of DNA or by synchronizing the cycle, usually by blocking the cells in a specific phase of the cycle by deprivation of specific nutrients or by chemicals. On removing the block, the cycle continues with many of the cells in the same phase. *In vivo* systems such as partial hepatectomy (where one lobe of the liver is removed) can be used to stimulate rapid regeneration of cell number. Cell sorting has shown *myb* expression to be cycle dependent. Stimulation from quiescence shows *fos* to be activated within minutes followed by a rapid decline, whereas *myc* expression appears later but is less transient. The liver regeneration experiments show that the major nuclear oncogenes, members of the kinase family, and *ras* are expressed during the highly proliferative phase. Thus, these results recapitulate our awareness that oncogenes are involved in normal proliferative responses, but with increased experimentation on these genes, the roles and pathways become yet more complex and circuitous.

9.6 Lessons learned from oncogenes

It should be clear from the discussion above that oncogenes are expressed in a plethora of cell types. Even the truly tumorigenic v-*onc* genes do not answer our queries. For example, the murine *abl*-containing virus causes immature B cell tumours in mice whereas the feline *abl* virus causes fibrosarcomas (Table 9.1). Is this owing to differences in the nature of the fusion proteins (between *abl* and viral genes) or to some inherent properties of the two animal species? Site-specific mutagenesis has shown that the gag portion of the mouse virus fusion protein is required for efficient transformation of cultured B lymphocytes, though it is dispensable for fibroblast transformation which may, in part, explain this discrepancy. Furthermore, many strains of mice are genetically resistant to leukaemogenesis by the virus, by a mechanism as yet unknown. We have to know more about the normal *abl* product. The highest level of *abl* mRNA in normal tissues occurs in the testes; haemopoietic tissues also express high levels. Is this significant with regard to aberrant transcription owing to translocation in CML? Other examples of these phenomena exist (see Tables 9.1, 9.2, and 9.10).

Understanding the role of the *myc* gene is certain to prove of central interest. The various v-*myc* genes are responsible for the induction of carcinomas, fibrosarcomas, and myeloid leukaemias, whereas hyperexpression owing to translocation or promoter insertion is observed in T and B cell leukaemias. Additionally, *myc* expression is apparent at low levels in most tissues, becomes elevated in cells responding to mitogens, and is very high in the most mature macrophages. There is also intriguing information from experimental manipulation of the gene. First, a new 'virus' was made by putting the cellular *myc* gene between viral LTRs from the MMTV genome and introducing it into fertilized mouse ova. The use of LTRs ensured that the gene could be incorporated into chromosomal (and germ line) DNA, and the resulting transgenic mice were examined for abnormalities of development. However, it was only in adult female mice that a change was seen: the animals developed mammary carcinomas as a heritable trait. In a similar way, a construct containing *myc* and the enhancer element from an immunoglobulin gene (from a rearranged gene in a mouse plasmacytoma, see above) induced a high incidence of B cell leukaemias in the transgenic mice, whereas other enhancers from a leukaemia virus LTR or SV40 virus were less efficacious in inducing tumours and showed different target specificities (a T cell lymphoma with the former, and lymphosarcoma, fibrosarcoma, and kidney carcinoma with the latter). These results emphasize the importance of specific promoter and enhancer elements for gene transcription in different cells and in neoplasia. Furthermore, the duality of function is emphasized from the studies on *p53* and *myc* as either can be an activator or a repressor of specific genes, and

can function as a cell cycle progression gene or stimulate apoptosis.

As discussed previously, oncogenes are relatively highly conserved evolutionarily in vertebrates. Indeed, structural and biochemical (functional) counterparts have been detected in yeast, slime moulds, fruit flies (*Drosophila*), and frogs (*Xenopus*). At the moment, the genes related to oncogenes in *Drosophila* provide a lot of interest because there exist many mutant flies that could throw light on the physiological function of oncogenes. Furthermore, it is also possible to induce mutations or to introduce mutant genes into the animals during embryonic development. As can be seen in Table 9.11, there are already identifiable mutations in *Drosophila* genes that are apparently related to mammalian oncogenes. While it is difficult to say that one such as *wingless* (the fly equivalent of *int-1*) has a direct functional homologue in primates, for example, it is interesting that a number of the oncogene counterparts are involved in overall body pattern formation. As another example, the mutation *sevenless* has been postulated to be a receptor defect and this would fit in very well with the idea that its relative *ros* is a receptor based on its structural counterparts in the tyrosine kinase family. Moreover, another gene called *bride of sevenless* encodes the ligand of *sevenless*; once purified and identified, this product should elucidate the nature of the ligand for mammalian *ros* and hence its functional role.

Over the years, a number of new techniques for introducing DNA into cells, other than calcium precipitation, have been devised and are discussed above; some have proved to be of greater value in cells of small size or those very sensitive to chemical treatment. One such improvement is the use of electroporation, in which uptake of exogenous materials

Table 9.11 Oncogene homologues in *Drosophila*

Oncogene	Homologue	Effect of mutation
rel	*dorsal*	Pattern development
ros	*sevenless*	Absence of eye segment
abl	*abl*	Lethal mutation (90% larvae and pupae)
ras	*ras*	Reduced viability and fertility; poor wing development; disordered eye structure
int-1	*wingless*	Absence of wings
erbB (EGFR)	*egfr*	Disordered eye structure

is facilitated during transient changes to cell membrane electrical potential. This method has been particularly useful in cells known as embryonic stem (ES) cells derived from the inner cell mass of early embryonic mice. ES cells are the closest type to pluripotential stem cells that can be cultured *in vitro* and *in vivo*; indeed they have the capacity to contribute to all three germ layers (endoderm, mesoderm, and ectoderm) of a developing embryo.

Homologous recombination is a term applied to the exchange of allelic, though not necessarily identical, genetic sequences from an exogenous source with the endogenous sequences of an organism. In this way, one might hope to substitute—with specificity—the allelic gene: (i) from a different species but having the same physiological function (a specific type of transgenic manipulation); (ii) from an intact gene copy to replace a defective endogenous gene (i.e. gene therapy); or (iii) from a defective gene to replace the endogenous normal gene. In the last case, if the defective gene was incapable of being expressed, the result would be the loss ('knockout') of the endogenous gene and hence absence of its biochemical function. All of the above alternatives are 'transgenic' experiments *per se*, and the chances are more likely that recombination at a non-homologous region should occur at higher frequency. It has thus been surprising that the actual frequency of homologous recombination is often quite high (up to 1 per 30 transgenic events), certainly much greater than anticipated; this result makes the experimental system much more attractive and efficacious for studying the importance of protooncogenes, oncogenes, and tumour suppressor genes, and their regulatory sequences on viability, development, and oncogenesis, as discussed above in relation to *RB1*, *p53*, and *myc* (Table 9.12).

We are looking through a small window at what is going on in a cell. The viral oncogenes have called our attention to the cellular counterparts and transfection assays and chromosomal aberrations have helped to identify further potentially important genes for neoplastic growth.

New modes of cancer therapy are suggested by the identification of novel oncogene products. For example, point mutations in *ras* genes contribute to the transformation process through constitutive transduction of growth-promoting signals. These oncoproteins are distinct from normal *ras* p21 in both DNA and protein sequences at specific sites. A high frequency of human cancers harbour point

Table 9.12 Comparison of oncogenes and tumour suppressor genes

Oncogene	Tumour suppressor gene
One mutation sufficient for cancer	One or generally two mutations required for cancer (e.g. *p53*, one mutation causes 'dominant negative' effect)
Gain of function 'dominant'	Loss of function 'recessive'
Somatic mutation	Germ line and somatic mutations
Altered gene involved in positive regulation of cell proliferation	Wild-type gene involved in negative regulation of cell proliferation
Transfection with altered gene causes malignant transformation of established fibroblasts	Transfection with wild-type gene causes suppression of malignant phenotype in tumour cells
Common mutations include point mutations, truncations, rearrangements, amplifications	Common mutations include deletions, point mutations

mutations in the *ras* gene at codon 12, where the normal Gly residue is substituted with either a Val, Asp, or Cys residue, generating 'neo-determinants' that could provide specific epitopes for T cell recognition in cancer immunotherapy (see Chapter 19). Other potential therapeutic targets could be the fusion oncogene products. Furthermore, antisense oligonucleotides have been shown to be efficacious *in vitro*; ways of delivering them direct to a tumour site might have a similar role *in vivo*.

Our sojourn into oncogenes has led to the conclusion that normal cellular genes can be diverted into neoplastic pathways by somatic mutations as diverse as single nucleotide substitutions to gross alterations involving translocations or amplifications. Underscoring these perturbations, there may be more subtle effects on expression in inappropriate cells, alterations in transcription rates or mRNA turnover, or stabilization of the gene products, and, in turn, their target substrates within the cell. Most of the changes observed have led to overexpression of the gene. But taking a cellular *onc* gene and putting it under the control of a strong promoter does not necessarily lead to oncogenic potential (indeed this works for *mos* but not for *src*). Overabundance of an oncogene product might also uncover cryptic activities normally absent when the protein occurs at some subthreshold dose.

Overall, cell metabolism and proliferation is an intricate and delicately balanced response to extracellular signals (e.g. mitogens), involving regulated transmission by effector molecules to the nucleus. Some of the known oncogenes already recapitulate a few stages of these mechanisms in their mimicry of growth factors and growth factor receptors. Others display functions suggestive of second messages or transmitters. And the nuclear oncogenes might be the ultimate effector molecules. Despite the formidable task ahead of identifying these interweaving pathways step by step, we have gained considerable insight within the last ten years. The identification of tumour suppressor genes has opened up another stratum of conceptualizing changes in tumorigenesis (see Table 9.12). Indeed, the studies on the first identifiable retrovirus oncogenes quickly aroused the interest of scientists in many areas of diverse research and showed how interrelated their endeavours had become. In the final analysis, oncogenes and tumour suppressor genes are just genes that, when perturbed, march to the tune of a different drummer.

References and further reading

Bishop, J. M. (1991). Molecular themes in oncogenesis. *Cell*, **64**, 235–48.

Bishop, J. M. (1995). Cancer: the rise of the genetic paradigm. *Genes and Development*, **9**, 1309–15.

Bodmer, W. F., Bailey, C. J., Bodmer, J., Bussey, H. J., Ellis, A., Gorman, P., Lucibello, F. C., Murday, V. A., Rider, S. H., Scambler, P. *et al.* (1987). Localization of the gene for familial adenomatous polyposis on chromosome 5. *Nature*, **328**, 614–6.

Boguski, M. S. and McCormick, F. (1993). Proteins regulating *ras* and its relatives. *Nature*, **366**, 643–54.

Bos, J. L. (1988). The *ras* family and human carcinogenesis. *Mutation Research*, **196**, 255–71.

Cooper, G. M. (1995). *Oncogenes*. Jones and Bartlett Publishers, Boston.

Friend, S. H., Bernards, R., Rogelj, S., Weinberg, R. A., Rapaport, J. M., Albert, D. M. and Dryja, T. J. (1986). A human DNA segment with properties of the gene that predisposes to retinoblastoma and osteosarcoma. *Nature*, **323**, 643–6.

Glover D. M. and Hames, B. D. (ed.). (1989). *Oncogenes*. IRL Press, Oxford.

Hartwell, L. H. and Kasten, M. B. (1994). Cell cycle control and cancer. *Science*, **266**, 1821–8.

Hesketh, R. (1994). *The oncogene handbook*. Academic Press, London.

Hinds, P. W. and Weinberg, R. A. (1994). Tumor suppressor genes. *Current Opinions in Genetics and Development*, **4**, 135–41.

Huang, H. J., Yee, Y. K., Shew, J. Y., Chen, P. L., Bookstein, R., Friedmann, T., Lee, E. Y. and Lee, W. H. (1988). Suppression of the neoplastic phenotype by the replacement of the RB gene in human cancer cells. *Science*, **242**, 1563–6.

Lane, D. P. (1992). p53, guardian of the genome. *Nature*, **358**, 15–6.

Oliff, A., Gibbs, J. B., and McCormick, F. (1996). New molecular targets for cancer therapy. *Scientific American*, **275**, 110–5.

Ruddon, R.W. (1995). *Cancer biology*, (3rd edn). Oxford University Press, Oxford.

Sidransky, D. (1996). Advances in cancer detection. *Scientific American*, **275**, 70–5.

Trichopoulos, D., Li, F. P., and Hunter, D. J. (1996). What causes cancer? *Scientific American*, **275**, 50–7.

Varmus, H. E. (1984). The molecular genetics of cellular oncogenes. *Annual Review of Genetics*, **18**, 553–612.

Varmus, H. and R. A. Weinberg. (1993). *Genes and the biology of cancer*. Scientific American Library (distributed by W.H. Freeman), New York.

Weissman, B. E., Saxon, P. J., Pasquale, S. R., Jones, G. R., Geiser, A. G. and Stanbridge, E. J. (1987). Introduction of a normal human chromosome 11 into a Wilms' tumor cell line controls its tumorigenic expression. *Science*, **236**, 175–80.

10

Chromosomes and cancer

DENISE SHEER

10.1 Introduction

Cancer arises from the accumulation of genetic changes that confer a selective advantage to the cells in which they occur. These changes consist of mutations, and numerical and structural chromosome aberrations. They usually occur in somatic cells, but certain genetic changes can be inherited and cause a predisposition to cancer.

Recurrent and sometimes highly specific chromosome aberrations are present in different types of cancer. Molecular genetic analysis of these aberrations has identified numerous genes that contribute to tumorigenesis, opening up new avenues of research into regulatory pathways in the cell. Chromosome aberrations are increasingly playing a role in the clinical management of cancer patients, since they can provide critical diagnostic and prognostic information. Tumour-specific chromosome aberrations act as tumour markers and can be used to monitor the effectiveness of therapy. These aberrations are also likely to provide novel targets for innovative cancer therapy.

Human somatic cells normally have 46 chromosomes and are described as diploid. Chromosome analysis is conventionally carried out on cells during the metaphase stage of mitosis (cell division) when the chromosomes become visible as distinct entities. After each chromosome in a cell is identified by its characteristic size, shape, and staining properties, a karyotype displaying the full chromosome complement of the cell is prepared (Fig. 10.1).

The first recurrent chromosome aberration to be described in a human tumour was the 'Philadelphia chromosome', an unusually small chromosome found in chronic myeloid leukaemia (CML) in 1960 by Nowell and Hungerford in Philadelphia. This discovery aroused considerable interest in cancer cytogenetics as it gave the first direct evidence for a consistent genetic alteration in a tumour. The search that followed for abnormalities in other tumour types was hampered by difficulties in defining chromosome aberrations using current staining methodology, by the apparent variation in chromosome abnormalities from one tumour to the next, and by the finding of aneuploidy (abnormal chromosome numbers) and multiple rearrangements (abnormal breakage and rejoining of chromosomes) in many tumours.

The introduction of chromosome banding techniques in 1970 revolutionized cancer cytogenetics. Consistent chromosome aberrations were shown in other types of tumours. Chromosome aberrations in different cells of a tumour were found to be related

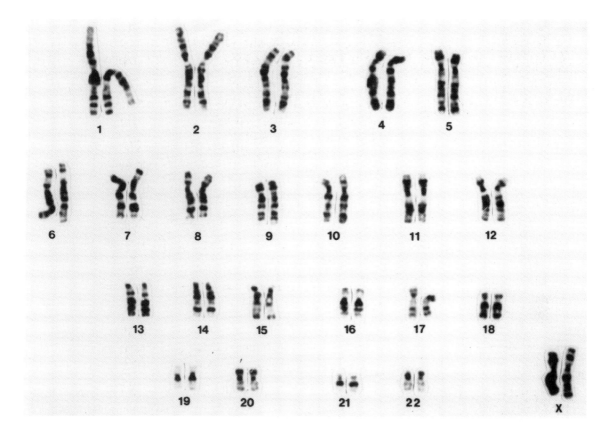

Fig. 10.1 G-banded karyotype from normal peripheral blood lymphocytes, prepared by incorporating BrdU into the chromosomes to give a late-replication banding pattern.

to one another, and further aberrations were shown to occur during tumour progression. Methods for improving yields of dividing cells and methods for high resolution banding of elongated chromosomes in the 1980s facilitated more precise definition of rearrangements as well as the identification of previously undetected rearrangements. Using these techniques, most tumour cells can now be shown to have some chromosomal defect.

Our current understanding of the significance of consistent chromosome aberrations in cancer will be reviewed below. Evidence that these aberrations are non-random has come from cytogenetic analysis of large numbers of human tumours. These have been documented by Felix Mitelman in a continuously revised database, the *Catalog of Chromosome Aberrations in Cancer*, which is an invaluable resource for all researchers in this area (Mitelman 1994).

10.2 **Methodology**

10.2.1 Cytogenetic analysis

Detailed methods and the theoretical background to the cytogenetic analysis of tumours can be found in Rooney and Czepulkowski (1992). Ideally cytogenetic studies are performed before a patient has undergone radiotherapy or chemotherapy as these treatments generate secondary genetic instability.

Leukaemias are analysed from bone marrow aspirates, or peripheral blood samples if the white cell count is high, by immediate processing (direct preparation), or after *in vitro* culture for 24–72 hours.

The cells in solid tumours often have to be physically or enzymatically separated and may have a low mitotic index. Direct preparations, short- or long-term cultures, and cell lines from solid tumours are all used as sources of metaphase spreads. Direct preparations are preferable, however, to avoid difficulties in distinguishing aberrations generated *in vivo* from those generated *in vitro*. Any period of *in vitro* culture may give rise to selective growth of certain cells that are well adapted to culture conditions.

Chromosomes are conventionally examined during or just prior to the metaphase stage of mitosis when they become condensed and can easily be seen under the microscope (Verma and Babu 1995). DNA replication occurs before mitosis so that each chromosome consists of two identical sister chromatids held together at the centromere. When making chromosome preparations, colchicine or a related agent is added to the tumour cells to arrest them in metaphase by disrupting the formation of the mitotic spindle fibres that normally separate the chromatids. The cells are then swollen in a hypotonic solution, fixed in methanol-acetic acid, and metaphase 'spreads' prepared by dropping the fixed cells on to microscope slides. Chromosomes are identified by one of several staining techniques which produce a characteristic series of bands along the chromosomes.

Cytogenetic analysis of cells in metaphase results in karyotypes with approximately 300 bands in the haploid chromosome set (22 chromosomes plus X or Y). It is often preferable to obtain less condensed chromosomes, i.e. with more, thinner bands, earlier in mitosis. One method used is to treat the cultures with methotrexate, a drug that blocks one of the metabolic pathways in DNA synthesis, so that the cells collect at one stage before mitosis. The block is released by thymidine so that large numbers of cells at the same stage of mitosis are produced. These cultures are said to be synchronized. After a brief exposure to colchicine, high resolution karyotypes can be obtained with up to 1200 bands in the haploid chromosome set, thus allowing the delineation of previously undetected chromosome aberrations.

10.2.2 Fluorescence *in situ* hybridization (FISH)

Fluorescence *in situ* hybridization (FISH) has become an essential tool for gene mapping and characterization of chromosome aberrations (Verma and Babu 1995). DNA probes that are specific for single loci, chromosomal regions, or whole chromosomes are chemically modified, usually by incorporation of biotin and/or digoxygenin, and are then hybridized to complementary sequences in denatured metaphase chromosomes. After

removal of unbound probe by washing, hybridized sequences are detected using avidin, which binds strongly to biotin, and/or antibodies to digoxygenin, coupled to fluorescein isothiocyanate (FITC), Texas red, or another fluorochrome. As the target DNA remains intact, unlike in molecular genetic analysis, information is obtained directly about the positions of probes in relation to chromosome bands (thus 'mapping' the probes) or to other hybridized probes. Chromosome aberrations can therefore be defined using differentially labelled probes which delineate particular chromosomes or chromosomal regions.

A major difficulty in tumour cytogenetics is the inability to obtain chromosome spreads from many types of tumours. FISH, however, can also be performed on interphase nuclei from tumour biopsies or cultured tumour cells, which enables cytogenetic aberrations to be visualized without the need for chromosome preparations. This procedure is called 'interphase cytogenetics'. Numerical chromosome aberrations can be detected using specific centromere probes which give two signals on normal nuclei but one signal when there is only one copy of the chromosome (monosomy) or three signals when there is an extra copy (trisomy). Chromosome deletions can be similarly detected using probes from the deleted region and counting the signals. FISH detection of translocations in interphase nuclei is based on the principle that adjacent probes give adjacent signals when cohybridized to normal interphase nuclei. When a translocation separates the probes, the signals on the nuclei become separated. Alternatively, probes that are close to specific translocation breakpoints on different chromosomes that become joined as a result of the translocation can be used. These probes are normally far apart in interphase nuclei but become joined in nuclei carrying the translocation. These procedures are particularly useful for rapid detection of aberrations that give diagnostic or prognostic information.

10.3 Terminology and types of chromosome aberrations in tumours

Karyotypes are described according to an International System for Human Cytogenetic Nomenclature (ISCN 1995). The total chromosome number is listed first, then the sex chromosomes, then gains and losses of whole chromosomes, and finally structural rearrangements. The short and long arms of chromosomes are represented by 'p' and 'q', respectively. Gains and losses of whole chromosomes are identified by a '+' or a '−' before the chromosome number. For example, 46,XY and 46,XX represent normal diploid male and female karyotypes, respectively. 47,XX,+8 represents a female karyotype with an extra copy of chromosome 8. Trisomy 8 is the most common aberration in myeloproliferative disorders.

Translocations are common structural chromosome aberrations in tumours and are derived from the interchange of segments from different chromosomes. They may be balanced (reciprocal) or unbalanced resulting in loss or gain of genetic material. Translocations are signified by a 't'; the chromosomes involved are enclosed within a first set of brackets and the translocation breakpoints are enclosed within a second set of brackets. For example, t(9;22)(q34;q11) represents a reciprocal translocation between chromosomes 9 and 22 at bands 9q34 and 22q11, respectively. This translocation generates the Philadelphia chromosome in CML (described further in Section 10.5.1). Other structural aberrations include deletions, which may be interstitial or terminal, inversions, and isochromosomes. Deletions are signified by 'del', followed by the chromosome in one set of brackets and the breakpoint(s) in a second set of brackets. Thus, del(5)(q13q32) represents an interstitial deletion of bands 5q13 to 5q32, with breakage and rejoining of these bands. del(5)(q32) represents a terminal deletion of chromosome 5 from band 5q32 to the telomere. Inversions are signified by 'inv', so that inv(16)(p13q22) represents an inversion within chromosome 16, with breakpoints occurring in bands p13 and q22. This inversion is present in acute myelomonocytic leukaemia with abnormal eosinophils (AML–M4Eo). Isochromosomes are derived from loss of either the long or the short arm of the chromosome with the duplication of the other arm. They are signified by an 'i'. Thus, an i(17)(q10) or i(17q) consists of the duplicated long arm of chromosome 17. This aberration is frequently seen in many types of tumours.

Amplified chromosomal regions often manifest as homogeneously staining regions (HSRs) or small acentric (centromere-lacking) chromosomes known as double minute (DM) chromosomes. Thus, hsr(2)(q31) in a karyotype represents a homogeneously staining region in band 2q31. Double min-

ute chromosomes are signified by 'dmin' after descriptions of other chromosome aberrations.

Only clonal chromosome aberrations are reviewed here. Clonal structural aberrations and chromosome gains are conventionally defined as being seen in at least two cells of a tumour. Clonal chromosome loss (monosomy) is defined as being seen in at least three cells. Although these may seem very few cells to be considered definitive, there may be normal cells within tumour preparations as well as difficulties in getting metaphase spreads from some tumour types.

10.4 Molecular consequences of chromosome aberrations in tumours

Rapid progress in molecular biology and gene mapping has greatly advanced our understanding of the significance of chromosome aberrations in cancer. We now know that they directly affect the functioning of two broad classes of genes: cellular oncogenes and tumour suppressor genes. Cellular oncogenes generally promote cell growth and division, inhibit differentiation, or block apoptosis (programmed cell death). They transmit signals to the genome by means of multiple regulatory pathways. When oncogenes become inappropriately activated, they stimulate cells to multiply relentlessly, forming a tumour. Tumour suppressor genes, on the other hand, normally constrain cell growth and division. Their removal or inactivation from the genome also results in relentless cell multiplication. The general principles of these mechanisms are given below and specific examples are described in Sections 10.5 and 10.6.

10.4.1 Activation of cellular oncogenes

Chromosome aberrations and mutations activate cellular oncogenes in a dominant fashion (Chapter 9). This means that only one activated oncogene is required to exert a tumorigenic effect. Cellular oncogenes often encode transcription factors, suggesting that abnormal transcription plays a major role in tumorigenesis.

There are three basic chromosomal mechanisms for activating oncogenes (Fig. 10.2):

1. Juxtaposition of the oncogene to regulatory elements in immunoglobulin or T cell receptor genes in B and T lymphocyte malignancies, respectively, leading to inappropriate expression of the oncogene.

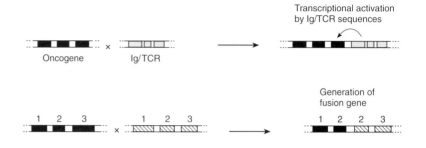

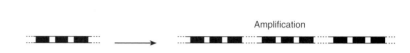

Fig. 10.2 Chromosomal mechanisms of oncogene activation.

2. Fusion of the oncogene with a second gene at a translocation or inversion junction generating a chimeric gene, mRNA, and protein. This mechanism has been found so far predominantly in leukaemias, lymphomas, and sarcomas.

3. Gene amplification, i.e. the generation of multiple gene copies, in DMs or HSRs, leading to overexpression. Gene amplification is a common feature of solid tumours, but is seldom found in haematological malignancies.

Examples of these mechanisms are given in Sections 10.5 and 10.6. An outstanding review of chromosome translocations in cancer can be found in Rabbitts (1994).

As HSRs and DMs are rarely present in the same cell (although tumour cell lines may have both HSR- and DM-containing cells), they are believed to represent alternate states of gene amplification. Various mechanisms have been proposed for the amplification process based on molecular analysis of amplicons in different cell types (Hahn 1993). Amplified regions are usually found in tumours at chromosomal sites that are different from the original locations of the genes involved, suggesting that the early steps occur either extrachromosomally or *in situ* at a new chromosome location. While tumour cells growing *in vivo* usually have DMs, when they are grown *in vitro* HSRs often form.

Gene amplification was first observed in rodent cell lines which became resistant to treatment with high levels of folic acid antagonists such as methotrexate. These cell lines produced elevated amounts of the enzyme dihydrofolate reductase (DHFR), owing to a large increase in the number of *DHFR*

genes. Amplification of the *MDR1* (multidrug resistance) gene, which encodes P-glycoprotein, prevents cellular accumulation of antineoplastic drugs, thus enabling tumour cells to become resistant. It is now apparent that oncogene amplification plays a major role in tumorigenesis, particularly in solid tumours (see Section 10.6).

10.4.2 Deletion of tumour suppressor genes

As described in Chapter 4, analysis of constitutional deletions of chromosome 13 associated with the inherited form of retinoblastoma led to the development of the 'two-hit' model of tumorigenesis (Knudson 1971). This model predicted that certain genes, now called 'tumour suppressor genes', exert a tumorigenic effect when both alleles become inactivated by mutation or chromosomal deletion. The first allele is inactivated either in the germ cells, where it confers dominant familial susceptibility to cancer, or in the somatic cells. The second allele is inactivated in the somatic cells. The mutation or deletion, which is inherited as a dominant trait, is thus recessive at the cellular level.

This model was validated for retinoblastoma when the *RB* gene was cloned and shown to be mutated in a wide variety of malignancies. The RB gene product is believed to be a negative regulator of the G1–S cell cycle transition, and is the main substrate for cyclin-dependent kinase-4 (CDK4)-cyclin DI mediated phosphorylation (Fig. 10.3) (reviewed in Cordon-Cardo 1995). Dephosphorylated RB binds and holds inactive a set of proteins that stimulate cell proliferation. RB is itself inactivated when phosphorylated.

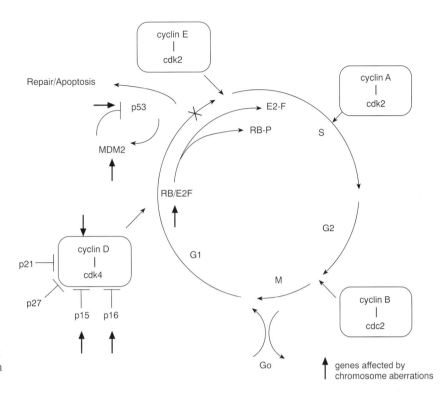

Fig. 10.3 Control of cell cycle progression (see text for details). Adapted from Cordon-Cardo (1995).

Molecular studies of chromosome deletions and regions showing loss of heterozygosity (LOH) in other hereditary and sporadic tumours have now enabled the isolation of other tumour suppressor genes (see Tables 4.4a and 4.4b in Chapter 4). It remains to be established whether recurrent chromosome deletions, LOH, monosomies, and isochromosomes involving a large number of other genomic regions in sporadic malignancies indicate the presence of many more tumour suppressor genes.

The *p53* gene, which is located at band 17p13, is frequently mutated or deleted in sporadic tumours. The p53 phosphoprotein is believed to play a central role in tumour suppression. It is normally expressed at low levels and has a short half-life. Following DNA damage, p53 appears to regulate the transcription of at least two sets of genes (reviewed in Hainaut 1995). One set induces G1 arrest to enable cells to undergo repair before DNA replication. The other set initiates apoptosis. When the *p53* gene is inactivated by mutations of its DNA-binding domain and/or by deletions encompassing band 17p13, genomic instability accumulates leading to tumorigenesis and tumour evolution. *p53* mutation often results in overexpression and can be visualized in tumour cells using immunohistochemical assays.

10.5 Leukaemias and lymphomas

Leukaemias and lymphomas usually have few chromosome rearrangements. Chromosome numbers are in the diploid range, except in Hodgkin's disease which usually has chromosomes in the triploid–tetraploid range. The chromosome rearrangements are therefore generally easy to define, especially when analysed using high resolution banding. Consistent and, in some cases, highly specific chromosome aberrations have been found in leukaemias and lymphomas (Tables 10.1–10.4) (Cotter 1993; Hogge 1994). These are being exploited as markers for detecting residual malignant cells after treatment, in order to improve clinical management (Campana and Pui 1995).

Translocations and inversions result in inappropriate activation of cellular oncogenes (see Section 10.4.1). The presence of recurrent chromosome deletions as the sole visible chromosome changes in these malignancies indicates the involvement of tumour suppressor genes as well (Johansson

Table 10.1 Recurrent chromosomal aberrations in myeloid malignancies

Malignancy	Chromosomal aberration	Affected genes
CML	t(9;22)(q34;q11)	*ABL* (9q34), *BCR* (22q11)
CML blast crisis	t(9;22)(q34;q11), +8, +Ph, +19, or i(17q)	*ABL* (9q34), *BCR* (22q11), *p53* (17p13)
AML-M1, -M2, -M4	t(8;21)(q22;q22)	*MTG8* (8q22), *AML1* (21q22)
APL-M3, M3V	t(15;17)(q22;q11.2)	*PML* (15q22), *RARA* (17q11.2)
AMMoL-M4Eo	inv(16)(p13q22) or t(16;16)(p13;q22)	*MYH11* (16p13), *CBFB* (16q22)
AMMoL-M4/M5	t(1;11)(p32;q23)	*eps15* (1p32), **MLL** (11q23)
	t(4;11)(q21;q23)	*AF4* (4q21), **MLL** (11q23)
	t(6;11)(q27;q23)	*AF6* (6q27), **MLL** (11q23)
	t(10;11)(p12;q23)	*AF10* (10p12), **MLL** (11q23)
	t(11;17)(q23;q21)	*AF17* (17q21), **MLL** (11q23)
	t(11;19)(q23;p13)	*ENL* (19p13), **MLL** (11q23)
	t(11q13 or q23)	**MLL** (11q23)
AMoL-M5	t(9;11)(p22;q23),	*AF9* (9p22), **MLL** (11q23)
	t(11q13) or (q23)	**MLL** (11q23)
AML-M7 (infants)	t(1;22)(p13;q13)	
AML	+8	
	7 or del(7q)	
	−5 or del(5q)	
	t(6;9)(p23;q34)	*DEK* (6p23), *CAN* (9q34)
	t(3;3)(q21;q26) or inv(3)(q21q26)	
	t(3;21)(q26;q22)	
	del(20q)	
	t(12p) or del(12p)	
Therapy-related AML	−7 or del(7q)	
	and/or −5 or del(5q)	
	der(1)t(1;7)(p11;p11)	
	t(3;21)(q26;q22)	
	der(5)t(5;7)(q11;p11)	
	t(9;11)(p22;q23)	*AF9* (9p22), **MLL** (11q23)

See text for references.
Genes in bold typeface are involved in multiple translocations.

Table 10.2 Oncogene activation by immunoglobulin loci in B cell malignancies

Malignancy	Activated oncogene	Immunoglobulin locus
B-ALL, Burkitt's lymphoma	c-*MYC* (8q24)	*IgH* (14q32)
pre-B ALL	*IL-3* (5q31)	
B-CLL	*CCND1* (11q13)	
	BCL3 (19q13.1)	
Follicular lymphoma	*BCL2* (18q21)	
B-ALL, Burkitt's lymphoma	c-*MYC* (8q24)	*IgL* κ (2p12)
B-ALL, Burkitt's lymphoma	c-*MYC* (8q24)	*IgL* λ (22q11)

Table 10.3 Oncogene activation by T cell receptor loci in T cell malignancies

Malignancy	Activated oncogene	T cell receptor locus
T-ALL	*TAL1* (1p32)	*TCRdα/δ* (14q11)
	c-*MYC* (8q24),	
	HOX11 (10q24)	
	RBTN1 (11p15)	
	RBTN2 (11p13)	
	LCK (1p34)	*TCRβ* (7q35)
	TAL2 (9q34)	
	TAN1 (9q34.3)	
	HOX11 (10q24)	
	RBTN2 (11p13)	
	LYL1 (19p13)	
T-CLL	*TCL1* (14q32.1)	*TCR-Cα* (14q11)

Table 10.4 Non-Ig or -TCR chromosomal rearrangements in lymphoid malignancies

Malignancy	Chromosomal aberration	Affected genes
Aberrations generating fusion genes		
pre-B ALL	t(1;19)(q23;p13.3)	*PBX1* (1q23), *E2A* (19p13.3)
pro-B ALL	t(17;19)(q22;p13.3)	*HLF* (17q22), *E2A* (19p13.3)
ALL	t(9;22)(q34;q11)	*ABL* (9q34), *BCR* (22q11)
	t(1;11)(p32;q23)	*eps15* (1p32), *MLL* (11q23)
	t(4;11)(q21;q23)	*AF4* (4q21), *MLL* (11q23)
	t(6;11)(q27,q23)	*AF6* (6q27), *MLL* (11q23)
	t(9;11)(q22;q23)	*AF9* (9p22), *MLL* (11q23)
	t(11;17)(q23;q21)	*AF17* (17q21), *MLL* (11q23)
	t(11;19)(q23;p13.3)	*ENL* (19p13.3), *MLL* (11q23)
	t(11;19)(q23;p13.1)	*ELL* (19p13.1), *MLL* (11q23)
	t(X;11)(q13;q23)	*AFX1* (Xq13), *MLL* (11q23)
Other aberrations		
CLL	+12, del(13q)	
ALL	del(6q), del(9p), del(11q), del(12p)	

See text for references.
Genes in bold typeface are involved in multiple translocations.

et al. 1993). Trisomies are sometimes the only visible aberrations, but the significance of these at a molecular level is not understood.

10.5.1 Myeloid malignancies

Virtually all patients with CML have the Philadelphia (Ph) chromosome in their leukaemic cells. In addition, approximately 80 per cent of patients entering blast crisis (see Chapter 13) show further chromosome abnormalities. These secondary changes are usually an extra Ph chromosome, trisomy 8, or an i(17q), suggesting that genes on these chromosomes confer a proliferative advantage to the cells carrying them. *p53* mutations are frequently associated with rearrangements of chromosome 17 in blast crisis of CML, although they are rarely seen in acute myeloid leukaemia (AML) or myelodysplasia (Feinstein *et al.* 1991). A change in karyotype is a grave prognostic sign, with death usually occurring within a few months.

Different subtypes of AML (Bennett *et al.* 1985) carry consistent, and in some cases highly specific, chromosome aberrations (Table 10.1). The prognostic implications are shown in Table 10.5. The most common change in AML is trisomy 8, occurring together with other aberrations in about 9 per cent of cases, and as a sole change in about 5 per cent. Some of the translocations are described below.

Both myelodysplastic syndrome (MDS) and myeloproliferative disease (MPD) can evolve to an

Table 10.5 Prognostic significance of chromosomal aberrations in myeloid and lymphoid malignancies

Malignancy	Prognosis		
	Good	Intermediate	Poor
CML blast crisis			+Ph, +8, i(17q) or +19
AML	t(8;21)	47–50 chromosomes	rearr. 3q21–26
	t(15;17)		−5 or del(5q)
	inv(16)		−7 or del(7q)
			t(6;9)
			+8
			t(11q23)
			del/t(12p)
			complex karyotypes
ALL	>50 chromosomes	47–50 chromosomes	<47 chromosomes
	dic(9;12)		∼ 96 chromosomes
	+4, +10		t(9;22)
			t(8;14)[1]
			t(1;19)
			t(11q23)
			t(4;11)(q21;q23)

Adapted from Hogge (1994) and Raimondi (1993).

[1] Although this translocation is a marker of poor prognosis, recent therapeutic advances have greatly improved the outlook for patients showing the translocation.

acute leukaemia indistinguishable clinically from *de novo* AML, but more refractory to treatment. Certain chromosome deletions are common to MPD, MDS and AML, reflecting the poor definition of boundaries between these conditions. MDS and AML can arise as a late complication of cytotoxic therapy. Deletions or monosomy of chromosomes 5 and/or 7 are present in the majority of secondary AMLs, compared with an incidence of only 16 per cent of patients with *de novo* AML. These deletions are also present in AML following exposure to pesticides and organic solvents (Cuneo *et al.* 1992). The region most commonly deleted in chromosome 5 is 5q23–32 and in chromosome 7 is 7q22–36 (Johansson *et al.* 1993). The putative tumour suppressor genes in these regions have not yet been identified.

The Philadelphia chromosome The t(9;22) (q34;q11),which generates the Ph chromosome in CML, results in the fusion of the 5′ region of the *BCR* gene at 22q11 with the 3′ region of the cellular oncogene, *ABL*, at 9q34 (Figs 10.4 and 10.5).

BCR is a large gene of 130 kb containing many exons. It encodes a serine kinase. The ABL protein is a nuclear tyrosine kinase that contains a DNA-binding domain. It appears to function as a negative regulator of cell growth, since overexpression causes cell cycle arrest. The translocation breakpoints in *BCR* usually occur in either of two introns within a small region, but they occur in *ABL* over a large distance of more than 200 kb. One of two alternative first exons normally used by the *ABL* gene becomes replaced by *BCR* sequences, generating a fused mRNA (8.5 kb, in contrast to the two normal ABL mRNAs of 6.0 or 7.0 kb, depending on which of two alternative first exons is used). The fusion 210 kDa BCR–ABL protein relocates from the nucleus to the cytoplasm, has greatly enhanced tyrosine kinase activity, and becomes a positive regulator of cell growth (Sawyers 1992). The Ph chromosome also occurs in ALL (see Section 10.5.2).

The role of the chimeric *BCR–ABL* gene in tumorigenesis has been studied by experiments in which irradiated mice were reconstituted with bone

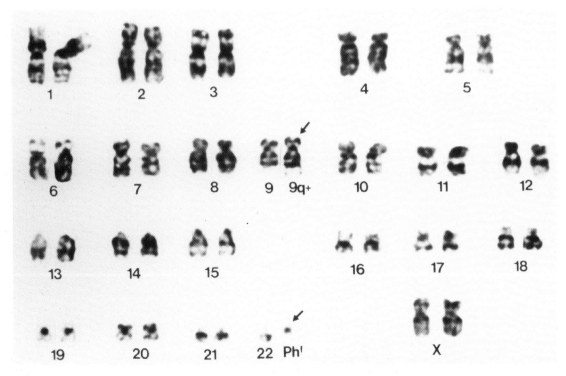

Fig. 10.4 Karyotype showing the Philadelphia chromosome in CML.

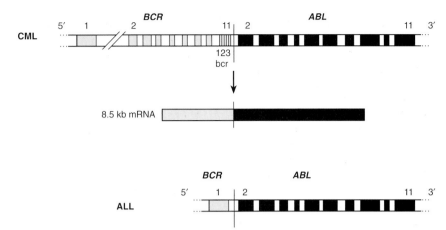

Fig. 10.5 Schematic representation of the *BCR–ABL* fusion arising from the t(9;22) in CML and ALL.

marrow containing a retrovirus encoding the 210 kDa BCR–ABL protein (Daley *et al.* 1990). Almost half the mice studied developed a haematological disorder similar to that of CML or ALL. These experiments provide evidence that the chimeric *BCR–ABL* gene in CML plays a central role in leukaemogenesis.

t(8;21)(q22;q22) This translocation occurs in approximately 12 per cent of all AMLs, predominantly in AML-M2, but also in AML-M1 and -M4. It has never been seen in any other malignancies. AML-M2 patients with the translocation have a higher remission rate than those without it. A chimeric gene is generated from the *AML1* gene at 21q22 and the *MTG8* gene at 8q22 (Ohki 1993).

The *AML1* gene is expressed constitutively in all haemopoietic cell lines studied so far, and in lung, heart, and spleen, but not in brain, liver, or kidney. The gene encodes a protein containing a region that is homologous both to the CBFA (PEBP2a) component of the mouse core-binding factor CBF, and to the *Drosophila* segmentation gene *runt*. CBF in the mouse binds to the core site of polyomavirus and to the enhancers of T cell receptor genes. The CBFA/runt domain appears to be a conserved protein- and DNA-binding motif, suggesting that the AML1 protein functions in transcriptional activation.

The *MTG8* gene is not normally expressed in myeloid cells. It has two putative zinc finger DNA-binding domains and a transcriptional activation domain. The *AML1–MTG8* fusion protein contains the runt domain of AML1 and the zinc finger domains of *MTG8*, and may therefore function in tumorigenesis by activating transcription of a novel set of genes.

t(15;17)(q22;q11.2–12) This translocation is only found in acute promyelocytic leukaemia (APL, AML-M3), and promyelocytic transformation of CML (Gillard and Solomon 1993). The translocation breakpoints occur within the retinoic acid receptor (*RARA*) gene on chromosome 17 and a gene designated *PML* (for promyelocytic leukaemia) on chromosome 15, and generate a chimeric *RARA–PML* gene. The RARA protein normally binds to retinoic acid, and also to DNA through a zinc finger region, thereby presumably activating a particular set of target genes. PML is also a DNA-binding, zinc finger protein with a leucine zipper motif. The translocation results in both the zinc finger- and the retinoic acid-binding domains of the *RARA* gene joining to the zinc finger and leucine zipper domains of *PML* on the derivative chromosome 15. The fusion protein thus retains important functional domains of both *RARA* and *PML*. The PML protein is normally tightly bound to the nuclear matrix, in discrete spherical bodies. These nuclear bodies become disorganized in APL, presumably owing to the presence of the RARA–PML fusion protein. A role for the PML protein in other oncogenic processes has recently been suggested by the finding that these nuclear bodies appear to be preferential targets for DNA tumour viruses (Carvalho *et al.* 1995).

A variant translocation, t(11;17)(q23;q21), fuses *RARA* to another zinc finger-containing gene designated *PLZF* (for promyelocytic zinc finger). The fusion protein similarly retains the important functional domains of *RARA* and *PLZF*. These findings suggest that the translocations may result in transcriptional activation of an aberrant set of genes in a retinoic acid-dependent manner. Interestingly, APL is responsive to treatment with retinoic acid, which appears to induce differentiation along the granulocytic pathway.

inv(16)(p13q22) and t(16;16)(p13;q22) Rearrangements involving chromosome bands 16p13 and 16q22 are present in most cases of AML-M4Eo (Liu *et al.* 1993). These usually consist of a pericentric inversion of chromosome 16 or a translocation between the two homologues of chromosomes 16. A fusion gene is generated between the *CBFB* gene at 16p13, and the smooth muscle myosin heavy chain gene, *MYH 11*, at 16q22. In the mouse, CBFB is a second component of the corebinding factor described above. The CBFB protein does not contain any known DNA-binding motifs or transcriptional activation domains, and the role played by *MYH 11* in the fusion protein is unclear.

Translocations involving the *MLL* gene at band 11q23 Over 25 different reciprocal translocations affecting chromosome band 11q23 are present in acute myeloid and lymphoid leukaemias (Djabali *et al.* 1992; Bernard and Berger 1995). These include secondary myeloid leukaemias in patients who have received chemotherapeutic drugs that inhibit topoisomerase II, such as etoposide, for a primary tumour. Analysis of these translocations at the molecular level is beginning to provide fascinating insights into the critical events of leukaemogenesis and may give us a handle for studying the interaction between chemotherapeutic drugs and DNA aberrations.

These translocations involve the *MLL* gene (myeloid-lymphoid leukaemia, also called the *ALL-1, HTRX* gene) which spans 100 kb at band 11q23 (Fig. 10.6). *MLL* encodes a transcription factor of 3968 amino acids containing AT hooks at the N-terminus, a transcriptional repressor region, and a region homologous to mammalian DNA methyltransferase (MT). A zinc finger region and a region homologous to the *Drosophila* trithorax protein are located at the C-terminus. The translocation breakpoints are clustered in an 8.3-kb region, such that the AT hooks and MT are retained in the chimeric protein. The zinc finger and trithorax regions of MLL are replaced by sequences encoded by the partner gene.

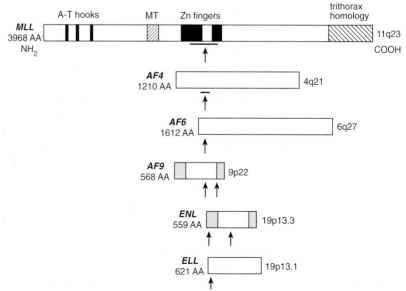

Fig. 10.6 Schematic representation of *MLL* translocations. Each translocation results in the NH$_2$ region of *MLL* combining with the COOH region of the protein encoded by the partner gene. Arrows indicate translocation breakpoints. Adapted from Bernard and Berger (1995) and Rabbits (1994).

AT hooks are believed to bind to the minor groove of the DNA double helix, possibly giving other transcription factors access to the DNA. The methyltransferase might affect transcription by alterating methylation status. Loss of the zinc finger region presumably abolishes specific DNA binding.

Several partner genes have now been characterized. None appear to be closely related at the structural and functional levels, except for *AF10* and *AF17* at bands 10q23 and 17q21, respectively, and *AF9* and *ENL* at bands 9p21 and 19p13.3, respectively. Most of the partner genes analysed so far encode putative transcription factors. The *ELL* gene at band 19p13.1 has been analysed in detail. It encodes an RNA polymerase II elongation factor, most of which is retained in the fusion protein (Shilatifard *et al.* 1996). Other genes encode proteins with different functions. The *eps15* gene at band 1p32 encodes a cytoplasmic target for the tyrosine kinase activity of the epidermal growth factor receptor, while *AF6* at band 6q27 encodes a cytoskeletal protein. This variety of partner genes makes it difficult to reach a unifying scheme of the molecular consequences of these translocations. One can hypothesize that the chimeric MLL proteins exert their tumorigenic effect by competing with normal MLL protein for DNA targets or by sequestering the normal MLL protein (Bernard and Berger 1995). A second scenario depicts the chimeric protein as a novel transcription factor which retains the AT hooks from MLL with a transactivating domain (still to be identified) from the partner gene. A third is that the partner gene provides a protein dimerization domain (Bernard and Berger 1995).

Several other interesting features have emerged from sequence analysis of the translocation breakpoints. For example, numerous Alu repeats are present between exons 5 and 11, where the breakpoints are clustered. These may be responsible for a DNA configuration that is amenable to translocation (Gu *et al.* 1994). Regions homologous to the heptamer-nonamer recombination recognition signals of the VDJ recombinase have been found in some t(4;11) near the breakpoints (Gu *et al.* 1992). It may be significant that topoisomerase II recognition signals have also been found at the breakpoints of two translocations, as *MLL* translocations are strongly associated with secondary leukaemia following chemotherapy using topoisomerase II inhibitors (Negrini *et al.* 1993).

Identical translocations have been found in lymphoid and myeloid lineages, indicating that the translocation partner is not always determined by the cellular phenotype. However, the t(4;11)(q21;q23) is found predominantly in lymphoid leukaemia with some myeloid features, while the t(9;11)(p22;q23) is found predominantly in myeloid leukaemia with some lymphoid features. These data suggest that rearrangements of the *MLL* gene affect a pluripotent progenitor cell that is capable of either myeloid or lymphoid differentiation.

10.5.2 Lymphoid malignancies

Many recurrent structural and numerical chromosome aberrations are present in lymphoid malignancies (Raimondi 1993) (see Tables 10.2–10.4). The structural aberrations consist mainly of translocations, inversions, and deletions. The translocations and inversions result either in the generation of chimeric genes or in oncogene overexpression induced by adjacent regulatory sequences from immunoglobulin or T cell receptor genes, which are normally highly active in lymphoid cells.

The prognosis for children with acute lymphoblastic leukaemia (ALL) has improved dramatically in the past 20 years, with at least 80 per cent of patients being cured with intensive therapy. Chromosome aberrations in ALL are of particular importance as they are clear indicators of prognosis in both adults and children (Table 10.5). A hyperdiploid karyotype (51–59 chromosomes) is usually found in young children with ALL. The prognosis in this category is good, with over 75 per cent of patients achieving long-term survival. Hypodiploidy in ALL is relatively rare but indicates a poor prognosis as do the translocations, t(9;22) (q34;q12), t(8;14)(q24;q32), and t(4;11)(q21;q23).

The chromosome regions that are most often deleted in acute lymphoblastic leukaemia owing to structural rearrangements are 6q15–27, 9p11–24, 12p12–13, and 19p13, while the most common monosomies are –X, –Y, –7, –20, and –21 (Johansson *et al.* 1993). None of the putative tumour suppressor genes in these regions has yet been identified except for the *CDKN2* (cyclin-dependent kinase-4 inhibitor, p16) gene at band 9p21 (Fig. 10.3), which is mutated or homozygously deleted in ALL and in non-Hodgkin's lymphoma (NHL) (Stranks *et al.* 1995).

The most common chromosomal aberrations in B cell chronic lymphocytic leukaemia (CLL) are trisomy 12, which is a marker of poor prognosis, and deletions involving chromosome band 13q14. Although these deletions often include the *RB* gene, a different gene, telomeric of *RB*, is believed to be the major target of these deletions (Newcomb *et al.* 1995). Translocations are occasionally found, including a t(11;14)(q13;q32), in which the *CCND1* gene (also known as *BCL-1* or *PRAD-1*), encoding the cell cycle regulatory protein cyclin D1 (Fig. 10.3), becomes activated by juxtaposition with IgH sequences as described below.

Aberrations generating chimeric genes Several recurrent translocations in ALLs result in the formation of chimeric genes as described in myeloid leukaemias above. A t(9;22)(q34;q12) identical to that seen in CML is present in 20 per cent of adult ALL and 5 per cent of childhood ALL. A chimeric *BCR–ABL* gene encoding a 190-kDa protein is generated, containing a smaller segment of *BCR* than in CML (Fig. 10.5).

A translocation occurring in approximately 30 per cent of childhood and 6 per cent of adult pre-B ALL is t(1;19)(q23;p13) (Secker-Walker *et al.* 1992). The translocation results in the DNA-binding homeodomain of the *PBX-1* gene on chromosome 1 fusing to the E2A transcription factor gene on chromosome 19, replacing the DNA-binding b-HLH (basic helix–loop–helix) motif of E2A. E2A normally binds specifically to the enhancer sequence of the *IgL* κ locus. *PBX-1* is not normally expressed in lymphocytes. The powerful positive transcription signal that normally stimulates the *IgL* κ locus thus becomes directed to the gene normally targeted by the PBX-1 protein, but in inappropriate cells. A variant translocation, t(17;19)(q22;p13), similarly generates a fusion gene in which the DNA-binding and protein-dimerization bZIP (leucine zipper) domain of *HLF* on chromosome 17 replace the DNA-binding domain of E2A.

Seventy per cent of infant ALLs have translocations involving the *MLL* gene at band 11q23 (see Section 10.5.1) (Chen *et al.* 1993). The most common of these is t(4;11)(q21;q23) which is found primarily in very immature, pre-B ALL in infants with an extremely high white cell count. These infants have a 15 per cent projected event-free survival at 46 months after diagnosis, compared with 80 per cent in infants with ALL without rearrangements of *MLL*.

Aberrations involving the immunoglobulin and T cell receptor loci Lymphocytes play a central role in the immune system. B lymphocytes are responsible for immunoglobulin (Ig)-mediated immunity. T lymphocytes play a role in cellular immunity after conditioning in the thymus. Helper and suppressor T cells also regulate B cells by either enhancing or reducing the Ig-mediated immune response, respectively. The various lymphoid malignancies correspond to maturation arrests at different stages of lymphoid differentiation (see Chapter 13).

During B lymphocyte maturation, somatic recombination of the Ig heavy (IgH) chain, and of the k and λ light chain loci precedes Ig production. Newly synthesized Ig molecules are retained in the cytoplasm and are expressed on the cell surface after further cellular maturation. The *IgH*, *IgL* κ and *IgL* λ loci map to chromosome bands 14q32, 2p12, and 22q11, respectively. The *TCRα/δ*, β and γ chain loci, which encode the T cell receptor (TCR) molecules, map to chromosome bands 14q11.2, 7q35, and 7p15, respectively.

In B and T cell malignancies, specific translocations and inversions result in inappropriate activation of cellular oncogenes by placing them under the control of regulatory elements from the *Ig* and *TCR* loci (Korsmeyer 1992). These aberrations appear to be facilitated by errors in the DNA processing by the recombinase enzyme during the process of normal recombination of the V, D, or J regions of the *Ig* and *TCR* loci in B and T cells, respectively. Most of the oncogenes activated in this way encode transcription factors, and it is believed that their activation leads to a cascade of aberrant, positive or negative, gene expression.

Burkitt's lymphoma is a B cell malignancy in which one of three translocations invariably occurs (Figs 10.7 and 10.8). These translocations are also present in a small proportion of B cell ALLs. The translocation t(8;14)(q24;q32), which is present in approximately 90 per cent of Burkitt's lymphoma juxtaposes the c-*MYC* gene at band 8q24 and the IgH chain locus. In the variant translocations, t(2;8)(p12;q24) and t(8;22)(q24;q11), c-*MYC* becomes juxtaposed to either the *IgL* κ or *IgL* λ genes, respectively. The consequence of each of these translocations is constitutive overexpression of c-*MYC* under the influence of the immunoglobulin regulatory sequences.

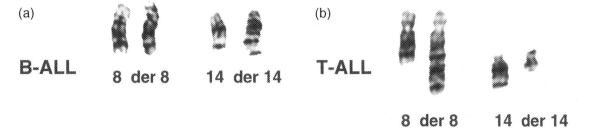

Fig. 10.7 Partial karyotypes of (a) t(8;14)(q24;q32) in Burkitt's lymphoma and B-ALL. (b) t(8;14)(q24;q11) in T-ALL. Courtesy of D. Lillington.

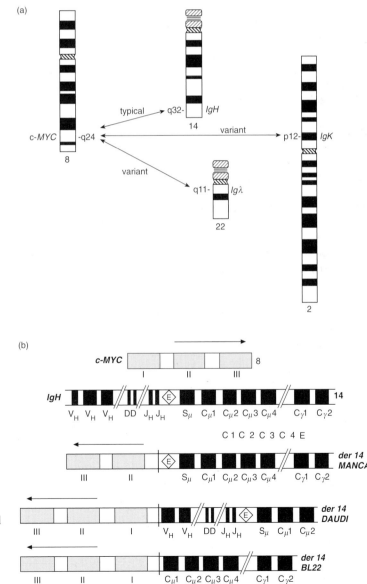

Fig. 10.8 (a) Schematic representation of translocations involving *Ig* loci in Burkitt's lymphoma and B-ALL. (b) Schematic representation of c-*MYC* and *IgH* genes, and the rearrangement of these genes at the translocation breakpoints in three cell lines derived from Burkitt's lymphoma with the typical t(8;14). Arrows indicate direction of transcription of c-*MYC*.

c-*MYC* encodes a nuclear protein which has a DNA-binding region, and basic helix–loop–helix and leucine zipper (ZIP) protein dimerization motifs (Koskinen and Alitalo 1993). The c-MYC protein dimerizes with a protein called MAX, which can bind to DNA and to two other proteins MAD and MXI1. MYC–MAX dimers function as transcriptional activators, while MAX–MAD and MAX–MXI1 dimers are repressors. Overexpression of c-*MYC* presumably disturbs the equilibrium normally maintained by these dimers, thereby altering the transcription of target genes that are involved in cell proliferation (see Chapter 11).

Approximately 85 per cent of follicular lymphomas have a translocation in which the *IgH* locus at band 14q32 juxtaposes with the *BCL-2* gene located at band 18q21, resulting in its constitutive overexpression. *BCL-2* encodes a small GTP-binding protein (GTP is guanosine 5′-triphosphate) located on the surfaces of the nuclear membrane and the mitochondria. The protein modulates apoptosis, apparently by regulating antioxidant pathways (Korsmeyer *et al.* 1993). Overexpression of *BCL-2* thus drives the cell through a continuous proliferative state. Transgenic mice with constitutive *BCL-2* expression develop B cell hyperplasia and B cell malignancies.

Other genes that are activated in B cell malignancies by translocation with the *IgH* gene include *CCND1* at 11q13, *BCL-3* at 19q13, and *IL-3* at 5q31. As described earlier, *CCND1* encodes cyclin D1, *BCL-3* encodes a transcription factor from the I kappa-B family, and *IL-3* encodes the growth factor interleukin-3.

In acute T cell leukaemias, specific translocations involving the *TCR* genes similarly result in inappropriate gene activation (Table 10.3, Figs 10.7 and 10.9). The oncogene c-*MYC* and two other genes encoding bHLH motifs, *TAL1/SCL* and *LYL1* at bands 1p32 and 19p13, respectively, are targeted by these translocations. T-ALLs in children show a t(1;14)(p32;q11) in which *TAL1* is activated by sequences from the *TCRα/δ* gene or they show rearrangements of *TAL1* (Bash *et al.* 1995). Other genes similarly activated are *HOX11*, *RBTN1*, and *RBTN2*. *HOX11* encodes a homeodomain protein with specific DNA-binding activity. *RBTN1* and *RBTN2* genes encode proteins containing two LIM domains which can function in protein-protein interactions (Sanchez-Garcia and Rabbitts 1993). The role of the RBTN1 and RBTN2 proteins in T cell tumorigenesis has been confirmed in experiments where transgenic mice with constitutive expression of these genes develop T cell leukaemias. The

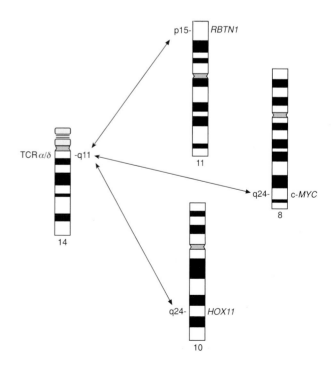

Fig. 10.9 Schematic representation of translocations involving the *TCRα* locus in T-ALL.

RBTN2 protein also plays a central role in mouse erythroid (red cell) differentiation.

10.6 Chromosomes in solid tumours

Identification of recurrent chromosome aberrations in solid tumours has lagged behind that of leukaemias and lymphomas, mainly because studies are hampered by low success rates and long processing times. When chromosomes are obtained, their morphology is usually poor and they may be grossly rearranged, especially in carcinomas. Nevertheless, data are beginning to accumulate showing distinct chromosome aberrations in different categories of solid tumours (Tables 10.6–10.8). These can be of direct benefit to the patient as their identification can enable accurate diagnoses to be made (Ilson *et al.* 1993; Sreekantaiah *et al.* 1994) and assignment of the tumour to a good or bad prognostic category.

10.6.1 Sarcomas

Sarcomas are a heterogeneous group of mesenchymal tumours that display differentiated features of the various supporting tissues of the body. Although they constitute only a small proportion of all malignant tumours, great interest has been shown in their cytogenetic aberrations (Table 10.6) (Sreekantaiah *et al.* 1994).

Several types of sarcoma have specific translocations that result in the formation of chimeric genes encoding transcription factors. A detailed evaluation of the consequences of these translocations is found in Sorensen and Triche (1996). As in leukaemias and lymphomas, the chimeric transcription factor often retains the DNA-binding domain from one of the translocated genes and the transcriptional transactivating domain from the other. Other sarcomas show recurrent chromosome aberrations preferentially affecting particular chromosomal regions. Some of these aberrations are described below.

Translocations involving the *EWS* gene at band 22q12 The *EWS* gene on chromosome 22 participates in specific translocations in several types of sarcoma (Fig. 10.10). In each translocation ana-

Table 10.6 Recurrent chromosomal aberrations in sarcomas

Tumour	Chromosomal aberration	Affected genes
Benign tumours		
Lipoma	t/inv/ins(12q15)	*HMGI-C* (12q15)
	del(13)(q12q22)	
Uterine leiomyoma	del(7)(q11.2-22q31-32)	
	t(12;14)(q15;q24)	*HMGI-C* (12q15)
	t(12;14), -22	
	+12	
Pleomorphic salivary gland adenoma	t/inv/ins(12q15)	*HMGI-C* (12q15)
Malignant tumours		
Ewing's sarcoma and pPNET	t(11;22)(q24;q12)	*FLI-1* (11q24), ***EWS*** (22q12)
pPNET	t(7;22)(p22q12)	*ETV1* (7p22), ***EWS*** (22q12)
	t(21;22)(q22;q12)	*ERG* (21q22), ***EWS*** (22q12)
Ewing's sarcoma	der(16)t(1;16)(q11–25;q11-24)	
Clear cell sarcoma	t(12;22)(q13;q12)	*ATF1* (12q13), ***EWS*** (22q12)
Intra-abdominal small cell sarcoma	t(11;22)(p13;q12)	*WT1* (11p13), ***EWS*** (22q12)
Extraskeletal myxoid chondrosarcoma	t(9;22)(q22;q12)	*CHN*(9q22), ***EWS*** (22q12)
Alveolar rhabdomyosarcoma	t(2;13)(q35;q14)	*PAX3* (2q35), *FKHR* (13q14)
Synovial sarcoma	t(X;18)(p11.2;q11.2)	*SSX1/SSX2* (Xp11.2), *SYT* (18q11.2)
Myxoid liposarcoma	t(12;16)(q13;p11)	*CHOP* (12q13), *TLS/FUS* (16p11)
	t(12;22)(q13;q12)	*CHOP* (12q13), ***EWS*** (22q12)

Genes in bold typeface are involved in multiple translocations.

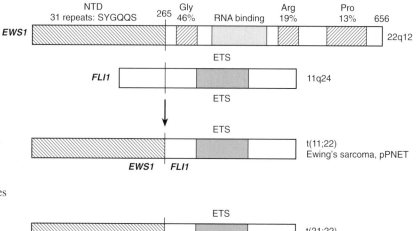

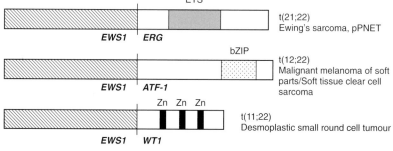

Fig. 10.10 Schematic representation of the *EWS* translocations. *EWS* encodes a glycine-rich protein (G-rich) with a glutamine–serine–tyrosine rich N-terminal domain (QSY). The RNA-binding domain of EWS is replaced in the resulting fusion protein by the DNA binding domain of each of the partner genes. Adapted from Rabbitts (1994).

lysed so far, the partner gene encodes a transcription factor. *EWS* itself encodes a transcription factor, consisting of two functional domains. The N-terminal region contains a putative transcriptional transactivation domain, while the C-terminal region contains an RNA-binding domain. The common theme in all these translocations is that a chimeric gene is formed containing the transcriptional transactivating domain of *EWS* and the DNA-binding domain of the partner gene.

The most common example is t(11;22)(q24;q12) present in virtually all Ewing's sarcomas and in peripheral neuroepitheliomas, also known as peripheral primitive neuroectodermal tumours (pPNET) (Figs 10.10, 10.11 and Plate 1). These malignancies, which affect children and adolescents, are believed to be of neuroectodermal origin and show varying degrees of neuronal differentiation. As a result of the 11;22 translocation, the *EWS* gene from chromosome 22 fuses with the *ETS*-related gene, *FLI*, on chromosome 11. A chimeric gene is formed retaining the transactivating domain from *EWS* and the specific DNA-binding domain from *FLI* (Delattre *et al.* 1994). The fusion EWS-FLI-1 protein functions as an aberrant transcription factor, and is able to trans-

form mesenchyme-derived NIH/3T3 cells (Lessnick *et al.* 1995). The EWS-FLI-1 protein is a transactivator of the c-*MYC* promoter, and may therefore be responsible for the overexpression of c-*MYC* often seen in Ewing's sarcomas (Bailly *et al.* 1994). Variant translocations are also present in a small proportion of pPNETs. In t(7;22)(p22;q12) and t(21;22)(q22;q12), the *EWS* gene fuses with the *ETS*-related genes *ETV1* (Jeon *et al.* 1995) or *ERG* (Sorensen *et al.* 1994).

Malignant melanoma of soft parts (MMSP), or clear cell sarcoma, occurs in young adults, and is also believed to have a neuroectodermal origin. In the majority of MMSPs, a translocation t(12;22)(q13;q12) combines the *EWS* and *ATF1* genes. The transcriptional transactivating domain of EWS and the bZIP domain, which is responsible for DNA binding and protein dimerization, of ATF1 are retained in the chimeric protein. The EWS–ATF1 protein acts as a strong activator of some promoters containing an ATF1 binding site and as a repressor of others (Brown *et al.* 1995).

Intra-abdominal desmoplastic small round cell tumour is another malignancy showing a specific translocation involving the *EWS* gene. In the

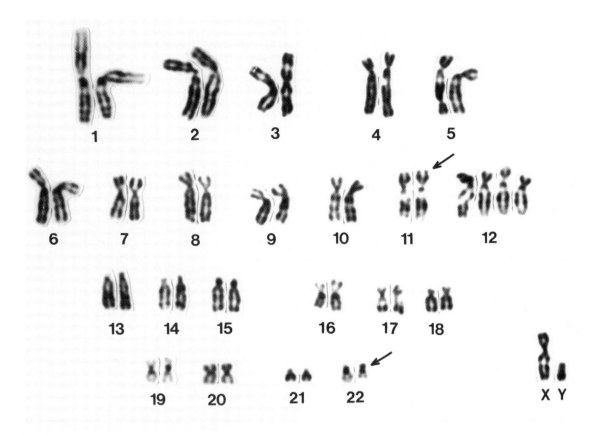

Fig. 10.11 Karyotype showing the t(11;22)(q24;q12) in Ewing's sarcoma.

t(11;22)(p13;q12), the *EWS* gene fuses with the *WT1* tumour suppressor gene, retaining the transcriptional transactivation domain of *EWS* and three zinc fingers from *WT1* (Gerald *et al.* 1995). The fusion protein is believed to modulate transcription of *WT1* target genes. Myxoid chondrosarcomas also have a recurrent translocation that disrupts the *EWS* gene, t(9;22)(q22;q11) (Gill *et al.* 1995).

t(2;13)(q35–37;q14) in alveolar rhabdomyosarcoma Alveolar rhabdomyosarcomas occur in adolescents and young adults. They usually contain either t(2;13)(q35;q14) or, occasionally, variant translocations such as t(1;13)(1p36.1;q14) (Fig. 10.12). In these translocations, the *FKHR* gene at 13q14, encoding a transcription factor belonging to the forkhead family, becomes juxtaposed with either the *PAX3* transcription factor gene at 2q35 or the *PAX7* gene at 1p36.1 (Galili *et al.* 1993). The resulting chimeric genes combine the transcriptional transactivating domain of *FKHR* and the DNA-binding domains of the *PAX* genes, presum-

ably encoding a fusion protein that inappropriately activates the *PAX3* and *PAX7* target genes (Fredericks *et al.* 1995).

t(12;16)(q13;p11) in liposarcoma Liposarcomas are the most common sarcomas in adults, usually occurring in the extremities. The most common form, myxoid liposarcoma, contains a recurrent t(12;16)(q13;p11) translocation, resulting in the entire coding region of the transcription factor gene *CHOP* on chromosome 12 fusing with the transcriptional transactivating domain of the *TLS/FUS* gene on chromosome 16 (Rabbitts *et al.* 1993). The resulting TLS–CHOP fusion protein is capable of transforming NIH/3T3 cells, but only if both the leucine zipper domain, which is required in C/EBP protein dimerization, and the DNA-binding bZIP domain of CHOP, are present (Zinszner *et al.* 1994).

t(X;18)(p11.2;q11.2) in synovial sarcoma Synovial sarcomas occur predominantly in adolescents and young adults and usually affect the extremities

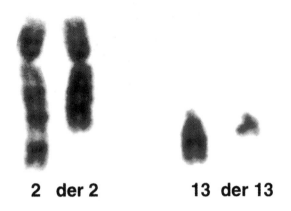

2 der 2   **13 der 13**

Fig. 10.12 Partial karyotype of t(2;13)(q35;q14) in alveolar rhabdomyosarcoma. Courtesy of J. Shipley.

near the joints. A specific translocation, t(X;18)(p11.2;q11.2), is present in almost all cases, and combines the 5′ region of the *SYT* gene on chromosome 18 with 3′ sequences of either the *SSX1* or the *SSX2* gene on the X chromosome (Crew *et al.* 1995). The function of the *SYT* gene is not yet clear. However, the *SSX1* and *SSX2* genes, showing 81 per cent sequence identity, encode putative transcription factors containing a Kruppel-associated box (KRAB) which is believed to act as a transcriptional repressor domain (Margolin *et al.* 1994). Because the KRAB is deleted from the *SYT–SSX* fusion gene, the fusion protein might function inappropriately as a transcriptional activator.

Other aberrations A variety of recurrent aberrations have been noted in other types of sarcoma. These include deletions within chromosome arms 3p, 6q, and 9p in malignant mesothelioma, t(12;19)(q13;q13.3) in haemangiopericytoma, and rearrangements involving bands 1p13–36, 1q32, 7p11–21, 13q14, and 14p11 in leiomyosarcoma (Sreekantaiah *et al.* 1994).

Several tumour suppressor genes are known to be affected, including *p53* and *RB*. The importance of *p53* in the development of sarcomas is emphasized by the occurrence of bone and soft tissue sarcomas in the Li–Fraumeni syndrome which arises from constitutional mutations of the gene (Malkin and Friend 1990, and see Chapter 4).

The *MDM2* gene, which maps to band 12q13, is frequently coamplified in sarcomas with several

other genes from this band, including *CDK4*, *GLI*, *SAS*, and *CHOP* (Table 10.8). Expression of the *MDM2* gene is controlled by p53. An autoregulatory loop is formed by the binding of the MDM2 protein to p53, thereby inhibiting the transcriptional regulatory activity of p53. Recent work indicates that the MDM2 protein regulates *RB* as well (Cordon-Cardo *et al.* 1994). Interestingly, overexpression of *MDM2* or *p53* in soft tissue tumours correlates with poor prognosis and short survival times (Cordon-Cardo *et al.* 1994). Other genes such as c-*MYC*, *SIS*, and *ERBB2* are amplified in these tumours (Maillet *et al.* 1992).

Benign mesenchymal tumours have various rearrangements involving band 12q15, in which the *HMGI-C* gene fuses with sequences from other genes (Schoenmakers *et al.* 1995). The *HMGI-C* gene normally encodes a High Mobility Group 1 protein that is involved in chromatin structure and function.

10.6.2 Carcinomas

There are several major obstacles to cytogenetic studies of carcinomas. For example, they often have relatively few dividing cells, and when chromosomes are obtained their morphology is often fuzzy and indistinct. Furthermore, in contrast to most of the malignancies described above, carcinomas often have gross aneuploidy, many chromosome rearrangements, and marked cytogenetic heterogeneity between cells. Carcinomas are usually examined after many cell divisions during which considerable cytogenetic variation may arise. It is thus important to karyotype substantially more cells than is necessary for other tumour types, and from different regions of the carcinoma if possible, in order to derive a representative profile of the tumour. These issues have been examined in detail by Pandis *et al.* (1994).

Despite these difficulties, data are now accumulating from carcinomas showing that, in general, the predominant recurrent genetic aberrations are chromosome deletions/LOH, chromosome gains, mutations, and gene amplification (Rodriguez *et al.* 1994). These are summarized in Table 10.7.

Recurrent translocations have been described so far in only a few carcinomas and adenomas. In papillary thyroid carcinomas, the tyrosine kinase domain of the *RET* oncogene at band 10q11.2 becomes fused with one of three genes (Fig. 10.13)

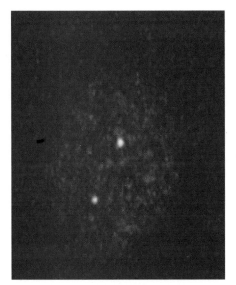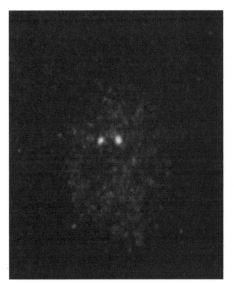

Plate 1 FISH detection of t(11;22)(q24;q12) in Ewing's sarcoma and pPNET. Probes flanking the EWS gene on chromosome 22 are differentially labelled and hybridized onto interphase nuclei. Nuclei containing two intact chromosomes 22, have two pairs of adjacent signals (left). If they contain a chromosome 22 with a translocation of the EWS gene, the signals from this chromosome become separated while those from the intact chromosome 22 give a pair of adjacent signals (right).

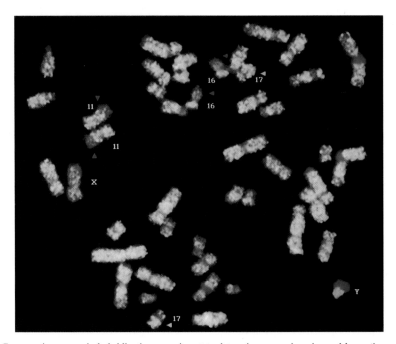

Plate 2 Comparative genomic hybridization experiment to determine genomic gains and losses in a primitive neuroectodermal tumour from a 2-year old boy. Tumour and female control DNA were labelled by DOP-PCR with FITC and Texas red, respectively. They were then competitively co-hybridized to normal male metaphase chromosome spreads. The experiment reveals gain of genomic material from the long arm of chromosome 17 (arrowed in green) and loss of genomic material from the long arms of chromosomes 11 and 16 (arrowed in red). The X-chromosome acts as an internal control as it appears red with apparent loss of genomic material when male DNA (green) and female DNA (red) are co-hybridized to male metaphase chromosomes.

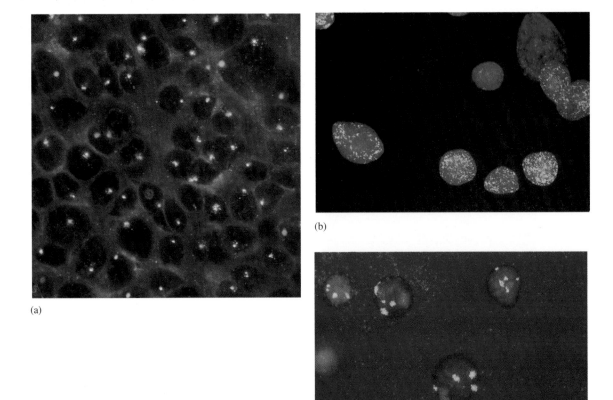

(a)

(b)

Plate 3 FISH detection of prognostic genetic markers in neuro-blastoma. (a) Deletion of 1p, using probe from band 1p36; (b) *NMYC* amplification; (c) ploidy, using probe from centromere of chromosome 8.

(c)

Table 10.7 Recurrent chromosomal aberrations in epithelial tumours

Malignancy	Chromosomal aberration
Benign tumours	
Colorectal adenoma	+8, +13, +14
	del(1)(p32–36)
Follicular thyroid adenoma	+5, +12
	t(2;3)(q12–13;p14–15)
Salivary gland adenoma	t(3;8)(p21–23;q12)
Malignant tumours	
Colorectal adenocarcinoma	+13, −14, −18, +X
	del(17)(p11–13)
	del(8)(p11-23)
	del(5)(q22-35)
	del(10)(q22-26)
Breast adenocarcinoma	del(3)(p14–23)
	del(1)(p13-36)
	del(16)(q21-24)
	del(6)(q21-27)
	DMs, HSRs
Ovarian adenocarcinoma	−13, −17, −18, −X
	del(6)(q15–25)
	del(11)(p11-15)
	del(1)(q21-44)
	del(1)(q31-36)
	del(3)(p13-23)
	del(9)(p22-24)
Wilms' carcinoma (kidney)	+12, +18
	del(11)(p13–15)
Non-papillary renal carcinoma	−14, −17
	del(3)(p11–22)
	del(5)(q22-35)
	t(3;5)(p13;q22)

Table 10.7 Recurrent chromosomal aberrations in epithelial tumours (contd.)

Malignancy	Chromosomal aberration
Papillary renal carcinoma	+17
	t(X;1)(p11.2;q21)
Small cell undifferentiated lung adenocarcinoma	−13
	del(3)(p14–24)
	del(1)(32-44)
	del(17)(p11-13)
	del(5)(q13-33)
	HSRs, DM
Non-small cell undifferentiated lung carcinoma	del(3)(p14–23)
	del(15)(p10-11)
	del(9)(p21-23)
	del(17)(p11-13)
	del(11)(p11-15)
	del(1)(p32-36)
	del(7)(p11-13)
	HSRs, DMs
Transitional cell bladder carcinoma	−9/del(9)(q11–34)
	del(11)(p11-15)
	del(6)(q21-25)
	del(3)(p14-21)
	del(10)(q24-26)
	i(5)(p10)
Papillary thyroid carcinoma[1]	inv(10)(q11.2q21)
	inv(10)(q11.2q11.2)
	t(10;17)(q11.2;q23)

Adapted from Rodriguez *et al.* (1994).

[1] These chromosomal rearrangements result in activation of the oncogene *RET* by gene fusion.

(Bongarzone *et al.* 1994). These are *ELE1*, also at band 10q11.2, the *D10S170/H4* locus at band 10q21, and the gene *PKA* encoding the regulatory subunit R1a of cAMP-dependent protein kinase A. Papillary renal cell carcinomas show a specific translocation, t(X;1)(p11.2;q21.2), involving a fusion of the *TFE3* gene, which encodes a transcription factor, with a novel gene designated *PRCC* (Sidhar *et al.* 1996).

The presence of recurrent chromosome deletions and regions showing LOH indicates the involvement of multiple tumour suppressor genes in carcinomas. In fact, all the cloned tumour suppressor genes that play a role in hereditary cancer have been found to be mutated in sporadic carcinomas as well, and their locations coincide with many of the documented deletions (Chapter 4). The finding that many dele-

tions and regions of LOH in carcinomas are very large, suggests that several tumour suppressor genes may be targeted.

Gene amplification is common in carcinomas (Table 10.8) and is often associated with advanced malignancy (reviewed in Rodriguez *et al.* 1994). For example, amplification of *ERBB2* and c-*MYC* has been correlated with poor prognosis in ovarian tumours. Chromosome band 11q13 contains several genes, including *HST1*, *INT-2*, and *CCND1*. These genes are coamplified in about 15 per cent of primary breast carcinomas, preferentially those expressing oestrogen receptor, where they also indicate a poor prognosis (Peters *et al.* 1995). *CCND1* overexpression occurs in about 40 per cent of breast carcinomas and can arise without amplification of the gene.

Table 10.8 Examples of gene amplification in cancer

Gene	Location of normal allele	Malignancy
c-MYC	8q24	Breast, colorectal, lung carcinoma, and many other solid tumours
MYCN	2p24	Neuroblastoma, retinoblastoma, small cell lung carcinoma
MYCL	1p32	Small cell lung carcinoma
PDGFRA	4q12	Glioblastoma
PDGFRB	5q33–35	Glioblastoma
EGFR	7p11–13	Squamous cell carcinoma, astrocytoma
IGFR-1	15q25–26	Breast carcinoma
MYB	6q22–23	Colorectal carcinoma
HRAS	11p15	Bladder carcinoma
ERBB-2	17q12	Breast, ovarian, gastric carcinoma, and many other solid tumours
CCND1	11q13	Breast, oesophageal carcinoma, squamous carcinoma, and many other solid tumours
HST-1		
GST		
SEA		
GLI	12q13	Soft tissue sarcoma, glioma
SAS		
CDK-4		
MDM2		
AR	Xq11–13	Prostate carcinoma

Of all the carcinomas, breast, colorectal, and ovarian carcinomas have been most extensively studied with respect to their cytogenetic changes. In a particularly thorough evaluation of a large series of primary breast carcinomas, Pandis *et al.* (1995) showed that eight aberrations are repeatedly found both as sole chromosomal aberrations and together with others. These are i(1)(q10), del(1;16)(q10;p10), del(1)(q11–12), del(3)(p12–13;p14–21), del(6)(q21–22), +7, +18, and +20. Interestingly, 27 out of 79 tumours with karyotypic abnormalities (34 per cent) showed cytogenetically unrelated clones. These findings support the authors' view that a substantial proportion of breast carcinomas are polyclonal, although the presence of submicroscopic mutations in single precursor cells cannot be ruled out. This question also needs to be clarified in other carcinomas with similar karyotypic patterns.

Given the propensity of carcinomas to genetic instability, it is not surprising that genetic aberrations besides gene amplification are associated with malignant progression. These have been studied in detail in colon carcinomas where the well-defined progression from premalignant adenomas to metastatic carcinomas correlates with distinct genetic aberrations (Fearon and Vogelstein 1990). These include mutations in the *APC*, *DCC*, *RASK*, *p53*, and DNA mismatch repair genes, some of which are also associated with chromosome aberrations (Bardi *et al.* 1995). Genetic aberrations associated with progression in bladder carcinomas may also facilitate predictions of clinical outcome (Reznikoff *et al.* 1993).

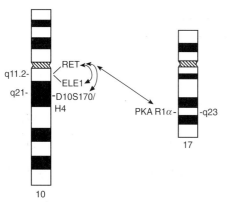

Fig. 10.13 Schematic representation of translocations involving *RET* in papillary thyroid carcinoma.

10.6.3 Brain tumours

Astrocytomas are the most common form of brain tumours in patients of all ages. They are classified according to the histopathological degree of malignancy. Adults tend to have anaplastic astrocytomas (grade III) or glioblastoma multiforme (grade IV), which are highly malignant and usually fatal despite aggressive treatment. Children tend to have juvenile pilocytic astrocytomas, which are low grade tumours with a more benign clinical course. As glioblastoma multiforme is occasionally present together with lower grade astrocytoma in the same patient, these grades may represent stages in malignant evolution.

Characteristic genetic aberrations accumulate with progression from low to high grade astrocytomas (James and Collins 1992; Westermark and Nister 1995). LOH is found on chromosomes 11, 13, 17, and 22 in all grades, and on 9p and 19p in anaplastic astrocytomas and glioblastoma multiforme. LOH on chromosome 10 occurs almost invariably in glioblastoma multiforme, but not in lower grade tumours. Detailed analysis of the sites of the chromosome 10 deletions indicates that at least two or three tumour suppressor genes on chromosome 10 may be targeted by the deletions. The target genes on chromosome 9 appear to be *MTS1* and *CDKN2* encoding the CDK inhibitors p15 and p16 (Fig. 10.3), respectively. When introduced into glioma cells that have no functional copies of the gene, p16 causes a marked suppression of cell growth (Arap *et al.* 1995). Many glioblastomas exhibit amplification of genes from band 12q13 (Reifenberger *et al.* 1994), and also of the *PDGFRA*, *EGFR*, *MET*, and *MYC* genes.

Meningiomas are usually slow growing, benign tumours. Monosomy or deletions of chromosome 22 occur in the majority of meningiomas, with non-random karyotypic changes superimposed during malignant evolution. These include LOH on the short arm of chromosome 1 (Bello *et al.* 1994).

Relatively few genetic studies have been performed on paediatric brain tumours, but they indicate that low grade paediatric astrocytomas might have different aberrations compared with their adult counterparts. High grade paediatric astrocytomas have recurrent deletions involving a tumour suppressor gene on 17p distal to *p53* (Willert *et al.* 1995). The most common change in primitive neuroectodermal tumours (PNETs), the other common category of paediatric brain tumour, is an isochromosome for the long arm of chromosome 17 Fujii *et al.* (1994) (Plate 2).

10.6.4 Neuroblastoma

Neuroblastoma is the most common extracranial solid malignant tumour of children. Patients fall into two broad prognostic categories which have been correlated with distinct clinical, biological, and genetic factors (Brodeur *et al.* 1992). Favourable prognosis neuroblastoma is associated with young age and early stage (1, 2a or 4s), triploid karyotype, absence of 1p abnormalities or *MYCN* gene amplification. This type has an excellent outcome with little or no therapy. Unfavourable prognosis neuroblastoma is associated with older age, advanced stage (2b, 3 or 4), pseudodiploid and tetraploid karyotypes, 1p deletions and *MYCN* amplification (Fig. 10.14 and Plate 3). The outcome is generally poor in these patients despite aggressive multiagent chemotherapy and, in some cases, marrow ablative treatment and bone marrow transplantation. The presence of del(1p), *MYCN* amplification, or pseudodiploidy/tetraploidy can thus be used at diagnosis to identify patients who need to be given intensive treatment. As less than 30 per cent of chromosome preparations from neuroblastomas are successful, and those that are can take several weeks to complete, highly efficient assays using FISH or PCR have been developed to identify these genetic markers (Taylor *et al.* 1994).

10.6.5 Retinoblastoma

The importance of the *RB* gene in inherited and sporadic retinoblastoma has been described in Chapter 4. Homozygous inactivation of the *RB* gene has been found in almost all retinoblastomas examined. Mutations of the *RB* gene are the predo-

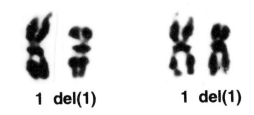

Fig. 10.14 Two partial karyotypes showing deletion of chromosome 1 in neuroblastoma.

minant mechanism for inactivation, as only < 25 per cent show cytogenetic lesions of chromosome 13. Additional copies of 6p, usually in the form of an isochromosome (6p), are the most common cytogenetic aberrations in retinoblastoma, and are mainly associated with an undifferentiated histology and invasion of the optic nerve (Cano *et al.* 1994).

10.6.6 Melanoma

Melanoma progression is characterized by recurrent cytogenetic deletions and/or LOH. The earliest and most common of these involves 9p (57 per cent of cases in one study), 10q (32 per cent), and 6q (31 per cent) (Walker *et al.* 1995). Deletions of 11q (26 per cent) and distal 1p (22 per cent) are associated with metastatic progression of melanomas. The *CDKN2* gene at band 9p21 is mutated constitutionally in certain families with inherited susceptibility to melanoma, and also in some sporadic melanomas. It is not yet clear whether the *MTS1* gene is also affected by these deletions.

10.6.7 Germ cell tumours

Approximately 80 per cent of adult testicular germ cell tumours in all histological subsets have an i(12p). Both gain of short arm sequences and loss of long arm sequences are believed to be critical in the development of these tumours. A detailed analysis of tumours lacking the i(12p) showed the presence of extra copies of 12p resulting from different aberrations. At the same time, LOH has been found in bands 12q13 and 12q22, identifying the sites of postulated tumour suppressor genes. Owing to the specificity of this aberration, its presence is indicative of a germ cell tumour in cases where a definitive diagnosis cannot be reached (Bosl *et al.* 1994).

10.7 Conclusions and future prospects

It is apparent that chromosome aberrations play a central role in tumorigenesis and tumour progression. Basic chromosomal mechanisms for oncogene activation and tumour suppressor gene inactivation have been identified from cytogenetic and molecular genetic analysis of large numbers of aberrations. These studies have been accompanied by functional analysis of these genes, revealing numerous regula-

tory pathways concerned with signal transduction, cell cycle control, differentiation, and apoptosis.

Major differences have emerged from these studies in the types of aberrations present in different malignancies. For example, leukaemias, lymphomas, and sarcomas generally have few aberrations with near-diploid karyotypes, whereas carcinomas often have many aberrations and gross aneuploidy. Leukaemias, lymphomas, and sarcomas often have translocations resulting in the generation of chimeric genes, whereas in carcinomas this mechanism has been confirmed so far only in papillary thyroid and papillary renal carcinomas. The extent of chromosomal instability may simply be hampering the identification of similar gene fusions in other forms of carcinoma. Amplification is a common feature of sarcomas and carcinomas, but has hardly ever been seen in leukaemias and lymphomas. The reasons for these differences are not yet known.

Two FISH-based approaches are bound to reveal novel genetic alterations in the future and may address some of these issues. Comparative genomic hybridization (CGH) enables genomic gains and losses to be identified by competitive hybridization of differentially labeled tumour and normal DNA to normal metaphase chromosomes followed by measurement of the relative fluorescence intensities along each chromosome (Plate 2) (Kallioniemi *et al.* 1994). Since it is not necessary to obtain chromosomes from the tumour, CGH is particularly useful for analysing tumours with a low mitotic index. 24-colour FISH allows chromosome rearrangements to be defined in tumours by simultaneous identification of each human chromosome using characteristic combinations of fluorochromes (Speicher *et al.* 1996; Schröck *et al.* 1996). Subtle translocations can thus be visualized easily, even when the metaphase preparations are sub-optimal.

There are several factors to consider when examining the aetiology of tumorigenic aberrations. Exposure to external or intracellular mutagens, such as cosmic radiation, dietary factors, or endogenous metabolites, is well known to play a major role in DNA damage. However, other factors also need to be considered, such as increased susceptibility resulting from an inherited DNA repair defect or an inactivated tumour suppressor gene. Presumably most genetic aberrations are not tumorigenic and are detected by p53 and/or other 'guardians of the genome' (Lane 1992) resulting in apoptosis unless they are repaired. Those aberrations that confer a proliferative advantage, and do not result in apoptosis (either because they are not detected by p53 or because p53 is not functional), allow clonal expansion of the cells carrying them.

Sequences that facilitate rearrangements at particular genomic regions are also thought to be important. These include heptamer–nonamer sequences, recognition motifs for VDJ recombinase at the breakpoints of translocations in lymphoid malignancies, and telomeric-type repeats and secondary DNA structures (reviewed in Bouffler *et al.* 1993). There is increasing evidence that genetic imprinting plays a role in genetic rearrangements in some types of cancer, including those in the Beckwith–Wiedemann Syndrome (Squire and Weksberg 1996).

As discussed above, a major function of *p53* is induction of apoptosis in cells that have sustained genetic damage. Inactivation of *p53* is found in most tumour types, suggesting a causative role for this event in tumorigenesis. One possible target for *p53* has been suggested to be defective telomere shortening in early tumorigenesis (Wynford-Thomas *et al.* 1995). Normal somatic cells are subject to progressive telomere erosion, as they lack the enzyme telomerase which replaces telomeric sequences in the early embryo. This process does not appear to take place in tumour cells, and telomerase activity has been detected in those tumours that have been examined so far. More research is needed before this theory can be substantiated.

Numerous examples have been given here of the clinical applications of cytogenetic aberrations. Treatment strategies for cancer are critically dependent on accurate diagnosis. In cases where conventional histopathology is insufficient to determine the tumour type, further investigations including cytogenetic analysis may then become necessary. For example, small round cell tumours of childhood, which include Ewing's sarcoma, pPNET, neuroblas-

toma, and rhabdomyosarcoma, may be difficult to distinguish from each other when they are undifferentiated, but, as described above, these tumours have distinctive chromosome aberrations that enable their precise diagnosis.

Identification of aberrations may also be important prognostically. The presence of those associated with poor prognosis may indicate that intensive therapy should be started as soon as possible to optimize the patient's likelihood of survival. On the other hand, the presence of those associated with good prognosis may indicate that less intensive therapy can be used or therapy even avoided altogether. Once the genetic aberrations in a tumour are identified, they can be used as tumour markers for serial sampling of blood or bone marrow, as in the case of leukaemia and lymphoma, to examine a patient's response to treatment and to monitor the clinical course in the longer term.

Future research on chromosome aberrations in cancer will undoubtedly focus on several issues. All the targeted genes have to be identified and their roles in normal and tumour cells understood. There is an urgent need to apply modern procedures to carcinomas, for which a disproportionately small number of cases has been examined so far. In addition, the significance of one of the most common aberrations, trisomy, has still to be understood at a molecular level. Another question is why certain translocations are so specific to particular tumour types. An improved understanding of lineage-specific transcription should emerge from functional studies of the abnormal genes generated by these translocations. These studies should give rise to fundamental knowledge of the biological processes that govern tumorigenesis and tumour progression, and hopefully lead to prevention of some cancers and the development of new, more effective forms of therapy.

References and further reading

Arap, W., Nishikawa, R., Furnari, F. B., Cavenee, W. K., and Huang, H. J. S. (1995). Replacement of the p16/cdkn2 gene suppresses human glioma cell growth. *Cancer Research*, **55**, 1351–4.

Bailly, R. A., Booselut, R., Zucman, J., Cormier, F., Delattre, O., Roussel, M., Thomas, G., and Ghysdael, J. (1994). DNA binding and transcriptional activation properties of the EWS–

FLI-1 fusion protein resulting from the t(11;22) translocation in Ewing sarcoma. *Molecular Cell Biology*, **14**, 3230–41.

Bardi, G., Sukhikh, T., Pandis, N., Fenger, C., Kronborg, O., and Heim, S. (1995). Karyotypic characterization of colorectal adenocarcinomas. *Genes, Chromosomes and Cancer*, **12**, 97–109.

Bash, R. O., Hall, S., Timmons, C. F., Crist, W. M., Amylon, M., Smith, R. G., and Baer, R. (1995). Does activation of the *TAL1* gene occur in a majority of patients with T-cell acute lymphoblastic-leukemia—a Pediatric-Oncology-Group study. *Blood*, **86**, 666–76.

Bello, M. J., de-Campos, J. M., Kusak, M. E., Vaquero, J., Sarasa, J. L., Pestana, A., and Rey, J. A. (1994). Allelic loss at 1p is associated with tumor progression of meningiomas. *Genes, Chromosomes and Cancer*, **9**, 296–8.

Bennett, J. M., Catovsky, D., Daniel, M.-T., Flandrin, G., Galton, D. A. G., Granlnick, H. R., and Sultan, C. (1985). Proposed revised criteria for the classification of acute myeloid leukemia. *Annals of International Medicine*, **103**, 626–9.

Bernard, O. A. and Berger, R. (1995). Molecular basis of 11q23 rearrangements in hematopoietic malignant proliferations. *Genes, Chromosomes and Cancer*, **13**, 75–85.

Bongarzone, I., Butti, M. G., Coronelli, S., Borrello, M. G., Santoro, M., Mondellini, P., *et al.* (1994). Frequent activation of *RET* protooncogene by fusion with a new activating gene in papillary thyroid carcinomas. *Cancer Research*, **54**, 2979–85.

Bosl, G. J., Ilson, D. H., Rodriguez, E., Motze, R. J., Reuter, V. E., and Chaganti, R. S. K. (1994). Clinical relevance of the i(12p) marker chromosome in germ-cell tumors. *Journal of the National Cancer Institute*, **86**, 349–55.

Bouffler, S., Silver, A., and Cox, A. (1993). The role of DNA repeats and associated secondary structures in genomic instability and neoplasia. *Bioessays*, **15**, 409–12.

Brodeur, G. M., Azar, C., Brother, M., Hiemstra, J., Kaufman, B., Marshall, H., *et al.* (1992). Neuroblastoma. Effect of genetic factors on prognosis and treatment. *Cancer*, **70**, (6, Suppl), 1685–94.

Brown, A. D., Lopez Terrada, D., Denny, C., and Lee, K. A. W. (1995). Promoters containing atf-binding sites are deregulated in cells that express the *EWS/ATF1* oncogene. *Oncogene*, **10**, 1749–56.

Campana, D. and Pui, C. H. (1995). Detection of minimal residual disease in acute leukemia: methodological advances and clinical significance. *Blood*, **85**, 1416–34.

Cano, J., Oliveros, O., and Yunis, E. (1994). Phenotypic variants, malignancy and additional copies of 6p in retinoblastoma. *Cancer Genetics and Cytogenetics*, **76**, 112–15.

Carvalho, T., Seeler, J.S., Ohman, K., Jordan, P., Pettersson, U., Akusjarvi, G., *et al.* (1995). Targeting of adenovirus E1A and E4-ORF3 proteins to nuclear matrix-associated PML bodies. *Journal of Cellular Biology*, **131**, 45–56.

Chen, C. S., Sorensen, P. H. B., Domer, P. H., Reaman, G. H., Korsmeyer, S. J., Heerema, N. A., Hammond, G. D., and Kersey, J. H. (1993). Molecular rearrangements on chromosome 11q23 predominate in infant acute lymphoblastic leukemia and are associated with specific biologic variables and poor outcome. *Blood*, **81**, 2386–93.

Clark, J., Benjamin, H., Gill, S., Sidhar, S., Goodwin, G., Crew, J., Gusterson, B. A., Shipley, J., and Cooper, C. S. (1996). Fusion of the *EWS* gene to *CHN*, a member of the steroid/thyroid receptor gene superfamily, in a human myxoid chondrosaroma. *Oncogene*, **12**, 229–35.

Cordon-Cardo, C. (1995). Mutation of cell cycle regulators. Biological and clinical implications for human neoplasia. *American Journal of Pathology*, **147**, 545–60.

Cordon-Cardo, C., Latres, E., Drobnjak, M., Oliva, M. R., Pollack, D., Woodruff, J. M., *et al.* (1994). Molecular abnormalities of mdm2 and p53 genes in adult soft-tissue sarcomas. *Cancer Research*, **54**, 794–9.

Cotter, F. E. (1993). Molecular pathology of lymphomas. *Cancer Surveys*, **16**, 157–74.

Crew, A. J., Clark, J., Fisher, C., Gill, S., Grimer, R., Chand, A., *et al.* (1995). Fusion of *SYT* to 2 genes, *SSX1* and *SSX2,* encoding proteins with homology to the kruppel-associated box in human synovial sarcoma. *EMBO Journal*, **14**, 2333–40.

Cuneo, A., Fagioli, F., Pazzi, I., Tallarico, A., Previati, R., Piva, N., *et al.* (1992). Morphologic, immunological and cytogenetic studies in acute myeloid-leukemia following occupational exposure to pesticides and organic-solvents. *Leukemia Research*, **16**, 789–96.

Daley, G. Q., Van Etten, R. A., and Baltimore, D. (1990). Induction of chronic myelogenous leukemia in mice by the p210$^{bcr/abl}$ gene of the Philadelphia chromosome. *Science*, **247**, 824–30.

Delattre, O., Zucman, J., Melot, T., Garau, X. S., Zucker, J. M., Lenoir, G. M., *et al.* (1994). The Ewing family of tumors — a subgroup of small-round-cell tumors defined by specific chimeric transcripts. *New England Journal of Medicine*, **331**, 294–9.

Djabali, M., Selleri, L., Parry, P., Bower, M., Young, B. D., and Evans, G. A. (1992). A trithorax-like gene is interrupted by chromosome 11q23 translocations in acute leukemias. *Nature Genetics*, **2**, 113–18.

Fearon, E. R. and Vogelstein, B. (1990). A genetic model for colorectal tumorigenesis. *Cell*, **61**, 759–67.

Feinstein, E., Cimino, G., Gale, R. P., Alimena, G., Berthier, R., Kishi, K., *et al.* (1991). p53 in chronic myelogenous leukemia in acute phase. *Proceedings of the National Academy of Sciences, USA*, **88**, 6293–7.

Fredericks, W. J., Galili, N., Mukhopadhyay, S., Rovera, G., Bennicelli, J., Barr, F. G., and Rauscher, F. J. (1995). The PAX3-FKHR fusion protein created by the t(2/13) translocation in alveolar rhabdomyosarcoma is a more potent transcriptional activator than PAX3. *Molecular Cell Biology*, **15**, 1522–35.

Fujii, Y., Hongo, T., and Hayashi, Y. (1994). Chromosome analysis of brain tumors in childhood. *Genes, Chromosomes and Cancer*, **11**, 205–15.

Galili, N., Davis, R. J., Fredericks, W. J., Mukhopadhyay, S., Rauscher, F. J., Emanuel, B. S., Rovera, G., and Barr, F. G. (1993). Fusion of a fork head domain gene to *PAX3* in the solid tumour alveolar rhabdomyosarcoma. *Nature Genetics*, **5**, 230–5.

Gerald, W. L., Rosai, J., and Ladanyi, L. (1995). Characterization of the genomic breakpoint and chimeric transcripts in the EWS–WT1 gene fusion of desmoplastic small round-cell tumor. *Proceedings of the National Academy of Sciences, USA*, **92**, 1028–32.

Gill, S., McManus, A. P., Crew, A. J., Benjamin, H., Sheer, D., Gusterson, B. A., *et al.* (1995). Fusion of the *EWS* gene to a DNA segment from 9q22–31 in a human myxoid chondrosarcoma. *Genes, Chromosomes and Cancer*, **12**, 307–10.

Gillard, E. F. and Solomon, E. (1993). Acute promyelocytic leukaemia and the t(15;17) translocation. *Seminars in Cancer Biology*, **4**, 359–68.

Gu, Y., Cimino, G., Alder, H., Nakamura, T., Prasad, R., Canaani, O., *et al.* (1992). The (4;11)(q21;q23) chromosome translocations in acute leukemias involve the vdj recombinase. *Proceedings of the National Academy of Sciences, USA*, **89**, 10464–8.

Gu, Y., Alder, H., Nakamura, T., Schichman, S. A., Prasad, R., Canaani, O., *et al.* (1994). Sequence analysis of the breakpoint cluster region in the *ALL-1* gene involved in acute leukemia. *Cancer Research*, **54**, 2327–30.

Hahn, P. J. (1993). Molecular biology of double minute chromosomes. *Bioessays*, **15**, 477–84.

Hainaut, P. (1995). The tumour suppressor protein p53: a receptor to genotoxic stress that controls cell growth and survival. *Current Opinions in Oncology*, **7**, 76–82.

Hogge, D. E. (1994). Cytogenetics and oncogenes in leukemia. *Current Opinions in Oncology*, **6**, 3–13.

Ilson, D. H., Motzer, R. J., Rodriguez, E., Chaganti, R. S., and Bosl, G. J. (1993). Genetic analysis in the diagnosis of neoplasms of unknown primary tumor site. *Seminars in Oncology*, **20**, 229–37.

ISCN (1995). *Guidelines for cancer cytogenetics. Supplement to an International System for Human Cytogenetic Nomenclature*. S. Karger, Basel.

James, C. D. and Collins, V. P. (1992). Molecular genetic characterization of CNS tumour oncogenesis. *Advances in Cancer Research*, **58**, 121–42.

Jeon, I. S., Davis, J. N., Braun, B. S., Sublett, J. E., Roussel, M. F., Denny, C. T., and Shapiro, D. N. (1995). A variant Ewings sarcoma translocation (7;22) fuses the *EWS* gene to the ETS gene, *ETV1*. *Oncogene*, **10**, 1229–34.

Johansson, B., Mertens, F., and Mitelman, F. (1993). Cytogenetic deletion maps of hematologic neoplasms: circumstantial evidence for tumor suppressor loci. *Genes, Chromosomes and Cancer*, **8**, 205–18.

Kallioniemi, O. P., Kallioniemi, A., Piper, J., Isola, J., Waldman, F. M., Gray, J. W., and Pinkel, D. (1994). Optimizing comparative genomic hybridization for analysis of DNA sequence copy number changes in solid tumours. *Genes, Chromosomes and Cancer*, **10**, 231–43.

Knudson, A. G. (1971). Mutations and cancer: statistical study of retinoblastoma. *Proceedings of the National Academy of Sciences USA*, **68**, 820–3.

Korsmeyer, S. J. (1992). Chromosomal translocations in lymphoid malignancies reveal novel proto-oncogenes. *Annual Review of Immunology*, **10**, 785–807.

Korsmeyer, S. J., Shutter, J. R., Veis, D. J., Merry, D. E., and Oltvani, Z. N. (1993). Bcl2/bax—a rheostat that regulates an antioxidant pathway and cell death. *Seminars in Cancer Biology*, **4**, 327–32.

Koskinen, P. J. and Alitalo, K. (1993). Role of *myc* amplification and overexpression in cell growth, differentiation and death. *Seminars in Cancer Biology*, **4**, 3–12.

Lane, D. P. (1992). p53, guardian of the genome. *Nature*, **358**, 15–16.

Lessnick, S. L., Braun, B. S., Denny, C. T., and May, W. A. (1995). Multiple domains mediate transformation by the ewings-sarcoma *EWS/FLI-1* fusion gene. *Oncogene*, **10**, 423–31.

Liu, P., Tarle, S. A., Hajra, A., Claxton, D. F., Marlton, P., Freedman, M., Siciliano, M. J., and Collins, F. S. (1993). Fusion between transcription factor CBFβ/PEBP2β and a myosin heavy chain in acute myeloid leukemia. *Science*, **261**, 1041–5.

Maillet, M. W., Robinson, R. A., and Burgart, L. J. (1992). Genomic alterations in sarcomas—a histologic correlative study with use of oncogene panels. *Modern Pathology*, **5**, 4101–4.

Malkin, D. and Friend, S. H. (1990). Germline p53 mutations in a familial syndrome of breast cancer, sarcomas, and other neoplasms. *Science*, **250**, 1233–8.

Margolin, J. F., Friedman, J. R., Meyer, W. K. H., Vissing, H., Thiesen, H. J., and Rauscher, F. J. (1994). Kruppel-associated boxes are potent transcriptional repression domains. *Proceedings of the National Academy of Sciences, USA*, **91**, 4509–13.

Mitelman, F. (1994). *Catalog of Chromosome Aberrations in Cancer* (associate editors, B. Johansson, and F. Mertens). 5th Edition. John Wiley and Sons, New York.

Negrini, M., Felix, C. A., Martin, C., Lange, B. J., Nakamura, T., Canaani, E., and Croce, C. M. (1993). Potential topoisomerase II DNA-binding sites at the breakpoints of a t(9;11) chromosome translocation in acute myeloid leukemia. *Cancer Research*, **53**, 4489–92.

Newcomb, E. W., Thomas, A., Selkirk, A., Lee, S. Y., and Potmesil, M. (1995). Frequent homozygous deletions of D13S218 on 13q14 in B-cell chronic lymphocytic leukemia independent of disease stage and retinoblastoma gene inactivation. *Cancer Research*, **55**, 2044–7.

Ohki, M. (1993). Molecular basis of the t(8;21) translocation in acute myeloid leukaemia. *Seminars in Cancer Biology*, **4**, 359–68.

Pandis, N., Bardi, G., and Heim, S. (1994). Interrelationship between methodological choices and conceptual models in solid tumor cytogenetics. *Cancer Genetics and Cytogenetics*, **76**, 77–84.

Pandis, N., Jin, Y. S., Gorunova, L., Petersson, C., Bardi, G., Idvall, I., *et al.* (1995). Chromosome analysis of 97 primary breast carcinomas — identification of 8 karyotypic subgroups. *Genes, Chromosomes and Cancer*, **12**, 173–85.

Peters, G., Fantl, V., Smith, R., Brookes, S., and Dickson, C. (1995). Chromosome 11q13 markers and D-type cyclins in breast-cancer. *Breast Cancer Research and Treatment*, **33**, 125–35.

Rabbitts, T. H. (1994). Chromosomal translocations in human cancer. *Nature*, **372**, 143–9.

Rabbitts, T. H., Forster, A., Larson, R., and Nathan, P. (1993). Fusion of the dominant-negative transcription regulator CHOP with a novel gene FUS by translocation t(12;16) in malignant liposarcoma. *Nature Genetics*, **4**, 175–80.

Raimondi, S. C. (1993). Current status of cytogenetic research in childhood acute lymphoblastic leukemia. *Blood*, **81**, 2237–51.

Reifenberger, G., Reifenberger, J., Ichimura, K., Meltzer, P. S., and Collins, V. P. (1994). Amplification of multiple genes from chromosomal region 12q13–14 in human malignant gliomas: preliminary mapping of the amplicons shows preferential involvement of *CDK4*, *SAS* and *MDM2*. *Cancer Research*, **54**, 4299–303.

Reznikoff, C. A., Kao, C. H., Messing, E. M., Newton, M., and Waminathan, S. (1993). A molecular genetic model of human bladder carcinogenesis. *Seminars in Cancer Biology*, **4**, 143–52.

Rodriguez, E., Sreekantaiah, C., and Chaganti, R. S. K. (1994). Genetic changes in epithelial solid neoplasia. *Cancer Research*, **54**, 3398–406.

Rooney, D. E. and Czepulkowski, B. H. (1992). *Human cytogenetics — a practical approach.* Vol. II. *Malignancy and acquired abnormalities.* Oxford University Press, Oxford.

Sanchez-Garcia, I. and Rabbitts, T. H. (1993). LIM domain proteins in leukaemia and development. *Seminars in Cancer Biology*, **4**, 349–58.

Sawyers, C. L. (1992). The bcr-abl gene in chronic myelogenous leukaemia. *Cancer Surveys*, **15**, 37–51.

Schoenmakers, E. F. P. M., Wanschura, S., Mols, R., Bullerdiek, J., Van den Berghe, H., and Van de Ven, W. J. M. (1995). Recurrent rearrangements in the high mobility group protein gene, *HMGI-C*, in benign mesenchymal tumours. *Nature Genetics*, **10**, 436–43.

Schröck, E., du Manoir, S., Veldman, T., Schoell, B., Weinberg, J., Ferguson-Smith, M. A., Ning, Y., Ledbetter, D. H., Bar-Am, I., Soenksen, D., Garini, Y. and Reid, T. (1996). Multicolor spectral karotyping of human chromosomes. *Science*, **273**, 494–97.

Secker-Walker, L. M., Berger, R., Fenaux, P., Lai, J. L., Nelken, B., Garson, M., *et al.* (1992). Prognostic significance of the balanced t(1;19) and unbalanced del(19)t(1;19) translocations in acute lymphoblastic leukemia. *Leukemia*, **6**, 363–9.

Shilatifard, A., Lane, W. S., Jackson, K. W., Conaway, R. C., and Conaway, J. W. (1996). An RNA polymerase II elongation factor encoded by the human ELL gene. *Science*, **271**, 1873–6.

Sidhar, S. K., Clark, J. Gill, S., Hamoudi, R., Crew, A. J., Gwilliam, R., Ross, M., Linehan, W. M., Birdsall, S., Shipley, J. and Cooper, C. S. (1996). The t(X;1)(p11.2;q21.2) translocation in papillary renal cell carcinoma fuses a novel gene *PRCC* to the *TFE3* transcription factor gene. *Human Molecular Genetics*, **5**, 1333-8.

Sorensen, P. H. B. and Triche, T. J. (1996). Gene fusions encoding chimeric transcription factors in solid tumors. *Seminars in Cancer Biology*, **7**, 3–14.

Sorensen, P. H. B., Lessnick, S. L., Lopez-Terrada, D., Liu, X. F., and Triche, T. H. (1994). A second Ewings sarcoma translocation t(21;22) fuses the *EWS* gene to another ETS-family transcription factor, *ERG. Nature Genetics*, **6**, 146–51.

Speicher, M. R., Gwyn-Ballard, S. and Ward, D. C. (1996). Karyotyping human chromosomes by combinatorial multi-fluor FISH. *Nature Genetics*, **12**, 368–75.

Squire, J. and Weksberg, R. (1996). Genomic imprinting in tumours. *Seminars in Cancer Biology*, **7**, 41–7.

Sreekantaiah, C., Ladanyi, M., Rodriguez, E., and Chaganti, R. S. K. (1994). Chromosomal aberrations in soft tissue tumors: relevance to diagnosis, classification, and molecular mechanism. *American Journal of Pathology*, 144, 1121–34.

Stranks, G., Height, S. E., Mitchell, P., Jadayel, D., Yuille, M. A., De Lord, C., *et al.* (1995). Deletions and rearrangement of CDKN2 in lymphoid malignancy. *Blood*, **85**, 893–901.

Taylor, C. P. F., McGuckin, A. G., Bown, N. P., Reid, M. M., Malcolm, A. J., Pearson, A. D. J., and Sheer, D. (1994). Rapid detection of prognostic genetic factors in neuroblastoma using fluorescence *in situ* hybridisation on tumour imprints and bone marrow smears. *British Journal of Cancer*, **69**, 445–51.

Verma, R. S. and Babu, A. (1995). *Human chromosomes.* McGraw-Hill Inc., New York.

Walker, G. J., Palmer, J. M., Walters, M. K., and Hayward, N. K. (1995). A genetic model of melanoma tumorigenesis based on allelic losses. *Genes, Chromosomes and Cancer*, **12**, 134–41.

Westermark, B. and Nister, M. (1995). Molecular genetics of human glioma. *Current Opinion in Oncology*, **7**, 220–5.

Willert, J. R., Daneshvar, L., Sheffield, V. C., and Cogen, P. H. (1995). Deletion of chromosome arm 17p DNA-sequences in pediatric high-grade and juvenile pilocytic astrocytomas. *Genes, Chromosomes and Cancer*, **12**, 165–72.

Wynford-Thomas, D., Bond, J. A., Wyllie, F. S., and Jones, C. J. (1995). Does telomere shortening drive selection for p53 mutation in human cancer? *Molecular Carcinogenesis*, **12**, 119–23.

Zinszner, H., Albalat, R., and Ron, D. (1994). A novel effector domain from the RNA binding protein TLS or EWS is required for oncogenic transformation by CHOP. *Genes and Development*, **8**, 2513–26.

11

Growth factor signalling pathways in cancer

ALASTAIR D. REITH AND GEORGE PANAYOTOU

An understanding of the mechanisms responsible for the control of normal proliferation and differentiation of the various cell types that make up the human body will undoubtedly allow greater insights into the abnormal growth of malignant cells. Particular attention is now focused on the signals that act as positive mediators and negative regulators of cell growth and function in both normal and abnormal cells. Such signals often take the form of secreted polypeptides that provide information essential for coordinated patterns of cell–cell communication. The perception of these environmental signals by the target cell is mediated by specific intrinsic signalling pathways, and the integration of information provided by these routes ensures an appropriate cellular response. Given this fundamental role in normal patterns of cellular regulation, it is perhaps not surprising to find that breakdown, or subversion, of intercellular signalling pathways is implicated in several disease states, including cancers. The last few years have seen major advances in our understanding of the molecular basis of growth factor signalling in cellular transformation and tumorigenesis. Here, we shall consider, briefly, our current understanding of the molecular mechanisms that mediate intercellular signalling in normal cells, the means by which oncogenes subvert these pathways, and how such information offers the prospect of rational strategies for therapeutic intervention.

11.1 Structural and functional diversity of growth factors

As a class of signalling proteins, polypeptide growth factors exert their various biological effects as a result of a primary interaction with specific receptors on the surface of a target cell. A given growth factor may be expressed by one or more of several different cell types and the expression of these receptors on target cells governs, at least in part, the cellular specificity of different growth factors. In contrast to signal molecules grouped together as hormones (see Chapters 14 and 15), polypeptide growth factor synthesis is not restricted to particular endocrine organs and can operate by one, or more, of several different routes (Fig. 11.1)

In the first system, termed *endocrine*, growth factor synthesis occurs in a specific tissue or organ, often at some distance from target cells that express the appropriate receptor. The factor may be subject to regulation by specific releasing factors that control the storage and secretion of the growth factor to the bloodstream, by which route it is delivered to the target cells. The second system is called *paracrine* and operates between cells in close proximity. In this case, one cell type synthesizes and secretes a growth factor for which the appropriate receptors are expressed on another cell type that is nearby. This contrasts with the third system, termed *autocrine*, in which the cell type that synthesizes the growth factor also expresses receptors that can elicit a cellular response to the factor. Given that some aspects of the cellular responses evoked by signalling pathways can involve changes in expression of other growth factors and receptors, it is apparent that combinations of these mechanisms can provide formidable regulatory systems to control cell growth and physiology.

While several polypeptide growth factors were identified initially through protein purification routes and the biological responses they elicit, the advent of DNA cloning strategies has greatly accelerated the identification of members of this class of signalling proteins. Morever, the cloning of genes encoding growth factors has enabled the production of bioactive recombinant growth factor proteins. These recombinant proteins provide both a more readily available source of growth factor and a purity that is often greater than can be guaranteed by isolation of the native protein from tissue sources. For these reasons, recombinant growth factors are of considerable value for ongoing research studies and some are proving to be of clinical value in disease management.

Analysis of growth factor structure has revealed several features that reflect not only the different routes by which they are delivered to target cells, but also additional regulatory mechanisms that serve to control the potent biological activities of these molecular signals (Table 11.1). For example, many growth factors are secreted as inactive precursors that require specific proteolytic cleavage events to achieve bioactivity. While several growth factor proteins are active as soluble molecules, some others are transmembrane proteins that signal in a

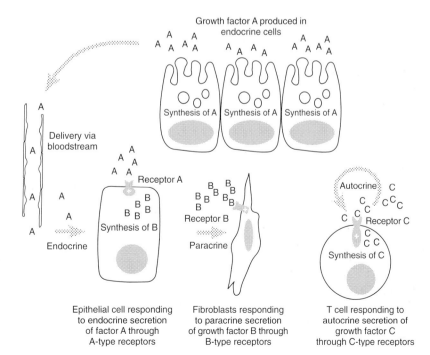

Fig. 11.1 Sites of release and action of growth regulators.

Table 11.1 Physiologic growth regulators

Regulator	Structures	Bioactivities	Receptors
EGF	130 kDa transmembrane active precursor. Soluble 6 kDa form results from proteolytic cleavage	Mitogenic for epithelial cells	EGFR RTK
TGFα	25 kDa palmitoylated precursor. Soluble 6 kDa form results from proteolytic cleavage	Mitogenic for epithelial cells	EGFR RTK
Amphiregulin	14–22 kDa glycoproteins	Mitogenic	EGFR RTK
HB-EGF	14–20 kDa active soluble protein. Transmembrane proforms subject to proteolytic cleavage	Mitogenic, chemoattractant	EGFR/ErbB4 RTKs
Betacellulin	32 kDa soluble glycoprotein. Membrane-bound precursor subject to proteolytic cleavage	Mitogenic for pancreatic and breast cells	EGFR/ErbB4 RTKs
Heregulins	42–59 kDa glycoproteins of at least 12 isoforms. Transmembrane proforms subject to proteolytic cleavage	Maintenance, differentiation, and maturation factors	ErbB3-4 RTKs
PDGF-A/B	30 kDa disulphide bonded homo/heterodimers. Proteolytic processing of prepropeptides to give 16–18 kDa (PDGF-A) and 12 kDa (PDGF-B) mature forms	Chemotaxis, hypertrophy mitogenesis	PDGFRα PDGFRβ
FGF1-9	17–30 kDa single chain secreted glycoproteins. Soluble and proteoglycan associated	Mitogenic, neurotrophic, angiogenic	FGFR1-4 RTKs
IGF-I IGF-II	7.5 kDa single chain secreted polypeptides	Cell proliferation, differentiation and survival	IGF-IR RTK INS-R RTK
NGF BDNF NT3 NT4	13–25 kDa active homodimers Inactive precursors	Mitogenic, differentiation, and survival factors for neuronal cells	trkA RTK trkB RTK trkC (trkA,trkB) RTKs trkB (trkA) RTKs
GDNF	20 kDa disulphide-linked homodimer, glycoprotein. Prepropeptide activated by proteolytic cleavage	Survival factor for neuronal cells	ret RTK
VEGF	34–46 kDa homodimeric glycoproteins. Heparin proteoglycan binding isoforms	Mitogenic for endothelial cells	Flt-1/Flk-1 RTKs
CSF-1	70–90 kDa homodimeric glycoprotein. Transmembrane and proteolytically cleaved soluble forms	Proliferation of macrophage/monocyte lineage. Embryo implantation	c-fms RTK
SCF	31–36 kDa glycoproteins. Transmembrane and proteolytically cleaved soluble forms	Proliferation, differentiation, migration, and survival of haemopoietic, melanogenic, and gametogenic cells	c-kit RTK
Flt-3L	Transmembrane form and soluble 30 kDa disulphide-linked homodimer	Proliferation/survival haemopoietic progenitor cells	flt-3 RTK

Table 11.1 Physiologic growth regulators (contd)

Regulator	Structures	Bioactivities	Receptors
HGF	Secreted inactive single chain precursor subject to proteolytic cleavage to active 60 kDa and 30 kDa disulphide-linked heterodimer	Motility and morphology of epithelial, endothelial cells	met RTK
MSP	Inactive precursor activated by proteolytic cleavage to 47 kDa and 22 kDa disulphide linked heterodimer	Motility and morphology of macrophages	ron RTK
ephrinA1-5	21–28 kDa soluble and GPI-linked forms	Axonal guidance, mitogenic, induced by proinflammatory cytokines	EphA1-8
ephrinB1-3	34 kDa transmembrane proteins		EphB1-6
gas6	75 kDa secreted protein	Mitogenic and survival factor	Axl RTK Sky RTK
Transforming growth factor (TGF)-β superfamily			
TGFβ1-3 BMP2-8 Activins/ Inhibins anti-Mullerian hormone	28-30 kDa disulphide-linked homodimers. Inactive precursors subject to proteolytic cleavage	Body plan organization, mesenchymal condensation, mesoderm induction, mesenchymal cell proliferation, Inhibition of epithelia, endothelial, haemopoietic cells	TβR-II, TβR-I BMPR-II, ActR-I ActR-II, ActR-I, ActR-IIB, ActR-IB
Tumour necrosis factor (TNF) superfamily			
TNFα	17 kDa transmembrane non-disulphide linked trimer	Mitogenesis, cytotoxicity, tissue remodelling, angiogenesis, apoptosis, cell adhesion	p55 TNFR p75 TNFR

paracrine fashion by direct contact with adjacent cells that express appropriate receptors.

The biological functions of growth factors include stimulation of cellular proliferation, differentiation, cell survival, and changes in cellular motility and morphology. Moreover, growth factors can act alone, or synergistically, to evoke cellular reponses and so the specific repertoire of growth factor receptors expressed by a target cell can influence growth factor function. These features, coupled with the expression of distinct growth factor isoforms and the formation of homo and hetero-dimeric proteins are also likely to contribute to the diversity of growth factor functions.

11.2 Structure and diversity of growth factor receptors

The various families of cytokine receptors are all membrane-spanning molecules, which serve to link extracellular ligand signals to the cytoplasm of target cells. This is achieved by specificity of receptor–ligand interactions, receptor activation, binding and activation of a repertoire of substrates and intracellular signalling pathways, and the integration of distinct signals. The discussion here is limited to three receptor classes, which reflect both the positive and negative growth regulatory roles of such pathways that are of relevance to transformation and tumorigenesis. G-protein coupled receptors are not considered here, while haematopoietins are discussed in Chapter 20.

11.2.1 Receptor protein tyrosine kinases (RTKs)

Members of this superfamily of membrane-spanning molecules, which act as high affinity receptors for a wide variety of growth factors, are characterized by an extracellular ligand-binding domain, a single transmembrane domain, and an intracellular region bearing a highly conserved tyrosine kinase catalytic domain. The catalytic domain is composed of an amino-terminal ATP-binding region and a carboxy-terminal phosphotransferase domain which, in some RTKs, are separated by a region of divergent sequence, the so-called kinase insert. Prototype members of this superfamily were identified as receptors for growth factors, purified, and cloned according to their biological activities, including epidermal growth factor (EGF), platelet-derived growth factor (PDGF), nerve growth factor (NGF), and hepatocyte growth factor (HGF). As discussed in Section 11.4.2, several receptor tyrosine kinases (RTKs) were cloned initially in aberrant form, either as transforming genes of oncogenic retroviruses, or through their ability to induce cellular transformation *in vitro*. More recently, many additional RTKs have been cloned by direct screening of cDNA expression libraries with antiphosphotyrosine antibodies, and polymerase chain reaction-based cloning approaches that utilize the highly conserved nature of amino acid motifs within the tyrosine kinase catalytic domain. In turn, the high affinity interaction between the extracellular domain of a RTK and its cognate ligand has been used in direct screens to identify, purify, and clone growth factor ligands for such 'orphan receptors'.

As shown in Fig. 11.2, RTKs can be categorized into distinct subfamilies according to a conserved organization of specific amino acid sequence motifs within the extracellular domain. For example, members of the PDGFR, FGFR, and flk-1 subfamilies are characterized by extracellular domains bearing five, three, or seven immunoglobulin (Ig)-like motifs, respectively. Fibronectin type III repeats, in unique combinations with Ig-like domains, characterize Eph, Axl, and Tek family RTKs (van der Geer *et al.* 1994). Most RTK ligands are secreted soluble proteins existing as disulphide-linked dimers, or in monomeric form. However, membrane-bound and extracellular matrix ligands are also known. The normal biological properties of ligand-activated receptor tyrosine kinases are diverse and can include differentiation, morphogenesis, motility responses, cell–cell adhesion, mitogenesis, inhibition of cellular proliferation, and cell survival. Moreover, the physiological responses of RTK signalling can vary according to the cellular context and this, together with synergism between signalling pathways, provides a means by which RTKs may help to determine the specificity and sensitivity of cellular responses essential for the coordinate development and function of many cell types.

From analysis of prototype RTKs a generally accepted model of RTK activation has emerged (Fig. 11.3). A steady-state equilibrium is thought to exist at the cell surface between inactive receptor monomers and active dimers. Ligand binding to the extracellular domain stabilizes dimers, so pushing the equilibrium in favour of dimer formation. Dimerization may be driven by either the dimeric nature of the ligand, which would provide binding sites for two receptor molecules, or through conformational changes in the ligand-binding domain that expose interaction sites between receptor monomers. One consequence of dimerization is juxtaposition of cytoplasmic domains that results in a transient activation of the tyrosine kinase catalytic domain, possibly induced by a conformational change. In turn, this results in transphosphorylation of specific tyrosine residues within the intracellular region of the RTK, most of which lie outside the catalytic domain. As discussed later (see Section 11.3.1), it is the specificity of autophosphorylation sites in the activated receptor that helps to maintain the integrity of the signal initiated by receptor/ligand interaction during transduction through the cytoplasm.

11.2.2 Receptor protein serine/threonine kinases

The TGF-β superfamily of growth factors presently comprises around 25 homologous proteins that share a common structure of 110–140 amino acid disulphide-linked homo- or hetero-dimers. They are synthesized as precursor proteins that dimerize and are then proteolytically cleaved to release the active C-terminal fragments. Members of this superfamily can be categorized into four subgroups; TGF-βs, activins/inhibins, BMPs (bone morphogenetic proteins), and anti-Mullerian hormone (see Table 11.1). While several of these factors are known to play key roles in normal development, the best understood in relation to cancer is the TGF-β family, of which three isoforms, TGF-β1, TGF-β2, and TGF-β3, have been identified in mammalian cells. All three isoforms have similar properties but by far the best characterized is TGF-β1, which can elicit a range of biological responses.

While stimulating mitogenesis in some cell types, in other cells TGF-β acts as an inhibitor of cellular proliferation. These contrasting growth regulatory properties can also occur within the same cell type,

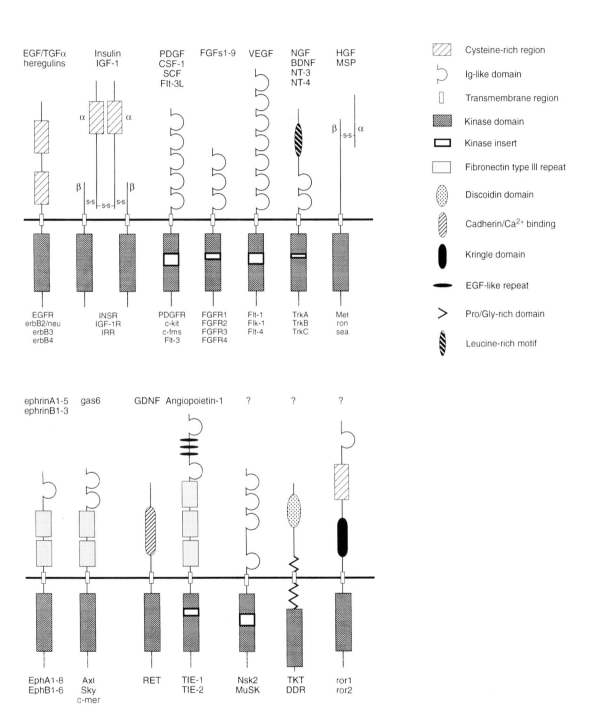

Fig. 11.2 The superfamily of receptor tyrosine kinases. RTKs can be classified into distinct subfamilies according to the structural organization of extracellular domain motifs and the presence of a kinase insert (see van der Geer *et al.* 1994, for review). Known growth factor ligands for members of each subfamily are shown. Specific extracellular ligands have yet to be identified for TKT, ror, and Nsk2/MuSK receptor subfamilies.

A. Receptor tyrosine kinases

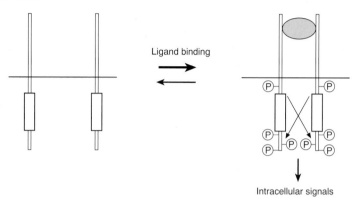

Intracellular signals

B. Receptor serine/threonine kinases

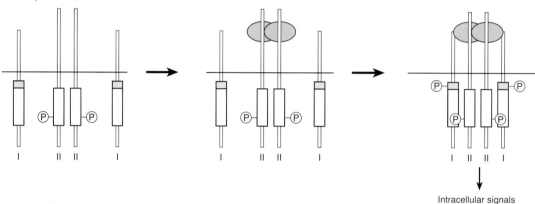

Intracellular signals

Fig. 11.3 Activation of receptor tyrosine kinases and receptor serine/threonine kinases. For both classes of receptor, ligand-mediated activation involves high affinity interaction between ligand and extracellular domain receptor motifs that serves to stabilize receptor aggregates. However, the mechanisms of receptor activation within such complexes are distinct (see text for details).

varying as a function of different culture conditions. There is some evidence to suggest that in mesenchymal cells the mitogenic properties of this growth factor are indirect. For example, in smooth muscle cells low concentrations of TGF-β induce expression of PDGF-α, whereas high concentrations of TGF-β are growth inhibitory in this culture system and correlate with inhibition of PDGFR-α synthesis. A distinct mechanism of growth inhibition may operate in epithelial cells, such as keratinocytes, which do not express PDGFR. Here, stimulation with mitogens leads to a rapid induction of c-myc protein while TGF-β1 rapidly inhibits both c-myc RNA and protein expression. In addition to regulating cell growth, a number of other properties of TGF-β are likely to be of significance in relation to tumorigenesis.

These include the promotion of angiogenesis, suppression of the effects of inflammatory cytokines on B and T cells, and inhibition of adhesion of neutrophils and T cells to endothelial cells.

Four classes of cell surface receptors for TGF-β have been described to date (Massague *et al.* 1994; Heldin 1995). Both type I (53 kDa) and type II (75 kDa) receptors are membrane-spanning molecules bearing a short N-terminal extracellular domain and an intracellular region that bears a serine/threonine catalytic domain. The TGF-β type II receptor exists as a homodimer in the absence of ligand and exhibits constitutive kinase activity. It can bind ligand directly, but kinase activity is unaffected and transduction of the signal requires the presence of the type I receptor. TGF-β type I receptors recognize ligand only when it is associated with the type II receptor, resulting in the formation of a stable ternary complex. Since type I receptor dimers can be detected following dissociation of type II receptors, a heterotetrameric signalling complex has been proposed (Fig. 11.3). Thus, in contrast to RTK signalling, ligand binding to the primary receptor (type II) would serve not to activate this molecule, but to mediate association between type II and type I receptors. As a consequence, the type I receptor is transphosphorylated by the type II receptor and it is this that transduces the signal to the cytoplasm. In this model, ligand specificity is determined by the nature of the type II receptor in the complex, possibly defined by the organization of cysteine residues in the extracellular domain, while specificity of intracellular signalling would be achieved by the type I receptor isoform that participates in complex formation. A further level of sophistication may be provided by the TGF-β type III receptor, a proteoglycan of more than 200 kDa, which can bind all three TGF isoforms. When complexed with type III receptors, TGF-β exhibits a higher affinity for binding to the signalling receptor. Moreover, soluble isoforms of the type III receptor have been identified that could sequester TGF-β in an inactive form, so acting as antagonists of TGF-β function. A fourth receptor type, endoglin (180 kDa) may play a similar role in some cell types.

11.2.3 Tumour necrosis factor receptor superfamily

Tumour necrosis factors (TNF)-α and -β (also known as LT-α) were among the first cytokines to be cloned at the molecular level and form the prototypes of an expanding family of related cytokines, currently comprising eight distinct members. Several potent normal cellular activities are associated with TNF signalling, including stimulation of cell proliferation, differentiation, cellular activation, and angiogenesis. Such pleiotropic functions vary according to the cell type, transformation status, and presence of other stimuli. However, it is the ability shared by TNF-α, LT-α, and FasL to activate a signalling pathway(s) that culminates in programmed cell death (apoptosis) that makes this family of major interest in relation to cancer.

TNF cytokines are transmembrane proteins in which a short amino-terminal intracellular domain precedes a single membrane-spanning region and an extracellular carboxy-terminal domain in which

homology between different members is shared. Structural studies suggest that most, if not all, members of this family exist as non-disulphide-linked trimers. Two distinct, but homologous, TNF receptors (p75 and p55) are known that are the prototypes for a superfamily of TNF receptors, comprising at least twelve members (Smith *et al.* 1994). Homology between receptors is found primarily in the extracellular domain that is separated from a short intracellular region by a single transmembrane domain.

Ligand-mediated activation of TNF receptors is thought to involve aggregation of receptor monomers in response to binding of the respective ligand trimer. X-ray diffraction studies of ligand-receptor complexes have revealed a receptor trimer to be bound with one ligand trimer such that each TNF subunit contacts two adjacent receptor molecules. The stabilization of receptor aggregates in this way is also likely to bring receptor cytoplasmic domains into close proximity, perhaps creating functional sites for interaction with intracellular signalling proteins. While second messenger pathways implicated in TNF signalling have been identified (Kolesnick and Golde 1994), the means of coupling to activated receptors is unknown. In contrast to the other classes of receptor discussed here, no catalytic domains are obvious in receptors of the TNF superfamily. However, a 65 amino acid sequence, weakly conserved between the cytoplasmic regions of p55 TNFR and Fas, has been defined that is necessary for the cell death signalling properties of these receptors. Novel binding proteins to these so-called death domains have recently been identified (Cleveland and Ihle 1995). Interestingly, these binding proteins also contain death domains, reflecting an ability of these motifs to dimerize that may be relevant to their function. In addition, a 15 amino acid negative regulatory 'salvation' domain at the C-terminus of Fas has been found to associate with a protein tyrosine phosphatase, suggesting the involvement of tyrosine phosphorylation in the Fas signalling pathway. The physiological significance of such interactions in relation to death signalling remains to be established.

11.3 Intracellular signalling by activated growth factor receptors

While the means by which activated TGF-β or TNF receptors stimulate intracellular signalling are largely unknown, the last few years have seen major advances in our understanding of the molecular mechanisms underlying the propagation of extracellular signals by activated tyrosine kinases. It has been known for some time that growth factor stimulation of receptor tyrosine kinases elicits autophosphorylation of specific receptor tyrosine residues in the intracellular domain of the receptor, but the functional relationship of such events to intracellular signal transduction remained elusive. It is now clear that receptor autophosphorylation is central for initiation of a series of protein–protein interactions and activations which together constitute signalling cascades that culminate in nuclear responses, including stimulation of cell growth.

11.3.1 Specific domains mediate interactions between signalling proteins

The tyrosine residues that become autophosphorylated following growth factor stimulation of receptor tyrosine kinases are located at various positions within the intracellular domain, and are specific for each receptor. For example, the EGF receptor sites are found near its C-terminus, whereas in the case of the PDGF receptor they are located in the kinase insert, juxtamembrane region and C-terminal tail. Distinct phosphotyrosine-containing peptide motifs, comprising the autophosphorylation site and amino acid residues immediately C-terminal to the phosphotyrosine (pTyr), act as specific and high affinity recruitment sites for downstream intracellular signalling molecules. A strict requirement for such protein-protein recognition events is the presence of distinct binding domains in the intracellular signalling molecules, which mediate recognition of specific tyrosine-phosphorylated sequences (Cantley *et al.* 1991; Cohen *et al.* 1995).

SH2 domain The src homology 2 (SH2) domain was so called owing to its initial discovery as a region of homology, approximately 100 amino acids in size, with a domain in the cytoplasmic tyrosine kinase $pp60^{c-src}$. It is found in many intracellular signalling molecules and has been shown to confer directly the recognition of specific phosphotyrosyl-containing motifs, including those of activated receptor tyrosine kinases (Pawson and Schlessinger 1993). SH2-containing proteins can be divided into two broad categories: (i) proteins that are enzyma-

tically active, including phosphoinositide (PI) 3 kinase (see below), phospholipase Cγ, members of the src family of non-receptor tyrosine kinases, and the ras–GTPase-activating protein (GAP). (ii) 'adaptor' molecules, such as GRB-2, crk, shc, and nck, which do not contain a catalytic domain but serve as linker proteins that can mediate association, and coordinate activation, of other signalling proteins.

The SH2 domains of all these molecules have been the focus of intense study in the last few years, both in terms of their functional properties and of the structural requirements for specific recognition of distinct pTyr-containing sequences. Several of these structures have been identified by NMR and crystallography and reveal an overall similarity in tertiary structure, in which a central antiparallel β sheet is flanked by two α helical regions with loops of variable sizes linking these elements (Kuriyan and Cowburn 1993). Determination of the structure of SH2 domains in complex with pTyr-containing peptides showed that the phosphotyrosine residue is located within a deep pocket that is clearly defined on the surface of an SH2 domain structure. Positively charged amino acid residues within this phosphotyrosine binding pocket are involved in intimate electrostatic contact with the negatively charged phosphate group of phosphotyrosine. Additional stability is provided by hydrophobic interactions between residues contributing to the pocket and the phenol ring.

Since the phosphotyrosine binding pocket is common to all SH2 domains, additional interactions with amino acids downstream from the pTyr are likely to mediate their unique binding specificities. Again, structural studies have defined the basis of this specificity, while complementary experiments involving screening of random peptide libraries have determined precisely the nature of amino acids within pTyr peptide motifs that bind particular SH2 domains. In many cases, the amino acid at position $+3$ from the pTyr has been shown to be the most important in determining specificity, although the $+1$ and $+5$ positions also contribute. In one case, that of the SH2 domains of GRB-2, the presence of Asn at the $+2$ position is the most critical. With regard to binding sites for these residues in SH2 domains, two distinct structural variations have been identified. In some cases, such as the src SH2, a clearly defined pocket is provided for binding the $+3$ amino acid. Together with the pTyr pocket, such SH2 domains resemble a socket for a two-pronged plug. In other SH2 domains there is no distinct second binding pocket, but additional interactions occur on a long 'groove' that extends from the pTyr binding pocket along the surface of the SH2 domain, providing interaction sites for up to five residues C-terminal to the pTyr. In either case, the combination of these interactions with the common pTyr binding pocket produces a high affinity, specific complex. Interestingly, evidence both *in vitro* and *in vivo* suggests that SH2 domain interactions are both transient and dynamic, displaying fast rates of association and dissociation. This has considerable implications for the regulation of complex formation, facilitating competition between different domains, and/or access to specific tyrosine phosphatases that may down-regulate the response.

PTB domain An interesting recent addition to the family of modules involved in growth factor signalling is the phosphotyrosine binding (PTB) domain (van der Geer and Pawson 1995). It essentially has the same function as the SH2 domain, binding pTyr within a specific amino acid context. However, it is structurally distinct and appears to require the presence of the motif Asn–Pro–X (where X denotes any amino acid) on the amino-terminal side of the phosphotyrosine, in contrast to SH2 domains that recognize carboxy-terminal residues. Although not yet identified in a large number of proteins, PTB domains seem to be used by important adaptor molecules that play a central role in growth factor and hormone signalling, such as Shc and the insulin receptor substrate-1 (IRS-1), in direct association with activated receptors. Interestingly, Shc also contains an SH2 domain, which may be used for recognition of pTyr-containing motifs in downstream signalling molecules. The existence of two distinct pTyr-binding domains emphasizes the importance of this recognition event in evolution and provides additional possibilities for regulation and fine-tuning of growth factor receptor signalling.

SH3 and PH domains While SH2 domains and PTB domains provide the crucial first recognition event in signalling by activated growth factor receptors, additional conserved recognition modules have been identified that mediate further downstream complex formation between signalling molecules. The best studied is the src homology 3 (SH3) domain, approximately 60–70 amino acids long with a predominantly β sheet structure, that specifically interacts with proline-rich (Pro-rich) regions in two different orientations (Kuriyan and Cowburn 1993). The region of contact between the left-handed Pro-rich helix and the SH3 is extended, with crucial interactions being provided by two prolines, while specificity is conferred by non-proline residues such as arginine and leucine. Many cytoskeletal proteins contain SH3 domains, implicating a more general recognition/localization role for this domain, not necessarily restricted to signal transduction. Moreover, in contrast to phosphotyrosyl–SH2 interactions, it is unclear if SH3 domain interactions are subject to rapid regulation, suggesting that they mediate more stable associations within the cell.

The pleckstrin homology (PH) domain is also conserved in a number of proteins that are directly or indirectly involved in signal transduction by growth factors (Shaw 1996). While primary amino acid sequence similarity between different PH domains is limited, much better conservation is observed at the level of tertiary structure. Despite advances in structure determination, the issue of the binding partner of the PH domains remains unresolved, although there have been suggestions that some of them may interact with βγ subunits of heterotrimeric G proteins or with specific phospholipids, thus facilitating the membrane localization of the proteins that contain them.

11.3.2 PI 3-kinase: a key mediator of growth factor signals

Prominent among the many signalling molecules recognized by activated growth factor receptors is phosphoinositide (PI) 3-kinase, which catalyses the addition of a phosphate group on the 3 position of phosphatidylinositol (PtdIns) and the phosphoinositides PtdIns(4)P and PtdIns(4,5)P2. Elevated levels of the products of this enzyme, especially PtdIns(3,4,5)P3, have been observed immediately following growth factor receptor activation and also in cells transformed by a variety of oncogenes. Originally, PI3K activity was found to coimmunoprecipitate with the polyomavirus middle T antigen–pp60^{c-src} complex from transformed cells, and later to participate in complex formation with a variety of growth factor receptors. The purification and cDNA cloning of this enzyme showed that it is a heterodimeric protein consisting of a regulatory p85 and a catalytic p110 subunit with molecular weights of 85 and 110 kDa, respectively. The regulatory domain consists of several distinct modules, including two SH2 domains, one SH3 domain and a region of similarity to the bcr gene product, flanked by two proline-rich motifs which are potential SH3 binding sites. The SH2 domains display a clear specificity in recognizing the motif pTyrXXMet (where X denotes any amino acid). The p110 catalytic subunit contains a kinase domain towards the carboxy-terminus which shares some similarity with, but is clearly distinct from, the protein kinases. The site of interaction with the p85 subunit is located towards the amino-terminus of p110, while the region of p85 responsible for association with the p110 subunit is located between the two SH2 domains. The primary function of the p85 subunit is to associate with activated receptors through its SH2 domains, thus bringing the p110 catalytic subunit into proximity with the plasma membrane where its substrates are available for phosphorylation. The precise functions of the other domains of p85 are unclear, but they could participate in additional regulatory interactions. There is some evidence to suggest that the Pro-rich motif in p85 can interact with the SH3 domain of src family protein tyrosine kinases and that the SH3 domain of p85 can bind focal adhesion kinase (FAK). The finding that ras in its active, GTP-bound form can bind to and stimulate the catalytic activity of the p110 subunit, suggests other interesting potential regulatory interactions involving p110 and provides a link between PI3K and another important regulator of intracellular signal transduction.

The availability of specific inhibitors and dominant negative mutants of PI3K has established that this enzyme is not only involved in growth factor-induced mitogenesis and oncogenic transformation, but can also mediate other physiological responses including cell survival, membrane ruffling, chemotaxis, the oxidative burst in neutrophils, oocyte maturation, platelet activation, and vesicular trafficking. These responses can be elicited by a wide variety of extracellular signals, often involving receptors other than tyrosine kinases, raising the question of the mechanism by which coupling to and activation of PI3K occurs. It is becoming clear that a family of structurally distinct PI3 kinases

exists, members of which may display different substrate specificities and couple through unique adaptor subunits to distinct receptor types. This diversity establishes PI3K activation as a key regulatory switch in metabolic pathways and cell growth.

11.3.3 A signalling pathway from the cell surface to the nucleus

A central role for the small GTP-binding protein ras (p21^{ras}) in intracellular signal transduction pathways and oncogenic transformation (see Chapters 8 and 9) has been appreciated for several years. Post-translational modifications at its carboxy-terminus localize ras to the inner aspect of the plasma membrane where it cycles between two alternate conformational states—an inactive GDP-bound form, and an active GTP-bound form. Only ras–GTP is capable of interacting with target molecules and transmitting signals in mammalian cells. The GDP-bound form is unable to activate a downstream target but can interact with upstream regulatory molecules. Conversion between these active and inactive states is achieved in two ways. The rate-limiting step in the conversion of inactive ras–GDP to the active ras–GTP is the dissociation of GDP from the GDP–protein complex, a reaction catalysed by guanine nucleotide releasing factors (GNRFs) such as Sos. Conversion of the active ras–GTP form to the inactive ras–GDP form and inorganic phosphate is mediated by the slow intrinsic GTPase activity of ras–GTP. This reaction is stimulated by interaction of ras–GTP with the SH2/SH3-containing p120–ras GTPase-activating protein (p120^{rasGAP}) (Fig. 11.4). In good agreement with these biochemical properties, p21^{ras} mutants with enhanced transforming activity exhibit either increased dissociation rates for ras–GDP or reduced GTPase activity.

A link between growth factor signalling and ras was suspected for many years. Stimulation of cells by a variety of growth factors, including insulin, EGF, and PDGF, results in increased levels of ras–GTP. Moreover, microinjection of anti-ras antibody into fibroblasts was found to inhibit PDGF- and EGF-mediated DNA synthesis. Similarly, constitutively high levels of ras–GTP were observed in fibroblasts transformed by oncogenic tyrosine kinases and such transformation could be blocked by microinjection of anti-ras antibodies. Recent data from several laboratories have now established the mechanistic details of a link between growth factor signalling and ras, and the nature of pathways downstream of ras that connect plasma membrane events to transcriptional regulation in the nucleus (Schlessinger 1993). A crucial role in this process is played by the SH2/SH3-containing adaptor protein, GRB-2 (Fig. 11.4). The SH3 domains of GRB-2 are in a complex with proline-rich motifs found on the nucleotide exchange factor, Sos. In contrast, the GRB-2 SH2 domain can bind activated growth factor receptors at autophosphorylation sites within a pTyr–X–Asn phosphotyrosyl-containing motif

(where X denotes any amino acid). As a consequence, GRB-2-associated Sos molecules are translocated to the plasma membrane, placing Sos in proximity to ras. Association between ras and Sos enhances the exchange of GTP for GDP, resulting in activation of ras. It should also be noted that $p20^{rasGAP}$ can also associate with activated growth factor receptors through phosphotyrosyl–SH2 interactions.

The events that follow ras activation have also been mapped in detail. The main downstream effector of ras is the serine/threonine kinase raf-1, the amino-terminal region of which binds selectively to

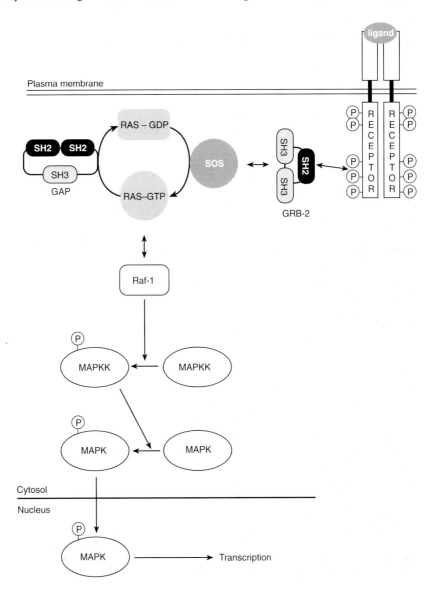

Fig. 11.4 A pathway from the cell surface to the nucleus. The SH2-containing adaptor protein, GRB-2, links ligand-activated receptor tyrosine kinases to the nucleus through activation of the ras-MAPK intracellular signalling pathway.

the GTP-bound form of ras. The resulting membrane localization of raf-1 also leads to its activation, although the precise mechanism remains unclear. Active raf-1 can then phosphorylate its substrate, mitogen-activated protein kinase kinase (MAPKK), initiating a cascade of phospho-transfer reactions. MAPKK is a dual specificity kinase and phosphorylates its substrate, MAPK, at a tyrosine and a threonine residue. In turn, activated MAPK is translocated from the cytoplasm to the nucleus, where it phosphorylates and activates specific transcription factors.

11.4 Oncogenic activation of signalling molecules

Over the last several years it has become clear that perturbation of signalling pathways that regulate normal cell growth is a frequent, and perhaps obligatory, event during the acquisition of the transformed phenotype. The strategies by which this is achieved are many and varied, involving both the subversion of proliferative signalling pathways and the inhibition of negative growth signals. Several oncogenes encode aberrant forms of normal signal transduction proteins, while the oncogenes of some transforming viruses encode distinct proteins that interact directly with components of normal signal transduction pathways.

11.4.1 Oncogenes encoding growth factors

It is now more than a decade since the first direct demonstration that the transforming genes of certain oncogenic retroviruses encode aberrant forms of proteins involved in growth control. This link between oncogene action and the regulation of growth control came from the realization that the amino acid sequence determined for the purified PDGF-B chain shared extensive homology with that predicted from the nucleotide sequence of the v-*sis* oncogene of the acutely transforming simian sarcoma virus (SSV) (Doolittle *et al*. 1983; Waterfield *et al*. 1983). Consistent with the origin of retroviral oncogenes as transduced forms of normal cellular genes, the c-*sis*-B chain protooncogene was subsequently found to encode a functional PDGF-like molecule expressed as a p28^{sis} homodimer. This finding suggested that the reduced requirements of certain transformed and tumour cell lines

for PDGF could be mediated by autocrine production of this factor in these cells. However, the precise mechanism by which autocrine action of v-sis transforms cells is not understood. The issue of whether receptors in this autocrine system are activated at the cell surface or intracellularly, a matter of significance in the design of potential antagonists of such interactions, is unclear. Cell surface interaction may seem unlikely since exogenous PDGF does not induce transformation of cell lines that are susceptible to transformation by v-sis. In good agreement, activated PDGF receptors are located within intracellular compartments in v-sis-transformed cells, whereas endogenous PDGF-A homodimers activate only cell surface forms of the receptor. However, it remains to be established whether such intracellular complexes are functional. Retention of v-sis to the early Golgi complex has been reported to block transforming ability (Hart *et al*. 1994), indicating that the point of autocrine action of this oncogene lies at some point on the secretory pathway distal to the early Golgi complex.

The bovine papilloma virus oncoprotein E5 provides a further example of cellular transformation mechanisms that involve intracellular activation of RTKs. This oncoprotein can cooperate with CSF1R and interacts directly with EGFR, but most commonly utilizes PDGFR. However, the E5 oncoprotein does not directly mimic the normal PDGF ligand, being predominantly an intracellular protein that localizes to the Golgi complex, where it forms complexes with intracellular forms of PDGFR. Recombinant E5 proteins retained in the early ER–cis Golgi are non-transforming, despite the formation of complexes with immature PDGFR, suggesting that transformation in this system also requires intracellular activation of PDGFR at more distal locations in the secretory pathway. For both v-sis and E5, the functionality of such complexes in relation to the location and activation of PDGFR substrates remains to be established.

The potential of growth factor receptor autocrine loops in cellular transformation has also been illustrated by members of the fibroblast growth factor (FGF) gene family. Activation of the *FGF3* locus (identified originally as *int-2*), as a result of proviral insertion, is frequently associated with the occurrence of mammary tumours induced by the mouse mammary tumour virus (MMTV) and can induce mammary gland hyperplasia in transgenic mice. Two further members of the family were identified from human tumour DNA in fibroblast focus formation assays. *FGF4* (also known as *Hst-1*, *KS3*, *kFGF*, or *HSTF1*) was cloned from Kaposi's sarcoma and gastric tumour DNA, while *FGF5* was isolated from bladder tumour DNA. In these cases, however, there is no evidence of a role for these factors in the genesis of the original tumours, and their isolation likely reflects the ability, shared by most members of the FGF family, to induce morphological change to fibroblast cell lines.

11.4.2 Oncogenes encoding mutated growth factor receptors

Soon after the relationship between v-sis and PDGF-B was established, the link between oncogene action and the regulation of growth control was strengthened further by the finding, by similar means, that the v-*erbB* oncogene of avian erythroblastosis virus (AEV) encodes an aberrant form of epidermal growth factor receptor (Downward *et al.* 1984). Subsequently, several other retroviral oncogenes were found to encode mutated forms of distinct members of the receptor tyrosine kinase superfamily, including v-fms, an activated form of CSF-1 receptor; v-kit, derived from the c-kit protooncogene, a receptor for stem cell factor; and v-ros, a mutated receptor tyrosine kinase, the growth factor ligand for which is currently unknown. Other RTKs such as trkA, met, and ret were identified initially as oncoproteins of chemically transformed cells, resulting from genomic translocations involving fusion of RTK sequences with novel unrelated genes.

The structural modifications that can convert protooncogene RTKs to oncogenes are diverse, but common features of such oncogenes include retention of the ability to dimerize and preservation of catalytic activity, concomitant with a loss of negative regulatory elements. This is consistent with the dominant nature of such oncogenes and suggests that the alterations to the receptor may result in the production of ligand-independent signals, which presumably provide misregulated second messenger signals to cells that express the mutated receptor. For the EGF receptor, insertional mutagenesis by avian leukosis virus leads to deletion of the ligand-binding domain resulting in erythroblastosis. Further truncation and mutation of the C-terminus in AEV erbB2 is associated with the generation of sarcomas. Mutations asso-

ciated with retroviral oncogenic activation in v-kit, v-sea (met family) and v-ryk/c-mer (axl family) also involve extensive deletions of extracellular domain coding regions, but additional mutations are required for full transforming activity. These can include activating mutations in nucleotide binding or phosphotransferase domains, and deletion of negative regulatory sites within the carboxy-terminal region.

In the cases of trkA, met, and ret RTKs, oncogenic activation involves chromosomal translocations that result in the expression of cytoplasmic fusion proteins in which extracellular domain regions are deleted but tyrosine kinase catalytic activity is retained. However, deletion of extracellular domains is not sufficient for transforming activity of these protooncogenes, indicating a requirement for novel amino-terminal regions of the fusion proteins in conferring oncogenicity. Consistent with this, sequences of the novel locus, *tpr*, are frequently found in oncogenic fusions involving both trk and met RTKs (Rodrigues and Park 1994). In common with the novel regions of many oncogenic fusion proteins involving protein tyrosine kinase catalytic domains, the *tpr* region encoded in trk and met fusions is predicted to form a coiled-coil structure, a leucine zipper motif in the case of *tpr*. Such structures most likely facilitate constitutive dimerization between oncoprotein molecules.

Oncogenic activation of RTKs can also occur as a result of more subtle mutations. The neu oncoprotein bears a single amino acid substitution in the c-erbB2 RTK in which a valine residue within the transmembrane domain is replaced by glutamate. This mutation confers constitutive receptor dimerization in the absence of ligand and analogous mutations confer ligand-independent activation in EGFR and insulin receptors. For the CSF-1 receptor, two distinct changes are required to form a fully transforming v-fms oncoprotein; firstly, a point substitution in the ligand-binding domain that activates the receptor, and secondly, a truncation at the C-terminus of the kinase domain which seems to remove a negative tyrosine phosphorylation regulatory site.

The examples of oncogenic activation described above have all come from experimental model systems or spontaneous tumours. A role for receptor tyrosine kinase mutations in familial predisposition to cancer has been demonstrated by the identification of germ line mutations in the ret protooncogene receptor tyrosine kinase that are associated with the autosomal dominant cancer syndromes multiple endocrine neoplasia (MEN) 2A and 2B (van Heyningen 1994). Individuals with MEN 2A or familial medullary thyroid carcinoma (FMTC) bear germ line mutations involving amino acid substitutions in one of five conserved cysteine residues within the extracellular domain of the ret RTK. It is likely that such mutations constitute a dominant gain of function since introduction of the most frequent mutations identified, $Cys^{635} \rightarrow$ Arg or Tyr, to normal ret molecules confers constitutive receptor dimerization and activation. Moreover, fibroblasts expressing these mutant receptors are morphologically transformed and produce tumours in xenograft models. Conversely, other germ line mutations in ret that may result in loss of kinase activity, are associated with Hirschprung's disease (HD), a condition not associated with tumorigenesis. Similarly, mice bearing germ line loss of function mutations in ret exhibit phenotypic similarities with HD patients.

MEN 2B patients have been identified that bear a distinct germ line mutation in ret compared with that in individuals with MEN 2A or FMTC, in which Met^{918} is mutated to threonine. This mutation has also been detected in some sporadic medullary thyroid carcinoma patients and is also likely to constitute a dominant gain of function. The occurrence of a threonine residue at this location within catalytic subdomain VIII of other classes of RTK, has led to the suggestion that this mutation in ret may alter its downstream signalling properties. However, the mechanism by which this mutation operates is unknown. How distinct mutations in ret relate to the differing abnormalities associated with MEN 2A, sporadic MTC, and MEN 2B remains to be established.

11.4.3 Oncogenes encoding intracellular signalling proteins

Given the identification of oncogenic forms of growth factors and receptors, it is perhaps not surprising that molecules participating in normal intracellular signal transduction events are also targets for oncogenic mutation. These include cytoplasmic protein tyrosine kinases, SH2/SH3 domain-containing adaptor proteins, and cytoplasmic serine/threonine kinases.

The product of the cellular src gene, $pp60^{c\text{-}src}$, was identified initially in an aberrant form as the onco-

gene v-*src* of a transforming avian retrovirus. $pp60^{c\text{-}src}$ is the prototype of a large family of related intracellular protein tyrosine kinases that contain one SH2, one SH3, and a carboxy-terminal tyrosine kinase catalytic domain. These cytoplasmic kinases can be recruited by activated growth factor receptors, such as the PDGFR, through the formation of a complex between the SH2 domain and specific receptor autophosphorylation sites. In addition, the SH2 domain of $pp60^{c\text{-}src}$ can also directly regulate the catalytic activity of this enzyme, through an intramolecular mechanism (Cantley *et al.* 1991). Tyrosine phosphorylation regulates $pp60^{c\text{-}src}$ activity not only in a positive manner, through autophosphorylation of Tyr^{416} in the catalytic domain, but also in a negative manner by the phosphorylation of Tyr^{527} in the carboxy-terminus of the molecule mediated by a distinct tyrosine kinase, Csk (Fig. 11.5). Phosphorylation of this negative regulatory site, Tyr^{527}, creates a binding site for the SH2 domain of $pp60^{c\text{-}src}$. This intramolecular interaction results in the positioning of the SH3 domain in such a way as to bind to the segment that links the SH2 and catalytic domains. Upon binding this segment adopts a polyproline type II helix (PP-II) conformation. This additional intramolecular binding event keeps the SH3 domain in contact with the small lobe of the kinase domain, thus inhibiting it. Dephosphorylation of Tyr^{527} reverses this series of events allowing autophosphorylation of Tyr^{416} and kinase activation. Further activation can occur by liganding the SH3 domain to an exogenous proline-rich sequence (Pawson 1997) (Fig. 11.5). Several oncogenes are known, which, through various strategies, block this negative regulation of c-src. For example, the v-src oncoprotein retains the catalytic domain but is deleted for Tyr^{527}, resulting in the expression of a constitutively active tyrosine kinase. In contrast, the polyomavirus middle T antigen complexes with normal $pp60^{c\text{-}src}$ in such a way as to prevent Tyr^{527} from becoming phosphorylated, resulting in the formation of a constitutively activated $pp60^{c\text{-}src}$ kinase.

The retroviral oncoprotein v-crk, consisting of one SH3 and one SH2 domain linked to viral gag sequences, may activate $pp60^{c\text{-}src}$ via a similar mechanism. The SH2 domain of v-crk can bind to $pTyr^{527}$, so competing with the c-src SH2 for this site and resulting in c-src kinase remaining in a constitutively active conformation. In turn, oncogenic activation of crk may occur by perturbation of a

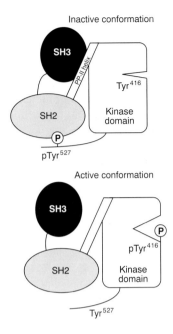

Inactive conformation

Active conformation

Fig. 11.5 Regulation of c-src tyrosine kinase activity. Phosphorylation of c-src residue Tyr^{527}, by Csk, negatively regulates c-src catalytic activity by facilitating an intramolecular phosphotyrosyl–SH2 interaction. Several oncogenes inhibit this negative regulatory reaction, by distinct mechanisms, to create a constitutively active src kinase in transformed cells.

similar negative regulatory event. v-crk differs from its normal cellular counterpart, a typical adaptor signalling protein, by a deletion encompassing an additional SH3 domain and a tyrosine residue (Tyr^{221}) in the linker region between the two SH3 domains. Phosphorylation of Tyr^{221} normally results in an intramolecular association with the SH2 domain of crk, rendering the molecule unable to recognize its targets (Feller *et al.* 1994). It is possible that this kind of intramolecular interaction may be a widespread mechanism of regulation for many SH2 domain-containing molecules.

Finally, it should be noted that although tyrosine phosphorylation plays an important role in signal transduction, serine/threonine kinases can also be directly involved. The v-raf oncoprotein is a mutated form of c-raf, a cytoplasmic serine/threonine kinase that acts in the ras signalling pathway. A further recent example is provided by akt, a widely expressed 55-kDa serine/threonine kinase that bears a catalytic domain, related to the protein

kinase C family, and a PH domain at its amino-terminus. Akt was originally identified as a retro-viral oncogene, v-*akt*, in which the entire normal akt amino acid sequence is expressed as a myristy-lated 105-kDa gag–akt fusion protein and displays a subcellular distribution distinct to that of c-akt. While the mechanism of oncogenic activation of akt is far from clear, recent data have implicated this Ser/Thr kinase as a potential downstream target of the activated PDGF receptor and PI 3-kinase (Franke *et al.* 1995). The activity of akt is stimulated in PDGF-treated cells, but not cells expressing PDGF receptors in which the pTyr residues responsible for recruitment of PI 3-kinase have been mutated. Moreover, inhibitors of PI 3-kinase also prevent activation of akt by PDGF. Interestingly, mutations within the PH domain also abolish the responsiveness of akt to PDGF stimulation, suggesting that the PH domain of akt could be a direct target for the 3′-phosphoinositide products of the PI 3-kinase.

11.5 Signal transduction pathways and cancer

The capacity of signalling proteins to mediate positive and negative growth control signals, together with the known oncogenic properties of some of these molecules, has identified these pathways as areas of major interest with regard to improvements in cancer treatment. Analysis of the expression of signalling proteins in tumours, combined with our understanding of the molecular mechanisms by which perturbed signalling contributes to cellular transformation, is providing a basis for the development of novel therapeutic strategies.

11.5.1 Aberrant expression of signalling molecules in cancers

While much of our current understanding of signalling pathways in oncogenesis has come from studies in experimental systems, both *in vitro* and in animal models, aberrant, or amplified, forms of signal transduction proteins are also frequently associated with human cancers and in some cases may be of prognostic significance.

The definition of distinct germ line mutations in *ret* associated with multiple endocrine neoplasias 2A or 2B, and a proportion of familial medullary thyroid carcinomas, offers the prospect of early identification of individuals within susceptible families that may be predisposed to these cancer syndromes. Currently, this is the only example of an inherited predisposition to cancer involving mutation of an intercellular signalling molecule. A much more common finding is aberrant expression of signalling molecules in patients with established tumours. Consistent with the involvement of *ret* in familial cancer syndromes, genomic rearrangements or point mutations at the *ret* locus have been identified in some sporadic thyroid carcinomas. The EGF receptor is often overexpressed in glioblastomas, breast carcinomas, and cancers of head and neck, pancreas, lung, and ovary. In some cases this is accompanied by production of TGF-α and/or EGF, suggesting potential autocrine signalling in such tumours. In cancers of the breast or ovary, over-expression of EGFR or the *erbB2* protooncogene correlates with poor prognosis, helping to identify individuals for which more aggressive therapy may be appropriate. PDGFR-α expression in ovarian cancers and expression of basic FGF in primary renal cell tumours have also been reported to correlate with poor prognosis in these cancer types.

11.5.2 Oncogenic subversion of signalling pathways

Both TNF and TGF-β have potent growth inhibitory properties and it is clear that several routes to oncogenic activation involve suppression of such activities. For example, overexpression of the receptor tyrosine kinase erbB2 confers resistance to TNF-mediated apoptotic cell death, while the growth inhibitory properties of TGF-β1 are sensitive to blocking by several DNA tumour virus oncoproteins, including SV40 T antigen, HPV16 E7, and adenovirus E1a. Although the molecular mechanisms underlying this inhibition are unclear, it is known that the ability to block TGF-β-mediated growth inhibition is lost in mutant oncoproteins deficient in binding to the retinoblastoma (RB) tumour suppressor. This suggests that TGF-β normally acts through RB, directly or indirectly, to suppress cell growth. A role for tumour suppressors in the growth inhibitory properties of TGF-β signalling is further supported by the finding that in colon carcinoma cell lines, loss of the chromosome containing the DCC tumour suppressor gene (see Chapters 9 and 10) correlates with loss of respon-

siveness to TGF-β-mediated growth inhibition. A similar effect is seen by inhibiting DCC expression by antisense techniques in cells that retain this chromosome. Moreover, a positive correlation exists between loss of responsiveness to TGF-β-mediated growth inhibition and TGF-β production in tumour cells. Thus, the acquisition of mutations that block the growth inhibitory signalling activity of this factor may allow transformed cells to utilize other properties of TGF-β signalling, such as stimulation of angiogenesis and modulation of immune responses, to promote tumour development.

The nature of mutations associated with oncogenic activation of growth factor signalling proteins generally suggests that their roles in cellular transformation reflect modifications of normal functions rather than loss of function mutations. One major role for aberrant growth factor signalling during tumorigenesis may lie in the inhibition of an apoptotic pathway of programmed cell death. While removal of growth factors from normal cells in culture results in the acquisition of a quiescent state, factor withdrawal from cells expressing nuclear oncogenes, such as c-*myc* or adenoviral E1A, results in apoptosis. However, apoptotic-mediated cell death can be blocked in this system by addition of exogenous IGF1 or PDGF (Harrington *et al.* 1994). Such a function would be consistent with the known activation of the IGF1 promoter and increased secretion of IGF1 by SV40 T antigen, and suppression of IGF1R expression by the Wilms' tumour suppressor protein in normal cells.

A direct demonstration of a role for IGF1R-mediated signalling in cellular transformation by certain oncogenes has come from studies using transgenic mouse models. Fibroblasts derived from mice homozygous for a null mutation at the IGF1R locus are refractive to transformation by SV40 T antigen or activated ras (Baserga 1994). A similar observation has been made concerning the HPV E6E7 oncogene and kit receptor tyrosine kinase signalling pathway. A transgenic mouse strain expressing the HPV E6E7 oncogene normally develops Leydig cell tumours of testis at a very high frequency. However, when crossed with Sl^d mice, which bear a loss of function mutation in the kit ligand, SCF, tumour incidence is markedly reduced, suggesting a requirement for signalling through the kit receptor tyrosine kinase in testicular tumorigenesis (Kondoh *et al.* 1995).

Another likely role for RTK-mediated signalling pathways lies in the promotion of tumour angiogenesis. The growth of solid tumours requires neovascularization, and several growth factors that utilize receptor tyrosine kinases, including PDGF, FGF and TGF-α, TGF-β, and TNF-α, are known to have chemotactic and mitogenic effects on endothelial cells *in vitro* (Folkman and Shing 1992). To date, the best candidate mediator of tumour angiogenesis *in vivo* is vascular endothelial growth factor (VEGF), an endothelial cell-specific mitogen for which the receptor tyrosine kinases flk-1 and flt-1 are high affinity receptors. While not expressed in low grade astrocytomas, VEGF is detected in high grade glioblastomas in which vascularization is an important diagnostic feature. Expression of both flk-1 and flt-1 RTKs is up-regulated in endothelial cells associated with the tumour, but not those of normal brain tissue, suggesting a paracrine mechanism for tumour angiogenesis. Further evidence implicating flk-1 in this process comes from use of a recombinant retrovirus expressing a dominant negative form of this RTK. When injected, together with tumour cells, into nude mice, the dominant mutant flk-1 virus confers a marked reduction in glioblastoma tumour size and vascularization (Millauer *et al.* 1994).

11.5.3 Signalling molecules as therapeutic targets

The diverse biological responses evoked by growth factors suggest that modulation of the signalling pathways utilized by these molecules may offer considerable hope for effective treatment of a variety of human disorders, including cancers. As discussed in Chapter 20, the use of cytokines in cancer treatment has focused largely on stimulation of immune responses to tumours and reducing toxicity associated with aggressive chemo/radiotherapy. Experience to date with negative growth regulatory factors, such as TNF, to inhibit tumour growth is not encouraging, perhaps reflecting the multifunctional nature of such factors, which greatly complicates their clinical use. An alternate rational approach to the design of novel antitumour agents is to utilize signal transduction proteins as targets to identify molecules that inhibit aberrant growth factor-mediated signalling pathways associated with cellular transformation and tumour development.

Blocking ligand–receptor interactions The cell surface location of receptor tyrosine kinases, and their frequent overexpression in some tumour types, makes these molecules suitable candidates for monoclonal antibody-directed therapy techniques (see Chapter 19). Monoclonal antibodies against extracellular epitopes of RTKs may also block receptor–ligand interaction, thereby inhibiting RTK-mediated signalling in tumour cells. Overexpression of the EGF receptor in several types of human malignancy (see Section 11.5.1) has made this RTK a target for such strategies, and several monoclonal antibodies raised against the extracellular domain of EGF receptor have been generated that inhibit ligand binding and receptor phosphorylation. Some monoclonals also inhibit the *in vitro* growth and transformation properties of squamous cell carcinoma cell lines that overexpress EGFR, and induce regression of tumours derived from such cells in athymic mouse models. Regression of tumours involves not only the appearance of necrotic areas, but also an increase in infiltrating host cells around tumour foci, suggesting the involvement of host effector functions. Treatment can also result in the appearance of cells expressing differentiated markers within the tumour. Anti-erbB2 monoclonal antibodies have also been found to be effective growth inhibitors of human tumour cell lines that overexpress this RTK when growing as xenografts in nude mice. Radioisotope-conjugated EGFR mouse monoclonal antibodies have been used successfully for tumour imaging in phase I clinical trials of patients with squamous cell lung carcinoma and no significant toxicity effects were reported, despite expression of EGFR in many normal cell types. It would appear that the monoclonal antibodies against RTKs that are most appropriate as potential therapeutic agents are those that block receptor activation, induce terminal differentiation, and activate host immune effector functions. The development of anti-rat or anti-mouse responses in treated patients may be circumvented by the generation of humanized versions of monoclonals directed against epitopes found to be effective in animal models (see Chapter 19). However, in xenograft models not all tumour cells are removed or subject to antibody-mediated growth inhibition, perhaps reflecting antigen modulation or antibody accessibility. An alternative approach, using anti-VEGF monoclonal antibodies to inhibit tumour angiogenesis, has also proved effective in inhibiting the growth of several human tumour cell lines in nude mice (Kim *et al.* 1993).

Efforts have also been made to develop chemical agents that block growth factor–receptor interactions. The polyanion suramin inhibits cell surface interactions between receptor and ligand, although the precise details of its mode of action remain elusive. Unfortunately, this reagent showed high toxicity in patients, and failed to have a significant antitumour effect in phase II trials of renal cell carcinoma patients. However, it may provide a lead for the development of analogues with greater efficacy.

Inhibitors of tyrosine kinase catalytic activity

Given the central role of tyrosine kinase activation in growth factor-mediated signalling pathways, identification and design of chemical agents that specifically block the catalytic activity of protein tyrosine kinases provides an alternative strategy for the development of novel potential antitumour agents.

A number of naturally occurring compounds isolated from fungal extracts act as inhibitors of tyrosine kinase activity, including genistein, herbimycinA, lavendustinA, querticin, and erbstatin. These molecules generally act as competitive inhibitors of ATP and/or non-competitive inhibitors with substrate molecules, but are of little use in themselves since they are broad range inhibitors and are effective only when used at high concentrations. However, they have proved valuable as models in the design of synthetic tyrosine phosphorylation inhibitors, known as tyrphostins, which exhibit greater specificity, activity, and efficacy in inhibiting tyrosine kinase activity and cell growth (Levitzki and Gazit 1995). Compounds are now available that are effective in the nanomolar to picomolar range and several also show marked selectivity of action for particular tyrosine kinases. For example, the quinoxaline tyrphostin AG1296 selectively inhibits the catalytic activity of PDGFR and reverts the transformed phenotype of fibroblasts expressing the v-*sis* oncogene, but not pp60^{src}-transformed cells. The 2-phenylaminopyridine class inhibitor CGP53716 also shows selectivity for PDGFR

and acts as a growth inhibitor of sis-transformed cells in xenograft models. Other tyrphostins are potent selective inhibitors of EGFR autokinase activity *in vitro*, and also show good efficacy *in vivo*, inhibiting the growth of squamous cell carcinoma cells in xenograft mouse models. However, like monoclonal antibodies, the effectiveness of these reagents is seen generally only when given at the time of tumour cell injection and they have little effect on established tumours.

11.6 Abnormal growth control in cancer—a summary

The availability and accurate perception of growth factors is a key regulatory mechanism in the survival and proliferation of normal cells. In contrast, transformed cells have reduced growth factor requirements as a consequence of strategies by which oncogenes misregulate normal growth factor-mediated signalling pathways. This is reflected in the identification of many oncogenes, either as mutated forms of normal signalling molecules, or as proteins that directly, or indirectly, perturb the functions of normal signalling proteins. The apparent requirement for subverted growth factor signalling to facilitate tumour cell survival and proliferation suggests that inhibition of such pathways is of potential therapeutic value in cancer treatment. Detailed knowledge of the molecular mechanisms underlying receptor tyrosine kinase signalling pathways is providing a rational basis for the development of such strategies, and several reagents are available that act as inhibitors of tumour growth, at least in experimental models. In addition to activation of growth stimulatory pathways, oncogenic strategies also involve suppression of negative growth regulatory signals. Major challenges remain, not only in deciphering the intracellular signalling pathways used by negative growth regulators, but also in understanding the molecular interplay between positive and negative growth signals in both normal and abnormal cells.

References and further reading

Baserga, R. (1994). Oncogenes and the strategy of growth factors. *Cell*, **79**, 927–30.

Cantley, L. C., Auger, K. R., Carpenter, C., Duckworth, B., Graziani, A., Kapeller, R., and Soltoff, S. (1991). Oncogenes and signal transduction. *Cell*, **64**, 281–302.

Cleveland, J. L. and Ihle, J. N. (1995). Contenders in FasL/TNF death signalling. *Cell*, **81**, 479–82.

Cohen, G. B., Ren, R., and Baltimore, D. (1995). Modular binding domains in signal transduction proteins. *Cell*, **80**, 237–48.

Doolittle, R. F., Hunkapiller, M. W., Hood, L. E., Devare, S. G., Robbins, K. C., Aaronson, S. A., and Antoniades, H. N. (1983). Simian sarcoma virus onc gene, v-*sis*, is derived from the gene (or genes) encoding platelet derived growth factor. *Science*, **221**, 275–7.

Downward, J., Yarden, Y., Mayes, E., Scrace, G., Totty, N., Stockwell, P., *et al.* (1984). Close similarity of epidermal growth factor receptor and v-*erb*B oncogene protein sequences. *Nature*, **307**, 521–7.

Feller, S. M., Knudsen, B., and Hanafusa, H. (1994). c-Abl kinase regulates the protein binding activity of c-Crk. *EMBO Journal*, **13**, 2341–51.

Folkman, J. and Shing, Y. (1992). Angiogenesis. *Journal of Biological Chemistry*, **267**, 10931–4.

Franke, T. F., Yang, S. I., Chan, T. O., Datta, K., Morrison, D. K., Kaplan, D. R., and Tsichlis, P. N. (1995). The protein kinase encoded by the Akt proto-oncogene is a target of the platelet-derived growth factor (PDGF)-activated phosphatidylinositol 3-kinase (PI 3-kinase). *Cell*, **81**, 727–36.

Harrington, E. A., Bennett, M. R., Fanidi, A., and Evan, G. I. (1994). c-Myc-induced apoptosis in fibroblasts is inhibited by specific cytokines. *EMBO Journal*, **13**, 3286–95.

Hart, K. C., Xu, Y-F., Meyer, A. N., Lee, B. A., and Donoghue, D. J. (1994). The v-sis oncoprotein loses transforming activity when targeted to the early Golgi complex. *Journal of Biological Chemistry*, **127**, 1843–57.

Heldin, C-H. (1995). Dimerisation of cell surface receptors in signal transduction. *Cell*, **80**, 213–23.

Kim, K. J., Li, B., Winer, J., Armanini, M., Gillett, N., Phillips, H. S., and Ferrera, N. (1993). Inhibition of vascular endothelial growth factor-induced angiogenesis suppresses tumour growth *in vivo*. *Nature*, **362**, 841–4.

Kolesnick, R. and Golde, D.W. (1994). The sphingomyelin pathway in tumor necrosis factor and interleukin-1 signalling. *Cell*, **77**, 325–8.

Kondoh, G., Hayasaka, N., Li, Q., Nishimune, Y., and Hakura, A. (1995). An in vivo model for receptor tyrosine kinase autocrine/paracrine activation: auto-stimulated KIT receptor acts as a tumor promoting factor in papillomavirus-induced tumorigenesis. *Oncogene*, **10**, 341–7.

Kuriyan, J. and Cowburn, D. (1993). Structures of SH2 and SH3 domains. *Current Opinions in Structural Biology*, **3**, 828–37.

Levitzki, A. and Gazit, A. (1995). Tyrosine kinase inhibition: an approach to drug development. *Science*, **267**, 1782–8.

Massague, J., Attisano, L., and Wrana, J. L. (1994). The TGF-β family and its composite receptors. *Trends in Cell Biology*, **4**, 172–8.

Millauer, B., Shawver, L. K., Plate, K. H., Risau, W., and Ullrich, A. (1994). Glioblastoma growth inhibited in vivo by a dominant-negative Flk-1 mutant. *Nature*, **367**, 576–9.

Pawson, T. (1997). New impressions of Src and Hck. *Nature*, **385**, 582–5.

Pawson, T. and Schlessinger, J. (1993). SH2 and SH3 domains. *Current Biology*, **3**, 434–42.

Rodrigues, G. A. and Park, M. (1994). Oncogenic activation of tyrosine kinases. *Current Opinion in Genetics and Development*, **4**, 15–24.

Schlessinger, J. (1993). How receptor tyrosine kinases activate ras. *Trends in Biochemical Sciences*, **18**, 273–5.

Shaw, G. (1996). The pleckstrin homology domain: an intriguing multifunctional protein module. *BioEssays*, **18**, 35–46.

Smith, C. A., Farrah, T., and Goodwin, R .G. (1994). The TNF receptor superfamily of cellular and viral proteins: activation, costimulation and death. *Cell*, **76**, 959–62.

van der Geer, P. and Pawson, T. (1995). The PTB domain: a new protein module implicated in signal transduction. *Trends in Biochemical Sciences*, **20**, 277–80.

van der Geer, P., Hunter, T., and Lindberg, R.A. (1994). Receptor protein tyrosine kinases and their signal transduction pathways. *Annual Review of Cell Biology*, **10**, 251–337.

van Heyningen, V. (1994). One gene—four syndromes. *Nature*, **367**, 319–20.

Waterfield, M. D., Scrace, G. T., Whittle, N., Stroobant, P., Johnsson, A., Wasteson, A., *et al.* (1983). Platelet-derived growth factor is structurally related to the putative transforming protein p28^{sis} of simian sarcoma virus. *Nature*, **304**, 35–9.

Stem cells, haemopoiesis, and leukaemia

MEL GREAVES

12.1 Introduction

The leukaemias, and related diseases lymphoma and myeloma, are all blood cell cancers. Because of the accessibility of this tissue, the relative ease of cell culture, and the availability of model systems with animal cells, knowledge of the cellular and molecular basis of these forms of cancer has often led the way and provided paradigms for cancer research in general. Leukaemias are different from other cancers in so far as their evolution and dissemination does not require the angiogenesis, architectural disruption, and metastatic processes that are critically involved in most other cancers. This distinction may, at least in part, account for the clinical sensitivity and curability of many disseminated leukaemias, particularly in children. Despite this important difference, leukaemias provide a particularly informative example of how multistep malignancy can be viewed as a parody or disruption of normal developmental processes. The key cell types in this process are those that serve as founders or stem cells for blood cell production. We refer to this process, overall, as haemopoiesis (or haematopoiesis) and it is often, for experimental or descriptive purposes, subdivided into its two major components, myelopoiesis and lymphopoiesis. The pathology of the leukaemias and associated tumours is described briefly in Chapter 1 (Section 1.10.3) and in detail in Knowles (1992).

12.2 Haemopoietic regulation

Blood cell production is initiated during embryogenesis, in the yolk sac (embryonic erythropoiesis), and

in the embryo body, in the so-called AGM (aorta, gonad, mesonephros) region. Subsequently, both myeloid and lymphoid cell production are housed in the fetal liver (first), bone marrow, and thymus (for T cells). During fetal life, haemopoiesis is seeded and then sustained by blood-borne stem cells. After birth and throughout life, haemopoiesis continues as a rapid and dynamic process in the bone marrow. Cell generation rates are prodigious—more than 10^{11} cells per day. This explosive rate of production can only be accommodated by an equivalent loss of cells.

Studies in mice in which individual cells can be genetically marked by unique (individual) chromosomal sites of retroviral insertion have provided convincing evidence for the existence of a class or population of multipotential stem cells that are the founders for all haemopoiesis. This provides us with the starting point for all haemopoietic lineage tree diagrams as shown in Fig. 12.1.

Within this lineage hierarchy, the different cell types can be distinguished by their phenotypic properties, which include some physical features (size, charge, adhesiveness), morphology (for maturing myeloid cells), enzymes synthesized by the cells, antigenic markers identified with monoclonal antibodies, and particular mRNA molecules expressed. Monoclonal antibodies have been especially important in this respect. Few of these individual properties are unique to any cell type but it is possible to identify *composite* phenotypes that are. The availability of these normal cell type markers has been extraordinarily useful, not only for experimental studies, but for practical, clinical purposes also, includ-

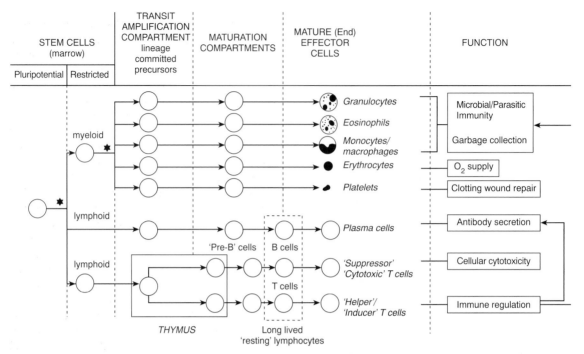

Fig. 12.1 Stem cell lineage hierarchy and cell function in haemopoiesis. The asterisks indicate that our understanding of developmental potentialities and the sequence or pattern of commitment at these apparent 'junctions' in the lineage tree are still very incomplete.

ing differential diagnosis of leukaemia, some therapeutic strategies (e.g. toxin-tagged antibodies, see Chapter 19), and for manipulation of stem cells for gene therapy and/or transplantation purposes.

Stem cells are the most critical cells in haemopoiesis and in other tissues with continual turnover or regenerative capacity. They are also believed to be the major cellular targets for leukaemogenesis. Tissue stem cells are usually defined as cells that have two particular properties (Fig. 12.2). Firstly, they can sustain their numbers after their brief embryological spawning, and throughout the lifelong postnatal period for which they are required. In haemopoiesis at least, this challenge is met by small numbers of stem cells taking turns at proliferation (called clonal succession), while most remain quiescent and out of cell cycle (G0). Also, proliferative cycles of stem cells can generate daughter cells that themselves have stem cell properties and can return to dormancy (so-called self-renewal cycles). Secondly, proliferating stem cells can generate daughter cells that undergo both substantial further cell cycling (referred to as amplification), and differentiation or maturation into functional, mature cells.

The divergent developmental 'options' or fates for a stem cell are illustrated in Fig. 12.2. Note that in addition to proliferation and maturation down a lineage, cells may have to choose to differentiate down one lineage out of several available, or may choose, or be persuaded, to opt out and die. The latter fatality occurs by an active or suicidal process usually referred to as apoptosis or programmed cell death. Apoptosis is a critical component of haemopoiesis helping to maintain, homeostatically, population numbers within appropriate limits, and, additionally in lymphopoiesis, to facilitate the process of stringent clonal selection that occurs both during the production of T and B lymphocytes and in subsequent immune responses. Apoptosis is now recognized as being an essential part of almost all developmental processes and many physiological responses. Two important corollaries are therefore not so surprising. Firstly, that multiple genes, mostly of ancient evolutionary origin as evidenced by studies in yeast and nematode worms, are involved in regulating cell death; and, secondly, that genes involved in apoptosis may be altered or mutated in leukaemia and other cancers. A further and perhaps

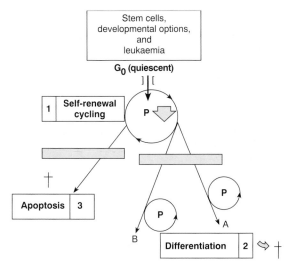

Fig. 12.2 Developmental options for stem cells. Haemopoietic stem cells normally reside out of mitotic cycle (in G_0 or quiescent). When activated to undergo proliferation (P), there are three developmental options: (1) self-renewal, (2) differentiation, and (3) apoptosis or cell death (†). Disruption of any one (or all) of these three pathways by loss of function (▭) or constitutive activation (⩔) can contribute to the development of leukaemia.

less obvious consequence of these developmental arrangements is that changes in the vulnerability to physiological cell death in leukaemic cells may have a major impact on the sensitivity of these cells to the common therapeutic agents that are given to patients (see Section 12.7, and Chapter 17).

12.2.1 Molecular rules of the game

We are still ignorant of some of the basic molecular processes in haemopoiesis, but remarkable insights have been gained in recent years. These are important since they may pin-point and help us to understand the molecular defects underlying leukaemias. With respect to DNA *replication* and *proliferation,* it is clear that the fundamental rules are laid down in a complex, multilayered, genetic circuitry occupied by interacting proteins and enzymes (predominantly kinases and phosphatases). These ground rules are of very ancient evolutionary origin, conserved and shared by different cell types and tissues. Primarily, what differs between cell types, other than some details of the circuit wiring, are the ligands and cor-

responding cellular receptors that regulate the process. In this respect each cell type lives in its own sensory world equivalent to the 'merkwelt' of an animal species! Similarly for *apoptosis,* a basic set of genes encoding particular proteins appears to have been invented early in evolution and, although the circuitry becomes elaborated and refined with further evolutionary developments, the ground rules remain largely intact. For apoptosis, key components for both haemopoietic and other cell types include a family of related proteins including bcl-2, BAX, and BCLx which form complexes that, depending upon their composition or stoichiometry, can impede or facilitate apoptosis. How they achieve this is not understood. Other critical proteins in apoptosis include a number that contribute to a cascade resulting in activation of a protease that degrades other proteins and cellular membranes, plus one or more endonucleases that can break up DNA to give the nucleosomal fragments, DNA-staining profiles, and nuclear morphology that are characteristic of apoptosis in both blood cells and most other cell types.

Differentiation is in one sense a lineage- or cell type-specific process, but even here there is common and evolutionarily conserved territory. The current view is that key differentiation decisions in haemopoiesis (and elsewhere) involve the initiation and stabilization of a unique programme of gene expression. Control of this process exists, in principle, at two levels. Firstly, the genes involved operate in sequential cascades with positive and negative feedback loops exercised by the protein products that they encode. Secondly, selective activation of genes, which is the key to the process, is believed to occur through the dynamic formation of stable transcription complexes. These are heterodimeric or polymeric assemblies of proteins which bind to DNA and, as a consequence, are able to modify chromatin or DNA structure, accessibility, and the enzyme-mediated process of gene transcription. Thirdly, cell surface receptors, interfacing with the cellular environment, regulate the process, often by initiating phosphorylation cascades that modify transcription factor complexes. Cell types in haemopoiesis come to exist and differ in their phenotypes as a consequence of their unique constellations of transcription factors empowered to regulate gene activity positively or negatively. This process is constrained by the ancestry of the cell (i.e. by prior genetic decisions) and is regulated by the cell's unique receptor profile—itself the product of a similar genetic decision making or differentiation process. Finally, as might have been anticipated, the processes of proliferation, differentiation, and apoptosis are integrated into a network as alternative pathways for cell fate. Many of these decisions operate during the G1 phase of the cell cycle and all are modulated or regulated by signals derived by means of cell surface receptors detecting changes in the local environment of the cells. Receptors may be triggered by soluble ligand released either locally or systematically, or by secreted ligands bound and compartmentalized by adjacent stromal cells and/or their cell surface-associated intracellular matrix components, such as heparan sulphate. Heterotypic cell–cell interactions between blood cells and vascular, lymphatic, and tissue stromal cells play a critical role in myelopoiesis and lymphopoiesis, regulating cell fate through the three major pathways alluded to above. In addition they control cell positioning and migration by selective adhesion (Fig. 12.3).

Discovering which particular transcription factors are involved in the derivation of particular cell types is difficult. Biochemical identification of proteins binding to control regions (promoters, enhancers, locus control regions) of genes that have lineage-specific expression (e.g. in haemopoiesis: haemoglobin, immunoglobulin, myeloperoxidase) provides candidates whose function can be further assessed by gene transfection assays. Gene knock-out (by homologous recombination) provides an alternative strategy for identifying essential transcription factors and the developmental stages at which they operate. Figure 12.4 is a summary profile of some of the key players in haemopoiesis identified by the knock-out approach. No doubt, more remain to be discovered and many transcription factors appear to have modulating, non-essential, or redundant functions in haemopoiesis.

12.3 Leukaemia as a clonal disorder of haemopoiesis

In common with other cancers, most leukaemias share a number of salient features (Table 12.1). *Proliferation* is usually continual or constitutive, though not necessarily at a fast rate in terms of cell cycle time. Very often, particularly in the acute leukaemias, *differentiation* appears to be blocked at an early stage of haemopoiesis. Cell death certainly

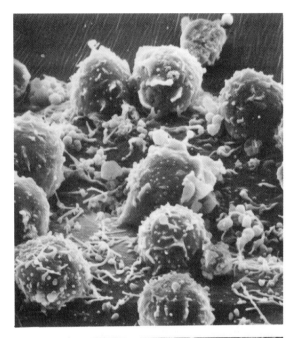
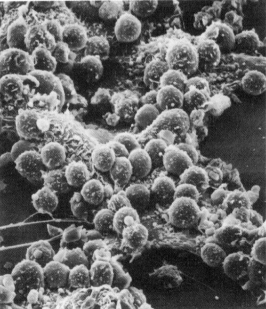

Fig. 12.3 Adhesive interactions with stromal cells regulate early haemopoiesis. Stereoscan electron microscopy images of T cell precursors binding to the surface of thymic epithelial cells. From an *in vitro* culture system believed to mimic developmental cell interactions in the thymic cortex.

occurs in leukaemia cell populations *in vivo* and *in vitro*, but leukaemic cells will often have an

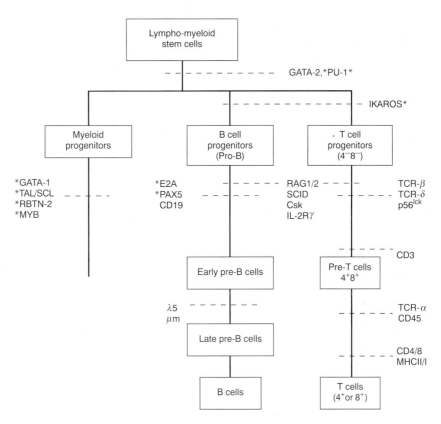

Fig. 12.4 Critical regulators of haemopoiesis can be identified by 'knock-out' experiments. The diagram lists transcription factors (*) or other proteins whose function is required for defined steps in early haemopoietic differentiation (at the level indicated by the cross-bar). Differentiation beyond the level indicated is aborted in transgenic mice in which the gene has been inactivated by homologous recombination.

Table 12.1 Consistent features of leukaemic cells

Monoclonal (single cell) in origin
Acquired gene mutations, visible or invisible by chromosome karyotype
Genetic instability, clonal diversification, and subclone selection
Dysregulation or uncoupling of critical cellular functions—proliferation, differentiation, cell death. Frequent differentiation arrest
Net growth advantages, clonal dominance, extravascular spread, and compromise of normal tissue functions

increased propensity to survive conditions of growth factor deprivation or stress that propel other cells into apoptosis. But first and foremost among these common features of leukaemia is monoclonality and its origin by means of mutation. In common with all but a few exceptional cases, leukaemias and other cancers are clonal diseases driven by mutation, i.e. the leukaemic cells of any one patient all derive from a *single* mutant progenitor cell. The conventional and probably correct interpretation of this feature is that the particular mutations required to give a clone a growth advantage sufficient to produce diag-

nostic symptoms and pathology are exceedingly rare, so rare that they only occur in a single cell amongst the extraordinarily high number of stem cell divisions that occur in a lifetime.

We assume that mutations occur all the time, but that the vast majority occur either in genes that cannot confer growth advantage and/or in irrelevant cells. We know that leukaemias are monoclonal by long-standing observations on chromosome karyotypes and by the application of a number of immunological, enzymatic, and molecular markers for clonal status (Table 12.2). The formation of a leukaemic clone through mutation is not equivalent to the activation of one faulty switch in the genetic circuit. Although one mutation does initiate the process, the resultant clone is seldom stable. Over time it will, in a Darwinian fashion akin to a species, diversify by further genetic change and will be subject to a competitive selection exercised by the body's own regulatory mechanisms or by therapy. This evolutionary process may be gradual or may involve relatively abrupt changes in cellular phenotype, cell behaviour, and disease pathology, as, for

Table 12.2 Markers of common clonal descent in leukaemia

X-linked gene polymorphisms (in females)[1]	
Glucose-6-phosphate dehydrogenase	(G6PD)
Hypoxanthine phosphoribosyl transferase	(HPRT)
Phosphoglycerate kinase	(PGK)
DXS255 locus	(M27β)
Androgen receptor	(HUMARA)
Immunoglobulin and T cell receptor gene rearrangements	
	IGH Igκ, λ
	TCR-α, -β, -γ, -δ
	Idiotypes
Acquired chromosome markers	
	e.g. Ph, t(9;22)(q34;q11)
Acquired molecular/DNA changes	
	e.g. RAS mutations
	MLL gene rearrangements
	p53 mutations
	Viral integration sites (HTLV-1)

[1] These methods all exploit the fact that during embryogenesis, progenitor cells destined to form various tissues, including mesodermal derivatives such as blood, randomly inactivate one of the two parental X chromosomes (the Lyon hypothesis). All descendant cells therefore express genes from one X chromosome, and a normal population of cells or tissue will be a mixture or mosaic of cells expressing either maternally or paternally derived X-linked genes. Differences or polymorphisms is parental and maternal copies of particular genes (alleles) can then be used as markers to determine which copy is active and hence whether a population of cells is polyclonal or derived from a single cell. The tests themselves exploit either electrophoretic mobility of the protein product (G6PD), polymorphism in enzyme restriction sites (HPRT, PGK), or variation in the number of tandem repeats (VNTR, M27β). Tests using HPRT, PGK and M27β as DNA clonal markers need to be adapted to distinguish active from inactive genes (since both alleles will be detected in heterozygous females at the DNA level). This is achieved by the use of restriction enzymes that are methylation-sensitive, exploiting the fact that the 5′ regions of X-linked genes that are expressed, as opposed to silenced, are methylated.

example, in the so-called blast crisis of chronic myeloid leukaemia. The development of leukaemic clones in this respect parallels the invariant feature of progression in cancer most clearly enunciated by the UK pathologist Leslie Foulds whose book on the subject remains a neglected classic. It also parallels what has been observed in experimental systems (e.g. virus-induced chicken erythroleukaemia, transformation of fibroblasts *in vitro*) where synergistic and complementary functions of two different oncogenes are necessary or optimal for malignant

transformation. If, as we suppose, multiple mutations in different genes encoding distinct, but complementary, functions (again as in species evolution) are an invariant or inevitable component of leukaemia, then it follows from the rarity of those events that mutations will be acquired *sequentially* over an unpredictable time period. The products of this dynamic process are successive waves of dominant subclones. These essential and combinational activities were in essence predicted from pathology by Foulds and they set the variable time-frame, pace, and course of disease evolution in terms of preclinical latency, progression, drug resistance, and, for solid tumours, metastasis.

12.4 Gene culprits

From what has been outlined above on the regulation of haemopoiesis, an astute student should have no difficulty in predicting what kinds or sets of genes would be involved in leukaemia as mutants. In principle, any gene that, when mutated, can give a clone a *net* growth advantage, can initiate and/or contribute to progression of disease. Since clonal population dynamics are determined by the interplay and balance of proliferation, differentiation, and cell death, it follows that lesions in any or each of these three circuits may participate in leukaemogenesis (Fig. 12.2). Furthermore, in view of their complementary functions, it is not surprising that single leukaemic clones, as they evolve to more aggressive phenotypes, may acquire mutations in two or all three of these circuits. Indeed, acquisition of a complementary set of mutations may not only be advantageous to the clone, but essential for its survival, if, as is currently believed, mutations in some oncogenes (e.g. c-*myc*) promoting constitutive proliferation simultaneously drive apoptosis when essential growth factors are limiting.

Although these pathological patterns are entirely predictable from first principles, it is only because the mutant genes have been cloned and sequenced and their protein functions uncovered in either a normal or abnormal context that we can present this scenario with some confidence. Table 12.3 categorizes some of the major gene alterations in leukaemia, their structural basis, the functions of their protein products, and leukaemia subtype associations. Note that some of these genes are involved in many forms of cancer (for example, as cell cycle regulators) and that others have leukaemia or leukaemia subtype specificity because of the functions they encode (e.g. differentiation regulation) and/or because of the other genes they fuse with (e.g. immunoglobulin or T cell receptor). Such a list illustrates the major genetic pathways involved in leukaemia, but it inevitably understates the remarkable diversity of mutation that can occur. For example, in one subtype of leukaemia, acute lymphoblastic leukaemia (the major cancer in children), over 200 different genetic abnormalities have been described; most are, however, relatively rare. This degree of diversity arises, we assume, because of the multiple points in the three control circuits that are rate limiting or able to perturb cell kinetics. Some changes are, however, much more common than others and these are the ones that have major clinical implications (see below).

The remarkable consistency with which some of these genetic lesions are associated with subtypes of leukaemia implies that they are critical if not essential components of the causal pathway of leukaemogenesis. The best evidence to support this comes from the demonstration that these same human leukaemia-associated genes, when cloned and transferred into the mouse germ line or into haemopoietic stem cells, generate biologically similar leukaemias in offspring or transplant recipients, respectively.

12.5 Origin of mutations and the natural history of leukaemia

Virtually all the described mutations in leukaemia are non-constitutive or acquired. They are assumed to arise either pre- or post-natally as a consequence of either random errors in DNA replication and recombination, perhaps under conditions of proliferative stress, or as a consequence of genotoxic exposure. Different leukaemias may well have distinct aetiologies in this respect and there is considerable epidemiological evidence to support the involvement of a variety of pathways or agents, including ionizing radiation, chemicals, and microbial infection (see Chapters 6–8 and references given at the end of this chapter).

Except in rare cases of known medical or industrial/occupational exposure that result in leukaemia after a period of some years, or even a decade or two, we have little insight into the detailed natural history of leukaemia. When, for example, do particular mutations occur in relation to the clinical emergence and diagnosis of disease? A rare exception to this state of uncertainty is in infant leukaemia. Here a particular gene (*MLL*) encoding an important transcription factor, related to the *Drosophila* developmental gene, *trithorax*, is involved in most cases. Rearrangements of this 'promiscuous' oncogene involving fusions with any one of very many (>25) partner genes are not constitutive and so, as in other cancers of very young children, one would anticipate that the mutation is acquired by the fetus *in utero*. Studies using *MLL* gene mutations as unique clonal markers in identical twin infants with leukaemia have shown that this is indeed the case (Ford *et al.* 1993). Intriguingly, similar rearrangements of the *MLL* gene are common in patients who, tragically, develop acute leukaemia as a consequence of prior exposure to cancer treatment with drugs (e.g. etoposide/VP-16) that operate through inhibition of the enzyme topoisomerase II (topo II). This enzyme is ubiquitously involved in the controlled breakage and resealing of DNA that is necessary to prevent tangling during DNA replication. Most drugs binding to topo II stabilize DNA in the form of a cleavable complex that usually precipitates apoptosis but could also result in inappropriate rejoining of broken DNA, resulting in the birth of illegitimate gene fusions as seen in *MLL* gene-associated leukaemias. These considerations have prompted current epidemiological studies on possible pregnancy exposures that might similarly compromise topo II activity and initiate leukaemogenesis.

Although most mutations characteristic of leukaemia and its subtypes are acquired rather than inherited, this does not rule out a contribution of inherited genetics to leukaemia aetiology. Firstly, a number of rare genetic syndromes involving chromosomal or DNA instability are associated with a very high risk of leukaemia (see Chapter 4). Secondly, inherited genetic factors may contribute indirectly to leukaemogenesis. There is evidence, for example, that genes in, or linked to, the HLA system are associated with an increased risk of leukaemia, and this has been interpreted as supporting an infectious aetiology.

12.6 Target cells in leukaemia

The morphology, immunophenotype, and mutant genes in leukaemic subsets provide an indication of the lineage and cell type that has been clonally selected in the disease. This information has, in principal, provided the framework for differential haematological and pathological diagnosis for almost a century, albeit with many biological refinements over the past two decades. But how does the leukaemic phenotype relate, developmentally within haemopoiesis, to the single 'target' cell whose transformation must have initiated clonal expansion and subsequent leukaemia evolution? Factors that need to be taken into account include the stringency of differentiation arrest and the possibility that some mutant genes may directly or indirectly produce an aberrant or misleading developmental phenotype.

The phenotype of leukaemic clones may generally reflect the developmental level or window of maturation arrest within the haemopoietic hierarchy. However, both the minority clonogenic stem cells driving or sustaining the disease, and the cell type that was initially transformed by mutation can lie anywhere antecedent or 'upstream' of the maturation arrest position. More insight can be gained into this issue by physical separation of clonogenic cells by means of their cell surface antigenic properties and such experiments have usually indicated that these cells have a more primitive phenotype than the bulk of their progeny, which must therefore undergo at least limited differentiation. Another strategy to identify the developmental level of clonal expansion is to evaluate, independently of the bulk population phenotype, what lineages contribute to the leukaemic population, as judged by a shared clonal marker. For this purpose, cells belonging to different lineages must be identified or sorted with appropriate markers (usually monoclonal antibodies) and then interrogated for the presence of one or more of the chromosomal or molecular markers that are available as indicators of common clonal descent (Table 12.2). When this type of analysis is performed, it is clear that many acute leukaemias, in which the population phenotype is dominated by one lineage or cell type, do, in fact, originate in dual or multilineage stem cells, with growth advantage and/or differentiation competence into different lineages being selectively expressed. The clearest example of this is with chronic myeloid leukaemia which has an overwhelmingly granulocytic lineage phenotype, but a multipotential lymphomyeloid stem cell origin (Fig. 12.5).

An interesting biological complication in these analyses is that leukaemic blast cells not infrequently appear to switch lineage during evolution or progression of disease, or may simultaneously express several markers indicative of different lineages—so-called lineage infidelity. The former phenomenon is explained in terms of a multipotential stem cell origin with different progeny cells having distinct differentiation potentials and acquiring preferential growth advantage at separate time points in the evolution of the disease. Again, the clearest example of this is with chronic *myeloid* leukaemia evolving into an acute phase of blast crisis in which the bulk or dominant population is now a subclone with immature *lymphoid* characteristics (Fig. 12.5). Simultaneous dual or multilineage gene expression of individual leukaemic cells has proved more of a puzzle to resolve. One view (*lineage infidelity*) is that mutant genes, e.g. hybrid or fused transcription factors, not only produce a partial differentiation block, but do this in part by corrupting differentiation signals leading to abortive entry into more than one lineage, or ectopic expression of inappropriate genes within a single lineage. This is certainly a possibility, although evidence supporting this position is limited to experiments in which cells committed to the B cell lineage can be converted into macrophages. An alternative interpretation (which I favour) is that normal multipotential stem cells have an inherent capacity for dual or multilineage gene expression prior to lineage commitment and that this property is amplified by differentiation arrest coupled with continual self-renewal in transformed stem cells. Recent evidence with normal murine stem cells supports this view of *lineage promiscuity*, but probably both mechanisms proposed contribute to leukaemic phenotypes.

Despite these complications and caveats, it is possible to draw up a lineage map that identifies the likely developmental origins of different types of blood cell cancers (Fig. 12.6). This analysis suggests that three 'tiers' of stem cell at risk exist in leukaemia and related disease: multipotential stem cells, lineage-restricted stem cells, and mature lymphoid stem cells. It is likely, though not formally proven, that most leukaemias and other cancers involve tissue stem cells responsible for embryonic morphogenesis (the paediatric tumours) or for sustained turnover (or regenerative capacity) in lymphomyeloid tissues, epithelial tissues, and endocrine organs. Mature lymphoid stem cells are, however, unusual. Despite being highly differentiated, they retain self-renewing stem cell properties and

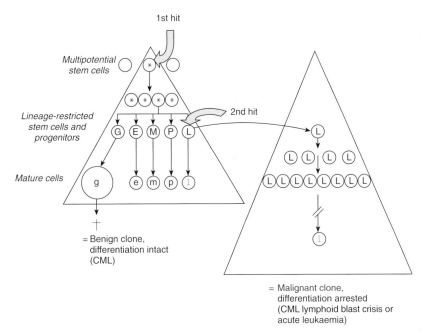

Fig. 12.5 Variable differentiation block and multilineage involvement and progression in stem cell leukaemia. Ph chromosome (bcr–abl)+ chronic myeloid leukaemia given as an example. First hit (mutation) (⊙), assumed to be the Ph chromosome formation. All cells within the left triangle are members of a single clone; subclones forming blast crisis (as a result of additional or second hit) are in the triangle on the right. Abbreviations: G/g = progenitor and mature granulocytic cells; E/e = progenitor and mature erythroid cells; M/m = progenitor and mature macrophage cells; P/p = megakaryocytic progenitors and platelets; L/l = progenitor and mature lymphoid cells.

may benefit from a decade or more life span (as a clone or as individual cells residing out of cycle) with extensive proliferative potential and differentiation competence, i.e. cytotoxic T cell function or antibody secretion (see Chapters 16 and 18). There are sound reasons of immunological economy why we should preserve, for a long time, clones of cells with a memory of antigenic or infectious exposure, but this arrangement does pose an unusual risk to mature cells that is seldom, if ever, found in other tissues that do not normally indulge in clonal selection and conservation.

Considerations of precise cellular origins may seem somewhat esoteric, but they do have practical implications. Clonogenic cells residing at the various developmental levels have different inherent sensitivities to cancer drugs and radiation. Attempts to purge leukaemic clones using differentiation-linked markers (e.g. antibody), either as a purging agent or as an indicator of efficacy of other agents, require that we can identify the position of most or all clo-ˈ nogenic leukaemic cells within the haemopoietic hierarchy.

12.7 Clinical and epidemiological implications of leukaemic cell and molecular biology

The remarkable insights that have been acquired into both normal haemopoiesis and leukaemia over recent years have found some immediate practical applications and have potentially profound implications for future clinical and epidemiological endeavours. Some of these applications and concepts merit special mention. Firstly, the molecular changes that drive the disease now provide specific diagnostic markers for disease subtypes. We already know for some of these, e.g. *bcr–abl*, *MLL* gene fusions and p53 alterations, that, independently of other features of disease, they have a strong association with very poor prognosis in the

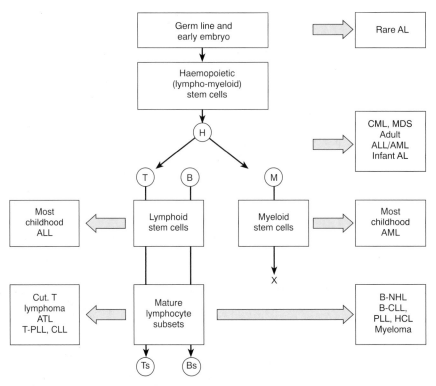

Fig. 12.6 Developmental origins of human blood cell cancers. The diagram illustrates a simplified haemopoietic lineage of the three major developmental stages (of stem cells) at which blood cell cancers may arise (arrow). Abbreviations: ALL = acute lymphoblastic leukaemia; AL = acute leukaemia; AML = acute myeloblastic leukaemia; CML = chronic myeloid leukaemia; CLL = chronic lymphocytic leukaemia; PLL = prolymphocytic leukaemia; HCL = hairy cell leukaemia; ATL = adult T cell leukaemia; MDS = myelodysplastic syndromes (preleukaemic clonal disorders of myelopoiesis with a high probability of evolving to AML); cut T = cutaneous T (lymphoma); H = haemopoietic stem cells; T = thymic or T lineage restricted stem cells; B = B lineage restricted stem cells; Ts = mature T cell subsets; Bs = mature B cell subsets; X = dead end of maturing myeloid cells.

context of currently applied therapeutic cocktails and regimes. Such cases are therefore being routinely identified and selected when possible for alternative therapies; for example, intensified chemotherapy and/or subsequent normal stem cell transplantation. Secondly, the molecular markers provide not only very *specific*, but very *sensitive*, clonal markers when identified using appropriate technology such as fluorescence *in situ* hybridization of interphase cells (i.e. cells without visible dividing, metaphase chromosomes), or, more especially, quantitative polymerase chain reaction (PCR)-based methods that can detect 10^{-4}–10^{-6} leukaemic cells. These latter methods have already provided clonal data that is predictive of the subsequent clinical course (i.e. continued remission or

relapse) for groups of patients and it is likely that in the future PCR will be used as an important aid to patient management guiding continuation, modification, or cessation of therapy.

Thirdly, and perhaps most significant, are the applications and implications for therapy itself. Somewhat contrary to pharmacological theory and expectations, it turns out that most cancer treatment agents, including genotoxic radiation and drugs, metabolic inhibitors, and corticosteroids eliminate leukaemic and other cancer cells, not by metabolic poisoning or direct toxic effects, but by eliciting suicidal apoptosis. From this follows a crucial consequence. As alluded to above, many genetic lesions in leukaemia and cancer effectively block apoptosis as a component of clonal advantage. An anticipated by-product of this function is that leukaemic cells can withstand therapeutic insults that would normally be lethal. Among the leukaemia-associated mutations that have this capacity (Table 12.3) are bcl-2 by rearrangement with *IgH* genes (the prototype example); bcr–abl kinase in Ph$^+$ leukaemias (CML and ALL), which has multiple functions including growth promotion, adhesion modulation, and apoptosis inhibition; and, most prominently in leukaemia, other blood cell malignancies, and cancer overall, p53. Not only does abnormal expression of these gene products rescue cells from apoptosis, but it may also facilitate the survival and future propagation of new mutants induced by the therapy itself, which damages DNA. These and other considerations suggest that the manipulation of apoptosis

should be a priority for future therapeutic research. The mutant genes and their mRNA or protein products provide an obvious specific 'Achilles heel' for therapeutic attack and much current work in both academic institutes and biotechnology companies is directed towards this goal.

Finally, the identification of unique molecular aberrations in particular leukaemias and lymphomas may aid epidemiological investigations into aetiological or causal mechanisms. We know that the causation of blood cell cancer can involve ionizing radiation, chemicals such as benzene, and, in two cases at least, viruses—HTLV-1 in adult T cell leukaemia (Fig. 12.7) and EBV in Burkitt's lymphoma. The cause(s) of most cases of leukaemia remain unknown although recent research has strongly,

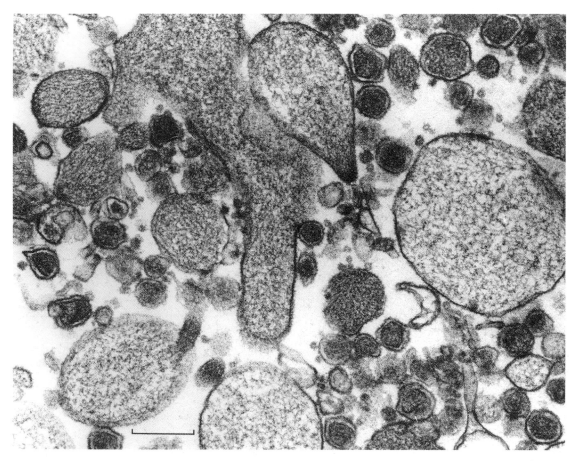

Fig. 12.7 Electron micrograph of human lymphotrophic retrovirus, HTLV-1 particles that are a critical component of the causal mechanism in adult T cell leukaemia. Horizontal bar = 0.2 mm. This form of leukaemia is relatively rare world-wide but is more common in regions where virus infection is endemic, e.g. Southern Japan, the Caribbean region, and South America (see Chapter 8).

Table 12.3 Diversity of molecular changes in leukaemia and related blood cell cancers

Abnormality/Genes	Function	Leukaemia/lymphoma subtype
Reciprocal chromosomal translocations		
(a) Dysregulation by juxtaposition to *TCR*-α, -β, -δ or *IgH*		
IgH–MYC	P	Burkitt's lymphoma
IgH–BCL-6	T	Diffuse (B) lymphoma
IgH–BCL-2	A	Follicular (B) lymphoma
TCR-δ–RBTN-1	T	T-ALL
TCR-β–HOX11	T	T-ALL
(b) Unique product by gene fusion		
BCR–ABL	P/A	CML, ALL
TEL–AML1	T	Bp ALL
AML1-ETO	T	AML
*PML–RARA*α	T	APML
Chromosomal deletions		
(a) Loss of function		
9p-(CDK4 INHIBITOR?)	P	ALL
5q-(?)	(?)	AML
(b) Hybrid gene formation		
TAL del = *SIL–TAL1* FUSION	T	T-ALL
Chromosomal inversions		
(a) Dysregulation by juxtaposition		
INV14 = TCR–TCL-1	T	T-CLL
(b) Unique product by gene fusion		
*INV16 = MYOSIN(MYH11)-CBF*β	T	AML
Ploidy changes		
Hyperdiploidy	?	Bp ALL
		Myeloma
+8		}AML
−7		
Point mutations		
N-*RAS*	P/A	Most subtypes
p53	P/A	Most subtypes

[1] P, proliferation regulation; T, transcriptional regulation of differentiation; A, apoptosis regulation; ALL, acute lymphoblastic leukaemia; AML, acute myeloblastic leukaemia; APML, acute promyelocytic leukaemia; T-ALL, thymic acute lymophoblastic leukaemia, Bp ALL, B cell precursor acute lymphoblastic leukaemia; CLL, chronic lymphocytic leukaemia; CML, chronic myeloid leukaemia.

albeit indirectly, implicated infection in childhood leukaemia and (as mentioned above) maternal–fetal exposures during pregnancy for infant leukaemia. It is unlikely that all leukaemias or lymphomas, or even large subgroups of these diseases, share a single common aetiology as suggested by the disease subtype associations of benzene (AML) HTLV-1 (mature CD4$^+$ T cell subset) and EBV (mature B subset). Defining molecular subtypes in the context of large-scale epidemiological studies is currently underway in the UK and US and is likely to pay dividends.

References and further reading

Adams, J. M. and Cory, S. (1991). Transgenic models of tumor development. *Science*, **254**, 1161–7.

Berardi, A. C., Wang, A., Levine, J. D., Lopex, P., and Scadden, D. T. (1995). Functional isolation and characterization of human hematopoietic stem cells. *Science*, **267**, 104–8.

Cleary, M. L. (1991). Oncogenic conversion of transcription factors by chromosomal translocations. *Cell*, **66**, 619–22.

Fisher, D. E. (1994). Apoptosis in cancer therapy: crossing the threshold. *Cell*, **78**, 539–42.

Ford, A. M., Ridge, S. A., Cabrera, M. E., Mahmoud, H., Steel, C. M., Chan, L. C., and Greaves, M. F. (1993). In utero rearrangements in the trithorax-related oncogene in infant leukaemias. *Nature*, **363**, 358–60.

Foulds, L. (ed.) (1995). *Neoplastic development.* Academic Press, London.

Greaves, M. F. (1986). Differentiation-linked leukaemogenesis in lymphocytes. *Science*, **234**, 697–704.

Greaves, M. F. (1993a). Stem cell origins of leukaemia and curability. *British Journal of Cancer*, **67**, 413–23.

Greaves, M. F. (1993b). A natural history for pediatric acute leukaemia. *Blood*, **82**, 1043–51.

Greaves, M. F. (1997). Aetiology of acute leukaemia. *Lancet*, **349**, 344–9.

Hall, P. A. and Watt, F. M. (1989). Stem cells: the generation and maintenance of cellular diversity. *Development*, **106**, 619–33.

Henderson, E. S., Lister, T. A., and Greaves, M. F. (1996). *Leukemia.* W. B. Saunders Company, Philadelphia.

Kinlen, L. J. (1995). Epidemiological evidence for an infective basis in childhood leukaemia. *British Journal of Cancer*, **71**, 1–5.

Knowles, D. (ed.) (1992) *Neoplastic haemopathology.* Williams and Wilkins, Baltimore.

Linet, M. S. (ed.) (1985). *The leukemias: epidemiological aspects.* Oxford University Press, Oxford.

Long, M. W. and Wicha, M. S. (ed.) (1993). *The hematopoietic microenvironment: the functional and structural basis of blood cell development.* The Johns Hopkins University Press, Baltimore.

Magrath, I. T. (ed.) (1994). *The non-Hodgkin's lymphomas.* Edward Arnold, London.

Metcalf, D. (1993). Hematopoietic regulators: redundancy or subtlety? *Blood*, **82**, 3515–23.

Müller-Sieburg, C. E. and Deryugina, E. (1995). The stromal cells' guide to the stem cell universe. *Stem Cells*, **13**, 477–86.

Nunez, G., Merino, R., Grillot, D., and Gonzalez-Garcia, G. (1994). Bcl-2 and Bcl-x: regulatory switches for lymphoid death and survival. *Immunology Today*, **15**, 582–8.

Oltvai, Z. N. and Korsmeyer, S. J. (1994). Checkpoints of duelling dimers foil death wishes. *Cell*, **79**, 189–92.

Pfeffer, K. and Mak, T. W. (1994). Lymphocyte ontogeny and activation in gene targeted mutant mice. *Annual Review of Immunology*, **12**, 367–411.

Pui, C., Crist, W. M., and Look, A. T. (1990). Biology and clinical significance of cytogenetic abnormalities in childhood acute lymphoblastic leukaemia. *Blood*, **76**, 1449–63.

Rabbitts, T. H. (1994). Chromosomal translocations in human cancer. *Nature*, **372**, 143–9.

Stamatoyannopoulos, G., Nienhuis, A. W., Leder, P., and Majerus, P. W. (ed.) (1994). *The molecular basis of blood diseases.* W. B. Saunders Company, Philadelphia.

Tomei, L. D. and Cope, F. O. (ed.) (1991). *Apoptosis: the molecular basis of cell death. Current communications in cell molecular biology.* Cold Spring Harbor Laboratory Press, New York.

Zucker-Franklin, D., Greaves, M. F., Grossi, C. E., and Marmont, A. M. (1988). *Atlas of blood cells function and pathology.* E. Ermes Publishers, Milan.

13

The molecular pathology of cancer

NICHOLAS R. LEMOINE AND GORDON W. H. STAMP

13.1 Introduction

Tumours are classified by their site of origin and their appearance under the microscope, the latter being a product of the neoplastic cells and their induced mesenchymal stromal elements (see Chapter 1). Over the years much effort has been expended in the standardization of the morphological analysis and classification of tumours to facilitate scientific study and, more importantly, selection of treatment. In the last twenty years, routine morphological examination has been extended by the application of biochemical, immunochemical, and nucleic acid techniques to whole cells or tissue sections. For example, labelled antibodies can be used to identify distinct antigens or antigen profiles on neoplastic cells allowing more sophisticated classification. Cytoarchitectural features reflect the genetic alterations that have occurred in the neoplastic cells, and we are now in an era where analysis of the DNA and mRNA from tumours can be performed on conventional tissue sections. These techniques will allow a more sophisticated analysis of cellular structure and function.

13.2 Morphological analysis of tumour tissue

The accuracy and relevance of molecular and cellular biological analysis is critically dependent on both accurate morphological classification and on selection of appropriate material.

13.2.1 Preparation and processing of tissues and cells

Optimal analysis of samples from human patients can only be undertaken if they are correctly handled. Fixation is the process whereby the structure of the cells and tissues is preserved to stabilize them for subsequent microscopy. In tissues this is generally done either by cross-linking the protein structure with fixatives such as formalin or by precipitating proteins with alcohol-based fixatives such as methacarn. Next, the sample is processed to remove lipids and dehydrate the tissue so that it can then be impregnated with paraffin wax for light microscopy, or in resin for ultrastructural study. Once the tissue is embedded in paraffin wax, it can then be cut on a microtome to produce a thin section of 3–4 μm, which is then counterstained conventionally with an acidic and a basic dye such as haematoxylin and eosin (H&E) which will highlight the nucleus and cytoplasm as well as showing up the extracellular matrix. Thinner sections can be cut from resin-embedded tissue for fine detail and for electron microscopy.

The tissues can also be snap-frozen in liquid nitrogen, which gives them sufficient rigidity for a slightly thicker section to be taken on a cryostat. Frozen tissue stored at $-80°C$ or in liquid nitrogen is also useful in that it is easier to extract nucleic acids from such tissue than from paraffin-embedded material, even though the latter can be analysed by use of techniques such as reverse transcription-polymerase chain reaction RT-PCR (see 13.5.1). In addition, some antigens that can be detected by immunohistochemistry can be better preserved using different fixatives. Fixation of samples in several different fixatives broadens the scope of potential investigation.

Cytopathology has an increasing role in the diagnosis of human tumours because it is now possible to place a needle into virtually any site in the human body with remarkable accuracy using advanced radiological techniques employing CT (computerized tomography) scanning, ultrasound, and nuclear magnetic resonance (NMR). Suction can be applied to a fine bore needle placed in a relatively inaccessible tumour and cells aspirated from it. For cytological analysis, the cells can either be fixed in alcohol or allowed to dry rapidly on a glass slide which enables the cells to adhere strongly. Fine needle aspiration biopsy offers considerable benefits in terms of cost and patient morbidity compared with open surgical biopsy, and it is possible to make an immunohistochemical analysis on the aspirated cells.

13.2.2 Morphological analysis by light microscopy

In most human tumours, histopathologists can establish an accurate diagnosis by looking at the H&E section. Subclassification of tumours along the lines outlined in Chapter 1 is mainly performed using conventional stains but, within each subset of tumours, even more complex classifications can be made by specialists. In certain cases, less common tumours, which have a better or worse clinical behaviour, can be identified and this may well modify the selection of therapy. In cases where there is limited

material, a rare or unusual tumour, or perhaps one that is poorly differentiated, other techniques such as histochemistry, immunohistochemistry, and, to a lesser extent, electron microscopy may be used.

13.2.3 Grading systems

As well as classifying and subclassifying tumours, morphological analysis can also give some prediction of behaviour based on the organization and appearance of the neoplastic cells themselves (see also Chapter 1). There are several systems to grade tumours which take into account a set of criteria that need to be highly reproducible between observers. This produces a fairly coarse subdivision, usually into groups of three or four, ranging from the best differentiated to the worst differentiated. These can then be compared with their clinical behaviour when adjusted for age, size, treatment, etc. One of the most familiar is the modified Scarff, Bloom, and Richardson grading system for breast cancer, which takes three parameters: (a) degree of tubule formation, (b) cellular pleomorphism, and (c) number of mitoses per unit area. This grading system has some clinical utility and is reasonably reproducible between different pathologists. Nevertheless, such a division serves to identify additional prognostic factors or markers within each subgroup. Other grading systems exist for different tumours, each having their own set of defined criteria.

Conventional morphological analysis identifies the type and subtype of tumour, the size, grade, and stage of progression; treatment selection is often based, at least initially, on these parameters. In the future, more defined information especially from biochemical, immunological, and genetic techniques applied at the cellular level will allow increased reproducibility and greater relevance of morphology to the biological behaviour of a cancer, by placing the molecular aberrations in the context of morphological subsets.

13.2.4 Histochemistry

Conventional histochemistry is an established but often neglected aspect of tumour diagnosis. As well as acidic and basic proteins, conventional histochemistry can highlight mucin subtypes which may be tumour specific, extracellular matrix components such as reticulin and interstitial collagen, muscle fibres, glycogen, and certain pigments, e.g. melanin, which can more accurately identify or subclassify a tumour. Neuroendocrine tumours (see Chapter 15) can be stained by a silver precipitation technique (Grimelius' stain) which highlights the dense core granules that typify these tumours. These can also be identified using electron microscopy, but this is a more time consuming and expensive option. Histochemistry is particularly useful for demonstrating the stromal architecture of a tumour by highlighting extracellular matrix structures and often the extent of spread.

13.3 Immunohistochemistry and immunocytochemistry

Immunohistochemistry (IHC) has had a major impact on the practice of histopathology. In principle, tissue sections or cell smears are treated with an antiserum to a specific protein and the binding site is identified by a marker which may be a coloured or fluorescent dye, a heavy metal (especially for electron microscopy), a radioactive label, or an enzyme. Markers are usually attached to the antibodies and may be visualized directly or by a subsequent reaction to identify the marker (see Chapters 16 and 19 and Colvin *et al.* 1996 for a fuller discussion). The technique allows the recognition of individual antigens on tissues and cells, which reflect both structural and functional features. From a practical aspect, the ability to recognize a poorly differentiated tumour or a few cells in a less than optimal sample enables an accurate diagnosis to be made. For instance, many high grade lymphomas were undoubtedly misdiagnosed as anaplastic carcinomas before the advent of immunohistochemistry. Since the response of high grade lymphomas to treatment is now very good, this is a critical distinction to make and relatively straightforward using a small panel of antibodies that recognize lymphoid-restricted antigens such as leucocyte common antigen or B and T cell markers on the cell surface or epithelial cell markers such as cytokeratin, epithelial membrane antigen, and epithelial glycoprotein. If necessary, a further subset of more restricted antigens can either confirm a tentative diagnosis or subclassify a tumour even further. This can be important as many tumours actually lose their high differentiation antigen during progression and may only retain a limited detectable phenotype.

Detection of certain antigens is highly dependent on fixation and processing, and the availability of multifixed tissues is valuable. The choice of an immunohistochemical or immunocytochemical technique depends on the location and nature of the target antigen. If, for instance, a fine linear target such as a membrane-associated or extracellular matrix component such as basement membrane requires highlighting, an immunoenzyme technique with a strong coloured label is ideal. Immunofluorescent techniques will also localize antigens that might be missed on transmitted light because of their low level or where the tissue is highly complex. On the other hand, if a particular target is poorly preserved after processing, or is present in a low amount, various amplification techniques can be used. This can be a help in looking for low abundance antigens in poorly differentiated cells or where there is a small amount of product in the cell, e.g. a secreted peptide or hormone. Immunohistochemical analysis can be performed in many ways. Some antigens can be uncovered by prior digestion of the sections with enzymes that will break certain protein linkages and expose the target epitope. Surprisingly, microwave treatment of sections that are boiled in a citrate buffer for a few minutes can allow detection of certain antigens hitherto only demonstrable on frozen sections.

Amplification techniques, while very useful to detect some low abundance antigens, can have problems in enhancing so-called non-specific staining from related molecules, or perhaps identifying a low level of a normal product constitutively expressed. For example, highly sensitive techniques combined with microwave treatment can reveal p53 immunoreactivity in both neoplastic and non-neoplastic cells, detecting both mutated and non-mutated product (see below).

13.3.1 Immunohistochemical analysis and tumour classification

Immunohistochemical analysis may allow the subclassification of tumours with a considerable degree of accuracy, where morphological diagnosis is unclear. The initial screen would use a broad range of differentiation antigens to classify tumours into epithelial, mesenchymal, and lymphoreticular/haemopoietic lineages, and, within these broad groups, sequentially subclassify with increasingly restrictive panels of antigens to determine the phenotype of the cells. One problem is that neoplastic cells may not only lose certain differentiation antigens but also acquire others during neoplastic progression. Examples of so-called aberrant expression, i.e. the detection of an antigen not expected in that particular lineage, are common. With the increasing application of immunohistochemistry, we can now find cytokeratin expression, for example, previously thought to be restricted to epithelial lineages, in a wide range of cell types including reticular cells in lymph nodes, chondrocytes, plasma cells, smooth muscle cells, rhabdomyosarcomas, and malignant fibrous histiocytomas, to name but a few. Markers of mesenchymal lineages such as vimentin, while strongly expressed in most sarcomas and malignant melanoma, may also be expressed in some carcinomas, especially those of renal and ovarian origin, and also in carcinomas that assume a spindle cell morphology.

The only antigen that is not expressed on other lineages is the leucocyte common antigen (CD45), which is restricted to lymphoid cells (although this expression may be lost in certain tumours such as large cell anaplastic lymphoma). Interestingly, some other antigens may be expressed on lymphoid cells that have previously been somewhat ignored; these may reflect a certain functional significance. One such example is the expression of MUC1 (epithelial membrane antigen) on plasma cells and some lymphoreticular cells and their neoplasms. These are but a few examples of unexpected aberrant expression, and for these reasons it is essential to assemble wide-ranging antibody screens with expected positive and negative results, preferably with more than one positive for each lineage or subtype. The resulting phenotype also has to correspond with a plausible clinical morphological interpretation. It also highlights the need for interpreting conservatively results from new reagents developed on a limited range of tissues. However, there are some lineage-specific or relatively specific antigens that can be detected that may identify a particular cell type with great accuracy. Examples of such antigens include thyroglobulin, parathormone, peptide hormones from neuroendocrine tumours such as calcitonin in medullary carcinomas of the thyroid gland, or endothelial antigens such as CD31, CD34, and Factor VIII-related antigen.

In addition to lineage markers, immunohistochemical analysis can also highlight structural alterations in neoplasia which can be useful in assessment of tumours. To give a basic example, staining of the basement membrane-restricted antigens type IV collagen, and laminin can delineate the basement membrane around *in situ* carcinomas. As tumours become invasive, they tend to lose the ability to form basement membranes (or it is degraded at the point of invasion) and thus, potentially, this analysis can distinguish between *in situ* and invasive cancers.

13.3.2 Interpretation of immunohistochemistry

One drawback of immunohistochemistry is that localization may well not give contributory information. It is, for instance, possible to localize TGF-β in both the secreted form and matrix-associated form but this gives very little additional data on behaviour or differentiation of tumours, possibly because the expression of the receptors and their response to receptor activation is far more important in respect of neoplastic cell differentiation and function.

In addition, immunolocalization may give paradoxical results on secretion and uptake of certain molecules. As an example, some matrix metalloproteinases associated with the invasive phenotype, such as 72 kDa type IV collagenase (MMP-2) immunolocalize to neoplastic cells but the mRNA can be localized to a completely different population (i.e. stromal fibroblasts) in most carcinomas. Thus immunolocalization can be complementary but, viewed in isolation, might give rise to the wrong interpretation of the actual cellular and molecular processes.

Another problem is that both monoclonal and polyclonal antibodies can recognize more than one epitope, or a similar epitope on related or unrelated molecules, which may give rise to cross-reactivity. So-called 'non-specific' staining may also arise when antibodies bind to other tissue components. These problems are encountered not infrequently, especially when antibodies raised to a particular target have only been investigated in a very restricted field. When applied in the wider sphere of diagnostic pathology, the antibodies being exposed to a whole range of potential targets in many complex tissues, problems with specificity may then become obvious. Unless one is aware of this potential problem (i.e. a knowledge of data on reactivity with a wide range of normal and neoplastic tissues), misinterpretation can arise.

There are also a whole range of potential artefacts owing to inappropriate fixation, endogenous pigments, endogenous enzymes activating the detection systems, and physical artefacts in the tissues or reagents that may give rise to false positive and false negative reactions. All of these problems can only be solved by experience and repetition of results with a whole range of appropriate controls, and in the case of a novel monoclonal or polyclonal antibody by corroboration with another antibody recognizing the same or a related molecule. Immunoblotting will provide additional data on the presence and relative abundance of a particular protein, and also give an indication of potential cross-reactivity if several bands are identified.

13.3.3 Immunohistochemistry in therapy

One more recent application of immunohistochemistry is to identify targets for potential treatment (see Chapter 19.5). It is possible to label monoclonal antibodies with radionucleotides or toxins which will bind to molecules that are either expressed at a relatively high density on neoplastic cell surfaces or are more accessible on tumour cells. Experimental and *in vivo* studies have been performed on free-floating neoplastic cells which can be found in neoplastic effusions (e.g. from an intra-abdominal malignancy-causing ascites). In theory, injected labelled antibodies should bind preferentially to neoplastic cells without significant binding to normal cells in the vicinity. A selection of the appropriate target can be made by prescreening tumour cell preparations with the intended antibody panels and selecting the ones with the broadest and/or the most intense reactivity. More recent proposals involve the use of bispecific or linked antibodies to activate T cells to induce cytotoxic tumour cell killing. In addition, it is now possible to identify the products of genetic abnormalities in tumours, which may serve as targets for gene therapy, such as ERBB2 (see later).

13.4 Nucleic acid changes using *in situ* hybridization

In situ hybridization (ISH) refers to the localization of a nucleic acid (either DNA or RNA) in cells or tissues. Previously, this technique was limited to specially selected, prepared, and fixed tissues, but now protocols have been developed that are sufficiently robust and sensitive to be applied to diagnostic surgical material and even old archival blocks. ISH

allows specific DNA or RNA sequences of interest to be localized to a particular cellular population, which is its main advantage over solution filter hybridization techniques. ISH is more technically demanding than IHC and certainly the applications in the diagnostic field are much more restricted. However, it is an invaluable technique in experimental pathology, demonstrating evidence of specific genetic changes or alterations in gene expression that will complement results from tissue cell or cell extracts and protein localization by immunohistochemistry.

13.4.1 In situ hybridization for DNA

DNA is relatively stable and preserved in tissues even after routine fixation, and, unlike mRNA, is not so liable to endogenous enzymatic degradation. To be detectable by ISH, DNA sequences should generally be in multiple copies in the target cells, or be a large target with a heavily labelled probe (e.g. for chromosomal markers); otherwise it is very difficult to get a signal. Thus DNA ISH is generally restricted to the analysis of amplified sequences or viral sequences and much work has been done on viruses such as HPV, HIV, etc., in human tissues and tumours (see Chapters 8 and 9). The extent and role of Epstein–Barr virus infection in neoplasia has also been clarified using *in situ* hybridization. In cases of viral infections, the large number of DNA or RNA copies enable more rapid but somewhat less sensitive non-isotopic labels to be used. The identification of particular subtypes of virus may have clinical significance as, for example, in human papillomavirus (HPV) infection where certain subtypes may be associated with specific tumours.

ISH is also of value in interphase cytogenetics, where probes may be used to localize sequences specific to individual chromosomes within cell preparations and establish the nature of translocations or the extent of deletions (see Chapter 10). This may be of particular value in certain tumours associated with specific translocations, and which may have a cytoarchitectural appearance simulating other tumours. Such examples may be in the field of soft tissue sarcomas or in certain lymphoma/leukaemias.

There are limitations to DNA ISH, such as point mutations or small deletions that cannot be detected, since probes of adequate length will strongly hybridize to a target even with a few mismatches. Delineation of clonal lymphoid populations by identification of common regions of T cell receptors or immunoglobulin gene rearrangements has been investigated and, although it is not practical for diagnosis, it may be possible to investigate regions with a limited number of potential combinations for future demonstration of clonality in lymphoproliferative disease.

13.4.2 In situ hybridization for mRNA

Identification of mRNA in tissues gives valuable topographic information on gene expression in tissues. It is less helpful in quantitative terms, but will complement data from Northern blot analysis (see Glossary). Formerly it was necessary to use very carefully prepared fresh frozen or fixed tissues, but now there are techniques for analysing mRNA expression in routinely fixed paraffin-embedded material. The technique is relatively straightforward but elaborate precautions have to be taken to avoid contamination by ubiquitous RNAses which rapidly degrade any RNA in tissues or sections. Maximal signal is detected on freshly cut sections mounted on autoclaved slides using molecular biology grade reagents throughout. An important part of the protocol is the use of high stringency washes to reduce background.

It is best to use the most sensitive method available for detection of mRNA, since much of the target is degraded even in optimally preserved material. Single-stranded antisense RNA probes (riboprobes) are the most useful, being generated by introducing a cDNA corresponding to the mRNA of interest into a plasmid vector containing a recognition sequence for RNA polymerase. The probe and target mRNA hybridize strongly and, after stringent washing, ribonuclease is added. This destroys unbound single-stranded probe, thus reducing background, and is the main advantage of using riboprobes in detection of mRNA.

cDNA probes are less efficient; however, a combination of labelled oligonucleotide probes can be used on occasion when there is abundant mRNA, even with a non-radioactive label such as digoxigenin or biotin.

We have observed on occasion that digoxigenin-labelled riboprobes or oligonucleotide probes will give rather paradoxical and unusual labelling, results that sometimes contradict results obtained

with ^{35}S-labelled riboprobes. The reason for this is unclear. The choice of methodology is often made in the light of the experience in the laboratory and available resources. There are many examples where localization of mRNA has provided significant complementary information to other studies involving extracts of protein or nucleic acid from tissue, and immunolocalization. As an example, biochemical and immunolocalization data indicated that certain matrix metalloproteinases were synthesized by neoplastic epithelial cells in carcinomas. However, *in situ* hybridization for the 72 kDa type IV collagenase, which is highly correlated with the invasive metastatic phenotype, clearly indicated that the stromal cells contained much of the mRNA. Following on from this, further studies have indicated that this enzyme binds to a factor on the cell surface and is there activated, where it exerts its action at the tumour stromal interface; presumably immunolocalization in neoplastic cell cytoplasm either reflects intake of enzyme or ingestion of breakdown fragments. There are numerous other examples whereby complex epithelial stromal interactions can be clarified by the use of *in situ* hybridization, such as growth factors and cytokines. The underlying message is that mRNA ISH is able to define where and when a gene is expressed within a complex cellular population *in vivo*.

Another situation where mRNA is of value is when a novel gene has been identified but no antibody is available to the gene product for localization. An example of this situation came with attempts to map the expression of the trefoil peptides in ulcerative disease of the gut, where it was possible to localize accurately the expression of human spasmolytic polypeptide and the pS2 protein to selective compartments in a novel gastrointestinal lineage, which appears on the margins of chronically ulcerated endodermal tissues. Further studies have indicated that these factors have a potential role in gastrointestinal ulcer healing, as well as in growth and function of neoplastic cells in the intestine, breast, and other sites. *In situ* hybridization may also localize gene expression where the product is rapidly secreted and exported, or present at very low levels and difficult to detect by immunohistochemical analysis. This may be relevant in the analysis of functional tumours such as those derived from neuroendocrine cells in the pancreas and gut.

13.5 Genetic abnormalities in neoplasia

The genetic basis of cancer, and the understanding of how multiple different events coincide to form the neoplastic programme, are expanded on elsewhere in this volume. The mass of new data in the last decade and the information emerging from the Human Genome Project will result in far more detailed profiles of genetic aberrations in tumours, which will radically alter the basis of classification and therapy. The following account deals with the major gross genetic abnormalities found in tumours and the essential methodologies used in their demonstration.

13.5.1 Microdissection and amplification of small amounts of nucleic acid

We now know that useful information can be derived from tissues fixed and embedded in paraffin wax which can be identified in surgical pathology archives, avoiding the need to collect specially selected tissues stored in liquid nitrogen in many cases. Thick histological sections taken on to cleaned glass slides can be 'mapped' from one stained section, and the areas or cells of interest can be removed from other unstained sections by a sharp needle or knife. The small amount of mRNA extracted from these cells is amplified by using the polymerase chain reaction and reverse transcriptase enzyme (RT-PCR) using exon-specific primers and is subsequently analysed for mutations. This technique requires considerable care to avoid cross-contamination by non-neoplastic cells and nucleic acids from other tissues, but is of great value in 'retrieving' data from stored tissues with small or subtle neoplastic alterations, not easily recognizable in frozen material.

13.5.2 Allelic imbalance

Loss of heterozygosity is a classic marker of potential tumour suppressor gene loci and its identification has been an essential tool for positional cloning of many of these genes. It was originally performed using Southern blotting to identify restriction fragment length polymorphisms (RFLPs) but with the advent of the polymerase chain reaction technique for DNA amplification, minisatellite and then microsatellite markers became useable. The density of coverage over the human genome continues to increase with progress in the human gene mapping project which greatly enhances their utility, as does the availability of fluorescently labelled primer sets that allow rapid, high throughput analysis in automated sequencing machines.

13.5.3 Assays of expression of cancer-associated genes

As with the analysis of gene structure and allelic imbalance, the original blotting and hybridization techniques to examine gene expression are being replaced with more rapid and potentially more sensitive techniques based on PCR amplification. mRNA is extracted from tissue samples, theoretically as small as individual cells, and reverse transcribed to produce complementary DNA, which can be amplified by the polymerase chain reaction with gene-specific primers. The amplified product can be detected by a variety of techniques, and can be quantified by parallel amplification of one or more control templates of known concentration. The development of combined amplification and fluorescent detection equipment has made this an approach that can be applied in a routine diagnostic setting and examples of gene products that are candidates for detection/quantitation in malignant disease are shown in Table 13.1.

13.5.4 Detection of cancer-specific gene rearrangements

There are a number of instances of genetic rearrangements that are characteristic of particular types of

Table 13.1 Genes expressed or overexpressed in human cancer

Gene product	Clinical situation
HIV and herpesvirus genes	AIDS, Kaposi's sarcoma
HPV-16/18 E6 and E7 genes	Cervical carcinoma
EBV	Nasopharyngeal carcinoma, ? others
ERBB2	Breast cancer
ERBB3	Breast cancer
BCR–ABL fusion gene	CML blast crisis
PML–RARA fusion gene	AML
EWS–FLI1/ETV1/ERG	PNET/Ewing's sarcoma
SYT–SSX1/SSX2	Synovial sarcoma
Mutant EGFR	Glioblastoma, ? others
N-MYC	Neuroblastoma
MDM2	Sarcomas

cancer, many of which are reviewed in Chapter 10. These can be detected even in very small biopsy specimens using conventional Southern blot and hybridization techniques or by gene-specific PCR approaches. The identification of these rearrangements can not only be helpful as an adjunct to pathological diagnosis but may be exploited for therapeutic targeting, a concept that will be increasingly important with the development of gene therapy for cancer. For instance, the identification of the precise sequence of the immunoglobulin gene rearrangement carried by the neoplastic cells in a B cell lymphoma allows the design of a specific anti-idiotype gene vaccine—an approach that is already in clinical trial—and the detection of characteristic rearrangements in the EGF receptor gene, which occur in glioblastoma multiforme, is useful for the selection of patients who are candidates for specific antibody-directed therapies.

It is now routine to use fluorescence *in situ* hybridization (FISH) to detect chromosomal rearrangements characteristic of particular forms of cancer, most commonly leukaemias and lymphomas, but also soft tissue tumours which can otherwise be difficult to classify. It is also possible to detect gene amplification using FISH not only in isolated cellu-lar chromosomes but even in tissue sections directly, which can be extremely helpful in the analysis of small neoplastic lesions such as ductal carcinoma *in situ* of the breast. The advent of multiplex FISH will increase the power of this technology for clinical application since it can be used for simultaneous recognition of each chromosome independently (Speichler *et al.* 1996). This can be very useful for monitoring the effects of therapy and detecting minimal residual disease or relapse, as well as identifying the origin of bone marrow cells following transplantation.

13.5.5 Detection of cancer-specific gene mutations

Activating mutations in oncogenes and inactivating mutations in tumour suppressor genes are extremely specific markers of neoplasia and the restricted pattern of some of them, such as those activating the RAS oncogenes, has led to the design of rapid and sensitive genetic tests that are suitable for clinical application. Examples of genes affected by mutation in malignancy and the tumour type where their detection may be particularly useful are shown in Table 13.2.

Table 13.2 Genetic mutations characteristic of cancer

Gene	Mutation	Tumour type
KRAS oncogene	Point mutation at codons 12 or 13	Colorectal neoplasms Pancreatic adenocarcinoma Lung adenocarcinoma
EGFR oncogene	Intragenic deletion	Glioblastoma multiforme
p53	Wide range of truncation or substitution mutations	Most solid and haematological malignancies
RB1	Wide range of truncation mutations	Retinoblastoma Breast cancer Osteosarcoma
APC	Truncation mutations at two hotspots	Colorectal neoplasms Ampullary cancers Stomach cancers
*h*MLH1/*h*MSH2/*h*PML1/*h*PML2	Range of truncation mutations	Colorectal neoplasms Many other solid malignancies
CDKN2 (p16)	Wide range of truncation mutations	Melanoma Pancreatic adenocarcinoma
SMAD4	Wide range of truncation and substitution mutations	Pancreatic adenocarcinoma Other solid malignancies
BRCA1 and *BRCA2*	Range of trunation mutations	Breast cancer Ovarian cancer

The fact that these mutations are found specifically in neoplastic cells and are often present early in tumorigenic development makes them good candidates for use in screening tests for early neoplasia and preneoplasia. Mutations in KRAS genes can be detected in stool samples in patients with colorectal neoplasia, and mutations of *p53* and *RAS* genes can be detected in saliva or urine of patients with head and neck cancer or bladder cancer, respectively.

There are a wide range of techniques available to detect mutations. Among the most useful for the analysis of frameshift and premature stop codon mutations (which are the most common type responsible for inactivation of tumour suppressor genes such as *APC* and *BRCA1*) is the protein truncation test in which a recombinant clone of the gene isolated from the tumour sample is translated *in vitro* and then detected immunochemically. Other useful techniques include altered band patterns after electrophoresis, heteroduplexing, and direct sequencing of the DNA segment carrying the mutation. Each of these has its own advantages and disadvantages with sequencing being the most widely used where automated facilities are available.

13.6 Tumour markers

There are relatively few instances whereby a distinction can be made between benign and malignant neoplastic cells on the basis of immunohistochemical evidence. In most instances there are relative differences in the expression which may be highlighted or detectable by immunohistochemical analysis. A prime example is p53 protein, whereby the mutated product commonly found in transformed neoplastic cells is far more stable than wild-type p53 and accumulates in cell nuclei, being relatively easily detectable. Nevertheless, there are exceptions to this inasmuch as mutations do not generally give rise to immunohistochemically detectable stable changes, and the already mentioned problem that enhancement and amplification techniques can detect overexpressed normal p53 in certain cells under the influence of various stimuli. Other potential markers include oncogene products such as ERBB2, which is rarely if ever expressed in non-neoplastic cells. This may be valuable in the analysis of intraductal proliferations of the breast, for instance, where ERBB2 is often expressed in the high grade intraductal carcinomas but rarely in the low grade *in situ* carcinomas. As well as protein markers detectable by immunohistochemistry many of the nucleic acid markers considered in the previous sections will eventually lead to new avenues in diagnosis and treatment.

References and further reading

Boyle, J. O., Mao, L., Brennan, J. A., Koch, W. M., Eisele, D. W., Saunders, J. R., and Sidransky, D. (1994). Gene mutations in saliva as molecular markers for head and neck squamous cell carcinomas. *American Journal of Surgery*, **168**, 429–32.

Colvin, R. B., Bhan, A. K., and McCluskey, R. T. (1996). *Diagnostic immunopathology*, (2nd edn). Lippincott-Raven, Philadelphia.

Dean, M. (1995). Resolving DNA mutations. *Nature Genetics*, **9**, 103–4.

Fitzgerald, J. M., Ranchuranen, N., Rieger, K., Levesque, P., Silverman, M., Libertino, J. A., and Summerhayes, I. C. (1995). Identification of H-ras mutations in urine sediments complements cytology in the detection of bladder tumours.

Journal of the National Cancer Institute, **87**, 129–33.

Murphy, D. S., Hoare, S. F., Going, J. J., Mallon, E. E., George, W. D., Kaye, S. B., *et al.* (1995). Characterization of extensive genetic alternative in ductal carcinoma in situ by fluorescence in situ hybridization and molecular analysis. *Journal of the National Cancer Institute*, **87**, 1694–704.

Naylor, M. S., Stamp, G. W. H., and Balkwill, F. R. (1990). Investigation of cytokine gene expression in human colorectal cancer. *Cancer Research*, **50**, 4436–40.

Roest, P. A., Roberts, R. G., Sugino, S., van Omman, G. J., and den Dunnen, J. T. (1993). Protein truncation test (PTT) for rapid detection of translation-terminating mutations. *Human Molecular Genetics*, **2**, 1719–21.

Sidransky, D., Tokino, T., Hamilton, S. R., Kingler, K. W., Levin, B., Frost, P., and Vogelstein B. (1992). Identification of ras oncogene mutations in the stool of patients with curable colorectal tumours. *Science*, **256**, 102–5.

Speicher, M. R., Ballard, S. G., and Ward, D.C. (1996). Karyotyping human chromosomes by combinational multifluor FISH. *Nature Genetics*, **12**, 368–75.

Stamp, G. W. H. and Poulsom, R. (1992). In-situ hybridization in pathology. *Surgery*, **10**, 202–3.

Wright, N. A., Poulsom, R., Stamp, G.W. H., Hall, P. A., Jeffery, R. E., Longcroft, J. M., *et al.* (1990). Epidermal growth factor (EGF/URO) induces expression of regulatory peptides in damaged human gastrointestinal tissues. *Journal of Pathology*, **162**, 279–84.

14

Hormones and cancer

M. G. PARKER AND L. M. FRANKS

14.1 Introduction

During the latter part of the eighteenth century the Scottish surgeon John Hunter established that removal of the gonads in animals led to a dramatic shrinkage in the size of the accessory sexual glands in both sexes. This glandular atrophy was particularly noticeable in the prostate in males and the breast and uterus in females. These observations showed that substances (hormones) produced in one organ had a profound effect on distant organs. We now know that specialized glands or cells produce different hormones that control differentiation, growth, and function in many organs and, in some, are associated with tumour development.

Hunter subsequently devised a remarkably sound system for the classification of human breast cancers and did a vast amount of work on their pathology; many of his specimens are still in the Hunterian Museum in London. Research began in earnest in 1889 when Schinzinger proposed a relationship between ovarian function and breast cancer. In clinical terms, the years 1894–6 were the watershed between speculation and reality. In this period, Beatson described the palliation of breast cancer in some patients after removal of the ovary (ovariectomy), and Rann and White advocated castration for the arrest of prostate cancer. Research in this area then gathered real pace with the purification and characterization of the principal steroid and polypeptide hormones. The synthesis of very active analogues and hormone antagonists has also had a profound effect on research, opening up possibilities for the successful treatment of cancer by hormonal means. For example, in 1941 Huggins and Hodges introduced the non-steroidal oestrogen, diethylstilboestrol, for the treatment of prostate cancer, a therapy still widely used today. In this chapter we consider modern concepts on the biology, mechanisms of hormone action, and responsiveness of these tumours in some detail. Our present knowledge of the molecular basis of hormone action and its genetic control gives us a clearer understanding of the process and should allow us to understand the role of hormones in the induction and growth of this group of tumours.

Cancer endocrinology is concerned with the role of hormones in cancer induction and their effects on tumour growth. Some tumours, particularly those that arise from hormone-responsive organs, may require hormones for their continued growth so that alterations in the concentration of these hormones can be exploited as a method of treatment.

14.2 Basic endocrinology

14.2.1 Types of hormones

As defined by Starling, a hormone (from Greek, to arouse) is a compound secreted by one organ to enhance the activity of other organs distant from the site of synthesis (endocrine). While still true in many respects, this definition needs qualification (see also Chapter 15). For example, testosterone has a direct effect on certain organs, such as muscle and testis, but in others it must be metabolized to a different end-product to produce a response; in the normal and neoplastic male accessory sex organs it must be converted into 5α-dihydrotestosterone. Non-hormonal substances may be converted into active hormones. Cholesterol is not a hormone but may be converted into the important steroid-like hormone, 1α,25-dihydroxycholecalciferol (the active metabolic form of vitamin D_3), by a sequence of reactions occurring in the skin, liver, and, finally, kidney. Many hormones have direct effects on their organs of synthesis, as in the case of sex hormones. Others work through second messengers, as originally proposed by Sutherland for cyclic-AMP (see Chapter 11). Lastly, hormones may activate or inhibit biochemical processes in their target cells; glucocorticoids, for example, kill T lymphocytes, granulocytes, and macrophages, and tumours derived from them.

Many hormone-like growth factors have been extracted and purified from serum in recent years; these are discussed in Chapters 11 and 20. This chapter will be concerned with those hormones secreted by the ovary, testis, adrenal cortex, and anterior pituitary. Chemically, these important hormones are either steroid or polypeptide hormones, but, in addition, other hormones, particularly the thyroid hormone, thyroxine, must be taken into account.

The secretion of all these hormones is regulated by precisely coordinated activity of the hypothalamus, pituitary, and the secretory (endocrine) glands themselves (Fig. 14.1). The hypothalamus is part of the central nervous system and controls the release of tropic hormones from the pituitary gland at the base of the brain. The pituitary has two parts, ante-

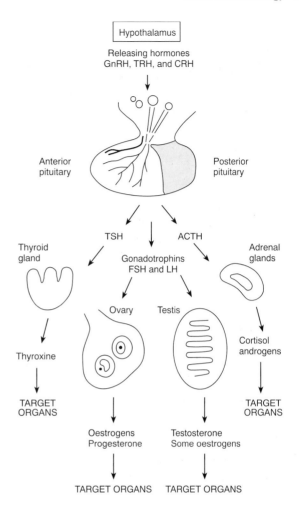

Fig. 14.1 The secretion of steroid hormones and thyroxine is controlled by the hypothalamic–pituitary axis. Under the control of specific hypothalamic-releasing hormones the anterior pituitary secretes thyroid stimulating hormone (TSH), follicle stimulating hormone (FSH), luteinizing hormone (LH), and adrenocorticotrophic hormone (ACTH), which in turn regulate the production of thyroxine and steroid hormones by endocrine glands.

rior and posterior, each of which produces different hormones. The regulatory system is a closed loop, requiring releasing hormones and stimulatory hormones or tropins; both of these classes of hormones are polypeptides. The crucial interaction is between complex nerve centres in the hypothalamus and the anterior pituitary which contains specialized cells responsible for the production of a distinctive tropin. In response to appropriate external and internal stimuli, the hypothalamus secretes releasing hormones into a system of veins that drain directly into the anterior pituitary and stimulate the selective synthesis of tropins. There are different releasing hormones for thyrotropin (TRH), corticotropin (CRH), and one for the two gonadotropins (GnRH), lutropin and follitropin. The gonadotropins stimulate the production of the female sex hormones (oestrogen and progesterone) from the ovary, or male sex hormones (androgens) from the testis. The tropins are secreted into the general circulation where they stimulate the synthesis of hormones from target cells. Thyrotropin stimulates thyroxine secretion from the thyroid. Corticotropin promotes the synthesis of the glucocorticoids, cortisol and cortisone, from the adrenal cortex together with a small but significant amount of testosterone.

There are two mechanisms to prevent excessive hormonal stimulation. Firstly, the steroid hormones and thyroxine are distributed strongly bound to specific transport proteins in serum; indeed, 0.5 per cent or less of free biologically active hormone may be available to the cells of the body. Secondly, there are powerful enzymes for steroid breakdown (catabolism) in the liver in both sexes. Should these latter control mechanisms fail, there is a dramatic rise in the concentration of free active hormone in serum with potentially dangerous consequences.

As well as the polypeptides already described, the anterior pituitary secretes two other polypeptide hormones, somatotropin and prolactin, in response to a variety of stimuli. Somatotropin promotes the growth of many cells and clearly may be important in the cancer process. Prolactin, as its name suggests, was originally identified by its powerful role in inducing lactation. Further research has shown, however, that prolactin has diverse functions and is certainly implicated in the carcinogenic process in many organs, notably breast and prostate.

A number of other hormones should also be mentioned. The mineralocorticoid steroid hormone aldosterone, is involved in maintaining the electrolyte balance and although its level in serum may rise enormously in Conn's syndrome (tumour in the zona glomerulosa of the adrenal cortex), it plays no significant part in the process of carcinogenesis. The hypothalamus also secretes two polypeptide hormones, oxytocin and vasopressin, along with carrier proteins known as the neurophysins, into the posterior pituitary; again, there is no proven involvement of either hormone in neoplasia.

All classes of steroid hormone circulate in the blood in association with specific transport proteins and have diverse effects on a wide range of target cells, but their most important feature as far as cancer is concerned is whether they can stimulate cell division. The oestrogens and androgens are powerful mitogens and promote growth and mitosis in many target organs, such as breast, uterus, and prostate; these are potentially dangerous hormones as can be demonstrated experimentally. By contrast, glucocorticoids and progestins are protective agents and generally inhibit cell multiplication; there are certain exceptions and these will be discussed later.

14.2.2 Receptors mediate hormone action

Steroid hormones, retinoids, and thyroxine Most of the responses to steroid hormones are mediated by specific and seemingly mobile receptor proteins; a few responses related to gluconeogenesis and secretion may be promoted by other means. Steroids enter all cells from the blood by passive diffusion, but there is some evidence that certain tumours may possess mechanisms for the facilitated or active transport of steroid hormones. In target cells, expressing the appropriate specific receptor, a high affinity hormone receptor complex is formed which is able to increase or decrease the rate of transcription of a subset of genes (Fig.14.2). We now know that these receptors are members of a much larger family of proteins that includes the receptors for thyroxin, produced by the thyroid gland, and a number of vitamins, including retinoids. Retinoids, unlike steroid and thyroid hormones, cannot be synthesized *in vivo*. Thus, animals require dietary vitamin A which is then converted in most, if not all, cell types into retinal, and subsequently retinoic acid. Concentration gradients of retinoic acid are thought to be critical in determining cellular responses and these are likely to be established partly by the activity of metabolizing enzymes and partly by the concentration of intracellular binding proteins.

There is usually only one form of receptor for each class of steroid hormone encoded by a unique gene, but there are multiple receptors for retinoids and thyroid hormone, encoded from distinct genes and further isoforms are generated by alternative splicing. Upon activation by hormone binding,

Fig. 14.2 Mechanisms of transcriptional regulation by nuclear receptors. In the classical type of response, receptors (R) bind directly to simple response elements associated with target genes as homodimers or heterodimers and stimulate transcription in the presence of ligand (L). Alternatively, the transcriptional activity of Fos (F)/Jun (J) family members bound to their cognate binding site AP-1 can be modulated either positively or negatively by receptors.

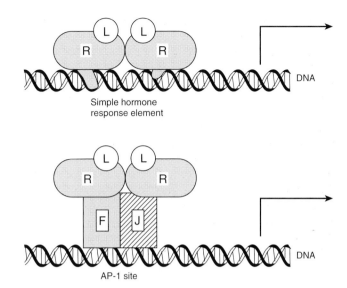

these receptors function directly as transcription factors by binding to regulatory DNA sequences, called hormone response elements, found in the vicinity of target genes (Fig.14.2). However, it has now become evident that nuclear receptors are also capable of regulating the transcription of genes that lack response elements, by modulating the activity of other transcription factors, such as the activator protein-1, AP-1.In these cases, proteinprotein interactions between the receptor and individual AP-1 family members are thought to be important, although direct DNA binding of the receptor to DNA also occurs on certain gene promoters.

The thyroid gland produces iodine-containing hormones, thyroxine (tetraiodothyroxine) and triiodothyroxine (T3). These have a profound effect on cell metabolism and the growth of many cells, including some tumours. A deficiency in infants leads to mental and physical stunting (cretinism). Iodine deficiency causes an overgrowth of the thyroid cells leading to the formation of tumour-like nodules (goitres) but these rarely become malignant. The receptors for triiodothyroxine are nuclear rather than cytosolic (see Chapter 9 for a discussion of the T3 receptor as a protooncogene).

Polypeptide hormones and growth factors Both these classes of compound have specific receptors as integral components of the outer surface of the plasma membrane. The receptors have a close structural and functional association with enzyme systems and ion gates capable of generating a wide range of second messengers (see Chapter 11). Oc-

cupation of the specific receptor sites enhances the synthesis or activity of second messengers, and since the subsequent steps are operational cascades, the hormonal signal is amplified and a few molecules of hormone can evoke a very pronounced effect. Some internalization of polypeptide hormones has been detected in the Golgi apparatus and lysosomes of target cells; this may represent a mechanism for their degradation but may be a more subtle reflection of a wider influence on cellular function.

There are defences against excessive hormonal stimulation. Excess polypeptides are degraded by proteases in the walls of arteries and capillaries. A long biological life for cyclic nucleotides is prevented by the ubiquitous presence of phosphodiesterases. Finally, there is evidence that protracted exposure of specific receptors to their appropriate hormone leads to a very significant decrease in the number of receptors (down-regulation); this phenomenon is being exploited in novel approaches to the hormonal therapy of certain tumours.

It follows from this general discussion that tumours may arise from hormone-producing or hormone-responsive cells (see Section 14.6).

14.3 Molecular mechanisms of hormone action: nuclear receptors

14.3.1 Nuclear receptor action

Steroid hormone action Steroid hormone receptors, after hormone binding, function directly as transcription factors by binding to regulatory DNA sites in the vicinity of target genes (for review see Parker 1993) (Fig. 14.3). In many cases, the sites are simple response elements consisting of inverted repeats that bind the receptor with relatively high affinity, while in other cases, at sites referred to as composite response elements, the receptor binds only in association with another transcription factor such as AP-1. Simple response elements for oestrogen receptors consist of inverted repeats of the sequence $^A/_G$GTCA, whereas the receptors for androgens, glucocorticoids, and progestins bind to inverted repeats of the sequence $AG^A/_G$ACA. The binding affinity of receptors for sites varies widely depending on their precise sequence and number. The majority of oestrogen response elements that have been characterized to date contain imperfect inverted repeats that function less well than the consensus sequence, but, in some promoters, there are several such sites which increases the oestrogen response.

In the absence of hormone, steroid hormone receptors exist as inactive oligomeric complexes containing a number of heatshock proteins, including hsp90 (Fig. 14.4), either in the cytoplasm (androgen and glucocorticoid receptors) or in the nucleus (oestrogen and progesterone receptors). The role of hsp90 appears to be to maintain the receptor in an inactive state in the absence of ligand and may also be important for folding of the receptor protein and/or transport across membranes. Following hormone binding, the oligomeric complex dissociates and the receptor either binds to DNA response elements in the form of homodimers or interacts with other transcription factors. Since the hormone-binding pocket is at or near the dimer interface it appears that dimerization is stabilized in the presence of the hormone on the basis of hydrophobic shielding.

Transcriptional activation by steroid receptors is mediated by at least two distinct activation regions, at least on simple response elements. One of these, referred to as AF-1, is located in the N-terminal domain and another, AF-2, is in the hormone-binding domain. In the oestrogen receptor, and probably in other receptors as well, their absolute and relative activities vary depending on the target promoter and the cell type. While the two activation domains have the potential to act independently, they appear to interact with one another in some ill-defined way in the intact receptor. It is generally accepted that the rate at which RNA polymerase initiates gene transcription depends on the formation of a preinitiation complex that includes a number of basic transcription factors, and that the role of transcriptional activators is to stabilize this complex. A number of activators, including steroid hormone receptors, have been shown to bind directly to basal transcription factors, but additional targets are suggested by cell-free transcription experiments.

It is likely that receptors often bind to DNA only in association with another transcription factor at sites called composite response elements. The best characterized example of this is the glucocorticoid control of proliferin gene transcription, which depends on the binding of AP-1 as well as glucocorticoid receptors. Glucocorticoids can either potentiate or inhibit transcription and this effect seems to

Steroid response elements (Inverted repeats)		Receptors			
AGAACAnnnTGTTCT	GRE	AR	GR	MR	PR
AGGTCAnnnTGACCT	ERE	ER			
Direct repeats					
AGGTCAnAGGTCA	DR–1	RXR/RAR			
AGGTCAnnAGGTCA	DR–2	RXR/RAR			
AGGTCAnnnAGGTCA	DR–3	RXR/VDR			
AGGTCAnnnnAGGTCA	DR–4	RXR/TR			
AGGTCAnnnnnAGGTCA	DR–5	RXR/RAR			

Fig. 14.3 Target DNA-binding sites for nuclear receptors. The receptors for androgens (AR), glucocorticoids (GR), mineralocorticoids (MR), and progestins (PR) bind to sites related to glucocorticoid response elements (GRE), while oestrogen receptors (ER) bind to oestrogen response elements (ERE). The retinoid X receptor and those for retinoic acid (RAR), vitamin D (VDR), and thyroxine (TR) bind to direct repeats (DR) consisting of half-sites separated by different spacings.

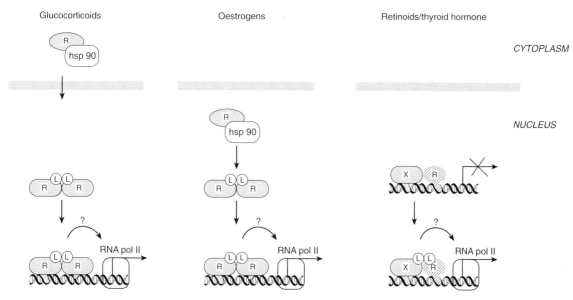

Fig. 14.4 Mechanism of nuclear receptor action. Steroid hormone receptors (R) are complexed with the heatshock protein (hsp 90) in the absence of hormone, but dimerize and bind to DNA upon ligand (L) binding. Retinoid and thyroid hormone receptors form heterodimers with retinoid X receptor (X) and bind to direct repeats, where they stimulate transcription upon ligand (L) binding.

depend on the composition of the AP-1 complex. Thus, glucocorticoid receptors stimulate AP-1 activity mediated by Jun homodimers but inhibit transcription mediated by JunFos heterodimers (Diamond *et al.* 1990). The oestrogen regulation of ovalbumin gene expression also seems to involve the binding of AP-1 to an oestrogen response element and may be a feature of many other hormone-sensitive genes.

Nuclear receptors can also modulate the activity of a number of transcription factors, including AP-1, without contacting DNA (Fig. 14.2). Such indirect effect of receptors are likely to be extremely important because AP-1 is implicated in many signalling pathways that regulate cell differentiation, proliferation, and transformation. The best characterized example of this is the ability of glucocorticoids to repress the transcription of the collagenase gene whose expression is induced by various growth factors, inflammatory agents, and phorbol esters through AP-1. Genomic footprinting suggests that the glucocorticoid receptor does not displace AP-1 from its binding site and probably acts without contacting DNA. The most likely mechanism involves interference with the transactivation potential of AP-1, mediated primarily by the DNA-binding domain of the receptor. AP-1 activity is also modulated by other steroid hormones and retinoids. For example, oestrogens enhance and antioestrogens inhibit growth factor-induced AP-1 activity in oestrogen receptor positive breast cancer cells (Chalbos *et al.* 1994). Since these effects cannot be accounted for by alterations in the levels of Fos or Jun it is likely that protein-protein interactions between the oestrogen receptor and AP-1 family members are involved.

Retinoic acid and thyroid hormone action The effects of retinoic acid and thyroid hormone are also mediated by receptors that act directly as transcription factors [Figs 14.2 and 14.4; and see review by Stunnenberg (1993)]. In contrast to steroid hormone receptors, there are multiple forms of these receptors. Thus retinoic acid receptors (RAR) are encoded by three distinct genes that generate additional isoforms by alternate splicing. In addition, there is a related family of receptors called retinoid X receptors (RXR) that do not bind all-*trans*-retinoic acid but the related ligand, 9-*cis*-retinoic acid. These receptors are also encoded by distinct genes that also generate multiple forms by alternate splicing. Initially, it was found that both the retinoic acid and thyroid hormone receptors could stimulate transcription of reporter genes from inverted repeats of the sequence AGGTCA with no gap between the repeats, and it seemed likely that the receptors were binding to these sites as homodimers. However, when binding sites were identified in natural target genes they were generally found to be direct repeats and not inverted repeats of this sequence. These sites are abbreviated as DR-1, DR-2, and so on, for sites in which the repeats are separated by one or two nucleotides, respectively (Fig. 14.3). Nevertheless the *in vitro* DNA-binding activity of the retinoic acid and thyroid hormone receptors to these sites was poor until it was found that RXR dramatically enhanced their DNA-binding activity by forming heterodimers. It appears that thyroid hormone receptors bind selectively to a DR-4, whereas retinoic acid receptors exhibit rather degenerate DNA-binding activity to a DR-1, DR-2, or DR-5. In each case, RXR was shown to occupy the upstream repeat. Nevertheless, it is doubtful whether these receptors exist exclusively as heterodimers in cells since there is preliminary evidence to suggest that the homodimer/heterodimer equilibrium is regulated, at least in part, by the bound ligand. In common with steroid receptors, there appear to be two activation regions, one in the N-terminus and one in the ligand-binding domain, whose activities are cell and promoter specific. Moreover, as with steroids, retinoids not only function as DNA-dependent transcription factors but also modulate AP-1 activity probably by protein-protein interactions.

Antioestrogens Antioestrogens have been developed to inhibit the transcriptional activity of the oestrogen receptor for a variety of clinical uses. To date, the most widely used therapeutic antioestrogen is tamoxifen but its action is far from straightforward, it being a mixed agonist/ antagonist. Thus, it is a fairly good antagonist in the mammary gland and effectively inhibits the growth of oestrogen-responsive breast cancer cells, but it is an agonist in the endometrium and in bone. The binding site for tamoxifen overlaps with that of the oestrogen-binding site and so it acts as a competitive inhibitor of oestrogen action. Transient transfection experiments suggest that tamoxifen binding allows the receptor to dimerize and bind to DNA with high affinity but blocks transcriptional activity mediated by the hormone-binding domain (Fig. 14.5). The agonist activity is thought to be derived primarily from AF-1 which appears to function

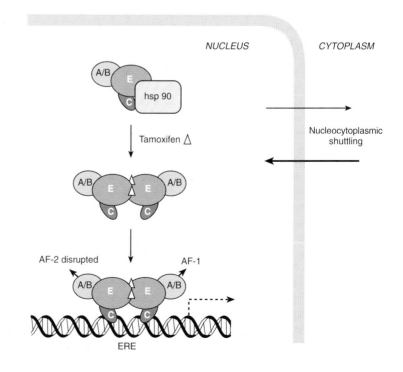

Fig. 14.5 Mechanism of action of antioestrogens with partial agonist activity. In the presence of the partial agonist tamoxifen receptors dimerize and the DNA-binding domain (region C) binds with high affinity to oestrogen response elements (ERE) in the vicinity of target genes. AF-1 in the N-terminal domain (regions A/B) is postulated to give rise to agonist activity, while the binding of tamoxifen to the hormone-binding domain disrupts the function of AF-2 (region E), which accounts for its antagonistic activity.

even when tamoxifen is bound to the receptor (see Dauvois and Parker 1993). Thus, tamoxifen has the potential to act as an antagonist when the transcriptional activity of the receptor is mediated by AF-2, but as an agonist on promoters where AF-1 is active.

Alternative antioestrogens have also been developed with less agonist activity, such as ICI 182780 which is reported to be devoid of oestrogenic activity (Wakeling 1992). ICI 182780 is currently being investigated as a potential second-line endocrine treatment for tamoxifen-resistant patients. The effectiveness of ICI 182780 as an antioestrogen depends on an alkylamine side chain at the 7α-position in the B ring in the steroid whose optimum length is 16–18 carbon atoms. One of the major effects of ICI 182780 is to cause a decrease in the cellular content of receptor protein by markedly reducing its half-life. The molecular basis for this increased turnover is not completely clear but it is accompanied by a block in nucleocytoplasmic shut-

tling (Fig. 14.6). In common with other steroid receptors the oestrogen receptor seems to be constantly diffusing out of the cell nucleus but is rapidly transported back into the nucleus in an energy-dependent step so that the receptor is predominantly nuclear under equilibrium conditions. In the presence of ICI 182780 nuclear re-entry does not occur and degradation takes place, probably in lysosomes.

An additional effect of ICI 182780 is that it might disrupt dimerization and, as a consequence, inhibit DNA binding. It seems likely that ICI 182780 binds to a similar if not identical site to that of oestradiol, which we have shown overlaps with a region involved in receptor dimerization so that the antioestrogen, by means of its 7α side chain, might sterically interfere with dimerization. This effect can be demonstrated *in vitro* but has yet to be confirmed *in vivo*. Finally, both tamoxifen and ICI 182780 modulate the response of AP-1 to growth factors, but the mechanism involved is completely unknown.

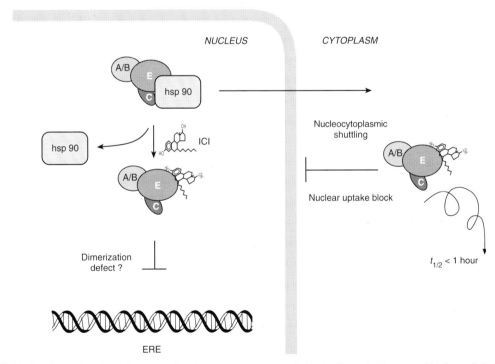

Fig. 14.6 Mechanism of action of pure antioestrogens. The pure antioestrogen ICI 182780 prevents nuclear uptake of the oestrogen receptor so that during the process of nucleocytoplasmic shuttling the receptor accumulates in the cytoplasm and is degraded. Within the cell nucleus dimerization of the receptor might be disrupted and this would reduce its DNA binding activity. For abbreviations see Fig. 14.5.

14.4 Hormones and carcinogenesis

The first hint that hormones were potential carcinogens came in 1932 when Lacassagne induced mammary tumours in male mice with the oestrogen, oestrone benzoate. Using a similar approach, Kirkman induced kidney tumours with oestrogens but only in hamsters. This unexpected finding showed that hormones may influence organs not usually thought to be hormone sensitive. The synthesis of the non-steroidal oestrogen, diethylstilboestrol, by Dodds in 1935, provided researchers with an extremely powerful research weapon. Of all the classes of steroid hormones, the sex hormones, and oestrogens in particular, are the most potent carcinogens. Work in this area is not without its controversies. There are often conflicting results when the effects of hormones are compared in different species. Of greater importance, data obtained from experimental animals often conflict with findings in humans. Taking an overall view, hormones can be carcinogenic under certain circumstances or can provide the means for the arrest of tumours. Our knowledge in this area is based on studies on animals, in humans, and on cells in tissue culture.

14.4.1 Animal studies

The literature on this topic is now vast and will be covered only briefly. In experimental animals prolonged exposure to oestrogens and their analogues, such as stilboestrol, results in cancer formation in many organs, but most commonly in reproductive organs, kidney, liver, and anterior pituitary, but there is a considerable variation between species. It has also been reported that protracted treatment of dogs with potent androgens may lead to prostate tumours. Concomitant administration of carcinogenic hydrocarbons, such as dimethylbenzanthracene, often enhances the tumour incidence achieved by hormones alone; in addition, hydrocarbons may help to induce tumours in organs normally insensitive to hormones. So far, tumours have not been consistently induced in experimental animals even by chronic treatment with polypeptide hormones including prolactin and somatotropin.

Two examples illustrate interspecies differences. Tumours of the uterine cervix can be induced in mice by extremely low doses of oestrogens; under similar dose-corrected conditions, all other species are refractory. Mammary tumours are common in some mouse strains and are often associated with a mammary tumour virus (see Chapter 8). Repeated pregnancies tend to increase the incidence of these tumours. In human breast cancer there is no evidence of a virus involvement and pregnancy tends to protect (see Chapter 3). Prostate tumours are very rare in most animals although common in humans. Such anomalies create problems when trying to assess the potential danger of hormones in humans. This problem was approached by Dunning in 1963. From a spontaneous rat prostate tumour, she developed a whole range of transplantable, androgen-sensitive and -insensitive tumours; these tumours are stable and can be grown in tissue culture.

While studies on experimental animals have taught us much about hormones and cancer, they have not shed any light on certain pressing human problems. For example, experimental studies have failed to explain why cancer is so prevalent in the human prostate, yet rare in adjacent accessory sexual glands which are in a similar hormonal milieu. Animal studies have failed to explain why the male dog is the only species to share a high incidence of prostatic cancer although at a much lower rate than in humans. Prostate cancer in humans is a disease of old age, and there have been some reports of spontaneous prostate tumours arising in aged AxC strain rats. The incidence of prostate tumours was raised to 70 per cent if the animals were exposed to exogenous androgens. While of considerable interest, these studies may tell us little about the human disease, because ageing men are unlikely to be exposed to exogenous androgens and the endogenous production of testosterone tends to decline with age.

The use of animals for testing potentially dangerous hormones has prompted many controversies. Perhaps the most notorious centres on synthetic progestins related to 17-hydroxyprogesterone. In beagle dogs, but not other animals, these compounds were found to induce mammary tumours. Despite lengthy debate, these synthetic progestins were banned from inclusion in contraceptive pills on the evidence obtained from one experimental species only.

14.4.2 Studies in humans

Evidence that hormones are carcinogenic in humans comes largely from clinical observations and epidemiological studies. Many relevant observations, still largely unexplained, have been made. For example, prostate cancer has never been recorded in eunuchs or castrati, and there is a high incidence of breast cancer in socially enclosed female communities, such as nunneries.

Hormones and cancer in women There is a rapidly growing body of evidence that prolonged exposure to sex hormones, especially oestrogens, results in a high incidence of several forms of human cancer. Women are more usually affected since they tend to take more hormone preparations, largely for obstetric and gynaecological reasons. None the less, androgen-containing formulations markedly increases the risk of hepatoma in men, and transvestites with oestrogen implants have a higher incidence of breast cancer than other men. The contraceptive pill (see Chapter 3) contains a combination of oestrogen and progesterone; the critical point in terms of potential danger is the relative proportions of the two hormones. While essential for contraceptive function, the oestrogen is the potentially threatening component, whereas the progesterone is protective or 'antioestrogenic'. Early preparations containing a high oestrogen to progesterone ratio have all now been banned because they markedly increased the risk of endometrial (uterine) cancer. Contraceptive preparations containing a very low oestrogen to progesterone ratio are currently considered safe and indeed may well provide protection against cancer of the ovary, breast, and endometrium. There have been cautionary reports of a high incidence of breast cancer in young women who have been taking oral contraceptives since just after the menarche. One recent survey in the UK shows an increase in the risk of about 40 per cent after four to eight years of pill use, and about 70 per cent after more than eight years' use. But researchers stressed breast cancer was still uncommon below age 36; even a 70 per cent increase in risk would put up the chances of developing breast cancer by this age only from one in 500 to one in 300. Fortunately, such dangers to health may be obviated in the future by the wider use of contraceptive implants containing only a synthetic progestin, levonorgestrol. These subdermal implants are effective, long lasting, and have a reduced risk of cancer.

Formulations containing oestrogens alone became fashionable for helping certain women through the undesirable psychological and physical aspects of the menopause. Many such preparations have now been withdrawn; although achieving the proposed objectives, patients also ran a higher risk of endo-metrial cancer and possibly breast cancer. Such postmenopausal treatments are ethically acceptable only if progestins are also included in the regimen. A most distressing and so far unexplained illustration of the dangers of hormones is provided in reports of vaginal cancer in young women whose mothers took stilboestrol during early pregnancy to prevent threatened abortion.

Extensive epidemiological studies have established the major risk factors for breast cancer (see Chapter 3). These include early menarche, late menopause, having close relatives with the disease, infertility, obesity, geographic location, and having the first pregnancy late in life. The current strategy is to try to explain these findings in terms of hormonal imbalance, but no unequivocal conclusions can yet be drawn. None the less, breast cancer is generally considered to result from overexposure to oestrogens and underexposure to progesterone. The risk associated with obesity can be partly explained by the ability of adipose cells to synthesize oestrogens, but impaired activity of detoxification mechanisms in the liver and elsewhere may also be implicated. The beneficial effect of having a child early in life could be owing to the high concentrations of progesterone-like hormones in pregnancy protecting the breast cells against oestrogens in the long term. The risks of early menarche and late menopause can be combined in that a high number of menstrual cycles may be dangerous in terms of the repeated surges of oestrogens ultimately providing the stimulus for malignancy. Raised concentrations of free oestradiol are present in the plasma of women with breast and endometrial cancer as compared with normal, age-matched controls. Similar measurements in other cancers could be vital in the future for diagnostic and prognostic purposes.

All of these epidemiological considerations apply equally forcibly to endometrial cancer. One possible clue, as with prostate cancer in men, is provided by studies on Japanese migrants to Western cultures. Breast and endometrial cancer increase in these women, possibly as a result of changing diet. Western foods tend to be richer in fat and this may cause subtle but significant changes in the hormonal milieu and even hormonal imbalance. This is considered in more detail in Chapter 3.

There is now evidence that genetic factors are also involved and specific chromosome and gene changes have been identified in 'Breast Cancer Families' in whom the risk of developing breast cancer is very high. The presence or absence of these genes and their relationship to sporadic breast cancers may lead to the development of diagnostic tests and also a possible approach to control and treatment. It seems likely that endocrine changes, diet, etc. may produce their effects by acting on cells that are pre-disposed to neoplastic development by genetic changes either transmitted *in utero* or induced by carcinogenic agents in later life [for a review see Fentiman and Taylor-Papadimitriou (1993)].

Hormones and cancer in men: prostate cancer The high incidence of prostate cancer in the human male remains an enigma and, as in so many cancers, we have no real idea why the incidence rises so sharply in old age (see Chapter 3). Certainly, the precise involvement of androgens remains to be defined. The only real clue so far is that the malignant prostate has a marked ability to form and retain elevated concentrations of 5α–di-hydrosterone; this androgen is a far more powerful mitogen than testosterone itself. The disease is associated with westernized, industrialized societies and remains relatively uncommon in Mongoloid races. In several studies, it has been shown that when Chinese and Japanese emigrated to California and Hawaii, their risk of developing prostatic cancer rose significantly. The formerly low incidence of prostate cancer in Japan itself is now gradually increasing, whereas formerly common cancers, especially of stomach, are gradually decreasing. While not a complete explanation, there is plausible evidence suggesting that the newly acquired risk is attributable to the adoption of social customs and particularly the diet more typical of the West.

In contrast to breast cancer, epidemiological studies on prostate cancer are much less extensive (see Chapter 3). In the United States, this cancer is more frequent in blacks than Caucasians and less so in Jewish immigrants. Throughout Europe, no relationship has been established between the high incidence of prostate cancer and socioeconomic status, marital status, fertility, social habits, hair distribution, and physical size. There are hints of a possible connection with recurrent prostatitis, repeated infections, and venereal disease. A remarkable connection has been drawn in several reports between prostate cancer and 'sustained sexual interest' and 'sex drive'. Needless to say, these terms are difficult to qualitate, let alone quantitate. Investigators have

used various parameters to measure sexual activity, and it remains possible that increased activity in some form is associated with prostate cancer.

Although a considerable literature has been amassed on the epidemiology of many human cancers, it is surprising that measurements of oestrogens and androgens in blood, urine, sebum, and even saliva, have so far failed to show that abnormalities in the concentrations of sex hormones are associated with the disease states. It should be stressed, however, that measurements in the past have been as total hormone concentrations. In biological terms, it is the concentration of free, unbound hormone that is important. As is the case in the breast, we now know that genetic changes are also involved, although studies are still in their early stages. Prostate cancer families have been identified and possible chromosome changes defined.

14.4.3 The actions of hormones on tumour cells in culture

Stable lines of tumour cells provide an invaluable approach for studying the direct effects of hormones. Such studies are expanding rapidly, because cells in culture, rather than in intact animals, have the advantages of easy manipulation, high biochemical activities, and ethical acceptance. Three experimental systems will be briefly reviewed.

Human breast cancer cells Because of the understandable concern about the present scale of the breast cancer problem, a great deal of effort has been directed at the establishment of such tumour cells in culture. The driving force behind these enterprises is the ability to screen the effects of hormones and other drugs on the tumour cells directly. Unfortunately, as noted briefly in Chapter 1, only a very small number of human tumours can be maintained in culture as permanent cell lines. We do not know why this should be but it does mean that those cell lines that have been established, particularly since most are derived from tumour metastases, are not representative of all tumours. Nevertheless, much useful work has been done on the direct effects and mode of action of hormones and their receptors as already discussed. Obviously these results apply to established tumours. A different technique is needed for studying the early stages of carcinogenesis. Most normal cells cannot be kept in tissue culture continuously but some workers have developed techniques that approach this aim. They separate normal epithelial cells from human breast tissue removed at operation to reduce the size of the breasts—although the fact that the breasts are abnormally large does raise a small doubt about their normality. Populations of epithelial cells grow out from cultures of this material and growing colonies are selected. These cells, like all normal cells in tissue culture, have a finite life span and go through a limited number of population doublings before they die. By treating these cells with chemical carcinogens and/or oncogenes and growth factors some cells can be immortalized. These systems are being used to study the molecular basis for cell differentiation, immortalization, and tumour development and have great promise.

Much valuable information has also been obtained from work on breast cancer cells in tissue culture. Somatic mutations have been mapped and changes in hormone and growth factor receptors and production have been identified. As well as increasing our understanding of the molecular basis for tumour development, measurements of these gene products are being used in an approach to early diagnosis, prognosis, and treatment, but the work is in its early stages. Although the results are valuable indicators we must remember that many have been established using highly selected tissue culture cell lines. We do not yet know whether all of these changes are to be found in human breast cancer patients [for a review see Fentiman and Taylor-Papadimitriou (1993)].

Prostate cells in culture Prostate cell cultures suffer from the same drawbacks as those found using breast tissue. Although a small number of human prostate tumour cell lines are available, normal epithelial cells cannot be kept for any length of time and few of the tumour or normal cells respond to hormones in the same way as do cells *in vivo*, probably because hormone action may also involve factors derived from the stroma. Using organ culture techniques (see Chapter 1), whole gland complexes, with epithelium in its normal relationship to its stroma, can be maintained for some weeks. A great deal of information on the direct effects of hormones was learnt in the past using organ cultures of rodent prostate (and breast). The method is still to be exploited fully using human tissues.

Rat lymphoma cells Powerful glucocorticoids are used in transplantation surgery to suppress the immune system and there is now some evidence that these steroids not only kill some lymphoid cells but may also act as a trigger for the development of some leukaemias and lymphomas.

Studies on rat lymphoma cell lines have provided explanations for the cytocidal effects of glucocorticoids, and also led to a better understanding of the mechanism of action of steroid hormones in general. This work has been expedited by the availability of powerful analogues of cortisol. Many of these analogues, such as dexamethasone, fluoprednisolone, and triamcinolone acetonide, contain substituent fluorine atoms at positions 6 or 9 of the steroid ring system. The halogen substitutions greatly potentiate the biological activity of these synthetic glucocorticoids because they do not bind to the transport protein, corticosteroid-binding globulin, in serum and also resist catabolism within glucocorticoid target cells.

The killing of B lymphocytes and tumours derived from them by glucocorticoids was first described by Daughaday in 1943. Subsequent research has shown that cell death is mediated by glucocorticoid receptors in the lymphocytes and lymphomas, and preliminary experiments suggest that this might involve the activity of the activator protein AP-1 (Helmberg *et al.* 1995). The hormone-induced cytolysis is clearly a complex process; certainly the uptake of life-maintaining glucose is completely suppressed, together with the intracellular accumulation of toxic fatty acids and DNAses.

Certain sublines of lymphomas have been found to be resistant to glucocorticoids and their study has been of fundamental importance. Resistance can be explained by several types of change in the receptor system for binding glucocorticoids. In the final analysis, however, these seemingly encouraging results on cultured tumour cells must be viewed with caution, tinged even with disappointment, when applied to the human equivalents of these cancers.

14.5 The mode of action of hormones in carcinogenesis

Because of their potential danger in ecological and industrial terms, a great deal of effort has been directed towards elucidating the general mechanism of action of chemical carcinogens. With a few exceptions, chemical carcinogens exist as precarcinogens which must be activated, usually in the target organ, before their carcinogenicity can be maximally expressed (see Chapter 6). Such activation is necessary with many naturally occurring carcinogens, including the aflatoxins, quercitin, and cycasin. In the latter activation is carried out by intestinal microorganisms. Before examining the carcinogenic properties of hormones in detail, it is useful to compare their mechanism of action with that of carcinogens (Table 14.1). It is clear that the mechanisms are very different except that both hormones and chemical carcinogens need dividing cells as targets for the malignant process to develop.

14.5.1 A comparison of hormones and chemical carcinogens

As described in Chapters 1 and 6 the original concept of Berenblum, that carcinogenesis consists of a first phase of initiation followed by various phases of promotion, is now widely accepted. With a few notable exceptions, hormones act as promoters or cocarcinogens (Moolgavskar 1986). There are only a few instances where they may be considered as genuine initiators, like the chemical carcinogens. Generally, hormones enhance the rate of initiation and development of tumours induced by all of the proven classes of initiators, such as chemical carcinogens, viruses, and ionizing radiations. A crucial point that argues against hormones being initiators is that they are not mutagenic, whereas almost all genuine initiators are powerful mutagens. Perhaps one case where hormones may act as genuine initiators is the vaginal cancer in young women whose mothers took stilboestrol during pregnancy. At various stages in development, human embryos are acutely sensitive to damage by a wide range of exogenous agents. In this case, traces of stilboestrol could pass through the protective barrier of the placenta and initiate carcinogenesis in oestrogen target organs such as the vagina, but why other target organs such as the uterus are not affected is not known. The cancer may only develop after birth under the promoting influence of oestrogens after puberty.

In acting primarily as cocarcinogens, hormones could exert their influence in any of three ways, namely in classical promotion, in accelerating tumour growth, or in sensitizing target cells to initiating agents. Dividing cells are prime targets for carcinogens. Both classes of sex hormone are powerful mitogens and promote division, and even hyperplasia, in certain of their target organs, including prostate, breast, and cervix. These hormones, therefore, increase the potential number of cells that will be at increased risk on exposure to initiating agents. This process may be termed sensitization. Hormones may also have a significant role in tumour progression (see Section 14.5.5).

14.5.2 Tumour promotion

There are many examples in experimental systems where hormones act as promoters and greatly increase the incidence of tumour development by initiators. Particularly good examples, although by different mechanisms, include the promoting influence of glucocorticoids, thyroxine and somatotropin on the induction of skin tumours in mice by methyl-

Table 14.1 A comparison of the mechanism of action of hormones and chemical carcinogens

Property	Hormones	Chemical carcinogens
Mutagenicity	Not mutagenic	Mutagenic
Site of action	mRNA and proteins	DNA
Latent period	Long	Short
Nature of tumours	Benign or locally invasive	Highly malignant and metastatic
Activation	Generally not necessary	Necessary
Species and sex dependency	Very marked	Barely relevant
Nature of repeated exposure	Prolonged	Single exposure may suffice
Expression of carcinogenicity	*In vivo* only	*In vivo* and *in vitro*
Regression after ceasing exposure	Regression	No regression
Need for cell division	Needed	Needed

cholanthrene and croton oil, and the activation of mouse mammary tumour virus by glucocorticoids.

Another good example is that of mammary tumours induced in rats by dimethylbenzanthracene (Russo and Russo 1986). This chemical is a potent inducer of breast tumours in the rat if it is administered at precisely 50 days of age; if administered at other times, its carcinogenicity to breast epithelium is markedly decreased (Table 14.2). Seemingly, the hormonal milieu and the developmental state of the cells at 50 days are optimal for tumour induction. Removal of the ovaries at any time reduces the induction of tumours and this may be reversed by administration of oestrogens. In hypophysectomized rats oestrogens are ineffective as promoters and it seems their influence is expressed through the hypothalamicpituitary axis by means of the accelerated secretion of prolactin. This may be an authentic example of prolactin-sensitive tumour induction. Progesterone has a complex influence in this experimental system. When administered before the initiating carcinogen, tumour incidence decreases, but when given after the initiator, tumour incidence increases. This paradox remains to be clarified. Certainly, it would be dangerous to extrapolate these findings to breast cancer in women. As emphasized before, data from animal work are not always consistent with clinical findings, and in this particular case, the very nature of the tumours may be fundamentally different.

The involvement of oestrogens in the development and course of endometrial cancer is much clearer, although it is difficult to draw an absolute distinction between initiation and promotion. Certainly, oestrogens promote the disease, after earlier phases of hyperplasia and preneoplasia, and these are all

countered by progesterone or synthetic progestins. While this is a striking example of tumour promotion in the human, it is surprising that oestrogens rarely induce endometrial cancer in experimental animals. The difference could be of some importance, because it could imply that induction of tumours by the sex hormones is not simply by evoking changes in cell proliferation and mitosis; other factors are almost certainly involved.

We know very little about the relationship between other hormones and carcinogenesis. Although it has been suggested that there is a close relationship between the androgens and tumour growth in the prostate, firm evidence that they play any role in tumour induction is lacking.

14.5.3 Tumour growth

In considering tumour growth, two aspects are particularly important. Tumour cells may divide more slowly than many normal cells, but are distinguished by their continued rather than their rapid growth. Secondly, an increase in tumour size occurs only when cell multiplication exceeds cell death; in the prostate and breast, it has been estimated that between 25 and 45 per cent of new cells soon die. From these considerations, hormones could exert an influence on tumour size by maintaining exponential growth or slowing cell death. Although hormones may affect tumour growth by direct action on the cells, indirect mechanisms may also play a part. The influence of hormones on the growth of common human tumours, such as prostate and breast, is complex. These tumours are composed of epithelium, stroma, and blood vessels. In the normal breast, oestrogens promote the proliferation of the endothelial cells in the capillaries and this may provide an indirect way in which these hormones modulate tumour growth by increasing the supply of nutrients. In the prostate, there has been a belief for many years that a close structural and functional interaction between the stromal and epithelial elements is mandatory for the coordinated normal growth of the organ. Prolonged exposure to androgens, especially 5α-dihydrotestosterone, could upset this delicate stromalepithelial interaction. Future research in this area has been given a strong boost by the successful maintenance of separated stromal and epithelial elements of human, dog, and rat prostate in culture; this breakthrough should provide new insights into the mechanism controlling prostate

Table 14.2 The influence of hormones on the induction of mammary tumours by dimethylbenzanthracene

Additional treatment	Number of tumours	Day of appearance of tumours
None	Many	90–94
Ovariectomy, 30–35 days	Few	106–110
Ovariectomy, 65–70 days	Few	106–110
Progesterone, 30–35 days	Few	106–110
Progesterone, 60–70 days	Very many	79–83

Dimethylbenzathracene was given through a stomach tube to female Sprague–Dawley rats of 50 days of age, either alone, with administration of progesterone, or to ovariectomized animals.

growth and the part played by the androgens in the process.

To study the mitogenic effects of hormones and growth factors a number of cancer cell lines have been developed, particularly from breast cancers but also from endometrial and prostate cancers. Some of these proliferate in response to steroid hormones but our understanding of the mechanisms involved is poor. This is partly because steroid hormones appear to regulate the expression of so many target genes implicated in cell proliferation that it is difficult to identify the crucial ones. It is quite possible that the concept of a single rate-limiting step is inappropriate to explain the effects of various mitogens, in which case steroid hormones might regulate several distinct steps in the cell cycle or different stages in the development of a tumour.

Autocrine growth control It has been suggested that tumour cells may themselves produce the growth factors necessary for maintaining cell proliferation and that these factors might function in an autocrine manner (see Glossary). Thus, steroid hormones might function as mitogens indirectly, by increasing the production of growth factors or possibly by reducing the secretion of growth inhibitory factors or by stimulating the expression of appropriate receptors (for reviews see Clarke *et al.* 1991; Roberts and Sporn 1992). A number of groups studying breast cancer cell lines have obtained support for this concept by demonstrating that oestrogens increase the expression of epidermal growth factor (EGF), transforming growth factor-α (TGF-α), platelet-derived growth factor (PDGF), and insulin-like growth factors (IGF) in different cell lines. However, in primary breast tumours, TGF-α is probably the best candidate for a growth stimulatory factor since the other growth factors are barely detectable in the majority of tumours. On the other hand, oestrogens have been found to decrease the production of the inhibitory growth factor TGF-β in several oestrogen receptor positive breast cancers. Moreover, since retinoids, which inhibit the growth of these cell lines, increase the production of this negative growth factor it has been suggested that TGF-β might also be an important mediator of nuclear receptors in cell growth. In addition to effects on growth factors, oestrogens have been shown to stimulate the expression of receptors for a number of growth factors including those for IGF-I and EGF.

Therefore, another effect of oestrogens might be to increase the sensitivity of cells to growth factors produced either by tumour cells themselves or perhaps by surrounding stromal cells, thereby regulating cell proliferation by a paracrine (see Glossary) mechanism (Clarke *et al.* 1991). Thus, according to these views, the major effects of steroid hormones and retinoids are indirect, stimulating cell growth by autocrine or paracrine control mechanisms.

In support of the autocrine hypothesis, oestrogen antagonists such as tamoxifen and the 'pure' anti-oestrogen ICI 182780 are capable of reversing most, if not all, of the oestrogen-inducible events described above. Thus, tamoxifen treatment reduces the expression of the growth factor TGF-α and increases the secretion of the growth inhibitor TGF-β consistent with its effects on cell growth. However, it is doubtful whether antioestrogens function simply by antagonizing the effects of oestradiol because they not only inhibit oestrogen-induced cell growth, but are also capable of blocking the mitogenic effects of growth factors such as EGF and IGF-1 (Chalbos *et al.* 1994). This observation indicates that antioestrogens elicit a growth inhibitory response in their own right. This might be achieved by its effects on TGF-β production or might involve the antagonism of other signalling pathways (see Section 14.3).

Direct effects of steroids on the cell cycle It has been found that steroid hormones function primarily in the G1 phase of the cell cycle. For example, oestrogens stimulate the recruitment of breast cancer cells into the cell cycle and shorten the length of their G1 phase. On the other hand, oestrogen antagonists reduce the proportion of cells in S phase supporting the suggestion that steroid hormones, like other growth factors, act within the G1 phase of the cell cycle to regulate cell proliferation. Of particular importance was the observation that oestrogen antagonists not only block the effect of oestrogens but also proliferation induced by other growth factors, suggesting that the antioestrogen–receptor complex functions as a growth inhibitor in its own right.

Many different types of genes are implicated in the G1 phase of the cell cycle, some of which are targets for steroid hormones. For example, the products of a number of immediate early response genes, including members of the Fos and Myc families, which are required for cell cycle progression, are increased in MCF-7 breast cancer tissue culture cells following oestrogen treatment. The expression of these immediate early response genes is transient and it is assumed that they in turn regulate the transcription of downstream target genes involved in cell proliferation. One such group are the cyclins and the cyclin-dependent kinases. The D-type cyclins may function at G1 control points and, interestingly, the expression of cyclin D1 mRNA and protein is regulated by steroid hormones in breast cancer cells (Musgrove and Sutherland 1994). The significance of these changes should soon become clearer because this has become a very active area of research.

Cross-coupling between nuclear receptors and other signalling pathways The transcriptional activity of the oestrogen receptor has been reported to be modulated by a number of other signalling pathways involving different protein kinase cascades. In some cases , the effect was oestrogen independent whereas in other cases the alternative

pathway modulated oestrogen-dependent transcription. One of the most striking observations is that the effects of oestrogen on the mouse uterus could be reproduced by administering epidermal growth factor (EGF) to animals and subsequent experiments with uterine cells indicated that the effects were mediated by the oestrogen receptor (Ignar-Trowbridge *et al.* 1992). EGF acts through several pathways, including protein kinase C and MAP kinase, and so it is possible that one of these directly phosphorylates the oestrogen receptor. Agents that increase intracellular cAMP levels and protein kinase A activity also increase the transcriptional activity of the oestrogen receptor (Fig. 14.7). This effect was first demonstrated by treating cells with the neurotransmitter dopamine, acting through the dopamine D1 receptor, which was found to stimulate the transcriptional activity of several steroid hormone receptors in the absence of cognate hormone (Power *et al.* 1991). Since steroid receptors do not appear to contain a consensus protein kinase A phosphorylation site

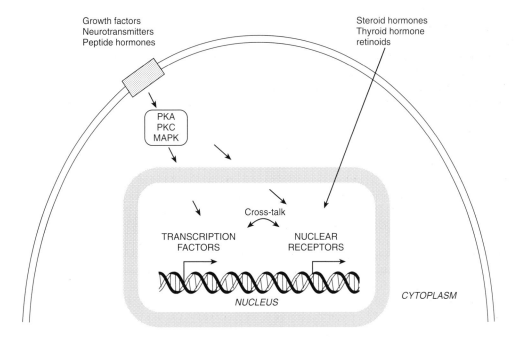

Fig. 14.7 Cross-coupling between nuclear receptors and membrane receptors. Growth factors, neurotransmitters, and peptide hormones activate a number of kinase cascades, including protein kinase A (PKA), protein kinase C (PKC), and the MAP kinase pathway, to stimulate the activity of specific transcription factors and also modulate the activity of nuclear receptors. In addition, the transcription factors and nuclear receptors interact directly with one another, either on or off DNA, to modulate transcriptional activity.

it seems likely that the effect of this kinase on transcriptional activity is indirect.

Finally, cross-coupling also occurs within the cell nucleus between receptors and other transcription factors whose activity is modulated by different signalling pathways, such as AP-1. AP-1 is implicated as a critical target for many signalling pathways that regulate cell differentiation, proliferation, and transformation (Vogt and Bos 1990; Angel and Karin 1991). Its importance as a target for growth factors, which stimulate the phosphorylation of Fos/Jun family members, is well established but it might also play an important role in growth regulation by steroid hormones and retinoids (Figs 14.2 and 14.7). In some cases AP-1 activity is increased and in other cases decreased, the differential response depending on the composition of the AP-1 complex. Thus, oestrogens, which stimulate the proliferation of MCF-7 breast cancer cells, increase growth factor-induced AP-1 activity, whereas retinoids and antioestrogens, which inhibit their growth, inhibit AP-1 activity (Chalbos *et al.* 1994; Fanjul *et al.* 1994). This might then explain how antioestrogens are capable of blocking the mitogenic effect not only of oestradiol but also certain growth factors.

14.5.4 Growth control by altered receptors

Oestrogen receptors There is no evidence to suggest that mutant oestrogen receptors are associated with the development or subsequent growth of either breast or endometrial cancers, but it is conceivable that alterations in the function of oestrogen receptors are associated with tamoxifen resistance. Despite the efficacy of tamoxifen treatment most breast cancer patients eventually develop drug resistance. In many cases this could simply result from the activation of other signalling pathways involved in cell growth that enable breast cancer cells to grow independently of oestrogen receptor activity. However, it appears that as many as 50 per cent of breast cancer patients still respond to an alternative form of endocrine therapy suggesting that in these cases the receptor is still required for optimum growth of the tumour. Thus, it seems reasonable to conclude that the function of the receptor in response to tamoxifen must have been altered.

Initially, it was thought that differences in tamoxifen metabolism or mutant receptor might be responsible. However, tamoxifen metabolites,

which could act as agonists rather than antagonists, have not been convincingly demonstrated, and mutations in the oestrogen receptor gene occur infrequently and have not been detected in the majority of tamoxifen-resistant breast tumours. On the other hand, receptor mRNA variants, formed as a consequence of aberrant RNA splicing, are relatively common and detectable in most oestrogen target cells . One of these, referred to as the exon 5 deletion (ERD5), has the potential to generate a receptor that lacks the hormone-binding domain, since RNA from exon 4 is spliced directly to RNA from exon 6 causing a frameshift mutation that results in premature termination of translation. In model systems, this variant receptor is incapable of binding tamoxifen and has been shown to stimulate transcription of target genes, but it is not clear whether it is expressed as a stable protein in tumours. Moreover, the variant mRNA is not found preferentially in tamoxifen-resistant tumours. Therefore, since neither tamoxifen or the oestrogen receptor itself seem to be altered in resistant cells, it is conceivable that changes in alternative signalling pathways might account for the change in sensitivity of the receptor to tamoxifen. For example, protein kinase A activation can increase the agonist effects of tamoxifen in model systems, but whether this occurs in primary tumours has yet to be demonstrated.

Retinoic acid receptors The importance of RAR in acute promyelocytic leukaemia was discovered independently by two groups using completely different rationales. The approach of Solomon and her colleagues (Grimwade and Solomon 1995), exploiting the observation that acute promyelocytic leukaemia is associated with a t(15;17) reciprocal translocation, was to map the breakpoint (Fig. 14.8). They found that the RAR-α gene on chromosome 17 had been fused to a gene on chromosome 15 that was subsequently called *PML*, for promyelocytic leukaemia. De The *et al.* (1991), on the other hand, predicted that RAR-α might be involved since it was known, firstly, that the RAR-α gene maps to chromosome 17q21 close to the t(15;17) translocation and, secondly, that retinoic acid stimulates the differentiation of primary bone marrow cells from patients with acute promyelocytic leukaemia into mature granulocytes. When they analysed the structure of the RAR-α gene they also found that the gene had been translocated to a locus on

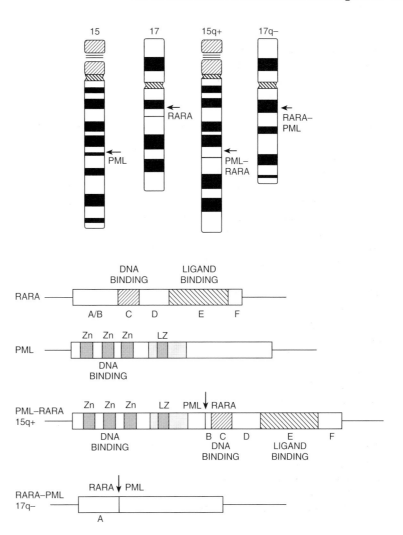

Fig. 14.8 Schematic representation of the reciprocal t(15;17) translocation observed in the promyelocytes in promyelocytic leukaemia (PML). Beneath is a schematic representation of the retinoic acid receptor α (RARA) and promyelocytic leukaemia (PML) showing functional domains. The RARA is subdivided into six regions A–F, and three potential zinc fingers (ZF) and a putative leucine zipper (ZIP) in PML are indicated.

chromosome 15 encoding PML. The translocation results in fusion genes that potentially encode two different fusion proteins, PML–RAR and RAR–PML. However, it is likely that PML–RAR rather than RAR–PML is associated with leukaemogenesis because it is the 15q and not the 17q derivative chromosome that is detected in the majority of the leukaemia cases. Moreover, most of the known functional domains in the two proteins are expressed in PML–RAR rather than RAR–PML (for reviews, see Grimwade and Solomon 1995 and De The *et al.* 1991).

RAR is clearly a ligand-dependent transcription factor but the function of PML is unknown. It contains a cysteine-rich region found in a number of DNA- and RNA-binding proteins and a potential

leucine zipper suggesting that it might be a transcription factor. The role of PML–RAR in leukaemogenesis is unknown but it appears to be behaving as a dominant negative oncogene that is antagonizing the action of either the normal RAR or PML. One model favours the suggestion that the differentiation of promyelocytes is under the control of RAR-α and that this is blocked by PML–RAR. There is no direct evidence for this but, interestingly, while the PML–RAR fusion protein retains its ability to stimulate transcription from retinoid responsive reporter genes it does display some promoter- and cell-specific differences from the wild-type retinoic acid receptor. It is therefore conceivable that these differences are related to its oncogenic activity. On the other hand it is also possible that cell differentiation is controlled by PML. An alternative model, therefore, is that the action of PML is blocked by the ligand-binding domain of the RAR but that this can be relieved upon ligand binding. Interestingly, the subcellular distribution of PML is perturbed in the fusion protein. The PML protein, which is ubiquitous, is normally detected as part of a macromolecular structure in the cell nucleus whereas the fusion protein is dispersed into a microparticulate pattern in APL cells. However, treatment of these cells with retinoic acid results in a reorganization of the fusion protein into a pattern resembling that of the wild-type PML protein (Dyck *et al.* 1994). This change is consistent with the clinical observation that retinoic acid treatment appears to restore the normal function of PML and the RAR. One of the major goals now is to identify target genes for PML and RAR-α that are involved in normal haematopoiesis in order to test whether they are aberrantly expressed in acute promyelocytic leukaemia.

Thyroid hormone receptors One of the best examples of a nuclear receptor that contributes to the malignant phenotype by interfering with cell differentiation is illustrated by the avian erythroblastosis virus (AEV). This retrovirus, which causes lethal erythroleukaemias and sarcomas in chicks, contains two oncogenes, v-*erbA*, a mutated form of the chicken thyroid hormone receptor α, and v-*erbB*, a truncated form of the chicken epidermal growth factor receptor (Beug and Vennstrom 1991). In erythroblasts, v-erbB stimulates cell pro-

liferation in the absence of erythropoietin while v-erbA arrests differentiation and promotes the effects of v-erbB. This arrest in erythroblast differentiation is reflected by the suppression of specific erythrocyte genes such as carbonic anhydrase, band 3, and the haem biosynthesis enzyme δ-aminolevulinate synthetase. In fibroblasts, v-erbB abrogates the requirement for mitogens and v-erbA seems to elicit only minor effects. The normal role of thyroid hormone receptor α in erythroid cell proliferation and differentiation is unknown but it seems quite likely that the normal pathway is a target for the oncogenic action of v-erbA. Finally, a role for these two receptors in human erythroleukaemias and sarcomas has not been reported but it is conceivable that similar target genes might be involved.

14.5.5 Tumour progression

Progression in tumours has been unequivocally demonstrated in many experimental systems and is supported by clinical observations. In general, hormone-sensitive tumours progress to an autonomous hormone-insensitive state, but whether this is owing to changes in the cells or to selection of resistant cells already present in the tumour is not known. A good example is seen in the BR6 mouse, which develops multiple mammary cancers very frequently. The tumours appear and grow rapidly during pregnancy and may regress after birth, but grow again at precisely the same site during the next pregnancy (Fig. 14.9). The tumours each behave independently.

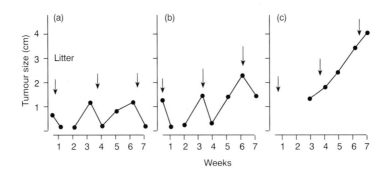

Fig. 14.9 Three mammary tumours with different properties in a single BR6 mouse. The tumours arise during pregnancy, and may disappear (responsive tumours) or persist (unresponsive tumours), after delivery of the litters, marked by arrows (data from Foulds 1969). (a) Left groin–pregnancy-responsive–complete regression. (b) Right axilla–pregnancy-responsive–incomplete regression. (c) Right neck–pregancy-unresponsive.

Some regress completely after pregnancy, others show incomplete regression and others become completely autonomous, i.e. they are no longer dependent on pregnancy-associated hormones for their growth (Foulds 1969). It should be stressed that progression is not invariably from normal hormone responsive to hormone unresponsive. Since the information given in Fig. 14.9 was taken from one mouse, it is clear that the hormonal responsiveness of a given tumour is intrinsic and not determined by the gross environment.

An observation of fundamental importance is that during progression of the Dunning prostate tumour, there are major changes in the complement of chromosomes, i.e. towards aneuploidy. Similar changes occur in other tumours but the precise gene changes involved have still to be discovered.

14.6 Types and nature of hormone-sensitive and hormone-producing tumours

From the earlier discussion it is clear that endocrine-associated tumours fall into two groups, hormone sensitive from target organs, and hormone producing from endocrine glands (see also Chapter 15).

14.6.1 Hormone-sensitive tumours

Tumours arising from target organs should be described as hormone sensitive rather than hormone dependent. This is not a semantic distinction. Hormone dependence implies that certain tumours could only persist during hormonal stimulation and would atrophy if the source of hormone was removed. Both clinically and experimentally this is rarely the case. All tumours are heterogeneous with respect to cell type, and it follows that some cells may be sensitive to hormonal manipulation whereas others certainly are not. By altering the hormonal environment of certain tumours, the disease may be checked in many cases; such tumours are best described as hormone sensitive. When considering hormone-sensitive tumours, it may well be that the future will hold some remarkable surprises. Traditional endocrinology has been set on its head over the last decade by the discovery of a bewildering array of polypeptide hormones, from coded neurotransmitters to growth regulators (see Chapters 11, 15, and 20). Few investigators would have anticipated the identification of the naturally occurring analgesics, the endorphins, or predicted that hormones classically associated with the gastrointestinal tract, such as gastrin, glucagon, and cholecystokinin, could also be synthesized within the central nervous system. Our traditional tenets of endocrinology are probably very insecure and many growth factors and hormones of great relevance to human cancer are now being isolated and characterized.

Steroid-sensitive tumours Tumours in the accessory sexual glands are among the most common forms of cancer in men and women and these tumours are rightly described as hormone sensitive. The aetiology of these diseases is clearly complex . At the turn of the century, for example, carcinoma of the uterus was the most common hormone-sensitive tumour in women, although at that time a clear distinction between carcinoma of the uterine cervix and cancers of the endometrium was not always recorded; since then the incidence of endometrial tumours has decreased but there has been a pronounced and increasing incidence of breast cancer. This could reflect hormonal changes resulting from improved hygiene, better contraception, and better medical care in general. This particular tumour highlights a major problem for modern investigators; it is clearly imperative to find a plausible explanation for such important changes, but early medical records are often wanting and experimental animal models are few. The only common animal equivalent for endometrial cancer is the rabbit, and even here the disease is endocrinologically and pathologically distinct from the human disease.

Breast cancer is a major threat to the health of the female population in all westernized societies. Benign tumours, fibroadenomas, are rare before puberty but represent the commonest form of breast tumour in the age span 25–30 years. Carcinoma of the breast is age associated, and becomes more common from about 30 years of age (see Chapter 3). There is a clear endocrinological basis for the disease and, as described later, this provides the rationale for clinical manipulation and arrest of the disease in many women. Tumours in other organs of the female reproductive tract, e.g. the vulva and vagina, are relatively rare, but may be induced by oestrogens under certain circumstances (see p. 283). In both cases, a hormonal imbalance, and particularly an excess of oestrogens, is involved.

In Western societies, cancer of the prostate is one of the most common male cancers. It usually appears in men of 60 years or older and increases in frequency with age. The tumours vary enormously from highly invasive, poorly differentiated tumours to relatively slow growing and well-differentiated forms. Cancers in other male accessory organs, such as epididymis and seminal vesicle, are rare. In all cases, there is likely to be a hormonal involvement. Cancer of the penis and scrotum are also very rare; a hormonal basis for these tumours is possible but not proven. Circumcision certainly is accepted as the prime defence against cancer of the penis; for reasons unknown, this cancer is particularly frequent in the stallion. No other animal shares this risk.

Polypeptide-sensitive tumours It is now clear that the cells of the body are continually exposed to many polypeptide hormones. Although many cells respond to somatotropin and virtually all cells respond to insulin by increasing uptake of glucose and amino acids, very few tumours seem to be sensitive to these polypeptide hormones. There is growing evidence for the involvement of prolactin in the induction and progression of certain tumours. The first indication of the involvement of prolactin in carcinogenesis came from studies on the growth of several lines of transplantable mammary tumours in the A×C rat. This hormone may also play a significant role in the growth of cancers in the breast and prostate; in the latter case, prolactin may enhance the uptake of androgens from the peripheral circulation. There are indirect indications, but little definite information, that polypeptide hormones of the pituitary may modulate the growth of certain tumours. The effects of other polypeptides are considered in Chapters 11, 15, and 20.

14.6.2 Hormone-producing tumours

All hormone-producing organs are potential sites for malignancy. Tumours, as well as producing effects by their size and position, may cause symptoms by interfering with the normal production of hormones by the organ; by overproduction of normal hormones, or by the production of hormones not normally produced.

Ovarian tumours most commonly occur in the age range 40–60 years. Benign conditions are also quite common. Ovarian cancers are of many different types. The most common tumours arise from the surface epithelium and have a wide range of structures; the second group are of germ cell origin; and a third rare group arises from sex cord stromal cells (these cells normally surround germ cells and are responsible for the production of ovarian steroid hormones). Tumours from these latter cells are likely to be hormone producing and may produce oestrogens or androgens.

Testicular tumours, although not common, are increasing in frequency and are the most frequent form of cancer in young men. As outlined in Chapter 3, there is strong evidence that hormonal changes *in utero* may be a factor in their development. As in the ovary, tumours may arise from the germ cells, or, much less often, from specialized androgen-producing interstitial cells or oestrogen-producing Sertoli cells. Some germ cell-derived tumours, for unknown reasons, may produce a hormone, human chorionic gonadotropin (HCG), normally produced by the human placenta.

The adrenal gland has two parts, an inner medulla and an outer cortex, each having a different embryological origin. The medulla can be considered as a neuroendocrine organ and its tumours are discussed in Chapter 15. The cortex produces steroid hormones, mainly gluco- and mineralo-corticoids, but it may also produce oestrogens and androgens. Tumours in the adrenal cortex have been widely investigated and have very interesting properties. Small, benign adenomas are quite common, but carcinomas are rare. The tumours show no age dependency and can occur from infancy to senility, but affect women more than men. The tumours are often well differentiated, with an almost normal glandular appearance, but in many cases they may grow to a remarkable size. The disease is usually fatal because of metastasis to vital organs, rather than a lethal deterioration in the synthesis of life-supporting glucocorticoids and mineralocorticoids.

The physiological outcome of cancer in steroid-producing organs can often be profound. Tumours may lead to overproduction or impairment of steroid secretion, either of hormones normally produced or of other steroids. In either event, the clinical consequences can be dramatic, often dangerous, and socially distressing. For example, certain adrenal tumours in women result in virilization owing to excessive secretion of androgens, with consequent psychological and physical disturbances such as abundant growth of bodily hair and voice changes.

Tumours in organs producing polypeptide hormones can also have dire consequences. In many pituitary tumours, the secretion of tropins is anomalous, with dramatic interference, for example, in sexual activity and fertility. Similarly, tumours of the pancreas can either curtail or overproduce the secretion of insulin and glucagon, with dangerous and even fatal consequences (see Chapter 15). Tumours of other endocrine organs, e.g. thyroid, can produce similar effects.

Human cancers can cause unexpected clinical difficulties. Some tumour cells may acquire the ability to synthesize hormones; for example, certain types of lung cancer actively secrete the pituitary hormone, adrenocorticotropin. This is generally referred to as ectopic hormone secretion. In women, tumours of placental origin (hydatidiform mole and choriocarcinoma) may secrete vast quantities of gonadotropins. The progression or cure of many of these cancers can be monitored by the cessation of abnormal hormone secretion.

14.7 Treatment of hormone-sensitive human cancers

From the overview of general endocrinology presented earlier (see Fig. 14.1), there are many opportunities for curtailing the supply of hormones to tumours. Some of the approaches are far more radical than others and in recent years ingenious and less stressful approaches have been explored. Means have also been found to reduce the harmful effects of many drugs and hormones on normal cells.

14.7.1 Hormonal manipulation

Endocrine treatment for prostate cancer has been used for more than 40 years. Huggins and Hodges argued that since the normal gland required androgens for its growth, antiandrogenic treatment might inhibit the growth of prostatic tumour cells. This can be done either by removing the main source of androgen—the testes—or by antagonizing androgens with oestrogens, usually by giving stilboestrol orally. In many cases this proved to be effective. About 80 per cent of all cases respond at first, but eventually most relapse. It was thought that this may have been owing to the production of androgens by the adrenals, perhaps stimulated by pituitary hormones produced in increased amounts as a result of castration or oestrogen treatment. Removal of the adrenals or pituitary was then used, but these operations are life threatening themselves and the results were not satisfactory. Most tumours eventually become hormone independent and continue to grow. The use and dosage of stilboestrol remains a very controversial issue. Certainly, it is accepted that only low doses should be used, to reduce the risk of breast enlargement, electrolyte and cardiovascular disturbances, as well as psychological problems. Obviously better forms of treatment are required.

Great thought has been given to the targeting principle in the therapy of tumours (see Chapter 19). The ideal is to deliver the drug selectively to the tumour itself, eliminating deleterious side effects on normal tissues. For example, thyroid cancers can be selectively and effectively killed by low doses of radioactive ^{125}I because thyroid cells concentrate this halogen, a property retained by many of the tumour cells. In the prostate a suggestion was to use phosphorylated forms of stilboestrol and oestradiol-1β. Until the phosphate groups are removed, the drugs have little if any biological activity; however, the prostate has a remarkably high activity of phosphatases, thus ensuring that the prostatic tumour will tend to concentrate and release the active drug component specifically, but the clinical results are still uncertain. Another approach of great promise is the development of drugs that selectively inhibit the enzyme 5α-reductase, responsible for forming the powerful mitogen 5α-dihydrotestosterone within the prostate tumour. A lot of effort has been applied to the development of antiandrogens which block the function of the androgen receptors. Many such compounds have been synthesized, including the steroid cyproterone acetate and the non-steroidal compound, flutamide. Clinically, neither have proved useful in curing prostate cancer, although they have been effective in individual cases. The most revolutionary proposal for the successful arrest of prostate cancer by hormonal means has come from research by Labrie and co-workers in Canada; suppression of androgen secretion in patients with prostatic cancer, by a drug combination of antiandrogens, such as flutamide or anandron, plus a powerful range of synthetic analogues of gonadotropin-releasing hormone (GnRH). The antiandrogens block the peripheral effects of any androgens while the GnRH analogues suppress the hypothalamic–pituitary axis and also reduce the gonadotropin receptors in the testis by down-regulation, thus effectively suppressing the secretion of androgens. This approach seems to be more effective than androgen treatment alone but after initial regression the tumours often recur. None the less, new approaches for the hormonal manipulation of prostate cancer are needed, because radical surgical removal of the prostate is now seen as a difficult and unsatisfactory procedure; metastases of the disease cannot be treated by surgical means.

Many of the considerations on prostate cancer are relevant to breast cancer in women. Methods are being sought to replace radical surgery on the breast or on the endocrine glands. Such practices as hypophysectomy and radical mastectomy of the breast tumour are much rarer now than in the past (see Chapter 17). As in the prostate, the normal breast and many of its tumours, respond to the relevant sex hormones, mainly oestrogens and progestins.

Two aspects of the research and management of breast cancer have been most encouraging. Firstly, it is now accepted that measurements of the concentrations of oestrogen and progesterone receptors are valuable in the successful management of individual patients. The measurement of progesterone receptors is based on sound evidence that they are oestrogen-induced proteins. If the tumour is receptor positive, r^+, then hormonal manipulation is advised; if r^-, then chemotherapy should be used. Secondly, there are several antioestrogens available now, and tamoxifen in particular has been of striking benefit in the treatment of many women; about 30 per cent of all patients had an objective response and a further 20 per cent showed some clinical improvement. The results are better in postmenopausal women. For premenopausal women, ablation of the ovary, either by surgery or X-rays, remains the first choice for reduction of oestrogen levels.

Synthetic progestins, of long biological life and which may be taken orally, are finding wide and successful use in the treatment of endometrial cancer. Antioestrogens may also have an important role to play here in the future.

Synthetic glucocorticoids, especially prednisone, prednisolone, and their fluorinated counterparts, have also been invaluable for the treatment of many types of lymphoma and leukaemia. Such approaches are only of value if the malignancy is r^+, containing receptors for glucocorticoids; this is not always the case. Even if cells are r^+, hormones alone will not eradicate the disease and additional chemotherapy is required (see Chapter 18). Novel

glucocorticoids that are more specific in their action on r^+ cells are currently under study. For example, triamcinolone acetonide 21-oic acid methyl ester is a potent glucocorticoid without the side effects of any of its structural congeners; in particular, it neither suppresses the secretion of natural glucocorticoids from the adrenal glands nor promotes involution of the thymus. A major problem in treatment of hormone-responsive tumours is the growth of hormone-independent tumour cells.

14.7.2 Chemotherapy

We have not yet explored all the possibilities for the successful treatment of breast and prostate cancer by hormonal means. Surprises and new opportunities may be in store. For example, there is a growing and impressive body of evidence that aminoglutethimide may be very valuable in the treatment of most hormone-sensitive tumours; this drug, like ketoconazole, is an inhibitor of enzyme complexes containing cytochrome P450 and thus provides a clinical means of suppressing steroid hormone synthesis. In both these tumours, the administration of pharmacological doses of steroid hormones, including glucocorticoids, has often been found to be beneficial. There is no plausible explanation for these observations in molecular terms. As mentioned earlier, the final arrest of hormone-sensitive human tumours will depend on a combination of hormonal manipulation and chemotherapy. There seems to be little doubt that tumours in hormone-producing and target organs are induced by the same agents that induce tumours in other organs and that their reaction to changes in the hormonal environment depends on the degree to which the tumour cells have retained some of their normal characters. Consequently they are also likely to respond to agents that control tumour growth in other organs.

14.8 Conclusions and future prospects

The only definite conclusions that can be drawn from experimental work and studies in humans are that specific hormones are associated with the development and growth of some human tumours, but their precise role is still uncertain. Now that the molecular mechanisms of hormone action and the role of receptors and their genetic control are being clarified we shall be able to relate the observed changes in human cancer to this new knowledge, and, in time, be able to design methods for the control of tumour growth.

In the last decade there has been tremendous progress in investigating the molecular mechanism of action of nuclear receptors. Since the nuclear receptor family is so highly conserved it was anticipated that they would function by similar mechanisms and this has certainly facilitated their characterization. Nevertheless, there are some striking differences between family members, most notably in the way that they dimerize with one another and bind to DNA. Given the relative ease of producing receptors and individual structural domains and the exponential increase in the number of protein structures that have been solved over the last few years, progress in solving the structures of a number of DNA- and hormone-binding domains should be fairly rapid and this should explain the molecular basis for some of the differences in dimerization and DNA-binding activity. The availability of purified receptors and the development of assay systems that discriminate different functions of the receptors should allow the identification of compounds, and ultimately drugs, with more selective actions and therefore fewer side effects.

While many advances have been made we still know remarkably little about the role of nuclear receptors in cell growth. Part of the problem, at least in the case of steroid hormones and retinoids, is that there are many target genes implicated in cell proliferation, whose expression is regulated by the ligand, so that it is extremely difficult to assess their relative importance. It would not be surprising if the immediate downstream targets for nuclear receptors were, in fact, other transcription factors that are responsible for regulating cell cycle progression, and candidates are becoming evident as more is learned about cell cycle genes themselves.

The role of nuclear receptors in cell differentiation is even less well understood than that in cell growth. In the case of acute promyelocytic leukaemia in humans, and erythroleukaemias and sarcomas in chicken, further progress depends on the identification of target genes for retinoids and thyroid hormone, respectively, that control differentiation of the appropriate precursor cells. This is not trivial since there are likely to be many such genes and it will be a major task to identify those that control, rather than those that are responding to changes in, cell differentiation.

We must also remember that the hormones may have no direct role in the actual process of carcinogenesis and that tumour cells are influenced by the endocrine environment only as long as they retain residual normal characters.

A final lesson to be learnt from endocrinological research—as well as research in other fields—is that many experimental observations are made using highly selected animals and tissue culture cells maintained under abnormal conditions. Great care is needed before the results can be applied directly to the situation in humans.

References and further reading

Angel, P. and Karin M. (1991). The role of Jun, Fos and the AP-1 complex in cell-proliferation and transformation. *Biochimica Biophysica Acta*, **1072**, 129–57.

Beug, H. and Vennstrom B. (1991). Avian erythroleukaemia: possible mechanisms involved in v-*erb*A oncogene function. In *Nuclear hormone receptors. Molecular mechanisms, cellular functions, clinical abnormalities* (ed. M. G. Parker), pp. 321–53. Academic Press, London.

Chalbos, D., Philips, A. and Rochefort, H. (1994). Genomic cross-talk between the estrogen receptor and growth factor regulatory pathways in estrogen target issues. In Seminars in Cancer Biology (ed. M. Parker), pp. 361–8. Academic Press, London.

Clarke, R., Dickson, R. B. and Lippman, M. E. (1991). The role of steroid hormones and growth factors in the control of normal and malignant breast. In *Nuclear hormone receptors. Molecular mechanisms, cellular functions, clinical abnormalities* (ed. M. G. Parker), pp. 297–319, Academic Press, London.

Dauvois, S. and Parker, M. G. (1993). Mechanism of action of hormone antagonists. In *Steroid Hormone Action* (ed. M. G. Parker), pp 166–85. IRL Press, Oxford.

de The, H. *et al.* (1991). The PML-RAR alpha fusion mRNA generated by the t(15;17) translocation in acute promyelocytic leukemia encodes a functionally altered RAR. *Cell*, **66**, 675–84.

Diamond, M. I., Miner, J. N., Yoshinaga, S. K. and Yamamoto, K. R. (1990). Transcription factor interactions: selectors of positive or negative regulation from a single DNA element. *Science*, **249**, 1266–72.

Dyck, J. A., Maul, G. G., Miller, W. H., jun., Chen, J. D., Kakizuka, A., and Evans, R. M. (1994). A novel macromolecular structure is a target of the promyelocyte-retinoic acid receptor oncoprotein. *Cell*, **76**, 333–43.

Fanjul, A., Dawson, M. I., Hobbs, P. D., Jong, L., Cameron, J. F., Harley, E., Gaupner, G., Lu, M.-P. and Pfahl, M. (1994). A new class of retinoids with selective inhibition of AP-1 inhibits proliferation. *Nature*, **372**, 107–11.

Fentiman, I. S. and Taylor-Papadimitriou, J. (ed.) (1993). Breast cancer. *Cancer Surveys*, **18**, Cold Spring Harbor Press, New York.

Foulds, L. (1969). *Neoplastic development*. Academic Press, London.

Grimwade, D. and Solomon, E. (1997). Characterization of the PML/RARa rearrangement associated with t(15;17) acute promyelocytic leukaemia. *Current Topics in Microbiology and Immunology*, (ed. F. J. Ragscher and P. K. Vogt), **220**, 81–112. Springer Verlag, Berlin.

Helmberg, A., Auphan, N., Caelles, C., and Karin, M. (1995). Glucocorticoid-induced apoptosis of human leukemic-cells is caused by the repressive function of the glucocorticoid receptor. *EMBO Journal*, **14**, 452–60.

Ignar-Trowbridge, D. M., Nelson, K. G., Bidwell, M. C., Curtis, S. W., Washburn, T. F., McLachlan, J. A. and Korach, K. S. (1992). Coupling of dual signalling pathways: epidermal growth factor action involves the estrogen receptor. *Proceedings of the National Academy of Sciences, USA*, **89**, 4658–62.

Moolgavskar, S. H. (1986). Hormones and multistage carcinogenesis. *Cancer Surveys*, 635–48.

Musgrove, E. A. and Sutherland R. L. (1994). Cell cycle control by steroid hormones. In *Seminars in Cancer Biology* (ed. M. Parker), pp. 381–9. Academic Press, London.

Parker, M. G. (1993). Steroid and related receptors. *Current Opinion in Cell Biology*, 5, 499–504.

Power, R. F., Mani, S. K., Codina, J., Conneely, O. M. and O'Malley, B. W. (1991). Dopaminergic and ligand-independent activation of steroid hormone receptors. *Science*, **254**, 1636–9.

Roberts, A. B. and Sporn M. B. (1992). Mechanistic interrelationships between two superfamilies: the steroid/retinoid receptors and transforming growth factor b. *Cancer Surveys*, **14**, 205–20.

Russo, I. H. and Russo, J. (1986). From pathogenesis to hormone prevention of mammary carcinogenesis. *Cancer Surveys*, **5**, 649–70.

Stunnenberg, H. G. (1993). Mechanisms of transactivation by retinoic acid receptors. *Bioessays*, **15**, 309–15.

Vogt, P. K. and Bos T. J. (1990). Jun: oncogene and transcription factor. *Advances in Cancer Research*, **55**, 1–3.

Wakeling, A. E. (1992). Steroid antagonists as nuclear receptor blockers. *Cancer Surveys*, **14**, 71–85.

15

The neuroendocrine system and its tumours

J. M. POLAK AND S. R. BLOOM

The classical view of endocrinology, meaning the study of hormone-producing glands and their disorders, has been challenged seriously following the discovery that many body tissues contain the so called 'diffuse neuroendocrine system' (Polak and Bloom 1983, Falkmer *et al.* 1984). The cells of this system produce 'regulatory peptides', capable of acting not only at a distance, as chemical messengers or hormones, but also locally as paracrine substances or as neurotransmitters/neuromodulators (see Fig. 15.1). The reason for this multiplicity of actions is that regulatory peptides are produced by two different classes of tissue cells. Active peptides can be produced by endocrine cells or by neural elements. The former release the peptide either into the bloodstream (circulating hormones) or locally, in a paracrine manner, whereas the latter release the peptide from the nerve terminal after neuronal depolarization to act as neurotransmitters/neuromodulators.

Peptide-producing endocrine cells are dispersed throughout the body, often intermingled with non-endocrine tissue. These cells were first recognized by Feyrter who called them 'clear cells' because of their weak histological staining, or cells of the 'diffuse endocrine system', in view of their dispersed localization and possible regulatory function. The special histochemical properties of these cells led Pearse to apply the term 'APUD' (amine precursor uptake and decarboxylation) to them whereas the morpho-

logical characteristics these cells share with neurones (i.e. dense core secretory granules) led Fujita to propose the term 'para-neurones'. The recognition that neural tissue, often anatomically closely associated with endocrine cells, is also capable of producing and secreting active peptides led to expansion of the diffuse endocrine system to the 'diffuse neuroendocrine system'.

Regulatory peptides are being discovered at an exponential rate, owing to advances in chemical extraction procedures and, in particular, to molecular biology. The latter approach has also been instrumental in the determination of the chemical structure of the pre-pro-molecules from which smaller active peptides are generated (Fig. 15.2).

It is beyond the scope of this short review to describe in detail the characteristics of each individual peptide. The reader is, however, referred to a number of extensive review articles and to Table 15.1.

15.1 Morphological features of peptide-containing endocrine cells and nerves

Endocrine cells are found scattered throughout the body and those located in hollow organs frequently possess microvilli extruded into the lumen (Solcia *et*

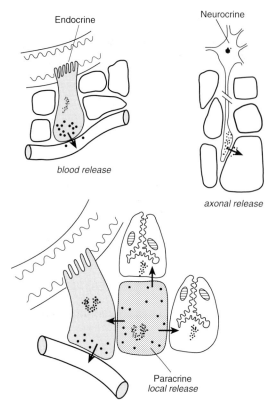

Fig. 15.1 Diagrammatic representation of the tripartite mode of action of the component cells of the diffuse neuroendocrine system.

al. 1987). The latter can be visualized better at the electron microscope level. Endocrine cells have intracytoplasmic secretory granules, the morphology of which, including their electron density and their limiting membrane and size, permits separation into various cell types. Secretory granules tend to be located at the basal pole of cells, close to the basement membrane and to the organ blood supply. Endocrine cells frequently display a cytoplasmic elongation along the basement membrane. The

arrangement of these features suggests functional properties: receptor functions are attributed to microvilli, peptide product is stored in secretory granules, and a cytoplasmic extension indicates a possible local or paracrine role for some of the peptide-containing endocrine cells.

Numerous neurotransmitters have been identified in the nervous system and these include not only the classical neurotransmitters, acetylcholine and noradrenaline, but also amino acid neurotransmitters and, in particular, peptide neurotransmitters. All can be identified in cell bodies, nerve fibres, and terminals by the use of specific antibodies.

15.2 Techniques for the visualization of the 'diffuse neuroendocrine system'

15.2.1 Light microscopy

General markers Secretory granules in the cytoplasm of endocrine cells have the ability to take up silver salts and precipitate them into a silver deposit with (argyrophilia) or without (argentaffinia) addition of a reducing agent. For amine-containing endocrine cells, argentaffin (Masson) silver impregnation is used, and, for other endocrine cells, a number of argyrophilic methods have been proposed. Among these, one of the most commonly used is the silver impregnation method of Grimelius. These techniques alsowork well in neuroendocrine tumour tissue.

Neurone-specific enolase (NSE) is an isoenzyme of the glycolytic enzyme enolase. Antibodies to NSE stain endocrine cells and their related nerves, and are useful for the demonstration of neuroendocrine differentiation in tumours, particularly poorly granulated neuroendocrine tissue (e.g. small cell carcinoma of the lung, Merkel cell tumours of the skin).

Chromogranins are a family of peptides originally extracted from the adrenal medulla. They have been

Fig. 15.2 Schematic representation of the pre-pro-glucagon molecule indicating the position of peptides of the glucagon family.

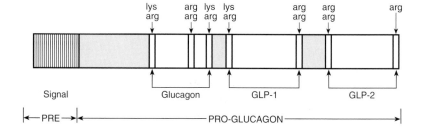

Table 15.1 Neuroendocrine regulatory peptides

Peptide	Distribution	Endocrine cells (C) Nerves (N)	Main known actions
Insulin	Pancreatic islets (β cells)	C	Blood sugar
Glucagon	Pancreatic islets (α cells)	C	Blood sugar
Enteroglucagon	Inestine	C	Trophic to gut
Secretin	Small intestine	C	Pancreatic bicarbonate secretion
Gastric inhibitory polypeptide (glucose dependent insulinotrophic peptide) (GIP)	Small intestine	C	Insulin secretion, gastric acid secretion
Vasoactive intestinal polypeptide (VIP)	Central and peripheral nervous system	N	Muscle relaxation, vasodilation, secretion
Peptide with histidine	Central and peripheral nervous system	N	Muscle relaxation, secretion
Growth hormone releasing	Hypothalamus	N	Growth hormone production
Gastrin	Pyloric stomach and small intestine	C	Gastric acid secretion
Cholecystokinin (CCK)	Small intestine	C	Gall bladder contraction, pancreatic enzyme secretion
CCK-8	Central and peripheral nervous system	N	Excitatory
Gastrin-releasing peptide (GRP) (see also Neuromedin (C)	Lung, central, and peripheral nervous system	C, N	Trophic, release of other regulatory peptides
(Bombesin)	Amphibian skin and gastrointestinal tract	C	
Neuromedin B, Neuromedin C (= GRP main form)	Spinal cord (porcine)	N	
Growth hormone-releasing factor (GRF)	Hypothalamus	N	Growth hormone production
Substance P	Central and peripheral nervous system	N	Sensory: vasodilation, muscle contraction
Dynorphin	(Anterior) and intermediate lobes of pituitary gland, central nervous system	C, N	Opioid
Enkephalin (met- and leu-)	Central and peripheral nervous system, adrenal medulla	C	Opioid
Vasopressin	Central nervous system (neurosecretory)	N	Antidiuretic
Oxytocin	Central nervous system (neurosecretory)	N	Contraction of uterus and let-down of milk
Thyroid hormone releasing hormone (TRH)	Hypothalamus	N	Release of TSH
Luteinizing hormone releasing hormone (LHRH)	Hypothalamus	N	Release of gonadotrophins
Coticotrophin releasing factor (CRF)	Hypothalamus	N	ACTH production
Growth hormone	Anterior pituitary gland	C	Growth
Prolactin	Anterior pituitary gland	C	Milk production
Placental lactogen	Placenta	C	Lactogenic trophic, lipoytic
Thyroid-stimulating hormone (TSH)	Anterior pituitary gland	C	Thyroid hormone production
Follicle-stimulating hormone (FSH)	Anterior pituitary gland	C	Ovarian follicle formation, spermatogenesis
Luteinizing hormone (LH)	Anterior pituitary gland	C	Ovulation, gonadal hormone
Chorionic gonadotrophin	Placenta	C	Luteotrophic
Various recently discovered peptides	Heart (atrium)	?C	Sodium excretion, diuresis, blood pressure

Table 15.1 Neuroendocrine regulatory peptides

Peptide	Distribution	Endocrine cells (C) Nerves (N)	Main known actions
Neurokinin A (= Substance K, Neuromedin L); Neurokinin B (Neuromedin K)	Spinal cord (procine)	N	
Pancreatic polypeptide	Pancreatic islets	C	Pancreatic enzyme secretion, gall bladder contraction
Peptide with C- and N-terminal tyrosine (PYY)	Intestinal system	C	
Neural peptide with tyrosine (NPY)	Central and peripheral intestinal tract	N	Vasoconstriction
Motilin	Small intestine	C	Gut motility
Somatostatin	Stomach, intestine, pancreatic islets, thyroid gland, central and peripheral nervous system	C, N	Release and action of many peptides; may be antitrophic
Neurotensin	Intestine, adrenal medulla, central nervous system	C	Vasodilation, gastric acid secretion
Parathyroid hormone	Parathyroid gland	C	Blood calcium
Calcitonin	Thyroid gland	C	Blood calcium
Calcitonin gene-related peptide (CGRP)	Central and peripheral nervous system	N	Vasodilation; sensory
Adrenocorticotrophic hormone (ACTH)	Anterior and intermediate lobes of pituitary gland; central nervous system	C, N	Production of adrenal corticosteroids
Corticotrophin-like intermediate lobe peptide (CLIP)	Intermediate lobe of pituitary gland	C	
Melanocyte-stimulating hormone (MSH) (α, β, γ)	(Anterior) and intermediate lobes of pituitary gland, central nervous system	C, N	Skin pigmentation
Endorphin (α and β)	Anterior and intermediate lobes of pituitary gland, central nervous system	C, N	Opioid
β-Lipotrophin	Anterior and intermediate lobes of pituitary gland, central nervous system	C, N	

classified as chromogranin A, B, and C. The pre-pro-chromagranin molecule gives rise to three different peptides which are separately expressed in tissues. These peptides are: pancreastatin, which is included in the structure of pro-chromogranin A; GAWK, included in the structure of chromogranin B; and a peptide found at the C-terminal end of chromogranin B, termed CCB (C-terminal of chromogranin B) (Fig. 15.3).

Synaptophysin is a molecule originally found in the membrane of a small secretory vesicle-type containing classical neurotransmitters, which is expressed differentially in the neuroendocrine system.

The occurrence of intermediate filaments, e.g. vimentin, keratin, and neurofilaments, is rare in neuroendocrine tumours (e.g. small cell carcinoma of the lung, Merkel cell tumour).

Peptide markers Immunocytochemistry, using antibodies specific to regions of regulatory peptides and their pre-pro-forms, has been used extensively.

15.2.2 Electron microscopy

Electron microscopy has been fundamental in determining the neuroendocrine differentiation of normal and tumour tissue. By electron microscopy, the presence of dense core secretory granules is easily dis-

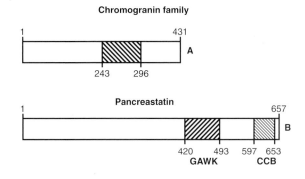

Fig. 15.3 Diagram showing the structure of chromagranins A and B. The positions of their derivative peptides pancreastatin (in chromagranin A), GAWK, and CCB (chromagranin B) are marked.

tinguishable (Fig. 15.4). Secretory granules are not destroyed by poor fixation, and thus can be distinguished in tissue fixed for routine pathology. In conventional osmium staining for electron microscopy, the limiting membrane of the granule is easily distinguishable and analysis of the size, electron density, halo, and characteristics of this membrane can thus be seen. These features are indicative, especially in normal tissue, of the production by a given cell of a particular peptide.

15.2.3 *In situ* hybridization

The use of cDNA probes, complementary to messenger RNA directing the synthesis of a given peptide in the technique of *in situ* hybridization, allows morphologists to visualize the biosynthetic events prior to peptide packaging in granules (Adams *et al.* 1987). A number of different methods for *in situ* hybridization exist, using radioisotope or biotin, and the end product is visualized by autoradiography or by methods permitting the visualization of biotin labels (see Chapter 10).

Table 15.2 summarizes the main applications of *in situ* hybridization. Figure 15.5 illustrates one of these applications, namely gene expression and site of synthesis. The latter application is particularly important in tumour pathology, since tumours may have an abnormally poor mechanism for peptide storage (low number of secretory granules), thus giving negative results with immunocytochemistry. Alternatively, the tumour may have receptors (binding sites) on the surface which are subsequently internalized, providing spurious false positive results with immunocytochemistry.

15.2.4 Receptor visualization

Peptide-binding sites can be visualized by autoradiography or by immunogold staining procedures. The techniques of *in vitro* autoradiography using tissue

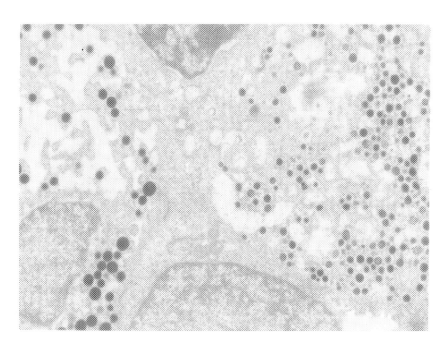

Fig. 15.4 Electron micrograph of human pancreatic glucagonoma showing two distinct secretory granule populations in neighbouring tumour cells. Glutaraldehyde fixation, uranyl acetate, and lead citrate counterstains. (×8600)

Table 15.2 Main applications of *in situ* hybridization in the study of the diffuse neuroendocrine system

1. Gene expression

   Sites of synthesis of hormones/neuropeptides are revealed by location of gene expression in tissues.

2. Rate of synthesis

   Physiological or pathological variations in hormone/neuropeptide synthesis are determined by monitoring changes in cells expressing specific genes.

3. Combination with other techniques

   Combination with, for example, immunocytochemistry gives more complete analysis of cellular function by allowing comparison of gene transcription with hormone/neuropeptide storage

4. Determination of cosynethesis of multiple messengers

   Coexistence of multiple regulatory peptides can be assessed by using multiple probes on a single tissue section

5. New taxonomy of normal neuroendocrine cells and tumours

   The previously unsuspected capacity of a neuroendocrine cell to synthesize a certain product provides the basis of new cellular/tumour classification

sections and emulsion-coated coverslips or sensitive film have been developed for the visualization of peptide-binding sites. Densitometric image analysis of these preparations is now being used for quantitation.

15.3 Neuroendocrine tumours

15.3.1 Nomenclature

Various terms have been used to describe tumours arising from the diffuse endocrine system, e.g. carcinoma, APUDoma; there is no consensus on nomenclature.

Immunocytochemistry and radioimmunoassay allow further characterization of these tumours in terms of their function. Neuroendocrine tumours frequently produce more than one regulatory peptide (mixed endocrine tumours), but often one circulating peptide is responsible for the associated clinical syndrome. In such cases the tumour is frequently referred to by the name of this active secretory product, e.g. gastrinoma and insulinoma. In view of these difficulties, we propose three levels of nomenclature. Firstly, 'neuroendocrine tumours' is to be used as a generic term to describe all tumours thought to be derived from the diffuse neuroendocrine system and showing the general histological, histochemical, and immunohistochemical features of such cells. Secondly, terms may refer to particular histological patterns at specific sites, e.g. islet cell tumour of pancreas or oat cell carcinoma of lung. Thirdly, an indication of the major peptide secretions of the tumour is included. In this system each level is complementary to the others and a full description of a tumour should include mention of all three.

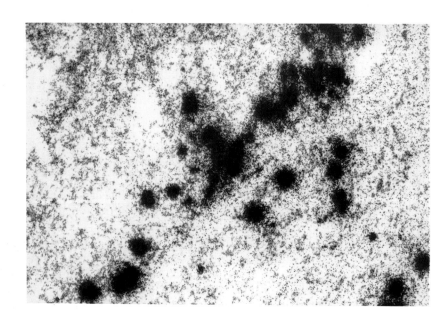

Fig. 15.5 Section of a small cell carcinoma of the lung with the sites of synthesis of human bombesin (gastrin-releasing peptide) marked by black silver grains. Haematoxylin counterstain. (×210)

15.3.2 General features of endocrine tumours

Clinical features It is difficult to assess the true incidence of endocrine tumours but well recognized, functioning tumours are clearly uncommon, with the exception of small cell carcinoma of the lung.

The clinical features of some functioning tumours may be obscured by the presence in the circulation of more than one regulatory peptide with counteracting effects. In addition to hormonal effects, non-specific manifestations, depending on site, size, and invasion, may be present. Clinical suspicion is usually roused when more common diseases have been excluded. This sometimes delays diagnosis, with adverse effects on the prognosis. High levels of secretion of a regulatory peptide may provide a useful assay, although circulating levels of active peptides can be elevated in diseases other than tumours. Many preoperative, non-invasive techniques are also widely used, including a series of stimulation and suppression tests for the particular hormone. Further, a series of localization techniques are used (see Chapter 17).

Biochemistry Highly sensitive specific radioimmunoassays for the measurement of regulatory peptides in blood and tissue are readily available and allow early diagnosis of functioning tumours. Thus, very small tumours may be diagnosed clinically and biochemically, but localization of the precise site of the tumour may still be a problem.

Histology Peptide-producing endocrine cells are frequently unevenly distributed within a tumour. It is therefore very important to sample a large number of specimens taken randomly throughout the tumour mass. The growth pattern of endocrine tumours is quite characteristic. Tumours are composed of uniform cells with few mitoses arranged in irregular masses, ribbons, or glandular structures. A glassy, amorphous degeneration of the tumour stroma (amyloid) is common and sometimes extensive. A more functional criterion of malignancy has recently been proposed. This is the production and release of alpha human chorionic gonadotropin (HCG) by many malignant endocrine tumours. This criterion is especially relevant for pancreatic endocrine tumours.

Electron microscopy Tumours have been found to contain variable numbers of secretory granules, but often peptide-producing tumour cells store less peptide than their normal counterparts. It is gener-ally accepted that a poorly granulated tumour reflects high secretory activity, and this frequently correlates with the presence of abundant ribosomes, rough endoplasmic reticulum, and prominent Golgi apparatus. Poorly granulated tumours are usually associated with significantly elevated levels of circulating hormone. This suggests that one of the metabolic defects in endocrine tumour cells resides in the control of hormone secretion.

15.3.3 Ectopic hormone production

By definition, ectopic hormones are produced by a tumour arising in an organ that does not secrete the substance normally. For example, Cushing's syndrome, caused by the overproduction of adrenal hormones, may develop as a result of the production of adrenal corticotrophic hormone (ACTH), a pituitary hormone that stimulates the adrenal glands, e.g. by neuroendocrine tumours of the pancreas or lung. Synthesis and sometimes secretion of a number of peptides by endocrine and non-endocrine tumours may be much more common than is realized. Symptoms of ectopic hormone secretion as tumour markers are important. Ectopic hormone production may occur in tandem with normal hormone secretion owing to abnormal regulation of DNA transcription, mRNA processing, or even, perhaps, defective post-translational modification of pre-pro-hormone.

15.3.4 Multihormonal tumours

Multiple hormone production may be caused by single or multiple endocrine neoplasia (MEN). The production of more than one hormone by a single endocrine tumour was thought to be uncommon. This was mainly owing to the fact that the effects of one secreted hormone were clinically predominant and thus obscured the presence of other less active peptides. It is now recognized that some patients have symptoms attributable to the simultaneous secretion of more than one hormone and may show a transition of effects from one to another, sometimes as a result of treatment (chemotherapy). In most instances the hormones are produced by separate cell types.

15.4 Individual tumours

15.4.1 Tumours of the pancreas and gut

Insulinomas β cells in the pancreatic islets secrete insulin, and insulinomas are one of the many causes of hypoglycaemia (low blood sugar). They constitute 70–75 per cent of all pancreatic endocrine tumours and are about equally common in both sexes. All patients with insulinomas should also be checked for other endocrine disturbances since β or non-β cell adenomas can be associated with other inherited endocrine neoplasms of the multiple endocrine neoplasia (MEN) syndrome. Clinical features (headaches, blurred vision, sweating, hunger, and palpitations) are almost always present, even with small tumours. Symptoms are usually intermittent and thus a patient can be misdiagnosed as having psychiatric, cardiac, or neurological disease. The highest incidence of insulinomas is found between ages 30–60. Virtually all insulinomas are localized in the pancreas. About 90 per cent of them are solitary and most (84–96 per cent) are benign.

Insulinomas, like most other endocrine tumours, produce different molecular forms of insulin, C peptide, and pro-insulin in variable proportions.

Tumours associated with the Zollinger–Ellison syndrome (gastrinomas) Gastrinomas represent 20–25 per cent of pancreatic endocrine tumours. They occur most often between 30 and 50 years of age and there is a slight male preponderance. The clinical features, as originally described by Zollinger and Ellison, are intractable gastric, duodenal, and jejunal ulceration, bleeding, and very high gastric acid secretion. These features are rarely found nowadays since the tumours are usually diagnosed at an earlier stage owing to increasing awareness and the availability of assays. Plasma gastrin levels are usually very high, but calcium stimulation of gastrin levels, a commonly employed diagnostic test, permits the distinction between a gastrinoma and other hypergastrinaemic conditions associated with recurrent peptic ulcers. Eighty-five per cent of gastrinomas are found in the pancreas. Extra-pancreatic gastrinomas are found, for instance, in the duodenum (13 per cent) and in other areas (1 per cent), including the stomach, upper jejunum, and bile ducts. This distribution in the frequency of anatomical sites for gastrinomas does not fit with the distribution of gastrin-containing (G) cells in normal tissue; in particular, G cells are not found in the adult human pancreas, but have been described in the fetal pancreas.

At least 60 per cent of gastrinomas are malignant. The tumours frequently metastasize, especially to the liver. Histologically these tumours have the typical appearance of neuroendocrine tumours, e.g. immunoreactivity for neurone-specific enolase, chromogranins, and various segments of gastrin and pre-pro-gastrin. Tumours producing gastrin frequently secrete other regulatory peptides, in particular pancreatic polypeptide.

Diarrhoeagenic (WDHA) tumour syndrome, VIPomas or PHMoma syndrome Certain patients with non-β islet cell tumours and severe diarrhoea do not meet the criteria for the diagnosis of gastrinoma. The absence of gastric acid hypersecretion in such patients has also beenreported. Since the discovery that vasoactive intestinal polypeptide (VIP) is produced frequently and in large concentrations by such tumours, the word VIPoma was coined. VIPomas represent 3–5 per cent of all pancreatic endocrine tumours. The syndrome is characterized by watery diarrhoea. Approximately two-thirds of patients complain of abdominal colic and some have intermittent high faecal fat output. There is often a significant weight loss. At operation, a high amount of alkaline secretion from the pancreas is found. Some patients may also suffer from occasional flushing attacks. Fifty to seventy-five per cent of tumours are malignant. The tumours are often quite large (2–7 cm). VIP is known to be produced both by endocrine and neural tumours and, histologically, tumours show either classical features of islet cell tumours of the pancreas or features of ganglioneuroblastomas.

Glucagonomas The typical clinical picture shows the following symptoms: a migratory skin rash localized to the lower abdomen, perineum, and legs; an abnormal glucose tolerance test; anaemia; a sore red tongue; angular stomatitis; severe weight loss; depression; tendency to develop overwhelming infection; and venous thrombosis (in about one-third of patients).

The characteristic skin rash gives a cutaneous marker of internal malignancy. Administration of zinc induces a fast remission of the skin rash. This led to the postulate that the skin condition may be due partly to zinc deficiency. The disease occurs most often between 40–70 years of age and appears to be slightly more common in women than in men. More than 60 per cent of glucagonomas are malignant. Pancreatic polypeptide-producing cells are found frequently, but also insulin-, somatostatin-, and gastrin-producing cells may be found.

Glucagon-producing pancreatic adenomas constitute part of the MEN type I syndrome.

Tumours producing pancreatic polypeptide (PP): PPomas Oversecretion of PP is one of the most frequent associations noted with well-defined, functioning neuroendocrine tumours. Tumours most frequently containing PP cells include VIPomas, glucagonomas, and insulinomas. Therefore, PP positive immunostaining in a metastasis of an endocrine tumour of unknown origin points to the possibility of the primary tumour being present in the pancreas.

Somatostatinomas The association of somatostatin production by endocrine tumours with a defined clinical syndrome remains in dispute. Most somatostatinomas are solitary and localized in the pancreas; fewer tumours have been described in the gut. Somatostatin-containing tumours are frequently malignant and their growth pattern is similar to that described for other neuroendocrine tumours.

Growth hormone releasing factor (GRF)-producing tumours, or GRFomas or acromegalic tumours Tumours of the pancreas associated with acromegaly have frequently been described in the literature, and GRF has now been found to be produced by pancreatic endocrine neoplasms.

Carcinoids and serotonin-producing tumours As the term carcinoid has been associated at various times with a morphological appearance, a clinical syndrome, and a biochemical feature (the production of serotonin), its usage has often been confusing. In this section, it is used to describe endocrine tumours of the gut whether or not they are associated with the clinical features of serotonin production. The typical carcinoid syndrome consists of episodes of flushing, hypertension, diarrhoea, cough, wheezing, and localized capillary dilation. Fibrosis, oedema, pellagra-like lesions of the skin, peptic ulcer, and abdominal fibrosis can also be present. The symptoms described above are particularly prominent once the tumour has metastasized to the liver, allowing the tumour products to enter the circulation. Seventy-five per cent of serotonin-producing tumours arise from the gastrointestinal tract. Unlike other endocrine neoplasms, the size of the tumour may be considered as a prognostic factor. When a tumour measures more than 2 cm in diameter it is considered malignant

and it is likely that metastases are already present. Frequently, carcinoids are multiple and sometimes associated with other malignant neoplasms. Serotonin is particularly prominent in midgut carcinoids but is usually absent from foregut and hindgut tumours. Apart from serotonin, carcinoid tumours of the bowel produce other regulatory peptides. Gastric carcinoids are a separate entity; these occur in association with mucosal atrophy (atrophic gastritis) and pernicious anaemia, or may occur in patients in which acid secretion has been blocked completely by newly discovered drugs for ulcer treatment.

Pituitary gland tumours In humans the pituitary is divided into two lobes, with the anterior lobe being known as the adenohypophysis and the posterior, or neural, lobe as the neurohypophysis. The former produces at least six hormones having major effects on metabolic processes and on other endocrine glands. Hormone production is stimulated or inhibited by hypothalamic factors and by feedback from the hormonal secretions of the target organs. The neurohypophysis is an extension of the brain containing a variety of peptides and amines, in addition to the main neurosecretory hormones, vasopressin and oxytocin.

Tumours of the pituitary gland are relatively frequent. Prolactin-secreting tumours are by far the most common and are followed by growth hormone-secreting tumours and then ACTH-secreting tumours. Gonadotropin- and thyrotropin-secreting tumours are infrequent. Mixed tumours, secreting more than one hormone, are a common finding. The cell of origin of all these tumours has been disputed but the frequent occurrence of 'mixed' pituitary adenomas might be thought to favour the existence of precursor cells that give rise to all tumour cell types.

Prolactin-secreting adenomas cause infertility and impairment of testicular function, milk secretion, and amenorrhoea. Tumours of this type are frequently poorly granulated. Thus, attempts to immunostain prolactin in an actively secreting, poorly granulated tumour may be unrewarding.

Pituitary tumours associated with Cushing's syndrome react with antibodies to various portions of peptides of the ACTH and related hormones.

Thyroid tumours Two classes of neuroendocrine tumour of the thyroid (medullary carcinoma) are now recognized: the sporadic and the familial types. The medullary carcinoma is one of the few malignant tumours with an inheritance of an autosomal dominant type with high penetrance (see Chapter 4). Twenty per cent of all cases of medullary carcinomas are thought to be genetically determined and these usually present with phaeochromocytomas (tumours of the adrenal medulla) and other tumours as part of the multiple endocrine neoplasia (MEN type 2) syndrome. The tumour arises from special calcitonin-producing cells (C cells) in the thyroid and C cell hyperplasia precedes and accompanies inherited medullary carcinoma. The defect is probably at the level of C cell hyperplasia and the development of the malignancy is possibly a secondary defect. It is, therefore, exceedingly important to screen relatives of a patient with inherited medullary carcinoma for the possibility of C cell hyperplasia, by measurement of plasma calcitonin. Furthermore, it is necessary to analyse the entire thyroid of sporadic medullary carcinomas for the possible presence of C cell hyperplasia and organize subsequent screening of relatives.

Calcitonin and its flanking peptide PDN-21, or katacalcin, are the peptides most frequently found in medullary carcinomas. Calcitonin gene related peptide (CGRP) is also often found. Other peptides or substances shown to be produced by medullary carcinomas are ACTH, neurotensin, bombesin, somatostatin, serotonin, prostaglandins, and substance P. The production of multiple hormones or other peptides may explain the bizarre clinical features often encountered in medullary carcinomas, including protracted diarrhoea.

Tumours of the adrenal medulla and paraganglia

Phaeochromocytoma is the most frequently found tumour of the adrenal medulla, but ganglioneuromatous differentiation can also be found. A phaeochromocytoma is clinically recognized in the following circumstances: as a familial case, hypertensive episodes, persistent hypertension with increased urine excretion of vanillyl mandelic acid, noradrenaline, or adrenaline.

The size of the tumour ranges from a microscopic lesion to over 2 kg in weight, but most are about 5–6 cm diameter and weigh an average of 9 g. Histologically, the appearance of phaeochromocytomas is quite bizarre, with very many irregular cells of variable size, structure, and arrangement. Many multinucleated, gigantic cells can be found which,

at the ultrastructural level, contain numerous distinctive electron dense secretory granules. Peptides of the enkephalin/dynorphin family, neurotensin, and, very recently, a novel peptide known to produce marked vasoconstriction, neuropeptide Y, are produced by both the normal and tumour tissue.

Phaeochromocytomas may be a component of the familial MEN type 2 syndrome, together with medullary carcinoma of the thyroid, parathyroid hyperplasia, or adenoma. Phaeochromocytomas are usually benign tumours but malignancy can occur when tumours are found bilaterally. They occur in adults between the ages of 25–55 years.

Tumours of paraganglia are called extraadrenal phaeochromocytomas in Europe, and paragangliomas in the US. These can occur all along the sympathetic chain and in the para-aortic bodies. Paraganglia form a widely disseminated system of small sensory and perhaps local neurosecretory organs that develop in fetal life, persist in infancy, and thereafter become smaller and more difficult to find in certain parts of the body, such as the fibrous tissue behind the peritoneum along the aorta. Several lie close to other major blood vessels, in or near nerves or ganglia, or are located in organs such as the lung or duodenum. The urinary bladder also contains paraganglia and phaeochromocytomas of the urinary bladder have been reported.

15.4.2 Respiratory tract tumours

The respiratory tract is also a common site for neuroendocrine tumours. One of the active peptides frequently produced by small cell carcinomas is bombesin/GRP (gastrin-releasing peptide) which is also present in normal mucosal endocrine cells. The structure of human pro-bombesin (gastrin-releasing peptide) from a small cell carcinoma of the lung has now been established using region-specific antibodies to various segments of the human pro-bombesin molecule. Antibodies directed to the C-terminal portion of human pro-bombesin are excellent, and possibly better than, antibodies to bombesin itself, for demonstrating the production of bombesin gene products by small cell carcinomas (Fig. 15.6). It is interesting that the small cell carcinoma is a poorly granulated neoplasm, suggesting that the tumour cell bypasses the secretory granule pathway.

Within neuroendocrine tumours of the lung, the carcinoid seems to represent the benign end of a continuous spectrum that ends in the small cell car-

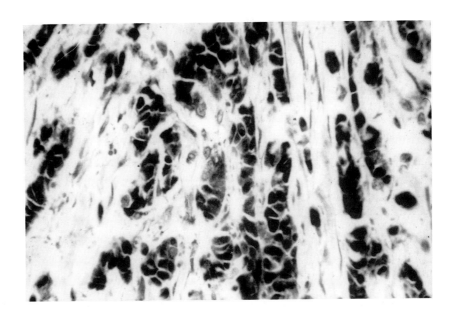

Fig. 15.6 Section of a small cell carcinoma of the lung densely immunostained (black) for the C-flamking portion of human pro-bombesin. (×262)

cinoma. The lung is a fairly frequent site of carcinoids, in fact 12 per cent of all carcinoids arise in the lung. However, carcinoids represent only 1 per cent of all lung tumours. The highest incidence of bronchial carcinoids occurs in the 31–40 year age group, with a slight preponderance in females (62 per cent). The tumour usually arises in the main bronchi but may be located in the lung periphery. Multicentric growth has been described and carcinoids may be part of a pluriglandular syndrome. Carcinoid tumours are generally well demarcated, grow slowly, and have a low malignant potential. Ultrastructurally, carcinoid tumours of the lung are frequently well granulated. Immunocytochemistry reveals a variety of products being produced by carcinoid tumours, in particular serotonin, bombesin PP, and, occasionally, ACTH, with or without overt clinical syndromes. Small cell carcinoma of the lung is the malignant counterpart of lung endocrine tumours. It is one of the most frequent neuroendocrine tumour types and comprises 20 per cent of all bronchial carcinomas. Small cell carcinomas are divided into two main types depending on cell size: (i) oat cell type, consisting of small oat-shaped cells with a finely granular chromatin pattern, no nucleolus, and very sparse cytoplasm; and (ii) intermediate cell type, composed of slightly larger cells with more abundant cytoplasm. There does not seem to be a correlation between the histologial subtype and patient survival. The best neu-

roendocrine marker for the characterization of small cell carcinomas is the non-granular marker neurone-specific enolase. Small cell carcinomas of the lung have long been associated with hormonal abnormalities, particularly Cushing's syndrome and inappropriate antidiuretic hormone secretion. Extensive data indicate that bombesin released from tumour cells of the small cell carcinoma acts in an autocrine (or paracrine) manner. The tumour cells release their product into the vicinity and in turn activate tumour cell receptors to enhance growth.

Small cell carcinomas of the lung are aggressive neoplasms, having the poorest prognosis of all lung tumours with an overall five-year survival rate of only 2 per cent. The tumour is generally extremely sensitive to combined chemotherapy and radiotherapy, whereas other lung tumours are more amenable to surgery.

15.5 Conclusions

Studies of the 'diffuse neuroendocrine system' are a new facet of endocrinology and expand the classical view of glandular endocrinology. Regulatory peptides are still being discovered and their role in the control of body functions is being firmly established. Advances in molecular biology make possible determination of the structure of peptide precursors and the use of region-specific antibodies to the various portions of the molecule are opening up new investigative areas of peptide neuroendocrinology. The application of other modern techniques now allows not only investigation of the stored peptide but of all intracellular steps leading to this peptide synthesis, including visualization of the mRNA. It is predictable that more functional studies will be forthcoming, analysing the quantities of messenger in relation to peptide biosynthesis. The site of action of regulatory peptide receptors can now be analysed and therapeutic agents are being developed to interact with particular regulatory peptides specifically, either at the site of their production or release or at their receptor level, and therefore new avenues for the treatment of this very interesting group of tumours are becoming available.

References and further reading

Adams, C., Hamid, Q. A., and Polak, J. M. (1987). In situ hybridisation with radio-labelled cRNA probes, using tissue sections and smears. In *Methods in molecular biology*, Vol. 5, *Tissue culture* (ed. J. Walker). Humana Press Inc., New Jersey.

Bloom, S. R. and Polak. J. M. (1981). *Gut hormones* (2nd edn). Churchill Livingstone, Edinburgh.

Eiden, L. E., Huttner, W. B., Mallet, J., O'Connor, D. T., Winkler, H., and Zanini, A. (1987). A nomenclature proposal for the chromogranin/secreto-granin proteins. *Neuroscience*, **21**, 1019–21.

Falkmer, S., Hakanson, R., and Sundler, F. (ed.) (1984). *Evolution and tumour pathology of the neuroendocrine system*. Elsevier, Amsterdam.

Hanley, M. R. (1989). Peptide regulatory factors in the nervous system. *Lancet*, **i**, 1373–6.

Havemann, K., Sorensen, G., and Gropp, C. (ed.) (1985). *Recent results in cancer research, peptide hormones in lung cancer*. Springer-Verlag, Berlin.

Polak, J. M. and Bloom, S. R. (1983). Regulatory peptides: key factors in the control of bodily functions. *British Medical Journal*, **286**, 1461–6.

Polak, J. M. and Bloom, S. R. (1985a). *Endocrine tumours*. Churchill Livingstone, Edinburgh.

Polak, J. M. and Bloom, S. R. (1985b). Pathology of peptide-producing neuroendocrine tumours. *British Journal of Hospital Medicine*, **53**, 153–7.

Polak, J. M. and Marangos, P. J. (1984). Neuron-specific enolase, a marker for neuroendocrine cells. In *Evolution and tumour pathology of the neuroendocrine*, Vol. 4. (ed. S. Falkmer, R. Hakanson, and F. Sundler), pp. 433–80. Elsevier, Amsterdam.

Polak, J. M. and van Noorden, S. (1983). *Immunocytochemistry practical applications in pathology and biology*. Wright, Bristol.

Polak, J. M. and Varndell, I. M. (1984). *Immunolabelling for electron microscopy*. Elsevier, Amsterdam.

Solcia, E. *et al.* (1987). Endocrine cells producing regulatory peptides. *Experientia*, **43**, 839–50.

Varndell, I. M. *et al.* (1984). Visualization of messenger RNA directing peptide synthesis by *in situ* hybridization using a novel single-stranded cDNA probe: potential for the investigation of gene expression and endocrine cell activity. *Histochemistry*, **81**, 597–601.

16

Immunology of cancer

PETER BEVERLEY

16.1 Introduction to the immune system

Animals or humans born without a properly functioning immune system suffer from multiple infections and usually die at an early age. These 'experiments of nature' are the best evidence of the importance of the immune system in defending the animal against pathogenic microorganisms. However it was proposed, as long ago as the turn of the century by Paul Ehrlich, that the immune system might also prevent, or at least delay, the growth of many tumours. This chapter examines Ehrlich's idea, but to do this it is necessary to explain how the immune system works.

16.2 Organization of the immune system

Many of the cells of the immune system (white cells or leucocytes) are found throughout the body because they circulate in the bloodstream and also migrate into tissues, particularly at sites of inflammation. Lymphoid cells are also found in specialized lymphoid organs, the thymus, spleen, and lymph

nodes (Fig. 16.1). The lymph nodes are widely distributed throughout the body. The tonsils and adenoids are specialized lymph node organs in the pharynx: the lymph nodes in the intestine are know as Peyer's patches. All the cells of the immune system originate from self-replacing stem cells in the bone marrow, as do red blood cells and platelets (see Chapter 12). In this chapter we shall be mainly concerned with the function of lymphocytes because these cells are responsible for specific immunity. In contrast granulocytes mediate non-specific protection, particularly against bacterial pathogens. Granulocytes and macrophages are attracted to sites where invading microorganisms are present and are able to ingest (phagocytose) and often kill the microorganisms. They lack the two major properties of lymphocytes: specificity and memory. Granulocytes are also short lived (hours) whereas lymphocytes are long lived (months or years). There are two main classes of lymphocytes. Bone marrow-derived (B) lymphocytes mature in the marrow and then migrate directly to the spleen and lymph nodes. They are then ready to react to foreign substances (antigens). Thymus-derived (T) lymphocytes migrate from the bone marrow to the

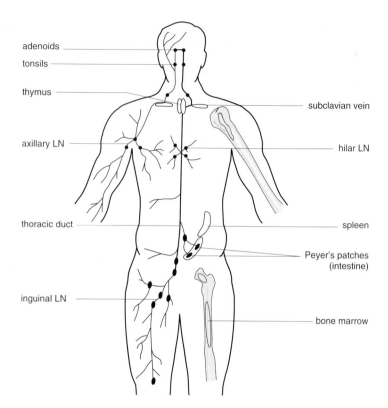

adenoids

tonsils

thymus

subclavian vein

axillary LN

hilar LN

thoracic duct

spleen

Peyer's patches
(intestine)

inguinal LN

bone marrow

Fig. 16.1 Lymphoid organs. The organization of the lymphoid organs is shown schematically. Afferent lymphatics drain the tissues and enter regional lymph nodes (LN). Efferent lymphatics from the lymph nodes drain into the thoracic duct which enters the venous system. The spleen, thymus, and bone marrow connect to other lymphoid organs mainly via the blood circulation (not shown in the figure).

thymus where they mature before migrating to the peripheral lymphoid organs (spleen and lymph nodes). These two types of lymphocyte, although morphologically very similar, can be readily distinguished by their differing cell surface phenotypes; that is, the array of glycoproteins carried in the lipid bilayer of the cell surface membrane. T and B lymphocytes also have very different functions although they interact during most immune responses.

16.2.1 B lymphocytes and antibodies

The principal function of B lymphocytes is to synthesize and secrete antibodies. When these cells are stimulated by encountering a foreign antigen, they first go through several cycles of cell division and then differentiate into specialized antibody-secreting cells called plasma cells. Antibodies are globular glycoproteins (hence immunoglobulins) found in the blood plasma. The general structure of an immunoglobulin molecule is shown in Fig. 16.2. It consists of two heavy (H) and two light (L) chains. The H and L chains are each divided

into two portions, the N-terminal portion (approximately 110 amino acids) being termed the variable part and the remaining portion (approximately 330 or 110 amino acids for H and L chains, respectively) being termed the constant part. The constant part of the heavy chain determines the biological function of the molecule, and differences in the amino acid sequence of the constant part of the H chain determine the class of the immunoglobulin molecule. There are five major immunoglobulin (Ig) classes, IgA, D, E, G, and M, with H chains designated by the Greek letters α, δ, ε, γ, and μ. The two light chain types, which also differ in their constant parts, are called κ and λ. Each class has different properties which are summarized in Table 16.1. IgM and IgD are found on the membrane of resting B lymphocytes and act as receptors for antigen. When B cells are stimulated they first secrete IgM. Secreted IgM is a pentamer of subunits joined by an extra polypeptide, the J chain. Later, most B cells switch to secreting IgG, A, or E. IgG is the main class present in the blood and is a monomer of the basic four-chain immunoglobulin molecule. In humans

Fig. 16.2 The structure of an antibody molecule. Heavy and light chains are linked by disulphide bonds (S–S). A further disulphide bond joins the two heavy chains. There are further intrachain disulphide bonds in each variable (V) and constant (C) domain of the protein. The symbol → denotes the site of carbohydrate attachment. The antigen-binding fragment (Fab) and crystallizable fragment (Fc) of the molecule are indicated.

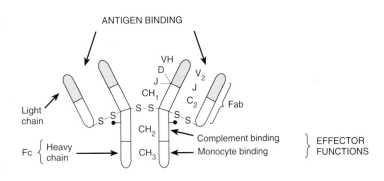

Table 16.1 Properties of human immunoglobulins

Property	IgG	IgM	IgA	IgD	IgE
Molecular weight (Da)	150 000	900 000	400 000	180 000	190 000
Concentration in serum (mg/ml)	10	1	2	0.03	<0.001
Relative amount in secretions	Low	Low	High	Very low	Low
Crosses placenta	Yes	No	No	No	No
Complement fixation	Yes	Yes	No	No	No
Transport across epithelia	No	No	Yes	No	Yes
Allergic responses	No	No	No	No	Yes
Fc binds to cells	Yes	Yes	Yes	No	No

there are four subclasses of IgG termed IgG1, IgG2, IgG3, and IgG4 which have closely related H chains. In the mouse and rat there are corresponding IgG subclasses called IgG1, IgG2a, IgG2b, and IgG3. IgA is specialized for protection of mucous membranes and can be transported across epithelia. IgE is a minor component of serum but plays an important role in allergic reactions. The function of IgD is not known.

It is a remarkable property of the immune system that it can produce specific antibodies (able to bind with high affinity) to almost any antigen encountered. This is possible because each B lymphocyte clone synthesizes and secretes a different immunoglobulin molecule. The molecules differ mainly in the variable part, and this variability is achieved by several mechanisms. These include selection from a large pool of variable (V) genes, random joining of V genes to minigenes coding for diversity (D) and joining (J) segments, random combination of heavy and light chains, and somatic mutation (Kocks and Rajewsky 1989, Schatz *et al.* 1992). This allows for the production of millions of different antigen-binding sites. Each combining site has a

unique structure (idiotype) and by immunizing an animal with homogenous Ig it is possible to raise anti-antibodies (anti-idiotypes) which react only with the immunizing Ig and not other Ig molecules (see Chapter 19).

Generally, when an animal encounters an antigen, for example a virus, many B cells are stimulated. Each B cell carries on its surface membrane immunoglobulin molecules with different antigen-binding sites. These act as the receptors and the secreted immunoglobulin of each cell has the same antigen-binding site (specificity) as the membrane-bound immunoglobulin. Each B cell will divide to produce a clone of daughter cells. During this clonal expansion somatic mutation occurs in the V regions of the heavy and light chains and cells secreting higher affinity antibody are selected so that antibody affinity increases during an immune response (Austyn and Wood 1993). Since many B cells bind the antigen the serum of the immunized animal will contain a mixture of the antibodies produced by many clones. A second contact with the same antigen elicits a greater and more rapid antibody response (immunological memory).

16.2.2 Monoclonal antibodies

Antisera made by animals in response to an antigen are the product of many different clones (polyclonal) of B lymphocytes and individual antibodies react with many different sites (epitopes) on the antigen. If the antigen is complex, as are bacterial or mammalian cells, it may be very difficult to determine exactly which molecules of the cell the antibodies are directed towards. For many years the complexity of cellular antigens hampered efforts to produce antibodies that would distinguish between tumour and normal cells, although in principle, the exquisite specificity of antibodies made this an attractive approach to understanding the changes occurring during malignant transformation. In 1975 Kohler and Milstein provided a solution to this problem when they published a method for immortalizing single antibody-secreting B lymphocytes by fusing them to cells from a plasma cell tumour (myeloma) to produce a hybrid cell (hybridoma). All the progeny of such a hybridoma cell produce identical (monoclonal) antibody molecules (for further details see Chapter 19). The ability to produce unlimited quantities of homogeneous antibody of any desired specificity has had a major impact in many areas of biology, including tumour immunology.

16.2.3 How T lymphocytes recognize antigen

Until recently the way in which T cells 'see' antigen was not understood. No T cell receptor for antigen was identified until 1983, but it is now clear that it consist of two protein chains rather similar to the light chains of immunoglobulin (Davis and Bjorkman 1988). Diversity of receptor specificity is generated by mechanisms similar to those found in B lymphocytes (described briefly in Section 16.2.1) except that there is no somatic mutation in T cells. In spite of the apparent similarities between the B and T cell receptors for antigen, the two cell types 'see' antigen in very different ways. While soluble antigen can bind to the surface immunoglobulin of B cells to stimulate a response, soluble antigen does not stimulate T cells. T cells always 'see' antigen in association with 'self': the phenomenon of genetic restriction.

This can be made clearer by describing one of the earliest experiments to demonstrate it. If an animal (or human) is immunized with a virus, for example influenza A, immune T cells from the animal are able to kill influenza A-infected cells but not unin-

fected target cells or cells infected with a different virus such as influenza B. The immune T cells are therefore specific for influenza A virus. The experiment, however, has a second part. The infected target cells must come from the same animal (or inbred strain) as the immune T cells or they cannot be killed. Thus the T cells do not recognize virus only; they appear to 'see' virus + self. Further genetic experiments showed that the 'self' components required were membrane glycoproteins coded in a region of the genome called the major histocompatibility complex (MHC) (see also Chapter 19). This name derives from older experiments which showed that the same gene products are responsible for the rejection of organ grafts, a reaction also known to be initiated by T lymphocytes. Thus, in both the response to foreign pathogens and to tissue grafts T lymphocytes recognize and respond to MHC antigens, although in one case it is foreign MHC and in the other self MHC+ antigen. T cells do not 'see' antigen as a whole protein molecule but rather as a small fragment consisting of as few as a dozen amino acids. These peptides lie in a cleft in the MHC molecules and the T cell receptor binds to the complex of MHC + peptide (Bjorkman *et al.* 1987). That only small fragments of antigens are recognized by T cells implies that larger molecules must be broken down (processed) before T cells can recognize them.

There are two distinct antigen processing pathways, which lead to initiation of very different types of T cell responses (Fig. 16.3). In the first, proteins produced within a cell are broken down by proteolytic enzymes to peptides. These are then transported into the endoplasmic reticulum (ER) where they become associated with newly synthesized MHC class I molecules and the complex is transported to the cell surface (endogenous processing). As far as is known all nucleated cells can carry out endogenous processing. The second type of antigen processing is carried out by specialized antigen presenting cells such as dendritic cells and macrophages. Antigens are taken up by these phagocytic cells and degraded in endosomes to peptides (exogenous processing). In a specialized postendosomal compartment the peptides bind to a different type of MHC molecule (class II molecules) and the newly formed complexes are transported to the cell surface.

Peptides presented by MHC class II molecules are recognized by T cells called helper cells, which carry

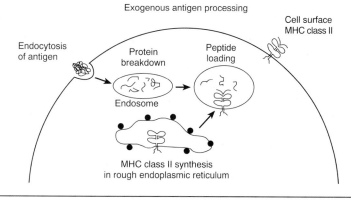

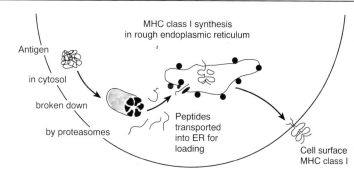

Fig. 16.3 Mechanisms of antigen processing. The top half of the figure (exogenous processing) shows how antigen taken up from the extracellular environment is broken down and how peptides derived from proteolysis become associated with newly synthesized MHC class II molecules for transport to the cell surface. The bottom half (endogenous processing) illustrates the way in which internal antigens are broken down in the cytosol before peptides are transported into the rough endoplasmic reticulum to become associated with MHC class I molecules.

the CD4 glycoprotein on their surface. This molecule acts as a coreceptor binding to MHC class II. In contrast, peptides bound to MHC class I molecules stimulate cytotoxic T cells, which carry a different coreceptor molecule, the CD8 glycoprotein, which binds to MHC class I.

16.2.4 The function of T cells

Like B cells, when naive T lymphocytes first encounter antigen they undergo clonal expansion, so that following the first exposure to antigen the frequency of antigen-specific T cells may increase by one to two logs, to as high as one in a few hundred cells. Unlike B cells there is no somatic mutation so that the affinity of the T cell receptor remains the same. T cell memory therefore resides in increased numbers of specific T cells. Memory cells are also qualitatively different from naive T cells.

In contrast to B lymphocytes, T cells do not appear to secrete their receptor in measurable amounts but mediate their functions by other means. Table 16.2 lists some activities of CD4 and CD8 T cells. Some of these are carried out by T cells alone and involve direct cell to cell contact. Typical

of this type of response is protection against virus-infected cells in which the infected cells, carrying peptide–MHC complexes derived from endogenous

Table 16.2 T lymphocyte functions

	Cells involved	
In vivo	CD4	CD8
Delayed type hypersensitivity	++	+/−
Graft rejection	++	++
Tumour rejection	++	++
Graft versus host response	++	++
Protection against viral and fungal infection	++	++
Protection against bacterial infection	++	+
In vitro		
Help for antibody responses	++	−
Mixed lymphocyte responses—proliferation	++	+
Mixed lymphocyte responses—cytotoxicity	+/−	++
Proliferation to mitogens	++	++
Proliferation to soluble antigens	++	−
Cytotoxicity against specific antigens (in association with MHC)	+/−	++
Production of cytokines	++	+

processing, are killed by CD8 cytotoxic cells. This type of T cell may also be important in the response to tumours.

Many other functions involve other cell types as well as the responding T cells. Very often these responses are immunoregulatory, i.e. the T cells control the responses of the other cell types. Most often these immunoregulatory functions are carried out by CD4 T helper cells. Thus, helper T cells can stimulate B lymphocytes to secrete antibody or macrophages to become phagocytic and cytocidal.

Many immunoregulatory functions are mediated by cytokines (Callard and Gearing 1994; see also Chapter 20). They have powerful effects on the growth and differentiation of their target cells and act as local hormones within the immune system. They are similar in many respects to the growth factors discussed in Chapter 11. Lymphokines are cytokines produced mainly by lymphocytes and Table 16.3 lists some of the better characterized as well as the monokine interleukin-1 which plays a role in the initial activation of T cells. One of the best characterized lymphokines is interleukin-2 (IL-

2) which is produced by activated T cells and can stimulate both the producing cell (autocrine stimulation) and other T cells (paracrine stimulation) to divide. Only T cells that have first been stimulated by contact with antigen express receptors for IL-2. The growth-promoting effects of IL-2 are very powerful and it is used to grow antigen-activated T cells *in vitro*. So potent a growth stimulus is IL-2 that it is possible to grow a large number of cells from a single T cell. This is known as an IL-2-dependent T cell clone. Such clones are being used to analyse the specificity and functions of T cells and are the T cell equivalent of monoclonal antibody-producing hybridomas.

In contrast to IL-2, which promotes T cell growth, other lymphokines induce differentiation into effector cells. Interleukins-4, -5, and -6 together regulate the proliferation of B lymphocytes after stimulation by antigen and their differentiation into high rate antibody-secreting cells. Although all T lymphocytes produce a multiplicity of cytokines, there is a tendency for CD4 T cells to produce larger amounts of those with effects on growth and differentiation such

Table 16.3 Functions and properties of cytokines

Cytokine	Main effects	Molecular weight (Da) and other properties
Cloned and characterized cytokines		
Interleukin-1α	Activation of T cells,	17 500 ⎱ Produced by many cells
Interleukin-1β	Pyrogenic response	17 500 ⎰
Interleukin-2	Growth of T cells	13 500, from T and NK cells
Interleukin-3	Growth of haemopoietic stem cells	18–30 000, T cell product
Interleukin-4	Growth and differentiation of T and B cells	15–18 000, T cell product
Interleukin-5	Effects on B cells and granulocytes	20–22 000, T cell product
Interleukin-6	B cell differentiation but many other effects also	21 000, produced by many cells
Interleukin-7	Growth of B cells	25 000
Interleukin-10	Inhibition of Th-1 cells	16–20 000, produced by Th2 cells
Interleukin-15	Growth of T cells	15 000, produced by many non-lymphoid cell types
Chemokines (e.g. IL-8, rantes MIP-1α)	Chemotaxis of lymphocytes, granulocytes and macrophages	8 000, a large family of peptides produced by many cell types
Interferon-α	Inhibition of viral replication	15 000, produced by many cells
Interferon-γ	Increase of MHC expression Inhibition of viral replication	38 000, T cell product
Tumour necrosis factor-α	Necrosis of tumours, pyrogenic	25 000 and multimers
Tumour necrosis factor-β	Cytotoxic *in vitro*	25 000 and multimers
Leukaemia inhibitory factor	Inducer of myeloid differentiation	20 000, produced by many cells
Colony-stimulating factors (see Chapters 11 and 20)	Promote growth and maturation of progenitor cells	Various

as IL-2, -3, -4, -5, and -6, while CD8 T cells produce more effector cytokines such as interferon-γ (IFN-γ). Interferons have complex effects but an important function is the induction of expression of MHC molecules, which increases the efficiency of antigen presentation.

Cytokine function is pleiotropic and redundant. Thus, cytokines act on many different cell types and frequently different cytokines may have very similar profiles of activity and may share receptors or parts of receptors. For example IFN-γ, in addition to induction of MHC classes I and II, is important in regulation of B cell immunoglobulin class switching, is cytostatic to many cell types, and can activate macrophages and cytolytic T cells. IL-2 and IL-15 have very similar effects on T cell growth and probably bind to the same receptor, although they are produced by different cell types.

There is specialization among T cells with regard to cytokine production. Thus, naive T cells produce mainly IL-2, while primed or memory T cells produce a wider range of cytokines. Among primed CD4 cells there are two major patterns of cytokine production. T helper-1 (Th-1) cells produce IL-2 and IFN-γ, while Th-2 cells produce IL-4, -5, and -6. While Th-1 cells are particularly effective at inducing macrophage activation and maturation of cytotoxic effector cells, Th-2 cells are most effective in inducing antibody production by B lymphocytes.

16.2.5 Self tolerance

Immune responses generate powerful effector mechanisms capable not only of combating microorganisms but also of causing acute tissue damage as is shown by the rapid destruction of foreign tissue grafts. There must therefore be mechanisms that prevent development of immune responses to self antigens (self tolerance). For T lymphocytes there is good evidence that induction of self tolerance occurs in the thymus. T cell precursors first express the T cell receptor in the thymus and if the receptor has a high affinity for self antigens expressed on thymic antigen-presenting cells, the developing T cells die. T cells that leave the thymus are therefore generally self tolerant but there are additional 'fail safe' mechanisms in the periphery which prevent the development of damaging autoimmunity (see Section 16.3).

The mechanisms of tolerance induction and maintenance in B cells are probably similar, with tolerance induction occurring during B cell development in the bone marrow and 'fail safe' mechanisms operating on mature B cells in lymphoid tissues.

16.3 The immune system and cancer

16.3.1 Immune surveillance

As the importance of the immune system in protection against infection became apparent, it was suggested that immunity to tumours might also be important. In 1909 Paul Ehrlich postulated that we might all die of tumours if the immune system did not remove 'aberrant germs' (nascent tumours). This idea led to many attempts to demonstrate immunity to tumours in which tumours were transplanted from one animal to another. The transplants were rejected and this was taken as evidence of immunity to the tumour. Only later was it recognized that these experiments demonstrated not tumour immunity but transplantation immunity directed against MHC antigens.

Only when genetically homogeneous inbred animals (mice) became available was it possible to carry out experiments on tumour immunity and it was then shown that if a growing tumour was excised from a mouse and the animal was challenged with a graft of the same tumour, the graft was rejected. A graft of a different tumour was not, showing that the animal was immune to the immunizing tumour and, furthermore, that immunity was tumour specific.

At about the same time as these early experiments on tumour specific immunity, Thomas, and later Burnet, restated Ehrlich's hypothesis of protection against 'aberrant germs' as the theory of immune surveillance against tumours. They proposed that tumours arose frequently and that the majority were eliminated by the immune system well before becoming clinically apparent. This hypothesis stimulated a great deal of experimental work in both humans and experimental animals because the theory made clear predictions that could be tested. In particular it suggested that tumours should differ antigenically from normal cells and that they would arise more frequently in circumstances when the immune response of the host is compromised. The theory also implied that it might be possible to use immunological means to detect tumours and perhaps to stimulate the immune system to destroy them (immunotherapy). The rest of this chapter discusses immune surveillance, the nature of tumour antigens, immunodiagnosis, and the potential of immunotherapy.

16.3.2 Evidence for and against immune surveillance

Burnet summarized his view of immune surveillance as follows. (i) Most malignant cells have antigenic qualities distinct from those of the cell type from which they derive; (ii) such antigenic differences can be recognized by T cells and provoke an immune response. If this view is correct it follows that, (iii) the incidence of malignant disease should be greatest in periods of relative immunological inefficiency, particularly in the perinatal period and old age; (iv) immunosuppression, whether genetic or induced by drugs, radiation, infection, or other causes, should increase the incidence of cancer; (v) spontaneous regression of tumours may occur and evidence of an immune response should be apparent in these cases; and (vi) large-scale histological examination of common sites of cancer should reveal a higher proportion of tumours than become clinically apparent. Burnet also suggested ways in which the theory of surveillance might be tested experimentally. Thus, immunosuppressive agents should facilitate the transfer of tumours, or damage to the T cell immune response produced by surgical removal of the thymus might lead to increased tumour incidence.

At first sight a variety of clinical and experimental data do seem to be in accordance with the surveillance theory. In humans some tumours show a higher incidence in the first few years of life than in early adulthood and the incidence, but of different tumour types, then rises progressively with increasing age (see Chapter 1). There is also compelling evidence in humans that the incidence of tumours is greatly increased in immunosuppressed individuals (Sheil 1992). This is true both in rare patients with inherited immunodeficiency and in the large number of kidney-grafted patients who are treated with immunosuppressive drugs to prevent rejection of the grafted kidney. However, a closer examination does not support the surveillance hypothesis.

The age incidence of tumours is as well explained by many other theories of cancer causation as by immunosurveillance. Tumours are caused by genetic changes in their cells of origin. These changes might be expected to occur either as errors during periods of rapid cell division (early life) or when external causes (carcinogens) have had time to take effect, as in later life.

The more persuasive data derived from immunosuppressed individuals are similarly less straightforward to interpret when examined more closely. Although there does seem to be a slight increase in the frequency of most tumours there is a disproportionate increase in a few tumour types (Table 16.4). The relative risk of suffering from some rare tumour types may be increased more than 1000-fold in immunosuppressed individuals.

Animal experimental data provide some clues to interpretation of the human data, but are equally confusing. In an early study using more than 15 000 nude mice, which lack a functional thymus and are therefore congenitally T cell immunodeficient, no tumours were seen. Unfortunately, in a later more closely investigated study (Sadoff et al. 1988), a group of nude mice with the nu/nu gene had a higer incidence of tumours; 19 lymphomas, 10 ovarian granulosa cell tumours, and 1 transitional cell carcinoma of bladder in 173 mice, while only 1 granulosa cell tumour was found in 53 heterozygotes (nu/+). The type of tumour probably reflects the specific tumour pattern of the parental NIH Swiss mouse strain (see Chapter 1). In contrast, when a large group of mice were treated from birth with antilymphocyte serum raised in rabbits, their T cell immunity was sufficiently depressed that skin grafts from another mouse strain were retained indefinitely. These mice did not develop spontaneous tumours but when they inadvertently became infected with polyomavirus (see Chapter 8), a number developed multiple tumours of a type character-

Table 16.4 Immunosuppression and tumours

Tumour type	Relative risk
Kaposi's sarcoma	>1000
Lymphoma—of the brain	>1000
—non-Hodgkin's	7.4
Endocrine tumours	320
Skin carcinoma	40
Liver carcinoma	30
Leukaemia	6.4
Cervix carcinoma	4.2
Digestive system carcinoma	2.6
Respiratory system carcinoma	2.1
Breast carcinoma	1.1

istically caused by this virus. Similarly, the lymphoid tumours seen in transplant recipients are commonly of B lymphocyte origin and have been shown to contain both DNA and proteins characteristic of the Epstein–Barr virus (EBV). This member of the herpesvirus family is implicated in the development of Burkitt's lymphoma, a B cell tumour seen in parts of Africa, and nasopharyngeal carcinoma (see Chapter 8). The virus can also immortalize normal human B lymphocytes *in vitro*. It is likely, therefore, that this virus is responsible for at least one step in the transformation of B lymphocytes into malignant lymphomas, which occurs in immunosuppressed individuals. These findings suggest, therefore, that the most important role of the immune system in tumour protection may be in preventing the spread of potentially oncogenic viruses.

This view agrees with experimental and clinical data on EBV, an ubiquitous infectious agent in human populations. More than 90 per cent of adults have evidence of past infection in the form of antibody to the virus in their serum. Infection may be symptomless but in young adults EBV causes infectious mononucleosis (glandular fever). Following either symptomless infection or mononucleosis the virus is carried lifelong and the individual also has lifelong immunity. Immune CD8 cytotoxic T lymphocytes can be demonstrated *in vitro*. Under normal circumstances there is thus a balance between virus production and the immune response, while in immunosuppressed individuals the immune system may be unable to prevent virus spread. The T cells of such individuals cannot kill EBV-transformed B cells *in vitro*, and virus can often be isolated from body tissues and secretions such as saliva.

Several viruses have now been implicated in the development of human tumours and the risk of acquiring these tumours is generally increased in immunosuppressed patients. In addition to EBV, hepatitis B virus is implicated in liver cancer and human papillomaviruses in genital cancer, while there is strong epidemiological evidence that Kaposi's sarcoma is caused by an unknown infectious agent. Skin tumours are the commonest tumours in immunosuppressed patients and here the position is less clear. Although warts and precancerous lesions of the skin contain papillomaviruses, the tumours that develop may not contain viral genes so that the role of the virus is less clear than for other tumours where viral genes are retained. Finally, what do the high incidences of

endocrine and ureteric tumours mean? One speculation is that so far unknown viruses may be involved.

If it is accepted that immune surveillance operates principally against oncogenic viruses, what is the role of the immune system in relation to other tumours? Evidence from experimental animals (see Sections 16.3.1 and 16.4.1) suggests that there are immune responses to many tumours and the slight increase of relative risk for tumours with no known viral involvement would support this (Table 16.4). However, the fact that most tumours grow and kill the host, would suggest that the immune response is probably a late event and in most cases is unable to prevent tumour growth. Nevertheless, that there is an immune response suggests that tumours do contain antigens recognized as foreign by the immune system. If this is the case it should be possible to boost immunity to them by deliberate immunization.

16.4 Cell-mediated immune responses to cancer

16.4.1 Tumour antigens detected by immune cells in animals

It has been demonstrated repeatedly that laboratory animals can be immunized against tumour cells. In the case of virus-induced tumours, immunity is usually cross-reactive so that animals immunized with a virus-induced tumour are generally immune to all other tumours induced by the same virus. Immunity can be transferred to other animals by immune cells but not by serum, and is mediated by T cells. In several such systems the target viral gene products have been identified. These results suggest that immunization against viral gene products should be a useful strategy for those human tumours where viruses are known to be involved.

In contrast, for experimental tumours induced by carcinogens, immunity is tumour specific (Section 16.3.1) and the nature of the tumour antigens remained obscure until the pioneering work of Boon and his colleagues (Boon *et al.* 1994). An established mouse tumour, which had become non-immunogenic by repeated passage in mice, was used for the experiments. Tumour cells were treated *in vitro* with a mutagenic chemical and variant tumour cell sublines obtained, which would no longer grow *in vivo* (unless very large numbers of cells were injected) because they induced a strong cytotoxic T cell response. Boon then set out to clone the tumour antigen of one such non-tumorigenic (*tum⁻*) subline, the P91A tumour, using the following strategy. Mice were immunized with P91A tumour cells and an IL-2-dependent cytotoxic T cell clone generated (see Section 16.2.4) which would kill P91A cells but not the parental (unmutated) P815 tumour. Parental tumour cells were then transfected with a DNA library from P91A and thousands of transfected cells tested with the cytotoxic T cells to determine which expressed the P91A tumour antigen. The transfected DNA was then recovered and subcloned until eventually a single gene coding for the tumour antigen was identified. The gene and its homologue in the parental tumour were then sequenced and found to differ by a single point mutation. This experiment firmly established that mutations in genes in a tumour cell can lead to a host immune response to the mutated gene product. This is an extremely important result since there is overwhelming evidence that the majority of human tumours contain several mutations and at least some of these might be expected to generate altered protein sequences, which would be immunogenic to the tumour-bearing host.

However, further experiments established a second important principle. Boon used the same strategy to clone the tumour antigens from several other similar mouse tumours. Surprisingly, in several of these the gene in the *tum⁻* variant tumour cells was found to be identical to that in the parental tumour line (or DNA from normal cells of the same inbred strain of mice). In this case the mouse appears to be responding to a completely normal self gene product. So far the evidence suggests that this is because the tumour antigen gene product is expressed at a higher level in the tumour cells than in normal tissues and can therefore stimulate an immune response.

16.4.2 Human tumour antigens detected by immune cells

Identification of human tumour antigens recognized by the host immune response is technically an even more demanding exercise than in experimental animals. This is because it is not possible in most cases to immunize humans deliberately against their own tumour, so that the frequency of primed T cells may be low. Even in animals deliberately immunized with an antigen, immunological memory or priming is usually detected by an *in vitro* boost. The immune T cells are stimulated *in vitro* with antigen and their response measured by a proliferative response or the production of cytokines such as IL-2 in the cultures; while CD8 cytotoxic effector cells, which develop during the cultures, can be assayed by their ability to kill appropriate target cells (Fig. 16.4). Furthermore, genetic restriction means that T cells can only be stimulated by MHC-matched antigen-presenting cells, and cytotoxic effectors only assayed on similarly matched targets.

These constraints have meant that most experiments in humans have taken a similar form (Fig. 16.4). Lymphocytes from peripheral blood, tumour draining lymph nodes, or extracted from the tumour itself (tumour-infiltrating lymphocytes or TILs) are cocultured with tumour cells, which have been X-irradiated or mitomycin treated to prevent their growth. Proliferation of CD4 T cells may be assayed by adding radioactive tritiated thymidine to the cultures and measuring its incorporation into DNA. After 7–10 days of coculture, T cells recovered from the culture can be assayed for their ability to lyse chromium-51-labelled tumour target cells. T cells can be cloned from these polyclonal populations by limiting dilution in the presence of antigen (tumour cells), antigen-presenting cells, and IL-2. The difficulty of obtaining lymphocytes and viable autologous tumour cells for this *in vitro* boosting procedure has dictated that most work has been carried out on tumours that can be disaggregated easily or grow well in tissue culture. In spite of these limitations evidence for a tumour-specific response of CD4 or CD8 T cells has been obtained for a number of human tumour types, including lung, ovary, and renal carcinoma, and melanoma. Perhaps because melanoma grows well *in vitro* and the tumours are often superficial and can therefore be biopsied, a great deal of work has been carried out on this tumour. Several target antigens have been identified.

The pioneering work was again carried out by Boon and his colleagues employing a similar strategy to that used for the cloning of murine tumour antigens (Boon *et al.* 1994). CD8 cytotoxic T cell clones specific for an autologous melanoma tumour cell line were generated following *in vitro* boosting. One of these was used to clone its target antigen. Repeated exposure of the autologous melanoma cell line to the cytotoxic T cells eventually generated a tumour variant lacking the target antigen, which

Fig. 16.4 *In vitro* boosting. CD4 and CD8 T cell responses can be revealed following an *in vitro* boost in which the antigen, in this case tumour cells inactivated by X-irradiation or mitomycin C, is cocultured with T cells and antigen-presenting cells. T cells recovered from the cultures may be assayed for cytotoxicity by isotope release from target cells or for proliferation or cytokine release after a further exposure to antigen. IL-2-dependent T cell lines or clones can also be derived from the cultures.

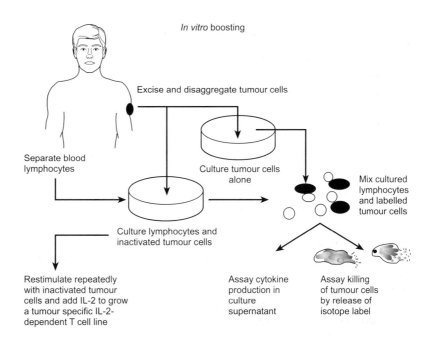

In vitro boosting

Excise and disaggregate tumour cells

Separate blood lymphocytes

Culture tumour cells alone

Mix cultured lymphocytes and labelled tumour cells

Culture lymphocytes and inactivated tumour cells

Restimulate repeatedly with inactivated tumour cells and add IL-2 to grow a tumour specific IL-2-dependent T cell line

Assay cytokine production in culture supernatant

Assay killing of tumour cells by release of isotope label

could not be killed by the cytotoxic T cells. A cosmid DNA library was then prepared from the original tumour and transfected into the tumour antigen negative variant. Thousands of transfectants were screened for the presence of the antigen using the cytotoxic T cell clone. From a transfectant expressing the tumour antigen, the cosmid was recovered and after further subcloning a previously unknown melanoma antigen gene (*MAGE*) was identified. The target epitope in MAGE is restricted by the MHC class I allele HLA-A1. The first *MAGE* gene has now been shown to be a member of a new gene family whose function is as yet unknown. *MAGE 1* has only been detected in the testis among normal tissues tested, but mRNA for *MAGE 1, 2,* or *3* are frequently detected in melanomas, lung cancers, and some other tumours. Interestingly the *MAGE 1* gene in melanoma cells is identical to that in non-tumour DNA of the patient. Several other antigens recognised by cytotoxic T cells have now been identified in melanoma and a number in other tumours (Robbins and Kawakami, 1996). In the majority of cases the antigens are identical in tumour and normal cells. The existence of T cell responses to these unaltered self antigens raises the question of why these self reactive cells have not been deleted in the thymus and why there is no response to MAGE or tyrosinase under normal circumstances. These questions cannot yet be answered but several factors may con-

tribute to the maintenance of tolerance unless a tumour expressing MAGE or tyrosinase develops. Most MAGE or tyrosinase reactive cells may be deleted in the thymus. Those that escape to the periphery may have low affinity for antigen so that they are only stimulated by the higher amount of antigen present in the tumour. Finally, the antigens may be poorly presented by normal cells which lack costimuli (see below) while the tumour cells, or antigen-presenting cells within the tumour, may process and present the antigens more effectively.

16.4.3 Unrestricted cytotoxicity

In early human experiments in which patients' lymphocytes were cultured with live tumour target cells, outgrowth of colonies of tumour cells was often inhibited (colony inhibition). In the early experiments the inhibition of growth appeared to be tumour type specific so that lymphocytes from a patient with lung cancer could inhibit the growth of all lung cancer cell lines but not that of other tumour types. When more extensive controls were included in the assays the specificity appeared less clear-cut and it emerged that lymphocytes from normal individuals were often as inhibitory to tumour cell lines as were those from cancer patients. Subsequent experiments suggest that two different types of cytotoxic activity may have been detected in the earlier experiments. Finn and colleagues have shown that T cells from breast cancer patients, repeatedly boosted *in vitro* with breast cancer cells expressing the polymorphic epithelial mucin (PEM) develop PEM-specific, but genetically unrestricted, cytotoxicity (Jerome *et al.* 1993). PEM has an extracellular domain mainly consisting of a 20 amino acid sequence repeated many times. It is suggested that because this is a large repetitive array, it may bind to the T cell receptor without the need for MHC presentation.

A second type of cytotoxicity detected in the early experiments is natural killer (NK) activity (Takasugi *et al.* 1973). Much effort has been expended in the identification of the cells responsible for NK activity, their relationship to other lymphocytes, their biological role, and identification of the antigens recognized by them on target cells. Only the first question can be answered with any confidence. NK cells have a characteristic phenotype. They are larger lymphocytes than most T and B cells and have characteristic cytoplasmic granules (large granular lymphocytes). They share surface antigens with T lymphocytes and also with monocytes but do not express the T cell receptor (TCR). There are also some surface molecules unique to NK cells. Just as their phenotype makes it difficult to determine their origin, so is it difficult to assign these cells a definite function, although various possibilities have been suggested; for example, that they regulate haemopoiesis or are an early non-specific response system for combating viral infections. Because they can kill many tumour cell lines, NK cells may also play a role in surveillance against tumours.

Irrespective of their exact function, NK cells make it difficult to study specific immune responses to human tumours using cytotoxicity assays. For this reason most experiments that have successfully used T cells to identify tumour antigens have employed T cell clones, since the cloning separates T cells from NK cells which may have survived during the initial *in vitro* boost.

16.5 Human tumour antigens detected by antibodies

A great deal of effort has been devoted to attempts to use antibodies to detect new antigens on human tumours (see also Chapter 19). A unique genetic change in a cell might lead to the expression of a new antigen unique to that tumour—a tumour-specific antigen. Such an antigen may provoke a host response but the development of antibodies to it may only be useful to the tumour-bearing individual because the same antigen is not found in other tumours, even of the same type. Most useful from the point of view of diagnosis or immunotherapy are tumour-associated antigens. These are antigens present on or in all tumour cells of a particular type but not found on normal cells. In tumours caused by viruses, proteins coded by the viral genome are effectively tumour associated because they are generally found only in very rare normal cells; for example, some lymphomas have EBV antigens and one type of T cell leukaemia has antigens of the human T cell leukaemia virus (HTLV-1). These are both rare tumours so we must now consider tumour-associated antigens of more common tumours.

Early attempts to reveal tumour-associated antigens used sera either from tumour patients or from animals deliberately immunized with human tumours. Both types of study have considerable problems. Sera from tumour patients might appear to be ideal reagents but in practice they often have in them antibodies capable of reacting with many types of cells. These include antibodies to blood group, and histocompatibility antigens and autoantibodies, which react with normal as well as tumour cells. To sort out a minor proportion of antibodies specific for tumour antigens is a complex task. It has usually been attempted by absorption analysis in which the serum is incubated with a succession of different normal cell types to remove antibody to them and then tested for reactivity with tumour cells. Such manoeuvres generally dilute the specific antibody and also lead to non-specific loss so that even if the resulting antiserum reacts only with tumour cells it may be so weak that it is difficult to use for identification and characterization of the antigens detected.

Antisera raised in animals, usually rabbits, present similar problems. The rabbit antiserum 'sees' many antigens on a human tumour cell but the majority of these are present on normal cells also. Such sera therefore require extensive absorption to render them specific for tumour cells and it is not surprising that reports of successful production of specific heteroantisera are few in number, nor have they in general been particularly useful in tumour diagnosis or therapy. Some exceptions are mentioned below.

When the hybridoma method for producing monoclonal antibodies was developed, many investigators realized that monoclonal antibodies might provide reagents for detecting molecular differences between cell types. This has indeed proved to be the case and, for example, mouse monoclonal antibodies can distinguish between human leucocytes and all other human cells, between T and B lymphocytes, or between different subpopulations of T lymphocytes. The molecules identified by these monoclonal antibodies are differentiation antigens (antigens present on one cell type but not another or expressed at a particular stage of maturation; see Chapters 12 and 19). In many cases they have been shown to be involved in functions associated with the particular cell type. These results suggested that it should be possible to produce monoclonal antibodies that could distinguish between tumour and normal cells, if differences existed. Differences have indeed been recognized but so far there is no convincing evidence of a specific tumour-associated antigen.

One of the few useful polyclonal heteroantisera was raised against acute lymphoblastic leukaemia (ALL) cells. After extensive absorption this serum could distinguish ALL cells from normal lymphocytes of bone marrow. Several monoclonal antibodies have been produced which react in a similar fashion and were therefore considered initially to identify a tumour-associated antigen of leukaemia cells (common acute lymphoblastic leukaemia antigen or CALLA). More careful examination of bone marrow showed that a small number of normal cells carried CALLA. Subsequent studies have shown that CALLA is a differentiation antigen transiently expressed on cells early in the B lymphocyte lineage. One category of antigens, which can easily be confused with tumour-associated antigens, are thus differentiation antigens expressed only on rare normal cells.

From the point of view of diagnosis and treatment, however, CALLA is a very useful antigen. CALLA positive cells are very rare in normal bone marrow (< 1 per cent) and are not found in peripheral blood, so their presence can be used to monitor disease. Furthermore, because CALLA is not present on stem cells, it is possible to remove CALLA positive cells from bone marrow without damaging the potential of the marrow cells to regenerate a functional haemopoietic system (see Chapter 12).

This, therefore, is an example of a normal differentiation antigen which, for practical purposes, may be regarded as a tumour-associated antigen.

Perhaps the most thoroughly studied tumour, from the point of view of tumour antigens, is melanoma, a tumour of pigment cells (Chapter 1). Over 40 different antigens have been defined in these tumours by monoclonal antibodies (Herlyn and Koprowski 1988). None of these are truly tumour associated, although some are only weakly expressed on normal cells in the adult. At least six categories of antigen have been described (Table 16.5). Several of these are likely to influence the behaviour of the tumour cells. For example, increased expression of growth factor receptors may lead to uncontrolled growth, while abnormal production or abnormal distribution of adhesion molecules will influence the ability of the cells to metastasize (Chapter 2). Several of these molecules may be potential targets for therapy because of their high expression on the tumour and low expression on normal pigment or other cells.

Another category of antigens that can appear tumour associated are those that are expressed in dividing cells only. Some monoclonal antibodies raised against tumour cell lines appeared initially to distinguish between tumour and normal cells. More extensive studies showed that these antibodies also detected an antigen present on normal cells when these were actively dividing. This antigen has now been shown to be the cell surface receptor for transferrin. Transferrin is a serum protein that transports iron required for cell division. The expression of the transferrin receptor is therefore correlated

Table 16.5 Melanoma antigens

Antigen	Comment
MHC antigens	Melanoma frequently expresses MHC class II as well as class I
Pigment antigens	Intracellular, sometimes of diagnostic value
Growth factor receptors	Receptors for EGF, TGF-α, TGF-β, NGF, and FGF
Adhesion molecules	Chondroitin sulphate proteoglycan, melanoma-associated adhesion molecule, gangliosides, intercellular adhesion molecule 1
Transport proteins	Melanotransferrin, S-100 calcium binding protein
Extracellular matrix proteins	Laminin and collagen

with the cell cycle, not with malignancy. The proportion of cells in a population that express transferrin receptors may therefore indicate how many cells are actively dividing. By no means all cells in a tumour divide, but in general the greater the percentage of dividing cells the more rapid will be the growth of the tumour. In a study of lymphomas it was indeed found that the more rapidly progressive tumours did have a higher proportion of transferrin receptor positive cells. The transferrin receptor is therefore useful in indicating the prognosis in tumour patients.

While the transferrin receptor is widely distributed on actively dividing normal cells, other differentiation antigens that appear on dividing cells are restricted to certain cell types. One example of this is the receptor for interleukin-2. This is expressed on T lymphocytes (and some B lymphocytes) after these have been activated by contact with antigen. Some T cell tumours express this receptor, and, as in the case of CALLA, for practical purposes it may be regarded as a tumour-associated antigen because normal T cells have been replaced by the malignant population. This has encouraged attempts to treat some patients with antibodies to the receptor or with IL-2 conjugated to a toxin.

Well before the advent of monoclonal antibodies, conventional heteroantisera were used to define a rather different category of tumour-associated antigens to which monoclonal antibodies have now been raised: these are differentiation antigens expressed at a high level during fetal life but only at a low level in the adult (oncofetal antigens). Certain tumours, however, re-express these antigens. Two examples have been studied particularly extensively: carcinoembryonic antigen (CEA) and α-fetoprotein (AFP). The former is found in fetal intestine and in colonic tumours, whereas the latter is found in fetal liver and adult liver tumours. Both antigens can be detected in the serum of tumour patients and sensitive immunoassays for their detection have been developed, but neither has proved satisfactory for diagnosis. In the case of CEA, this is because it is difficult to establish normal and abnormal levels since, in contrast to earlier data, more recent results have shown that many different tumours produce CEA and that levels may also be raised in a variety of non-malignant conditions. In the case of AFP, raised levels are associated with liver cancer but also with other liver diseases and false negative results are sometimes obtained. Both

CEA and AFP are probably most useful in monitoring the effects of treatment on CEA- or AFP-producing tumours. A fall in the serum level occurs following successful treatment and a rise may be detectable before clinical recurrence of tumour. Antibodies to both CEA and AFP have also been used in studies of tumour localization and immunotherapy (see Chapter 19).

Although the foregoing discussions suggest that tumour cells only express normal differentiation antigens this is not quite the case as at least some antigens detectable by monoclonal antibodies on tumour cells are altered. Tumour cells often show abnormal glycosylation with shorter and less branched carbohydrate side chains, often lacking terminal sialic acid residues. The abnormal carbohydrates are detectable with monoclonal antibodies and although not confined to tumour cells are certainly more highly expressed on them. Many epithelial cells and tumours express heavily glycosylated molecules known as a mucins. In the case of the breast-associated PEM, the altered glycosylation of the molecule on breast tumour cells reveals epitopes of the protein core of the molecule detectable by monoclonal antibodies. Like the altered carbohydrates, these epitopes of the protein backbone are relatively tumour associated. Antibodies to PEM are being used in immunodiagnosis and may eventually be useful for tumour therapy.

It is notable that there are no solely tumour-associated antigens, but studies of cellular oncogenes suggest that tumour cells do express altered proteins (Chapters 9 and 11) so that tumour-associated antigens should exist. Why then are they not detected? Several explanations may be offered. Firstly, if the genetic changes in a tumour are unique to that tumour the antigen would be tumour specific. While this might provoke a host response, the specific antibody in a polyclonal antiserum may be difficult to detect especially as it would only react with that particular tumour. Secondly, attempts to detect tumour antigens with heteroantisera or monoclonal antibodies are likely to be difficult because of the large number of foreign proteins seen by the immunized rabbit or mouse. In spite of this there have been some reports of detection of human tumour-specific antigens with monoclonal antibodies. These are of course difficult to confirm because the antibody reacts only with the immunizing tumour. Such antibodies are of use for diagnosis or therapy only in the original patient and may be most useful in studying genetic changes in tumour cells. In the foreseeable future the most useful antibodies are likely to be those against differentiation antigens with a restricted distribution, which are also expressed on tumour cells. How these can be exploited is discussed in Chapter 19.

Attempts to generate human monoclonal antibodies from cancer patients have not so far proved very useful. It has been difficult to generate stable hybridomas producing high yields of antibody and those antibodies that have been produced have shown a disappointing lack of specificity. Most appear to react with internal cellular antigens present in tumour and many normal cells. Similar antibodies can be generated by immortalizing B cells from normal individuals as well as cancer patients. In future this problem may be overcome by expressing libraries of human heavy and light chains in phages and using sensitive assays to screen for desired antibody specificities.

16.6 Immunodiagnosis

16.6.1 Immunodiagnosis *in vitro*

Ideal reagents for immunodiagnosis or immunotherapy would discriminate absolutely between tumour and normal cells. In addition they would distinguish between benign and malignant tumours. However, as discussed earlier, most if not all antibodies raised against tumours identify differentiation antigens. Nevertheless, antibodies can be useful in cancer diagnosis just because they identify differentiation antigens and thus the origin of a cell. Panels of monoclonal antibodies are finding a role in pathology and haematology laboratories where they are used to improve the identification and classification of tumours. For example, in the diagnosis of acute lymphoblastic leukaemia (see Chapter 12) antibodies have allowed clear distinctions to be made between T and B cell forms of the disease, each of which have a very different prognosis and respond differently to conventional chemotherapy. Identification of bad prognosis patients is important because it is sensible to try new forms of therapy in individuals with little chance of survival with current treatment.

Monoclonal antibodies are also useful in identifying the origin of tumour cells when this is difficult by conventional histological methods: antibodies to differentiation antigens (Table 16.6) can usually identify the origin of metastatic tumour cells even if these

Table 16.6 Antibodies for indentification of undifferentiatied tumours

Tumour type	Tissue of origin	Antibody specificity
Carcinoma	Epithelia	Cytokeratins
Sarcoma	Connective tissue	Vimentin
Neuroblastoma	Nervous tissue	Neurofilaments
Glioma	Glia	Glial fibrillary acidic protein
Myosarcoma	Muscle	Desmin
Leukaemia/lymphoma	Leucocytes	CD45

are cytologically undifferentiated. This has important implications for the management of the patient because secondary carcinoma is often chemotherapy resistant while lymphoid tumours are often chemotherapy sensitive.

Monoclonal antibodies are also being used in attempts to localize tumours *in vivo* (see Chapter 13).

16.7 Immunotherapy and immune escape mechanisms

16.7.1 Introduction

Immunotherapy is treatment by immunological means. In active immunotherapy the tumour bearer's own immune system is stimulated to respond to the tumour, while in passive immunotherapy, immune cells or their products are given. Table 16.7 summarizes the possibilities. The aim of treatment in cancer is to eliminate the tumour without harming the host. Because immune responses are highly specific, immunologists have long hoped that immune cells or antibodies might be used in this way. Unfortunately, as discussed earlier, few cells or antibodies are truly tumour specific so that some side effects on normal cells must be expected. Nevertheless, many experiments have been carried out. Since the use of monoclonal antibodies is discussed in detail in Chapter 19, only other means will be considered here.

16.7.2 Active immunization

Early attempts to treat human tumours by active immunization with tumour, or the administration of immunostimulating agents, met with little success. However, many of these experiments predated present understanding of the way in which antigens are processed and presented to T cells. Furthermore,

Table 16.7 Immunotherapy

Approach	Method	Agent
Non-specific		
Local, active	Intratumour injection	BCG,[1] viruses
Systemic, active	Immunostimulants	BCG, MER,[1] *C.parvum*,[1] levamisole
Systemic, passive		Mediators or thymic factors, lymphokines, interleukins, interferons
Specific		
Systemic, active	Immunization	Tumour cells, DNA, recombinant antigens, +adjuvant
Systemic, passive	Serotherapy	Specific factors
		Polyclonal or monoclonal antibodies, coupled to drugs, radioisotopes, or toxins
	Cells	*In vitro* grown specific T cells, LAK[1] cells, genetically altered lymphocytes
Ex vivo	Bone marrow purging	Antibodies + complement or antibodies coupled to magnetic beads or toxins

[1] BCG, Bacille Calmette–Guerin, a non-pathogenic strain of tubercle bacillus; MER, the methanol extraction residue of BCG; *C.parvum*, *Corynebacterium parvum*. BCG, MER, and *C.parvum* all have adjuvant activity. LAK, lymphokine-activated killer.

little was known of the importance of costimuli in initiation of immune responses. Over the last few years it has become clear that, in addition to interaction of the T cell receptor (TCR) with MHC molecules on antigen-presenting cells, many other interactions between the two cells occur (Fig. 16.5). These costimuli are crucial for successful activation of the T cell (Swain and Reth 1994). Among them, the interaction between CD28 on the T cell and its counter receptor B7 on the APC appears to be essential. Indeed ligation of the TCR in the absence of CD28–B7 interaction may deliver a negative signal leading to T cell anergy (Fig. 16.5(a)). Optimal costimuli are provided by specialized dendritic cells (Fig. 16.5(c)), but most tumour cells lack some or all of the costimulatory molecules and may therefore present tumour antigens inefficiently or to one T cell subset only (Fig. 16.5(b)). This has led to experiments designed to make tumour cells more immunogenic by introduction of genes coding for costimulatory surface molecules or cytokines. In animal experiments tumour cells transfected with the genes for B7 or cytokines such IL-2, IL-4, IFN-γ, or GM-CSF, grow poorly *in vivo*. When normal and transfected cells are injected together the growth of normal cells may be inhibited (bystander effect) and when animals immunized with transfectants are challenged with normal cells they may be protected. However, when tumour-bearing animals are immunized with transfected tumour cells there is seldom regression of the untransfected tumour. Clearly, the latter experimental protocol is more akin to that of

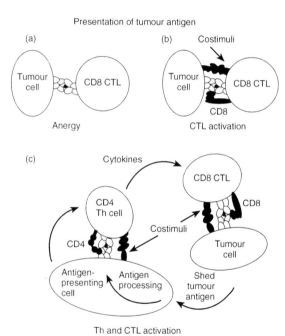

Fig. 16.5 Presentation of tumour antigen. Effective presentation of antigen is highly dependent on costimuli. In (a) a CD8 lymphocyte recognizes antigen on a tumour cell that does not express costimulatory molecules and a negative signal is delivered to the T cell. In (b) the tumour cell both presents antigen and some costimuli leading to T cell activation, while in (c) both CD4 and CD8 T cells are activated, a situation that should lead to optimal expansion of T cell clones and development of effector cells.

human cancer patients who might be treated by immunotherapy. Although the lack of effect of immunotherapy on established tumours is disappointing, the experiments are at an early stage and many variables remain to be worked out so that it is reasonable to expect that this sort of therapy may have some effect in some patients in the future.

One drawback of this form of immunotherapy is that it requires autologous tumour cells to be transfected with a costimulatory gene and reinjected. In many cases it may be difficult to obtain tumour cells so that alternative strategies are being developed. One is the use of recombinant protein antigen or peptides when tumour antigens such as MAGE have been identified. Alternatively, DNA coding for tumour antigens and costimuli can be injected. Surprisingly, naked DNA does induce immune responses to the antigens for which it codes but experiments with tumour antigen genes are at an early stage.

16.7.3 Passive immunization with cells or cytokines

When lymphocytes from tumour patients (or normal individuals) are cultured with high doses of the lymphokine IL-2, effector cells are produced that are able to kill many different tumour targets *in vitro*. These lymphokine-activated killer (LAK) cells have been reinfused into tumour patients who are also given high doses of IL-2 (Rosenberg *et al.* 1994). Regressions have most frequently been observed in melanoma and renal carcinoma, but in most cases the improvement is temporary and the tumours eventually recur. LAK therapy with high dose IL-2 is toxic and it is not clear whether both components are required for therapeutic effect. Current trials are exploring the use of IL-2 alone and at lower doses.

An alternative to LAK cells is the use of tumour-specific cytotoxic T cells. Since tumour-specific cells can sometimes be obtained from TILs and grown *in vitro* with IL-2, they could, in principle, be reinfused as immunotherapy. In animal models such cytotoxic T cell clones can cure tumour-bearing animals. In humans the difficulty of obtaining tumour for *in vitro* boosting and the necessity of obtaining large numbers of specific T cells means that this is a technically demanding (and expensive) procedure. Nevertheless, very large numbers of virus-specific T cells have been grown *in vitro* and given to patients following bone marrow transplantation, and experiments with TILs are under way. TILs may be made more effective by introducing into them genes coding for toxic molecules, for example, the cytokine TNF-α. Early experiments with marker genes have demonstrated that some of the transfected TILs do home to tumour sites.

Although the use of immune cells for immunotherapy has not progressed very far, many of their secreted products (lymphokines) have now become available. The techniques of molecular biology have made it possible to produce a sufficient quantity for *in vivo* studies of these substances, which are normally secreted in minute quantities during immune responses. So far the most extensively studied lymphokines are the interferons, a family of glycoproteins which were first identified because they inhibit the replication of viruses. Interferons also inhibit cell division and stimulate NK activity. Interferon-γ also induces expression of MHC class I and II molecules, thereby improving antigen presentation. All of these properties suggested that interferons might have therapeutic effects on tumours. A number of clinical trials on different types of tumour have been carried out and it is clear that interferons are not strikingly effective antitumour agents for treatment of most tumours. Some effects have been documented for certain rare tumours (for example, hairy cell leukaemia) and in experimental models; however, it may be that further research will better define when interferons can be useful and how they should be combined with other treatments. So far the antitumour effects of other lymphokines have not generally been particularly impressive, but IL-2, tumour necrosis factor, and lymphotoxin have been tested in clinical trials. As mentioned earlier, IL-2 may be effective against melanoma and renal carcinoma in a proportion of cases. Much further work remains to be done with cytokines however, before discarding them as therapeutic agents. So far, most trials have employed pharmacological doses given systemically. However, physiologically, cytokines act locally in lower doses, so that the optimum way of using them needs to be explored.

16.7.4 Escape mechanisms

Most spontaneous tumours grow and eventually kill their host if left unchecked, so that it is clear that they must escape from immune control. Several mechanisms probably contribute to tumour escape.

The possibility that many tumours present antigen poorly has already been alluded to (Section 16.7.2). In experimental models, delivery of an activation signal by means of the TCR in the absence of appropriate costimuli can lead to a state of T cell anergy. Although the mechanisms are not fully understood, there appears to be interference with the normal regulation of the IL-2 gene so that the T cells are unable to divide or function normally. T cells isolated from tumours sometimes exhibit signs of anergy and components of the TCR signal transduction complex may be down-regulated. In addition to a lack of cell surface costimulatory molecules, tumours may also produce cytokines, capable of interfering in immune responses. Tumour growth factor-β (TGF-β), produced by some epithelial cells and tumours, is such a factor known to have immunosuppressive activity.

In addition to difficulties at the induction stage of immune responses, tumours also exhibit changes that should make them resistant to immune effector mechanisms. The most striking is the loss of expression of MHC class I. Both total loss of class I and loss of single alleles are often seen and one or other of these changes may occur in more than half of all tumours. Clearly, loss of these molecules would make the tumour cells unable to present tumour antigen peptides and the cells would be resistant to CD8 cytotoxic T cells. Changes in the surface expression of other antigens have also been described which may give the cells a selective advantage. In melanoma, for example, increased expression of the adhesion molecule ICAM-1 is correlated with penetration of the tumour through the basement layer of the skin and metastatic spread. It has been suggested that expression of ICAM may partially protect the cells against attack by antibody and complement, and may also allow the tumour cells to migrate away from the skin. Changes in the splicing pattern of another adhesion molecule, CD44, are associated with metastasis in a rat tumour model.

16.8 Conclusions

The advent of the hybridoma technique for production of monoclonal antibodies has provided reagents to identify and purify molecules present in lymphocytes, other normal cells, or tumour cells. The techniques of molecular biology make it possible to isolate the genes coding for these molecules, to

sequence them, and, if required, to produce the molecule *in vitro*. These are powerful techniques for investigating the function of the immune system and for attempting to define how tumour cells differ from normal cells.

In the immediate future the use of monoclonal antibodies in immunodiagnosis and immunotherapy is likely to expand. For therapy, human monoclonal antibodies would be advantageous since rodent antibodies provoke antibody responses to the foreign protein, limiting the duration of treatment. So far it has proved difficult to produce human antibodies of a desired specificity with any regularity and in large quantities. However, genetic engineering methods should now overcome this problem. Murine monoclonal antibodies may be made chimeric, so that all but the variable part of the molecule is derived from a human antibody molecule, or further engineered to humanize them (see Chapter 19). In this case all but the antigen-combining sites are replaced by human sequences. Alternatively, completely human antibodies may be produced in bacteria using phage libraries of heavy and light chains. These methods will undoubtedly reduce the immunogenicity of monoclonal antibodies in humans and allow their wider and more prolonged use. Initial results of trials with monoclonal antibodies, particularly against minimal residual disease, are encouraging (Riethmuller *et al.* 1994).

Harnessing cell-mediated responses is more difficult. While cytokines have powerful effects on host responses, so far they have been largely disappointing. Whether combining cytokines or other costimuli with tumour cells, recombinant antigens, or DNA, for use as vaccines, will lead to effective immunotherapies remains to be seen. The frequent development of escape mechanisms in tumours suggests that immunotherapy will always be a race against time.

I have left until last an area in which immunology may well contribute to cancer treatment, or rather prevention. It is clear that a number of viruses play a role in the induction of tumours. These include hepatitis B virus in liver cancer, EBV in Burkitt's lymphoma and nasopharyngeal cancer, human papillomaviruses (HPV) in genital tumours, and HTLV-1 and -2 in some lymphoid tumours (see Chapter 8). Prophylactic immunization against these and perhaps other as yet undiscovered agents is likely to prevent or reduce the incidence of these tumours. Already hepatitis B vaccine is available and under trial; much effort is also being expended on vaccines for EBV and HPV. As in the case of infectious disease, prophylactic immunization rather than treatment may be the immunologist's most direct contribution to the reduction of cancer mortality.

References and further reading

Austyn J. M. and Wood K. J. (1993). *Principles of cellular and molecular immunology* (1st edn), Oxford University Press, Oxford.

Boon, T., Cerottini, J.-C., van den Eynde, B., van der Bruggen, P. and Van Pel, A. (1994). Tumour antigens recognised by T lymphocytes. *Annual Review of Immunology*, **12**, 337–66.

Bjorkman, P. J., Saper, M. A., Samraoui, B., Bennet, W. S., Strominger, J. L. and Wiley, D. C. (1987). Structure of the human histocompatibility antigen, HLA-A2. *Nature*, **329**, 506–12.

Callard, R. E. and Gearing, A. (1994). *The cytokine factsbook*, Academic Press, London.

Davis, M. M. and Bjorkman, P. J. (1988). T-cell antigen receptor genes and T-cell recognition. *Nature*, **334**, 395–402.

Herlyn, M. and Koprowski, H. (1988). Melanoma antigens: immunological and biological characterization and clinical significance. *Annual Review of Immunology*, **6**, 283–308.

Jerome, K. R., Domenech, N. and Finn, O. J. (1993). Tumor-specific cytotoxic T cell clones from patients with breast and pancreatic adenocarcinoma recognize EBV-immortalized B cells transfected with polymorphic epithelial mucin complementary DNA. *Journal of Immunology*, **151**, 1654–62.

Kocks, C. and Rajewsky, K. (1989). Stable expression and somatic hypermutation of antibody V regions in B cell differentiation. *Annual Review of Immunology*, **7**, 537–60.

Riethmuller, G., Schneider-Gädicke, E., Schlimok, G., Schmiegel, W., Raab, R., Höffken, K. *et al.* (1994). Randomised trial of monoclonal antibody for adjuvant therapy of resected Dukes' C colorectal carcinoma. *Lancet*, **343**, 1177–83.

Robbins, P. F. and Kawakami, Y. (1996). Human tumour antigens recognised by T cells. *Current Opinion in Immunology*, **8**, 628–636.

Rosenberg, S. A., Yang, J. C., Topalian, S. L., Schwartzentruber, D. J., Weber, J. S., Parkinson, D. R. *et al.* (1994). Treatment of 283 consecutive patients with metastatic melanoma or renal cell cancer using high-dose bolus interleukin 2. *Journal of the American Medical Association*, **271**, 907–13.

Sadoff, D. A, Giddens, W. E., jun., DiGiacomo, R. F., and Vogel, A. M. (1988). Neoplasms in NIH type II athymic (nude) mice. *Laboratory Animal Science*, **38**, 407–12.

Schatz, D. G., Oettinger, M. A. and Schlissel, M. S. (1992). V(D)J recombination: molecular biology and regulation. *Annual Review of Immunology*, **10**, 359–98.

Sheil, A. G. R. (1992). Development of malignancy following renal transplantation in Australia and New Zealand. *Transplantation Proceedings*, **24**, 1275–9.

Swain, S. L. and Reth, M. (1994) Lymphocyte activation and effector functions. *Current Opinion in Immunology*, **6**, 355–489.

Takasugi, M., Mickey, M. R. and Terasaki, P. I. (1973). Reactivity of lymphocytes from normal persons on cultured tumor cells. *Cancer Research*, **33**, 2898–902.

17

The local treatment of cancer

IAN FENTIMAN

17.1 How tumours present

Most patients with cancer seek medical help because of symptoms arising directly or indirectly from local invasion or metastasis. Invasion through the basement membrane into the surrounding stroma elicits a fibrous reaction and this scar tissue produces the hard irregular lump that is characteristic of a cancer. As scar tissue contracts this can produce strictures or complete obstruction in tubular organs such as the oesophagus and colon. Direct invasion of surrounding blood vessels gives rise to haemorrhage so that a patient with bladder cancer may pass blood-stained urine, or in the case of lung cancer may spit blood. Local invasion of lymphatic vessels is one route whereby cancer cells metastasize, but may also give rise to local lymphatic obstruction so that if these lymphatics drain the overlying skin there is local skin oedema (peau d'orange) which can be a presenting sign in women with breast cancer. It is important to realize that all these symptoms may result from non-malignant causes but they are signals to the clinician that further investigation is necessary, and sometimes may lead to the earlier diagnosis of malignancy.

By the time that a cancer becomes clinically detectable, which in superficial lesions might be at a volume of 1 ml, there are approximately 1×10^9 cells in that mass with a moderate probability of tumour metastasis. Thus, to increase the chances of cure, cancers need to be diagnosed at earlier stages, or better still, before invasion through the basement membrane (*in situ* carcinoma).

17.2 Screening

Although, theoretically, early detection by screening should be of value in improving the results of treatment for common solid tumours, in reality the cost-benefit ratio is acceptable for only a few types of cancers. Examples of success in screening are cancers of the uterine cervix and the breast. It is now established that screening for cancer of the cervix by examination of cervical smears leads to a reduction in mortality in those countries with extensive programmes.

For cancer of the breast the situation is more complex. Figure 17.1 shows the effect on mortality in four screening trials in which patients were randomized to mammographic screening or to serve as unscreened controls. What these studies show clearly is a substantial (about one-third) reduction in deaths from breast cancer in women aged over 50 who were

RANDOMIZED TRIALS OF MAMMOGRAPHIC SCREENING

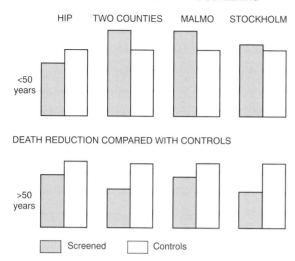

Fig. 17.1 Randomized trials of mammographic screening for breast cancer.

screened. However, for women less than 50 years, although the original Hospital Insurance Plan (HIP) Study, from New York, showed a slight reduction in deaths after some years, all other studies reported an increase in breast cancer deaths among the screened group. The reasons for this increase are not known.

These results may furnish important clues on the biology of breast cancer. The encouraging reduction in mortality in screened women aged over 50 (predominantly post-menopausal) arises for at least two reasons. Firstly, approximately one-fifth of the cancers diagnosed by screening are non-invasive (ductal carcinoma *in situ*). This particular form of malignancy is not in itself a life-threatening condition but is associated with up to a 50 per cent chance of developing invasive breast cancer subsequently in that breast. In the past, treatment was by mastectomy, but studies are now under way to determine whether, after complete excision of screen-detected ductal carcinoma *in situ*, the risk of progression to invasive breast cancer can be reduced by either breast irradiation or use of the hormonal agent tamoxifen. Secondly, lives may be saved by mammography screens, not just by detection of smaller cancers, but because those smaller cancers are less aggressive. Evidence is increasing that screen-detected cancers are of a less aggressive type and that with breast cancers in general, the larger they

are the less differentiated and more aggressive they are likely to be.

As a result of proven reduction in mortality after mammographic screening, this is now offered to women aged 50–64 in the UK. For women aged over 64 there is no call–recall system, which is to be regretted since approximately 50 per cent of all breast cancers will present in those aged 65 years or more.

For other cancers there are less compelling data on efficacy. Attempts to screen populations for colorectal cancers by testing for traces of blood from the tumour in the faeces (faecal occult blood) have been unsuccessful because of the high incidence of false positive results, particularly in older individuals who are more likely to have other bowel diseases, particularly diverticular disease of the colon. A new approach has been proposed in which 120 000 normal individuals between the ages of 55 and 60 would be offered flexible rectosigmoidoscopy (an endoscopic examination). Colonic polyps would be removed (polypectomy) and only 5 per cent with larger polyps would require further surveillance.

Other screening methods depend on the detection of tumour markers in the blood or other body fluids. Unfortunately no tumour-specific substances have yet been isolated (see Chapters 12, 13, 16, and 19), but the presence of abnormal tumour-associated proteins or normal tissue-specific proteins not usually present in the blood may be detected. Abnormal amounts of hormones in the blood may also suggest the presence of tumours of the endocrine system (see Chapters 14 and 15). None of these markers is sensitive enough or sufficiently specific to be used for the detection of cancers in patients without symptoms of disease, but, in some cases, particularly in prostate, ovarian, and testicular cancers, they are useful in predicting prognosis and monitoring the response to treatment.

For some testicular cancers and also the rare disease choriocarcinoma, which can arise after a hydatidiform mole in pregnancy, the detection of some hormones in the blood can be diagnostic. Furthermore, it is possible to detect cancer of the prostate gland using prostate-specific antigen (PSA). However, this is less useful than it would appear. Many elderly men have histological evidence of malignancy at autopsy although they do not develop clinical evidence of disease during their lifetime so that an intervention would represent unnecessary treatment. Furthermore, no proven surgical or endocrine procedure is available to treat screen-detected prostate cancer. Thus, at present screening, for common cancers is limited in efficacy.

17.3 Diagnosis

Clinical examination alone may enable a diagnosis of cancer to be made and confirmed after histological or cytological examination. Thus cancers of the tongue, skin, breast, and thyroid may be detected by either inspection or palpation. Certain other cancers, particularly those arising in the pelvis (such as prostate, rectum, uterus, and ovary), may be detected by internal digital examination. For other internal organs, cancers may be detected endoscopically using a variety of instruments. Thus, bladder, lung, and gastric cancers may be detected using a cystoscope, bronchoscope, or gastroscope, respectively. More deeply located organs such as the pancreas may require a variety of imaging techniques before they can be demonstrated. This is a burgeoning field, for detection of both primary and recurrent malignancy.

17.3.1 Radiography

A diagnosis of primary or secondary cancers of bone and lung may be suggested because of differences in density seen on plain X-rays of these sites. Additionally, plain X-rays of the breasts can be useful in making an early diagnosis of breast cancer, but their value is largely restricted to women over the age of 50. The reason for this is because breast tissue in younger women can be too dense for signs of malignancy, e.g. owing to microcalcification, or an irregular mass may be undetectable.

To assist in the diagnosis of cancers of the upper and lower gastrointestinal tract, radio-opaque mixtures are used, in the form of barium meals or enemas. Tumours may be recognized by the presence of strictures (narrowings), ulcers (craters), or filling defects (regions of the gut lumen from which radio-opaque material is excluded).

For certain cancers it is necessary to administer contrast medium (often containing iodine) through a needle (either intravenously or intra-arterially). Cancers of the urinary tract (kidney and bladder) may be seen after an intravenous urogram in which a radio-opaque dye is injected. The dye is concentrated by the kidneys and excreted in the urine and sequential radiographs of the kidneys, ureters, and bladder are taken. In order to visualize directly a renal cancer (hypernephroma), dye may be injected intra-arterially to show the vascularization of the tumour.

These techniques can be very useful but involve radiation exposure together with a small but definite risk of an allergic reaction to the injected dye. Furthermore, contrast media can produce tissue damage at the injection site if not given properly (extravasation) and arterial puncture may lead to haemorrhage on rare occasions. For these reasons a lot of work has been carried out to develop new methods of imaging in oncology.

17.3.2 Computerized tomography (CT) scanning

The accuracy of both diagnosis and monitoring of patients with known or suspected cancers has been improved considerably since the advent of CT scanning. Although it is relatively expensive and exposes the patient to relatively high radiation levels, it is of great value in imaging the brain when intracranial primary tumours or metastases are suspected, to image the lungs and intrathoracic organs in the pre-operative work-up of patients with lung cancer, and to assess the significance of bone abnormalities when metastatic tumour is suspected. Brain metastases may be imaged to determine the number and extent, since sometimes surgical resection may be possible. Similarly, when surgery is contemplated in a patient with a clinically operable lung cancer, subtle lymph node changes rendering the patient inoperable may be found thereby saving the patient an unnecessary and painful thoracotomy.

When patients have been treated by a combination of surgery and radiotherapy, it may be impossible to determine clinically or with plain X-rays whether changes are a result of treatment or recurrence of disease, and CT scanning may sometimes be helpful.

17.3.3 Ultrasound scanning

Because ultrasound depends upon reflection of sound waves, it does not involve any radiation exposure and thus can be repeated as often as necessary to monitor lesions and measure response to treatment. Ultrasound can detect abnormalities as small as 5 mm in diameter and is particularly useful for imaging the liver and distinguishing between benign gallstones and malignant secondaries in patients with liver function abnormalities or clinical evidence of jaundice. Another useful application is in screening and assessing gynaecological malignancies. Ovarian cysts can be detected and if necessary drained under ultrasonic control so that the fluid can be examined cytologically for the presence of malignant cells. Also, using a transvaginal ultrasound probe, the endometrium can be imaged and, if there is evidence of thickening, a biopsy can be taken to find out whether this is caused by hypertrophy or carcinoma. A particular use of ultrasound is to distinguish between cystic and solid lesions and this is of value in determining the nature of mammographic opacities picked up on routine screening. Demonstration that the lesion is cystic means that the patient is saved further investigation and can be safely reassured.

17.3.4 Magnetic resonance imaging (MRI)

This relatively new technique does not expose the patient to ionizing radiation. The patient is placed in a high magnetic field after which a short radiofrequency pulse is applied. This results in the emission of signals that can be transformed into images. Signals from tumours may differ from those emitted by normal tissues and can be characterized by two constants, the longitudinal and transverse relaxation times. Thus far, MRI has proved particularly useful in imaging midline structures such as the brain, spine, pelvis, and neck. Development of new coils and use of contrast media such as gadolinium diethylenetriamine pentacetic acid dimeglumine (GdDTPA) has meant a new approach to breast imaging has evolved which can be useful for distinguishing between fibrosis and recurrence after breast conservation therapy (Fig. 17.2). As more experience is gained, it may be possible to use contrast-enhanced MRI to follow young women at increased risk of breast cancer because they have inherited a mutated *BRCA1* or *BRCA2* gene (see Chapters 3 and 4).

17.3.5 Positron emission tomography (PET) scanning

This new technique may have important applications in tumour imaging. A radioisotope that emits positrons is injected into the patient; emitted positrons leave the nucleus and after a few millimetres collide with an oppositely charged electron, resulting in mutual annihilation and release of 511 keV

gamma rays, which can be detected by a positron camera and transformed into images of the region of isotope accumulation. By incorporating fluorine-18 into the glucose analogue ^{18}F-fluoro-2 deoxy glucose, the accumulation of the isotope in regions of increased metabolism can be detected.

The technique is sensitive but not specific and can provide an opportunity to study the biochemistry of tumours *in vivo*. PET does not provide structural images, but in combination with MRI may enable more accurate staging of disease and also elucidation of the nature of equivocal radiological changes. Recurrences as small as 4 mm in diameter can be found by PET, and again this may be useful when prior treatment may have obscured possible relapse. Additionally, since PET can examine tumour growth rates, it may be used to monitor response of malignancy to chemotherapy enabling effective or ineffective drugs to be identified so that they can be discontinued and the patient spared unnecessary treatment and toxicity.

17.3.6 Cellular diagnosis

Before any treatment for cancer can be instigated, it is essential that a cellular diagnosis is made. Without this, rational treatment cannot be planned, nor can therapies be compared, and a meaningful prognosis cannot be given. All the clinical signs of cancer can be mimicked by benign inflammatory conditions and even the most experienced clinicians may sometimes be misled. Only under the most exceptional circumstances should a patient be treated for suspected cancer without pathological proof of malignancy. This information is obtained from either cytological or tissue specimens.

17.3.7 Cytology

For the interpretation of cytological specimens, great experience is required and at present there is a national shortage of trained cytopathologists in the UK. Cells are removed from the suspected or potentially malignant site, smeared on a slide, and/or collected in normal saline, spun, fixed, and examined by the pathologist. Malignant cells are recognized by alterations in their size and shape, together with changes in nuclear morphology (see Chapter 1).

Exfoliative cytology This is the examination of shed cells and has been used most widely in screening for cancer of the uterine cervix. A cervical smear is taken painlessly with a special spatula

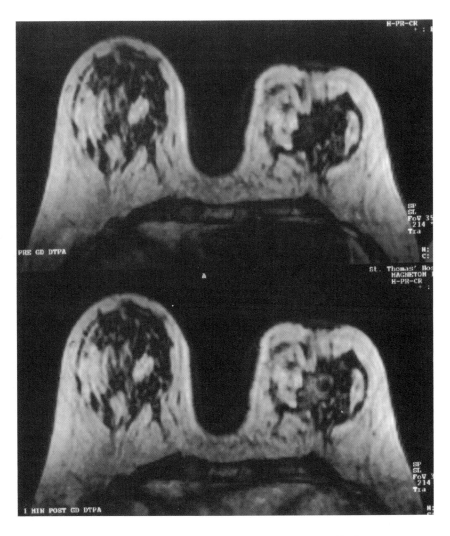

Fig. 17.2 MRI scan showing enhancement of a breast cancer using GdDTPA

twisted around the cervix and the shed cells are smeared on to a microscope slide, fixed, stained, and examined. Other uses are monitoring the urine of aniline dye workers who are at increased risk of urinary tract malignancy, and sometimes in testing sputum from smokers to diagnose lung cancer. Any body fluids can be examined cytologically; cerebrospinal fluid (CSF) for meningeal metastases, pleural effusion for primary or secondary lung cancers, and ascitic fluid when intraperitoneal malignancy such as ovarian cancer is suspected. The fluid is centrifuged and the pellet smeared, fixed, and stained. Identification of malignant cells is an indication for further investigation.

Fine needle aspiration cytology (FNAC) This is a more invasive procedure which may be uncomfor-

table and involves aspirating cells from a suspect lesion through a fine needle attached to an ordinary syringe. The technique is most suitable for relatively superficial lumps such as in the thyroid gland and the breasts. For suspect breast lesions, which have been detected mammographically and are impalpable, FNAC may be carried out after stereotactic localization of the abnormality.

Although a seemingly simple technique, experience is required by both the operator and the cytologist in order to maximize the accuracy of the procedure. Occasionally false positive FNAC reports are encountered, particularly after irradiation of an organ. Additionally, FNAC cannot distinguish between non-invasive (*in situ*) and invasive (infiltrating) cancers since single cells and clumps, rather than tissue architecture including basement membrane, are examined. The treatment of these two types of cancer is different and sometimes it is necessary to obtain a histological diagnosis before definitive treatment can be discussed with the patient.

17.3.8 Histopathology

This remains the cornerstone of diagnosis of malignancy, and apart from providing confirmation that cancer is present, the pathologist can distinguish between *in situ* and invasive disease, comment on the presence or absence of vascular invasion, and give an indication on the differentiation of the tumour (grade) (see Chapter 1). By marking the edges of the excised specimen with indian ink, the completeness of tumour excision may be determined.

Various types of specimen are examined by the histopathologist and these include needle biopsy, incision biopsy, and excision biopsy. Needle biopsy is particularly useful for making an outpatient diagnosis of malignancy suspected in the breast, prostate, and liver. After injection of local anaesthetic into the skin, a core of tissue is removed from the suspect organ using either a Trucut or Bioptycut needle. A definitive diagnosis of malignancy can be made in 80–90 per cent of cases. If the needle biopsy does not show the presence of cancer it is then necessary to proceed to an open biopsy to confirm or refute the clinical diagnosis.

The aim of an incision biopsy is to take a representative sample of the tissue, particularly when a large lesion is present, so that excessively radical surgery is not performed for what subsequently proves to be a benign condition. In contrast, an excision biopsy is intended to remove completely the suspect lesion. The specimen can be processed by the pathology laboratory in two ways, paraffin section and frozen section. Commonly, the former method is used and the specimen is first fixed in formalin, which can take up to 24 hours, after which it is dehydrated, embedded in paraffin wax, sliced with a microtome, dewaxed, and stained. The entire procedure takes about 48 hours and is the optimal preparation of material for examination by the pathologist. The delay involved in waiting for the results of the paraffin section has no impact on the patient's prognosis. In the past, great reliance was placed on frozen section for diagnosis of malignancy, particularly in women with suspected breast cancer. With the patient under a general anaesthetic, a biopsy was taken of the breast lump which was sent to the laboratory immediately and quickly frozen in solid carbon dioxide. The tissue was then rapidly sectioned, examined by the pathologist, and if cancer was confirmed the surgeon was notified (within 15–20 minutes) and then definitive surgery, usually mastectomy, was carried out immediately. However, there are disadvantages associated with frozen section diagnosis. The pathologist is being asked to make a hurried diagnosis on a suboptimally prepared specimen, and may both under- or over-diagnose cancer. Distinction between *in situ* and invasive disease may not be possible. Furthermore, a women with suspected breast cancer, would not know whether she would wake up from the anaesthetic with two breasts or one, and this might exacerbate postoperative psychological morbidity. Thus, whenever possible it is best to allow the patient time to come to terms with the diagnosis of cancer and the possible treatment options. Frozen section should be confined to cases with suspected recurrence of cancer in which preoperative tests have failed to make a definitive diagnosis and when the patient has been fully informed about the consequences of the frozen section confirming relapse of disease.

New approaches The basic histopathological evaluation of specimens depends upon the morphology and topography of the tissue, but important changes in protein translation and gene expression may be present without any morphological alteration. These can now be studied using techniques such as *in situ* hybridization, and immunohistochemistry is yielding important information about the behaviour of cancers, some of which may have prognostic implications. Another area where molecular biology has been of use to the clinician is the use of monoclonal markers to distinguish between morphologically similar, poorly differentiated cells of unknown origin, and to determine whether the tumour is a carcinoma, melanoma, or lymphoma. This may be particularly important when a malignant lymph node has been excised from the axilla or groin and when the primary site is unknown. The pathology laboratory can also serve as the link between the clinical and experimental domains of cancer research, providing tissue for study of tumours at a cellular and molecular level. Basic studies of steroid and growth factor receptors have yielded information that can now be used in selection of appropriate therapy. As an example, elderly patients with breast cancer who have tumours expressing epidermal growth factor receptor (EGFR) will not respond to the agent tamoxifen, and require surgical treatment for long-term control of the disease. Another area of collaborative research is in flow cytometry. This enables the determination of both ploidy and S phase fraction in both fresh and archival specimens. Patients with diploid tumours carry a better prognosis than those with aneuploid lesions. These new techniques are considered in Chapter 13.

17.4 Staging

17.4.1 Clinical staging

The idea of staging tumours is to select the most appropriate method of treatment, separate patients into prognostic categories, and make possible the comparison of results from different hospitals. Staging can be carried out rather crudely on a clinical basis but becomes more accurate when combined with information from both pathological and imaging investigations. The accuracy of clinical staging will depend upon a variety of factors including the location of the primary tumour, the physical characteristics of the patient, and the experience of the examining clinician. Even under the most favourable conditions the disease is often under or over staged. A good example of this is clinical evaluation of the axillary lymph nodes in women with breast cancer. These are the main site of first metastasis, but it has been found consistently that there is a 30 per cent false negative and a 30 per cent false positive rate among the most experienced clinicians. Unfortunately, lymphangiograms (see Glossary) are not a good way of examining the axillary lymph nodes and so surgical removal is necessary for staging to be accurate. In patients with testicular tumours the locoregional lymph nodes are in the para-aortic chain and these will be impalpable unless gross enlargement has occurred, and thus CT scanning is required to stage the disease accurately.

Despite these drawbacks, clinical staging remains the most widely used system since it does allow international comparison of cases and treatments under circumstances where sophisticated staging techniques may be unavailable. Several staging systems have been devised for different tumour types but the main international classification is the TNM system (Table 17.1). Broadly, this comprises an assessment of the tumour size (T), nodal status (N), and presence or absence of distant metastases (M). Extensions of the system can become very complex and may not be fully understood by many cancer clinicians.

Viewed simplistically, patients with stage 1 and 2 tumours are deemed operable and are treated by surgery and/or radiotherapy, sometimes with adjuvant systemic therapy. Stage 3 cancers are inoperable but can be encompassed by a radiotherapy field. Patients with stage 4 carcinomas are almost invariably incurable and receive appropriate palliative treatment with systemic therapy, radiotherapy, and sometimes surgery.

17.4.2 Other staging investigations

Selection of the most appropriate staging investigations will depend upon the primary site and nature of the tumour, together with a knowledge of the likely pattern of metastatic spread from the cancer. The way in which cancers metastasize is a reflection of both the biology of the individual tumour and the topographical anatomy of the organ involved. Gastrointestinal cancers spread to local lymph nodes and, because venous drainage from the bowel is through the portal vein to the liver, tumour deposits in the liver are common. Breast cancers less commonly metastasize to the liver but, because of relatively early vascular invasion, may produce metastases in bone and lung. Primary lung cancers often invade the pulmonary vein and spread to many organs throughout the body including the brain. Indeed, the commonest cause of a brain tumour is a metastasis from a pulmonary primary.

An essential form of investigation is a blood test to measure haemoglobin concentration together with the white cell count. This is required as part of the evaluation of fitness for anaesthesia, but also to exclude the presence of bone marrow metas-

Table 17.1 TNM staging

Stage	Clinical manifestations
I	Small localized tumour
II	Spread to local lymph nodes
III	Large local tumour and/or spread to further lymph nodes
IV	Presence of distant metastases

tases which can manifest as leucoerythroblastic anaemia (see Glossary). A test of greater sensitivity is a bone marrow aspirate from the sternum or iliac crest, which can detect bone marrow metastases and is particularly used when staging patients with lymphomas.

Another simple and inexpensive test is measurement of blood electrolytes and bone- and liver-derived enzymes that can be elevated in response to metastatic disease. For almost all patients, a chest X-ray is carried out to exclude gross disease of the lungs, pleura, and ribs. In patients with cancers of the lung, prostate, thyroid, kidney, and breast, it was common practice to carry out extensive X-rays of the skeleton, but this has been superseded by radioisotopic bone scans. However, even these are no longer used routinely in asymptomatic patients with early breast cancer.

17.4.3 Radioisotopic scans (scintiscans)

These scans produce images derived from gamma ray emission of isotopes tagged to compounds that are taken up selectively by particular organs. The presence of either filling defects or areas of increased uptake may suggest the presence of metastatic tumour. Bone scans of patients with metastases usually show areas of increased uptake (hot spots), although this is a non-specific finding whenever there is bone damage or turnover, so that confirmatory plain X-rays or CT scans may be needed when the pattern of hot spots is atypical for the suspected tumour.

Isotopic scans of the thyroid gland are particularly useful when investigating patients with thyroid tumours in order to determine the extent and function of the malignant nodule. PET scans have brought another dimension to radioisotopic imaging but radionuclide scans are still used to investigate the lung, liver, and brain. However, lung and brain lesions are usually demonstrated better by CT scanning. When hepatic metastases are suspected, the most effective and least invasive investigation is a liver ultrasound.

17.4.4 Lymphangiography

To visualize the lymph nodes draining tumours, it is possible to cannulate a fine bore lymphatic vessel and inject an iodine-containing contrast medium. This is a technically difficult procedure but does enable the visualization of intralymphatic metas-

tases from certain tumours. It is used particularly for patients with tumours of the prostate gland, testes, or bladder, and, in such cases, a lymphatic vessel in the foot is cannulated. Unfortunately, lymphangiography of the breast is insufficiently specific although it has been used to demonstrate the internal mammary lymph nodes so that they can be incorporated in the radiotherapy field. For most common tumours, the present techniques are of little practical use and research continues to examine monoclonal antibodies that might be used for lymphoscintigraphy, and to evaluate Doppler ultrasound for detecting increased blood flow through lymph node metastases.

New techniques of lymph node visualization would be of particular value in patients with breast carcinoma because, if it could be confirmed preoperatively that there were no axillary metastases, these patients could be spared an unnecessary clearance operation.

17.4.5 Operative staging

Although some tumours can be staged preoperatively, in the majority of cases this information is available only after a full pathological examination of the surgical specimen. For a tubular organ (oesophagus, stomach, colon, or rectum), it can be determined whether the cancer has penetrated through the wall. Furthermore, since the operation will usually have cleared the surrounding tissue, the presence or absence of local and regional lymph node metastases can be ascertained. This then enables a more accurate prognosis to be given, and in some cases identifies those patients who might benefit from additional (adjuvant) treatment with either systemic therapy or radiotherapy. An example is carcinoma of the rectum where the Dukes staging system is used (Table 17.2). Patients with Dukes

Table 17.2 Dukes staging system for cancer of the rectum

Stage	Description	Proportion of patients (%)	Crude five-year survival (%)
A	Cancer not infiltrating through rectal wall	15	80
B	Tumour spread through rectal wall	35	60
C	Spread to local lymph	50	25

stage A have disease that has not infiltrated through the rectal wall and 80 per cent of these will be alive five years later. Of those patients with Dukes stage B, who have tumour spread through the rectal wall, only 60 per cent will be alive at five years. For those with Dukes stage C, who have tumour spread to lymph nodes, there is a poor survival with only 25 per cent alive at five years.

For patients with operable breast cancer, it has been found that there is a direct arithmetical relationship between the number of axillary lymph nodes containing metastases and the risk of recurrence of disease, as shown in Table 17.3. Thus, knowledge of the axillary lymph node status forms an essential part in the staging and treatment of early breast cancer.

17.5 Treatment

It is important to stress that many patients with cancer are curable by local therapy, and many do not require toxic systemic therapy. However, as the tendency increases towards less invasive and extensive treatments, it has to be understood that the potential for cure must not be compromised by inappropriate attempts to carry out less than adequate surgery or radiotherapy in the hope that the situation can be salvaged by systemic therapy. Nevertheless, since undetectable micrometastases may be present at the time of surgery, or even caused by this event, there is an increase in the use of systemic therapy to augment the efficacy of surgery and radiotherapy.

17.5.1 Which cancers are curable?

At present there are two major groups of cancers that are almost invariably cured by local treatment. The first group comprises *in situ* cancers such as those of the breast and cervix. The former can be detected at an asymptomatic state as microcalcifications on mammograms and the latter by cervical screening followed by colposcopy or cervical conization.

Other potentially curable cancers are those that are locally invasive but have not metastasized. The commonest example is the basal cell carcinoma (rodent ulcer) of the skin, which typically arises on the facial area and is curable by either surgery or radiotherapy. Another example of tumours with locally aggressive behaviour but minimal metastatic potential are fibromatoses (desmoid tumours). This deceptively benign-looking tumour can affect any organ and provided that it is adequately excised, cure is possible. However, failure to achieve local clearance or destruction of the lesion results in an inexorable ulcerative process as invasion produces surrounding tissue destruction.

Sacral chordoma, a rare tumour of the spine, is another example of a locally invasive cancer that does not usually metastasize. Unfortunately, because of its pelvic location and propensity to invade surrounding nerves and viscera the tumour may only be curable by very extensive surgery, the procrustean measure of hemicorporectomy. Although this may result in a clinical cure the end result will daunt most patients. This extreme case illustrates one of the most difficult aspects of cancer surgery. What is the patient prepared to accept in order to have a high probability of cure? Thus Dukes stage A rectal cancers may be cured by excision of the rectum and anus leaving the patient with a permanent colostomy, but for some this may be unacceptable so a non-curative but anal sphincter-conserving procedure may be performed.

Although there are patients who can be cured in most solid tumours, our present methods are insufficiently precise to determine those that will be cured by local treatment. For most solid tumours, those that are histologically better differentiated are most likely to be cured by local therapy.

Table 17.3 Recurrence of breast cancer in relation to the number of axillary lymph nodes containing metastases

Number of positive nodes	Recurrence at 5 years (%)
0	19
1	33
2	40
3	43
4	44
5	54
6–10	63
11–15	72
16–20	75
21+	82

From Nemoto *et al.* (1980).

17.5.2 *En bloc* resection

This remains the fundamental principle of cancer surgery. The aim of *en bloc* resection is to excise the entire tumour together with the surrounding lymphatics and lymph nodes. In this way it is hoped that the entire tumour-bearing field can be removed with the underlying assumption that there is progression from local invasion into lymphatics with subsequent retention of tumour cells within lymph nodes and eventual blood-borne spread. While this situation does occur, vascular invasion may be an early event so that sometimes the presence of metastases in lymph nodes may be a marker of metastatic disease rather than just the local extent of tumour spread.

To achieve an *en bloc* resection for some gastrointestinal cancers requires technically difficult reconstructive surgery, with formation of anastomoses, which is associated with risk of leakage, haemorrhage, and death. In experienced hands, the mortality rate after colonic surgery can be reduced to very low levels. In contrast, cancers of the head of the pancreas, presenting as obstructive jaundice, are rarely cured by extensive surgery. The very high complication rate and associated mortality are such that for the majority of patients a curative procedure is not possible and better palliation is achieved by a simpler bypass procedure to relieve the obstructive jaundice without striving to excise the cancer.

17.5.3 Radiotherapy

There has been a great change in both medical and patient attitudes towards radiotherapy in recent years. Originally regarded as a palliative treatment for inoperable or incurable cancers, it is now perceived as a partner and partial replacement for surgery in the curative treatment of cancers of the skin, larynx, breast, and cervix. Advances in both technology and technique have meant that radiotherapy can be delivered accurately to the cancer with minimal damage to surrounding normal tissue. The mechanism of action of radiotherapy is incompletely understood but all dividing cells are particularly sensitive to radiation damage and, consequently, rapidly proliferating tumour cells are especially vulnerable. One of the drawbacks of radiation treatment is that therapeutic doses may also kill dividing cells in normal tissues.

There are two main techniques for delivering radiotherapy, external or interstitial. External beam radiation is either megavoltage treatment from a linear accelerator using photons or electrons, or low energy X-rays or gamma rays from a cobalt source. The latter are used to treat relatively superficial lesions such as basal cell carcinomas or recurrences within the skin. High energy radiation is used to treat deeply located cancers such as prostatic tumours without delivering an excessive dose to adjacent normal tissue. Radiation treatment is painless and is usually given for a few minutes a day in several fractions to maximize tumour killing and minimize extraneous damage to normal tissues.

Interstitial (implant) irradiation gives a high local dose to the tumour from sources such as radium, iridium, and caesium in the form of needles or wires implanted in or around the cancer. This technique is widely used in the treatment of head and neck cancers to give a high local dose without irradiation to sensitive organs such as the lens of the eye or the spinal cord. Sometimes interstitial irradiation is used to treat both the tumour and the surrounding, potentially malignant, field in patients with breast cancer. Insertion of the radioactive sources may be carried out under general anaesthesia, or tubes to take the isotopes may be inserted under anaesthesia and the sources introduced subsequently (after-loading). This technique has been used for implants in the breast or uterus.

17.5.4 Laser treatment

The interaction of lasers and tissue can have useful applications in many aspects of surgical treatment of cancer. Firstly, the effect can be ablative, with vaporization of tissue water producing a cut around the cancer. This can be used to destroy tumours in the oesophagus or colon so that obstruction is relieved. This can be achieved through an endoscope, avoiding a large skin incision. Secondly, there is a thermal effect which can be applied to metastases in the liver, avoiding the major morbidity that can occur after hepatic surgery. Introduction of laser filaments through stereotactically placed needles might have future application for treatment of some screen-detected breast cancers without leaving a surgical scar. Additionally, lasers can have a photodynamic effect whereby a photosensitizing agent can be bound to a tumour-specific marker and the laser used to destroy selectively the malignant tissue. This might have an application in individuals with genetic predispositions to malignancy, such as the *BRCA1* gene, where affected females have an 80 per cent chance of developing breast cancer. Photosensitization might be used to ablate the mammary epithelium at risk without destroying the surrounding stromal tissue. This might avoid the need for bilateral mastectomy, which is, at present, the only sure way of avoiding the disease for those at high risk.

17.5.5 Microinvasive surgery

To diminish the morbidity of surgery, great advances have been made in 'keyhole' surgery (laparoscopy) and this has some use in the treatment of certain cancers. Access to the thorax can be gained using a thoracoscope and some oesophageal cancers can be resected, particularly those of the middle and lower third of the oesophagus. This has the advantage of a reduced blood loss and less postoperative pain. The technique is still experimental and no controlled clinical trials have yet been conducted. Cancers of the stomach can be resected through a laparoscopic approach, and a gastrectomy performed. Limited experience suggests that there is less pain for the patient, faster postoperative mobilization, fewer complications, and a shorter period of hospitalization. Laparoscopic colorectal surgery has also been used with initially promising results, although the long-term aspects of recurrence-free and overall survival have not yet been evaluated. Another potential use for microinvasive surgery is in palliation in patients with inoperable obstruction of the common bile duct or duodenum from cancer of the pancreas, so that a very ill individual is spared the major morbidity of a laparotomy.

17.5.6 Combined approaches

To give effective treatment for cancer and spare the patient excessive disfigurement, combined approaches have been developed using surgery and radiotherapy, often with chemotherapy. Because of this multidisciplinary approach, many more patients with cancer are now being treated in specialized cancer centres. One example is the management of Hodgkin's disease, a lymphoma that was previously incurable but can now be cured in many cases. The diagnosis is made after biopsy of a pathologically enlarged lymph node, often from the neck.

Determination of the exact nature of the disease may require an experienced pathologist. Part of the staging investigations may include a laparotomy, with removal of the spleen, and biopsy of the liver and intra-abdominal lymph nodes. In females the ovaries are fixed with clips behind the uterus to diminish their risk of being included in the subsequent radiotherapy field. Following this a treatment plan can be formulated, with local radiation when the disease is localized or chemotherapy when the lymphoma is widespread, sometimes with local radiation to areas of bulky disease.

Another example of a combined approach is in the treatment of follicular carcinoma of the thyroid gland. After histological confirmation of the diagnosis, a total thyroidectomy is performed but with attempted preservation of the calcium-controlling parathyroid glands. This is followed by a thyroid scan using iodine-131, which is taken up selectively by thyroid tissue. If residual functional thyroid tissue is identified, this is subsequently ablated with a therapeutic dose of iodine-131. Next, thyroxine is given, both to prevent symptoms of hypothyroidism and to inhibit any further thyroid activity.

One of the most important combined approaches has been in the management of early breast cancer. Twenty years ago the standard treatment was a mastectomy, often followed by radiotherapy. This was believed to be the most effective way of achieving local control of disease and also offered the best chance of cure. However, this was effected at the cost of mutilation which was unacceptable to many patients and may have been one of the reasons why some delayed consulting their doctor with a breast lump. Now, however, the majority of women with early breast cancer can be treated by a breast-conserving technique. This has occurred because clinical trials conducted in Europe and the US demonstrated conclusively that combined techniques are as effective as mastectomy for patients with single breast cancers measuring up to 4 cm in diameter. The tested techniques involved a combination of tumour removal, axillary clearance, and subsequent breast irradiation. A good or excellent cosmetic result can be achieved in up to 80 per cent of patients treated by breast conservation. Research continues to examine ways of diminishing or even abolishing the need for irradiation in some patients but, at present, radiotherapy forms an intrinsic part of breast-conserving therapies.

17.5.7 Palliation

Although the main aim of treatment is to achieve cure of disease whenever possible, there are circumstances in which patients present with advanced disease or develop recurrences and cannot be cured by local treatment. However, surgery or radiotherapy can play an important part in palliation of those with distressing symptoms. Surgery can relieve obstruction of the bowel, jaundice, haemorrhage, and ulceration. Chronic haemorrhage and bone pain can be treated with external radiotherapy. Patients with bone metastases can be relieved of pain and have a reduced risk of pathological fractures. Sometimes, when a pathological fracture occurs in a weight-bearing bone or to prevent this occurrence, it is necessary to perform an orthopaedic procedure, with internal fixation so that the patient can become mobile once more.

Another common site of metastatic disease is the pleural cavity, particularly in patients with primary tumours of the lung, breast, and ovary. Pleural deposits give rise to a collection of serous fluid (pleural effusion), which, by compressing the underlying lung, causes shortness of breath. Immediate relief can be obtained by simple drainage of the fluid but in the majority of cases there is subsequent reaccumulation. Good long-term relief can be obtained by introducing sclerosing compounds into the pleural space. One of the most effective techniques is the use of sterile talc, which stimulates a fibrous reaction and obliterates the pleural space preventing any reaccumulation of fluid and thereby giving long-term palliation.

Intra-abdominal accumulation of serous fluid (ascites) after recurrence of cancers of the large bowel or ovary can lead to abdominal distension, discomfort, and vomiting. These symptoms can be relieved by inserting a peritoneovenous shunt. This device collects the ascitic fluid from the peritoneal cavity and delivers it through a non-return valve into the superior vena cava.

Tumours of the breast and prostate gland are often dependent upon steroid hormones for their continued growth. Significant remissions may be obtained in patients with advanced disease by removing the source of these hormones. In the case of breast cancer, metastases may regress after ovarian ablation (oophorectomy), and for men with prostatic cancer, testicular excision (orchidectomy) may relieve symptoms. Further remissions can occur after removal of the adrenal and/or pituitary gland but such procedures are now rare because similar effects can be achieved using a variety of hormone or antihormone drugs (see Chapter 14).

17.6 The problem areas

The standard of surgical training in the UK is exceedingly high so that throughout the country patients have access to good surgical advice and treatment. Unfortunately, not all surgeons have close working relationships with radiotherapists, and not all conduct joint clinics. This is one reason why cancer centres have been set up in most major cities to develop combined approaches to treatment. Now that breast cancer screening has been set up, there is quality assurance of surgery and this is going to improve greatly the standard of treatment for both screen-detected and symptomatic cases.

As part of the process of change, healthy individuals need to be educated in recognition of warning signs of cancer, together with modification of their diet and life style to reduce their risk. Useful screening such as mammography for women over 50 needs to be promoted. Pressure has to be exerted so that funding is available for a call–recall system for all women over 50, not just those up to 64.

The accelerating advances in molecular biology are already having an impact on clinical practice. Thus, the identification of the *BRCA1* gene on chromosome 17 means that women at high risk of breast cancer can be identified.

As more knowledge of the fundamental changes of malignancy is acquired, tumour markers will be identified and used for imaging, staging, and possibly for therapy. Refinements in surgical technique should enable treatments to become more user friendly, which in itself may prompt more individuals to present at earlier stages of disease.

At present, some improvements in health could be obtained by wider dissemination of available techniques among both the medical profession and the public. However, for major improvements to occur, a combination of patient education, screening, and close links between basic and clinical scientists will be required.

References and further reading

Atkin, W. S., Cuzick, J., Northover, J. M. G., Whynes, D. K. (1993). Prevention of colorectal cancer by once only sigmoidoscopy. *Lancet,* **341,** 736–40.

Fentiman, I. S. (1990). *Detection and treatment of early breast cancer.* Dunitz, London.

Fentiman, I. S. and Taylor-Papadimitriou, J. (1994). Breast cancer. *Cancer surveys,* Vol. 18. Cold Spring Harbor Laboratory Press, New York.

Guillou, P. J., Townsend, C. M., and Monson, J. R. T. (1993). Laparoscopic surgery for cancer. *Surgical Oncology,* **2** (Suppl 1).

Miki, Y., Swensen, J., Shattuck-Eidens, D., Futreal, P. A., Harshman, K., Tautigian, S. (1994). A strong candidate for the breast and ovarian cancer susceptibility gene BRCA-1. *Science,* **266,** 66–70.

Nemoto, T., Vana, J., Bedwani, R., Baker, H. W., McGregor, F. H., Murphy, G. P. (1980). Management and survival of female breast cancer: results of a national survey by the American College of Surgeons. *Cancer,* **45,** 2917–24.

Niewig, O. E. (1994). Potential applications of positron emission tomography in surgical oncology. *European Journal of Surgical Oncology,* **20,** 415–24.

18

Chemotherapy

J. S. MALPAS

18.1 Introduction

Chemotherapy is a relatively new method of treating cancer. Surgery has been used for treating localized disease for more than a century, and radiotherapy was also being widely used a quarter of a century before the first chemotherapy was given to a patient.

The modern era of chemotherapy begins with the introduction of nitrogen mustard (methylchloramine) by Wilkinson in the UK and Gilman and Goodman in the US. Significant clinical benefit was seen in patients with Hodgkin's disease even when the condition was widely spread throughout the body. This, together with the successful use of stilboestrol by Dodds and steroids by Hickman and Kendall in disseminated prostatic cancer and lymphoid tumours respectively, ushered in a new era of cancer treatment.

Within two years, a treatment for acute leukaemia was devised by Seeger and given a clinical trial by Farber and his colleagues. They used aminopterin, an antimetabolite, to produce remission of acute leukaemia in children. There rapidly followed a golden age for anticancer therapy, with Hitchings and Elion synthesizing purine and pyrimidine antagonists, and Heidelberger the drug 5-fluorouracil.

Introduction of the drug into the clinic had now to be carried out in an orderly manner with the trial drug progressing through a series of tests. Initially its toxicity and the effects on various organs had to be established in experiments on small animals. Toxicity in the liver or kidneys, for example, could be assessed, and these features looked for carefully when it was first administered to patients. The sequence of events in clinical trials is given in more detail later, but, essentially, phase I studies of drugs establish the dose, route of administration, excretion pattern, and salient toxic features. Once this information is available, phase II studies are carried out in which patients with a variety of malignancies receive the drug and the spectrum of tumours that are sensitive to the agent can be defined. More advanced studies, sometimes called phase III studies, allow for in-depth evaluation of patients; usually the drug being tested in one form of malignancy only, in which the new drug plus the best established previous method of treatment is compared with a control group of patients in a randomized manner, the control group having the previously most successful form of treatment. Some of the difficulties, errors, and constraints on the introduction of new drugs is discussed in more detail at the end of this chapter.

18.2 Classification of chemotherapeutic drugs

Using this approach, a whole range of clinically effective drugs was made available over the next two decades. Some of these act directly on tumour cells whereas others must be activated by metabolic processes, either in the tumour cells or in organs such as the liver. A list of the most important drugs is given in Table 18.1. Increasing knowledge of the mechanism of cell division was being gained at the same rate as the introduction of these agents, in the hope that greater knowledge of how these agents worked would enable them to be used more effectively, clinically. Questions as to whether they were active on the dividing cell and, if this was so, whether they were acting at a particular stage of cell division, became of great interest.

It is possible to divide drugs into those that are active on both dividing and non-dividing cells, those that are active on dividing cells and affect a very particular phase of cell division (phase-specific drugs), and those that affect all or most of the phases of the cell cycle (Table 18.2). The particular phases where some of these drugs act are shown in Fig. 18.1. Whatever the mode of action of the chemotherapeutic agent, a very important finding is that it destroys malignant cells according to first-order kinetics; in other words, the same proportion of cells is killed for each dose of the agent.

It is very important to recognize that chemotherapeutic drugs damage normal tissues as well. Indeed, if they were non-toxic to normal tissues, cancer would have been cured long ago. The only reason that chemotherapy is feasible is that normal tissues may recover fully, sometimes more rapidly than the tumour cells. It is on this narrow difference in behaviour that practical clinical chemotherapy rests.

From the point of view of the practising clinician treating patients, the contribution that the knowledge of the kinetics of cancer cells and the effect of drugs on the cell cycle has made has been disappointing, probably because human tumours are very different in their behaviour from the rapidly growing experimental animal tumours in which the proportion of dividing malignant cells in the tumour is very high.

A classification, based on the mode of action of particular groups of agents, is probably of more immediate help (Table 18.3). The remarkable feature about this table is the wide variety of sources for

Table 18.1 Anticancer drugs

Classification	Drug
Alkylating agents	Mechlorethamine
	Busulphan
	Chlorambucil
	Cyclophosphamide
	Melphalan
	Thiotepa
Antimetabolites	Methotrexate
	6-Mercaptopurine
	Thioguanine
	5-Fluorouracil
	Cytosine arabinoside
	5-Azacytidine
Plant alkaloids	Vinblastine
	Vincristine
	VP-16
Antibiotics	Actinomycin D
	Doxorubicin
	Bleomycin
	Daunorubicin
	Mithramycin
	Mitomycin C
Nitrosoureas	Carmustine
	Lomustine
	Semustine
	Streptozotocin
Enzymes	L-Asparaginase
Random synethetics	cis-Platinum diammine dichloride
	Dacarbazine
	Dibromomannitol
	Hexamethylmelamine
	Hydroxyurea
	Mitotane
	Procarbazine

Table 18.2 Phase- and cycle-specific drugs

Phase specificity	Acts on	Drug
S phase specific	DNA synthesis	Methotrexate
		Cytosine arabinoside
		Hydroxyurea
Relatively S-phase specific	DNA, RNA, and protein synthesis	5-Fluorouracil
		6-Mercaptopurine
Cycle specific	DNA at all phases of cycle	Nitrogen Mustard
		Nitrosourea
		Cyclophosphamide

chemotherapeutic agents. Some were produced deliberately on the basis of interfering with metabolic pathways, but many were discovered by pure chance. Vincristine, for example, was discovered in

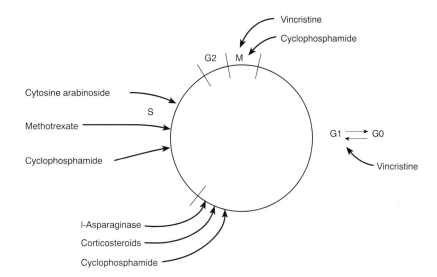

Fig. 18.1 Cell cycle showing the site of action of some phase-specific drugs.

Table 18.3 Groups of chemotherapeutic agents

Class of compound	Examples	Tumours against which drug is most active
Antifolic compounds	Methotrexate	Acute leukaemia Choriocarcinoma
Antipurines and pyrimidines	6-Mercaptopurine 5-Fluorouracil	Acute leukaemia Breast cancer
Alkylating agents	Melphalan Cyclophosphamide Busulphan	Myeloma Lymphoma Chronic myeloid leukaemia
Sex hormones	Oestrogens Androgens	Prostate cancer Breast cancer
Steroids	Corticosteroids	Leukaemia Lymphoma
Antitumour antibiotics	Actinomycin Anthracyclines Daunorubicin Doxorubicin Mitomycin	Wilms' tumour Leukaemia Lymphoma
Plant extracts	Vinblastine Vincristine Vindesine	Hodgkin's disease Leukaemia

the search for a new antidiabetic agent, procarbazine in the development of a tranquillizing drug, and the antitumour antibiotics were often discovered in the search for new antibacterial agents. The source of these drugs gives very little indication of the likelihood of activity against a particular tumour.

18.3 Pharmacokinetic principles

Before considering the main classes of anticancer drugs, it is necessary to consider the ways in which these drugs achieve their effects, and factors that govern their absorption, distribution, and excretion; in other words, their pharmacokinetics. Pharmacokinetics has been defined as what the body does to the drug, and pharmacodynamics as what the drugs do to body cells. An anticancer drug given orally may be wholly or partially absorbed from the intestinal tract into the intestinal blood vessels, which carry it through the liver into the general circulation. The blood level of the drug rises rapidly but in passage through the liver it may be metabolized, i.e. so-called 'first pass metabolism'. Various metabolites start to circulate, some of which may be excreted in the urine. The level reached in the blood will give some indication of exposure of the tumour. If the level in the blood is studied over the course of time, until it is all excreted, a curve is formed, and the area under this curve is an indication of the level of exposure of the body cells with time. This area ('area under the curve' or AUC) is a very important pharmacokinetic measurement. There are some instances where the AUC is not a helpful guide to tumour exposure; for example, if the tumour is in the brain occupying what is called a sanctuary site, it is protected from the systemic levels of drug by the so-called blood–brain barrier, and consequently will not be affected. The blood–brain barrier is not absolute, but varies with the drug; only some may pass through.

Bioavailability is another important concept, and is approximately the measure of the area under the curve following oral administration, compared with the level under the curve of drug concentration following an intravenous injection.

Toxicity is also related to the area under the curve and a high blood level may be toxic, for example, to the bone marrow, kidneys, liver, or other organs. Some drugs are excreted or broken down to inactive metabolites by the kidneys. If these organs are not functioning properly, then a very high maximum level of drug with a very slow fall in concentration may severely damage susceptible tissues, such as the bone marrow, and this may be fatal.

18.4 Pharmacology of the main classes of agents

18.4.1 Alkylating agents

Nitrogen mustard is the parent substance of this group of drugs. It contains an ethylamine CH_2CH_2Cl group, which is highly reactive, combining with nucleophilic elements in a wide variety of biological molecules. In particular, it binds to the seventh nitrogen atom in the guanine molecule which makes up the helix of DNA (see Chapter 5).

The ability to form bridges and cross-links impairs the replication of DNA at mitosis. A number of substitutions in the molecule of nitrogen mustard has led to less toxic but effective substances such as phenylalanine mustard (melphalan) and chlorambucil, which can be safely given by mouth. Cyclophosphamide, another very effective agent, is changed to the active metabolite 4-hydroxycyclophosphamide on first pass metabolism. These agents have been useful in the treatment of acute and chronic leukaemias, Hodgkin's disease, non-Hodgkin's lymphoma, and myeloma. Cyclophosphamide has also been found to be effective in solid tumours such as breast cancer and lung cancer.

18.4.2 Antimetabolic drugs

Methotrexate was one of the most successful of a number of analogues synthesized by Seeger. It works by irreversibly and tightly binding to the enzyme dihydrofolate reductase, which stops the production of reduced folic acid thereby inhibiting thymidylate synthesis and halting DNA production,

which, of course, is necessary for cell replication. Its action can be reversed by leucovorin or folinic acid. Methotrexate can be administered safely by a wide variety of routes, including intrathecal injection. It was shown to be possible to cure experimental leukaemia in mice and is an important component of modern antiacute leukaemia therapy. Other antimetabolites acting on acute leukaemia are 6-mercaptopurine and 6-thioguanine, but probably the most important antimetabolite introduced is cytosine arabinoside. This proved to be effective in the otherwise completely incurable adult form of leukaemia, adult myelogenous leukaemia.

5-Fluorouracil is an antimetabolite that was specifically synthesized by Heidelberger to be effective against solid tumours, and indeed proved to be useful in the management of gastric and colon cancer. Exploiting new knowledge of its metabolism, it can be shown that its activity can be enhanced by concomitant administration of folinic acid.

18.4.3 Drugs derived from natural sources

Many potent drugs have been derived from natural sources: doxorubicin, daunorubicin, actinomycin D, and bleomycin from bacteria; vinblastine and vincristine from the Madagascar periwinkle plant; etoposide and teniposide from the mandrake plant, which produces epipodophyllotoxin; and, more recently, taxol and taxotere from yew tree bark.

Doxorubicin and daunorubicin are anthracyclines, which were originally thought to have their effect by intercalating with DNA. It now seems most likely that they achieve their effect by binding with the enzyme topoisomerase II, which produces strand breakage and resealing. When topoisomerase II levels fall, anthracycline activity is inhibited. The anthracycline also produces superoxide, which, in conjunction with iron, has the ability to cause damage to heart muscle. This may produce cardiac failure in adults given a cumulative total dose of more than 550 mg/m^2. Doxorubicin is effective in a wide variety of haematological malignancies and breast and other solid tumours. Daunorubicin has a limited range of activity being effective only in acute myeloid and acute lymphoblastic leukaemia.

The vinca alkaloids, vincristine and vinblastine, and the other plant-derived anticancer agents listed above, work by poisoning the microtubule that is formed during the process of mitosis, and along which the daughter chromosomes move to the two poles of the dividing cells. These anticancer agents prevent microtubule assembly as their main action, but etoposide and teniposide also affect topoisomerase II.

All these agents are effective in haematological malignancies, but have also achieved great importance in the management of testicular and other germ cell tumours, and, more recently, small cell lung cancer. Taxol is being investigated for its activity in ovarian cancer.

18.4.4 Other agents

One heavy metal, *cis*-platinum, must be mentioned as it has been of great value in the management of testicular and ovarian cancer. Some 125 years after Lisauer showed the effect of inorganic arsenic on tumours, Rosenberg showed that the fluid surrounding platinum electrodes had antigrowth activity against bacteria. Later it was shown that platinum compounds also inhibit the growth of animal cells and thus *cis*-platinum and its analogue carboplatin are establishing themselves as curative drugs for testicular cancer.

18.5 Drug toxicity

Information on toxicity is most useful to the clinician when considering the choice of chemotherapeutic agents. Toxicity can be divided into that occurring shortly after administration, that which is somewhat delayed, and the very long-term toxic effects. Before a drug or combination of drugs is administered to a patient, the gain in terms of clinical benefit must be balanced against these toxicities, examples of which are shown in Table 18.4. This table has been arranged to show the common nonspecific toxicities that may be encountered with most therapeutic agents. Specific toxicities are shown on the right-hand side of the table. The clinician must know in detail the general and specific toxicities of all the chemotherapeutic agents that he uses.

18.6 Principles of chemotherapy

It is important to be quite clear about the reason for giving a cytotoxic drug or combination of drugs. From experience we now know that it is possible for chemotherapy to cure various malignancies. Children with acute leukaemia, Wilms' tumour, sarcomas, lymphomas, and other tumours may be cur-

Table 18.4 Drug toxicity

Common	Special
Immediate (within hours)	
Nausea and vomiting	Haemorrhagic cystitis (cyclophosphamide)
Phlebitis	Radiation recall (actinomycin)
Hyperuricaemia	Fever (bleomycin)
Renal failure	
Early (days to weeks)	
Reduction in white blood cells (leucopenia)	Paralytic illness (vinca alkaloids)
Reduction in blood platelets (thrombocytopenia)	Pancreatitis (asparaginase)
Hair loss (alopecia)	Cerebellar disorders (high dose cytosine arabinoside)
Diarrhoea	Ear toxicity (platinum)
Delayed (weeks or months)	
Anaemia	Peripheral nerve damage (vinca alkaloids)
Aspermia	Inappropriate ADH (cyclophosphamide)
Liver cell damage	Jaundice (6-mercaptopurine)
Fibrosis of lung	Adrenal deficiency (busulphan)
Late (months to years)	
Sterility	Liver fibrosis (methotrexate)
Testicular or ovarian atrophy	Brain damage (methotrexate)
Second malignancies	Bladder cancer (cyclophosphamide)

able. Adults with acute myelogenous leukaemia, lymphoblastic leukaemia, non-Hodgkin's lymphoma, Hodgkin's disease, teratoma of the testis, and choriocarcinoma are potentially curable. Drugs, therefore, have to be given to the limits imposed by toxicity, on a definite schedule, which may have to be tailored around other methods of treatment such as surgery or radiotherapy.

In some tumours, cure may not be possible but effective drugs or drug combinations may be able to extend useful life considerably. Good examples are breast carcinoma, ovarian carcinoma, small cell carcinoma of the bronchus, and myeloma. More recently, the use of α-2-interferon has extended the overall survival of chronic myeloid leukaemia patients.

There are some forms of malignant disease where it is known that there has been no improvement in the duration of survival since chemotherapy was introduced, but the quality of life has been immeasurably improved. In chronic lymphatic leukaemia, the judicious use of steroids and/or chlorambucil has relieved the sweating, fever, loss of weight, and general debility that is a feature of this condition. Patients lead normal lives during most of the course of the disease, and the benefit of this palliative therapy is immense.

Finally, there are occasions when chemotherapy may be used as an effective palliative agent in a tumour that has been previously treated with radiotherapy or surgery. The bone pain associated with disseminated breast cancer may be rapidly relieved and the fearful symptoms of strangulation (respiratory obstruction) occasioned by a large carcinoma in the region of the trachea may be dispelled in a few hours by the injection of nitrogen mustard. These beneficial effects should not be underrated.

18.7 Administration of chemotherapeutic drugs

18.7.1 Combination chemotherapy

A good example of the beneficial effect of combination chemotherapy is the use of vincristine and prednisolone for the treatment of childhood acute lymphoblastic leukaemia. Either drug was able to produce remission in about half the patients treated when given singly. When the two drugs were combined, the rate of remission rose to over 90 per cent. Furthermore, as the two drugs had very different toxicities, this was achieved without great hazard; the antitumour effect doubled, but the toxicity did not.

The addition of even more drugs was found to be effective in some tumours, and a good example of where four drugs were shown to be better than single agents alone is Hodgkin's disease. Hodgkin's disease would respond to single agents but was rarely if ever cured by either the single alkylating agent vinblastine or procarbazine therapy. When four drugs were combined in the programme, using nitrogen mustard, Oncovin (vincristine), procarbazine, and prednisolone, there was not only an improvement in response but a marked improvement in durable remissions and many patients were cured. The latest adult tumour to show sensitivity to this approach is teratoma of the testis, the most common tumour in young men between the ages of 20 and 35. They can be cured even when it is disseminated by a combina-

tion of vinblastine, bleomycin, and *cis*-platinum. These combinations prevent the emergence of drug-resistant strains of tumour cells (see below).

18.7.2 Adjuvant chemotherapy

This form of chemotherapy was first introduced into the treatment of Wilms' tumour, a tumour of the kidney in young children, on the assumption that metastases were already widely disseminated when the patient was first seen. This hypothesis considered that these so-called micrometastases are composed of a few cells, which have an increased mitotic rate and a good blood supply, so that although they are not detectable, they are nevertheless very susceptible to the action of drugs. More recently, this degree of sensitivity has been queried, but nevertheless, when this hypothesis was tested in Wilms' tumour, it was shown that survival has increased considerably. With surgery and radiotherapy, survival was seen in only about 40 per cent of patients. When children were given adjuvant therapy, i.e. treatment directed at the micrometastases, from the time of presentation of the tumour, there was a marked increase in survival, and in many clinical series this proved to be 85–95 per cent.

This principle has been applied, with considerable success, to other childhood tumours. It has been much less successful in adult solid tumours, but this is only to be expected, since the response to chemotherapy of most carcinomas affecting adults is much less satisfactory.

18.7.3 Sanctuary sites

A major problem in the administration of anticancer agents is that they may not always be distributed throughout the body. This was mentioned earlier in discussing the pharmacokinetics of anticancer drugs. An example of a sanctuary site is that seen in children with acute lymphoblastic leukaemia. The drugs vincristine and prednisolone, which could produce a systemic response leading to a normal bone marrow and a normal blood picture, were not able to destroy leukaemic blast cells in the meninges surrounding the brain and spinal cord. This was responsible for the high frequency of relapse seen in these children, who, until the early 1970s often developed meningeal leukaemia, and following that systemic relapse, and died.

At that time, radiotherapy to the brain and spinal cord was the best way of preventing meningeal relapse. Subsequently, the use of very high doses of agents, such as methotrexate, which do pass through the blood–brain barrier in tumoricidal doses, has been a satisfactory alternative. Other sanctuary sites have been recorded, such as the testis in boys with acute leukaemia and occasionally the ovaries of girls with acute leukaemia.

18.7.4 Principles of high dose therapy

Studies on experimental tumour systems have shown that for some drugs, alkylating agents for example, the number of tumour cells that are killed is directly related to the dose of the drug that is given. There is also evidence that the emergence of drug resistance is related to the intensity of the initial drug therapy, and that resistance is far less likely to develop if effective drugs are given in high dosage early in the course of the disease. Drug resistance, which will be discussed later, most often develops if repeated small doses of the anticancer agent are given over a long period of time. The range of drugs that can be used in the clinic for high dose therapy is limited. There are two kinds: one in which there is a specific antidote to the drug (for example, methotrexate, where the patient may be rescued by the use of a specific agent, citrovorum factor or folinic acid) and the other in which the dose-limiting toxicity is such that the patient can be supported through the period of acute damage to normal tissues produced by the drug. An example of the latter is the use of the alkylating agent melphalan, which in normal circumstances is very toxic to bone marrow but has no other deleterious effects, even when given in quite high doses. If the bone marrow is removed and stored before the drug is given, it can be replaced as soon as the drug has been excreted. Repopulation of the bone marrow follows and the patient's blood count recovers rapidly.

Other drugs that may be useful in high dose therapy include cyclophosphamide, cytosine arabinoside, and busulphan. The use of these drugs in the clinic is still at a relatively early stage, but it appears that increased response rates and possibly increased duration of survival may occur in both low and high grade lymphomas, aggressive subgroups of both lymphoblastic and myeloblastic leukaemia, and myeloma.

High dose chemotherapy or a combination of this procedure and whole-body irradiation is being explored in a number of haematological and solid tumours, including breast cancer. It is theoretically important to consider the removal of any contamination of the reinfused bone marrow with malignant cells, and various methods have been devised. One technique includes the use of magnetic beads covered with specific antitumour antibodies which attach themselves to the contaminating malignant cells, and can then be removed by passing the cell suspension through a magnetic field. In another technique, a toxic material, ricin, is coupled to specific monoclonal antibodies directed against the phenotype of the lymphoblastic or lymphoma cell so that the drug is delivered only to the tumour cells (see Chapter 19), or such antibodies may be coupled to complement. Yet another approach is to use the drug 4-hydroxyperoxycyclophosphamide. This is related to cyclophosphamide, but, unlike its parent compound, it does not require activation by passage through the liver *in vivo*, but can be safely incubated with human bone marrow cells *in vitro*.

Until quite recently, the best way of achieving sufficient numbers of haemopoietic stem cells was to harvest the bone marrow. More recently, the use of peripheral blood stem cells has been introduced. In this technique, bone marrow suppression is induced by combination chemotherapy, and then following this, during the rebound phase, a cytokine such as G-CSF (see Chapter 20) is administered over a four-day interval, providing a very rapid increase in the number of progenitor stem cells bearing the CD34 phenotype in the peripheral circulation. One or, at most, two leucophoreses (removal of white blood cells from circulating blood) can achieve cell collections of 1.5×10^8 cells/kg which is sufficient for safe reconstitution of the bone marrow.

These procedures have been safely pioneered and, in small non-randomised institutional studies, have apparently shown benefit in a number of different tumours. They are now being explored, usually by randomized control studies on a larger scale, and the results of these trials are awaited.

18.8 Drug resistance

It is generally agreed that biochemical resistance to chemotherapy is a major cause of failure to cure cancer. If the resistance to agents in common use could be abolished, cancer would be curable. Tumours are either initially resistant to chemotherapy or after a period acquire resistance. Examples of intrinisically resistant tumours are melanoma, renal cell carcinoma, and non-small cell lung cancer. Acquired resistance is seen in breast cancer and small cell lung cancer. Although this is a useful guide to the clinician, it is theoretically possible that all tumours are initially sensitive.

Goldie and Coldman's hypothesis states that the more cells there are in the tumour, the greater the chance that some will have become resistant to cancer chemotherapy. Since the progeny of these cells will continue to divide while sensitive cells are eliminated, tumours eventually consist entirely of resistant cells. This can be taken further by the discovery that many tumours shed dead cells so that they grow very slowly. Although the tumours are small when they are discovered, they will nevertheless have had many cell divisions and opportunities for resistant clones to replace the sensitive tumour cells. This may explain why some solid tumours like colon cancer, although relatively small, are nevertheless composed almost entirely of cells that do not respond to common chemotherapeutic agents. It appears that cell resistance is not acquired in one step, as was originally thought, but in stages. It is also true that there are a large number of ways in which a tumour cell can become resistant.

Some of these mechanisms are specific to a particular drug, such as the amplification of the gene responsible for dihydrofolate reductase formation in the process of resistance to methotrexate. The amplification of the multidrug resistance gene *MDR1* which produces P-glycoprotein 170, is responsible for eliminating a large number of naturally derived drugs such as actinomycin D, doxorubicin, daunorubicin, etoposide, mitoxanthrone, taxol, teniposide, vinblastine, and vincristine.

In summary, the main causes of drug resistance are:

- the drug is actively pumped out of the cell by the P-glycoprotein in the cell membrane;
- the drug fails to cross the cell membrane adequately;
- having entered the cell, the drug fails to be activated, or;
- having been activated, it is rapidly deactivated before it can become effective;
- the damage it does is rapidly repaired;
- the drug target is rapidly increased so that the metabolic block is bypassed;

- alternative biochemical pathways are opened;
- there is a decrease in topoisomerase II and DNA breaks.

Many of these mechanisms may coexist which makes the problem of combating drug resistance in the clinic very difficult.

It can be shown that drug resistance is conveyed from one cell generation to the next. Further evidence is provided by the fact that transfection of an amplified 'resistance' gene into a non-resistant cell conveys the capacity of that cell to be resistant.

Resistance to methotrexate is a good example of the multifactorial nature of resistance. Methotrexate may pass through the cell membrane by passive diffusion, or by an energy-dependent mechanism. Once the drug is in the cell, it is polyglutamated and thus cannot diffuse out. Mutations leading to impaired uptake or failure of polyglutamation will lead to resistance. Methotrexate may then meet varieties of the enzyme dihydrofolate reductase that have arisen by mutation and with which it does not bind so avidly, allowing thymidylate synthesis to resume and hence DNA formation to proceed. Finally, as mentioned above, the gene for dihydrofolate reductase production may be amplified; once only a few molecules of dihydrofolate reductase enzyme are present, cell division can proceed.

The other area of drug resistance of great interest is the multidrug resistance gene first found in Chinese hamster ovary cells that were selected for resistance to colchicine. It was noted that these cells were also resistant to a wide range of naturally derived antitumour antibiotics and plant alkaloids, and that the resistance was conveyed by the P-glycoprotein 170 in their walls. Two genes have now been identified that control multidrug resistance, *MDR1* and *MDR2*, and these genes are amplified in human multidrug resistance. P-Glycoprotein forms an energy-dependent pump with two ATP sites on the molecule. Strenuous efforts have been made in the clinic to reverse this resistance—with disappointing results so far. Verapamil, a calcium-blocking agent, and cyclosporin, an immunosuppressant, have met with only very limited success. Derivatives of cyclosporin are now being introduced for clinical trial, and it is hoped that these may prove to be more useful. The main difficulty is that drug resistance is multifactorial, and that simply dealing with one mechanism is quite inadequate.

18.9 Clinical trials

The vast array of synthetic and non-synthetic compounds that might be effective in cancer chemotherapy has led to the definition of some common sense principles of assessment, so that time, expense, and other resources are not wasted.

The introduction of a new agent, whether it has been developed in the pharmaceutical industry or university laboratory, is preceded by a time consuming and expensive series of toxicity trials in animals. A phase I trial in humans is designed to determine the best route of administration, the features of the pharmacokinetics such as the routes of excretion and rapidity of excretion, details of toxicity such as dose-limiting toxic side effects, and the range of toxic effects that may occur. Many patients may have previously had all the conventional treatment available, so that the response may be minimal. Even so, a response in one patient in a consecutive series of, say, 14 or 15 patients who have been previously treated, would encourage a phase II study.

Phase II trials concentrate on the clinical responses, as defined in Table 18.5. These trials are used to determine the spectrum of activity of the agent, and the drug will be given as defined in the phase I studies to a variety of patients with different tumours. The response rates will be noted and a picture of the drug's clinical efficacy will be built up. Phase III studies are used to introduce drugs into clinical practice. This is usually done by adding the drug into an arm of a programme in which the control arm is the best previous drug regimen. Careful planning of these studies is necessary. The degree of benefit expected must be estimated. After this, the number of patients that will be needed in the trial can be determined. Knowing the number of patients available each year will give an estimation of the duration of the study and hence how long it will have to go on before a positive result is achieved.

Table 18.5 Criteria for response in solid tumours

Response	Criteria
Complete response	Complete disappearance of all demonstrable disease
Partial response	More than 50 per cent reduction in the sum of the products of the longest perpendicular diameters of tumour with no disease progression elsewhere
No response	No change or less than 50 per cent reduction
Progression	Increase in size of tumour at any site

It is very tempting in this case to turn to comparing results with historical controls (see Chapter 21), but it is very difficult to conclude that the historical controls are ever matched adequately. If nothing else has changed, the physician will have improved his ability to manage the condition under investigation (or at least one would hope so). Criticisms about variation in the general supportive care, ancillary services such as blood transfusion, treatment of bacterial infections, etc. are valid, but are less likely to be true in the case of a unit that admits a lot of patients suffering from one particular disease, and where the supportive care is relatively unchanged over a number of years. Any marked improvement in response or survival is then probably a true finding, and has the advantage that any new modification can be built into the therapeutic programme quite rapidly. However, the safest way of evaluating any new introduction is by the randomized clinical trial (see Chapter 21).

18.10 Supportive care

One of the major improvements in the last few years in the supportive care of patients being treated with chemotherapeutic agents is the introduction of the potent serotonin antagonists, also known as 5-HT3 antagonists, of which ondansetron is one of the first members to be introduced for clinical trial; granisetron, tropisetron, and dolasetron are now in various stages of clinical development. These have reduced the marked emesis (vomiting) seen in the administration of agents such as *cis*-platinum to a minor level, and because of this have enabled chemotherapeutic programmes to be continued without interruption. This is very likely to be reflected in an improved overall response and survival rate; their value cannot be underestimated.

18.11 Conclusion

It will be seen that the agents currently employed in the treatment of cancer are imperfect, achieve their effects by methods that are often poorly understood, and may produce lasting damage to normal tissues. Despite this, the number of patients who are being cured of their cancers as a result of chemotherapy is increasing gradually every year. This is a remarkable achievement when it is remembered that it has occurred within the space of one professional lifetime.

References and further reading

Balkwill, F. R. and Fiers, W. (ed.) (1989). Biological response modifiers. *Cancer Surveys*, **8** (4).

Burchenal, J. H. (1977). The historical development of cancer chemotherapy. *Seminars in Oncology*, **4**, 134–43.

Calman, K. C., Smyth, J. F., and Tattersall, M. H. N. (1980). *Basic principles of cancer chemotherapy.* Macmillan Press, London.

Calvert, H. (ed.) (1989). A critical assessment of cancer chemotherapy. *Cancer Surveys*, **8** (3).

Chabner, B. A. and Collins, J. (ed.) (1990). *Cancer chemotherapy: principles and practice.* J. B. Lippincott Company, Philadelphia.

Erlichman, C. (1993). The pharmacology of anticancer drugs. In *The basic science of oncology*, (2nd edn) (ed. I. F. Tannock and R. P. Hill). Pergamon Press, New York.

Goldstein, L. J., Krystal, G., Hartley, D. *et al.* (1989). Expression of a multidrug resistance gene in human cancers. *Journal of the National Cancer Institute*, **81**, 116–23.

Ling, V. (1989). Does P-glycoprotein predict response to chemotherapy? *Journal of the National Cancer Institute*, **81**, 84–5.

Monfardini, S. (ed.) *Manual of cancer chemotherapy*, (3rd edn), UICC Technical Report Series, Vol. 56. UICC, Geneva.

Potmesil, M. and Ross, W F. (ed.) (1987). *Topoisomerases in cancer treatment,* NCl Monograph No. 4. National Cancer Institute, Bethesda.

Skeel, R. T. and Lachant, N. A. (1995). Handbook of Cancer Chemotherapy (4th edn.). Little Brown & Co., New York.

Stark, G. R. and Calvert, H. (ed.) (1986). Drug resistance. *Cancer Surveys*, **5** (2).

van der Bliek, A. M. and Borst, P. (1989). Multidrug resistance. *Advances in Cancer Research*, **52**, 165–204.

Workman, P. and Gram, M. A. (1993). Pharmacokinetics and cancer chemotherapy. *Cancer Surveys*, **17**.

For detailed information on specific topics, consult the following specialist review series:

Seminars in Oncology. Grune and Stratton, New York.

Journal of the National Cancer Institute. Public Health Service, National Institutes of Health, Bethesda.

19

Monoclonal antibodies and therapy

PHILIP E. THORPE, EDWARD J. WAWRZYNCZAK, AND FRANCIS J.
BURROWS

19.1 Introduction

Antibodies are proteins made by higher animals when infected with bacteria, viruses, or other foreign substances. They are secreted into the blood by plasma cells as part of a complex immune response against the invading 'organism' (see Chapter 16).

Animals in the laboratory produce antibodies against a wide range of foreign molecules that need differ only slightly in structure from the animal's own molecules to be immunogenic. Thus, homologous proteins even from closely related species may stimulate antibody production. Tumour cells often bear surface molecules that are immunogenic in the natural host or in other animal species. By immunizing animals with preparations of tumour cells, antisera can be raised that contain antibodies recognizing the various antigens found on the tumour cell surface. Antibodies that bind to normal cells can then be removed from the antiserum by suitable absorption procedures leaving behind those antibodies that react strongly with tumour cells.

Attempts to use such antibody preparations for cancer therapy have been disappointing. This is partly because the antiserum contains many antibodies with different specificities, which increases the likelihood of cross-reaction with normal cells, and partly because the antitumour antibody is diluted with a large excess of antibodies with irrelevant specificity. In addition, the antitumour antibodies are often difficult to purify in adequate quantities and preparations from different animals are not equally effective. These problems were largely overcome by the technique devised by Kohler and Milstein (1975) for immortalizing and cloning individual antibody-forming cells. Each clone of cells produces a single type of antibody called a 'monoclonal antibody' having a single type of antigen-binding site. These cells can be grown up in large numbers allowing the reproducible manufacture of the monoclonal antibody in essentially unlimited amount and in a highly pure state. Such antibodies have a number of important uses in the diagnosis and therapy of cancer (see Chapters 12, 16, 17, and 18).

One application of monoclonal antitumour antibodies is to identify the type of malignant cell by analysing the tumour cells with a panel of monoclonal antibodies against different antigens. This helps the clinician to decide the most appropriate course of treatment. Antibodies can be used to measure the levels of soluble antigens that some tumour cells shed into the blood (see Chapters 15, 16, and 18). Antitumour antibodies can also be injected into the patient and may selectively concentrate within the tumour tissue. If the antibodies are radiolabelled, then it is possible to identify the sites of the primary tumour and large metastatic deposits within the body from the radiation that they emit. Moreover, antitumour antibodies injected into a patient can exert specific therapeutic effects by stimulating the various defence systems of the body to attack the tumour. Similarly, powerful cell poisons can be attached to the antibody which then carries the poison to the tumour cells and kills them. Lastly, monoclonal antibodies can be used to remove malignant cells or T lymphocytes from bone marrow *ex vivo* as part of the treatment of leukaemia and other malignant diseases. Here, we review the present and possible future applications of monoclonal antibodies in the treatment of cancer.

19.1.1 Antibody structure and function

As discussed in Chapter 16, the antibody molecule, in its simplest form, consists of four polypeptide chains linked by disulphide bonds: two identical 'heavy' chains and two identical 'light' chains (Fig. 19.1). Each heavy chain consists of a variable domain and three or four constant domains, whereas the light chain consists of a variable domain and a single constant domain. The variable and constant domains of one light chain fold over the variable and first constant domain of one heavy chain to give an 'Fab' arm which contains a single antigen-binding site and, hence, each antibody molecule has two reactive sites (i.e. is bivalent). The other constant domains of the heavy chain constitute the 'Fc' portion which mediates the effector functions of the antibody according to the immunoglobulin (Ig) class to which it belongs (Fig. 19.2).

The variable region domains contain 'framework' regions and 'hypervariable' regions. Framework regions of the primary sequence are very similar in antibodies of the same class and are believed to include amino acid residues that are concerned with maintaining the three-dimensional structure of the domain. Within hypervariable regions there is much greater diversity of the amino acid sequence between antibodies of the same class. It is principally the spatial distribution of these amino acid residues that determines the individual antigen-binding specificity of an antibody molecule. The antigen-binding sites of antibody molecules constitute unique structures that can be distinguished immunologically and are called 'idiotypes'.

Immunoglobulin classes are defined according to the kind of heavy chain the molecule contains. There are five major types of heavy chain, γ, μ, δ, α, and ϵ, which differ in their constant domains, and two types of light chain, κ and λ. The most abundant immunoglobulin in the bloodstream is IgG. It exists as a monomer with two γ chains and either two κ or two λ chains, which have a combined molecular weight of 150 kDa. In humans, there are four IgG subclasses, IgG1, IgG2, IgG3, and IgG4, which have closely related constant domains encoded by different genes. In the mouse and rat, the subclasses are IgG1, IgG2a, IgG2b, and IgG3. IgM (containing μ

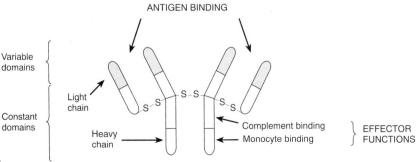

Fig. 19.1 The structure of IgG.

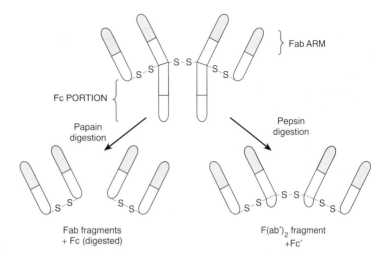

Fig. 19.2 Proteolytic fragments of IgG.

chains) exists in the bloodstream as a pentamer of subunits linked by the J chain and having a combined molecular weight of 900 kDa. Each of the subunits resembles an IgG monomer except for the presence of an extra constant domain on the heavy chain to which the J chain attaches. IgD (together with IgM) is present on the surface of B lymphocytes and acts as a receptor for antigen. IgD, IgA, and IgE are minor components of serum.

Antibodies of different classes and subclasses activate different effector mechanisms in the animal and may differ in their activity as antitumour agents against any particular tumour. Since it is the Fc portion that activates the effector arm of the immune response, the intact antibody molecule is usually used for immunotherapy. For radioimaging or targeting of cytotoxic agents, however, only the antigen-binding portion of the antibody is needed and so it is possible to use Fab or F(ab')$_2$ antibody fragments made by the proteolytic action of papain or pepsin respectively (Fig. 19.2). Advances in recombinant DNA technology now make it possible to produce a range of novel immunoglobulin forms, including the smallest antigen binding fragments, Fv, comprising just the V_H and V_L domains of the parent antibody and scFv, where the V_H and V_L are joined into a single polypeptide chain (see Section 19.1.5).

19.1.2 Monoclonal antibodies

When an antigen binds to a B lymphocyte bearing surface immunoglobulin that recognizes the antigen (in the presence of macrophages, helper T cells, and their soluble products), it triggers B cell proliferation and gives rise to a clone of cells all of which, when mature, secrete the same antibody. A single antigen usually stimulates many different B cells. Thus, an immunized animal produces many different antigen-specific antibodies. Since normal B lymphocytes soon die out in culture, it was important when Kohler and Milstein ingeniously preserved the specific antibody-producing characteristics of individual B lymphocytes by converting them into continuously growing clonal tumour cell lines. Their procedure has three stages (see Fig. 19.3).

In the first stage, a suspension of lymphocytes is prepared from the spleen of a suitably immunized animal, usually a mouse or rat. These lymphocytes are mixed with myeloma cells in the presence of an agent such as polyethylene glycol, which causes the cells to fuse together (a myeloma is a malignant plasma cell tumour whose cells secrete immunoglobulins). The myeloma lines used for fusion are variants that have been selected for a number of useful characteristics including resistance to 8-azaguanine, inability to synthesize or secrete immunoglobulin encoded by the endogenous genes, high fusion rates, and stable growth in culture or in rodents. The fusion of a splenic B lymphocyte with a myeloma cell gives rise to a hybrid cell called a 'hybridoma'. This hybrid inherits both the capacity of the myeloma partner for continuous proliferation and the capacity of the B lymphocyte partner to synthesize and secrete a specific antibody.

In the second stage of the protocol, hybridoma cells are isolated by drug selection. This step is necessary because myeloma cells often divide more rapidly than hybridoma cells and would soon out-

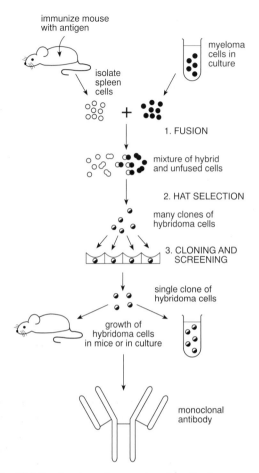

immunize mouse
with antigen

myeloma
cells in
culture

isolate
spleen
cells

+

1. FUSION

mixture of hybrid
and unfused cells

2. HAT SELECTION

many clones of
hybridoma cells

3. CLONING AND
SCREENING

single clone of
hybridoma cells

growth of
hybridoma cells
in mice or in culture

monoclonal
antibody

Fig. 19.3 Production of monoclonal antibody.

phocytes do not grow in culture, only the hybridoma cells persist when cultured continuously in the HAT selection medium.

Finally, the mixture of purified hybridoma cells is screened to identify and isolate individual hybridoma clones which secrete an antibody that binds the antigen of interest. This is usually done by diluting suspensions of hybridoma cell mixtures into individual wells of plastic microtitre plates so that each well contains, on average, less than one cell. Clones of cells are allowed to grow and the cell supernatant fluids are assayed for the presence of specific antibody by immunochemical techniques. Cells of clones that secrete such an antibody can be recloned by the same limiting dilution procedure and rescreened until truly monoclonal cell suspensions are obtained.

Hybridoma cell lines can be grown up in large numbers either in tissue culture or in the peritoneal cavity as ascitic tumours in mice or rats. IgG monoclonal antibodies can be purified by a combination of ion exchange and size exclusion chromatography or by affinity chromatography on absorbants containing the IgG-binding *Staphylococcus aureus* proteins, Protein A or Protein G. IgM monoclonal antibodies are purified by ion exchange and size exclusion chromatography or by affinity chromatography on absorbants containing mannose-binding protein. These and other methods of antibody purification are described in detail in a popular laboratory manual (Harlow and Lane 1988).

19.1.3 Human monoclonal antibodies

One factor that limits the usefulness of rodent monoclonal antibodies for cancer therapy in patients is that the antibodies themselves are immunogenic in humans. Human monoclonal antibodies would be less immunogenic because they would have the same constant domains as normal human immunoglobulins. However, the hypervariable region of human antibodies may still be immunogenic because it is complementary in structure to the antigen and may itself be recognized as foreign. The production of human monoclonal antibodies is more difficult than that of murine monoclonal antibodies for a number of reasons. Firstly, mouse myeloma cell lines are not ideal fusion partners for human B lymphocytes because mouse:human hybrid cells tend to lose the human chromosomes encoding the antibody molecule during prolonged growth in culture.

grow them in culture. Normally, myeloma cells cannot grow in the presence of 8-azaguanine. However, the variant myeloma cells used for fusion are resistant to this drug because they lack hypoxanthine phosphoribosyl transferase (HPRT), an enzyme that catalyses a step in the synthetic pathway from hypoxanthine to purines (see Chapter 6). These resistant myeloma cells use alternative synthetic pathways for DNA synthesis and replication. Accordingly, the cell mixture is grown in medium containing hypoxanthine, aminopterin, and thymidine (HAT). Aminopterin blocks the main pathway of purine and pyrimidine synthesis so that the myeloma cells (lacking HPRT) are unable to grow. The hybridoma cells divide normally since they have HPRT activity contributed by the parental splenic B lymphocyte and can use hypoxanthine as a substrate for DNA synthesis. As unfused splenic B lym-

Secondly, there are at present few human myeloma cell lines that fuse with human B lymphocytes to produce hybridomas that secrete monoclonal antibodies in useful amounts. Thirdly, immune B lymphocytes are difficult to obtain from humans although such cells may be extracted from within and around tumour sites in patients. This problem may be solved by the techniques now being developed for immunizing human B lymphocytes with the antigen *in vitro*. Finally, not all human–human hybrid cells grow as tumours even in immunologically deficient mice. Other ways of immortalizing human antibody-forming cells are being sought; for example, B lymphocytes can be transformed into continuously growing cell lines by infecting them with viruses such as the Epstein–Barr virus. All these methods are likely to be superseded by emerging technologies where monoclonal antibodies are produced from mice whose entire immunoglobulin gene repertoire has been replaced with a human immunoglobulin gene repertoire. Alternatively, phage display libraries may be used (see Section 19.1.5).

19.1.4 Humanized antibodies

Genetic engineering techniques have been used to construct vectors with human or partly human immunoglobulin genes. When a suitable non-producing mouse myeloma cell is transfected with one of these vectors, it expresses the manipulated genes and is able to secrete the modified antibody. Thus, it is possible to create antibodies in which the variable region domains of both heavy and light chains are encoded by genes of a mouse antibody-secreting myeloma and the constant region domains are encoded by human genes. These 'chimeric' antibodies have the antigen-binding specificity of the antibody produced by the parental mouse myeloma and effector functions determined by the Fc portion of the human molecule. In a development of this approach, the six hypervariable regions from the heavy and light chain variable domains of a rat antibody recognizing a widely distributed leucocyte surface antigen (CDw52) on human lymphocytes were successfully 'grafted' on to the framework of a human immunoglobulin molecule (Fig. 19.4). The refashioned human antibody proved more effective than the parent rat antibody at inducing the lysis of target cells because it more effectively recruited human effector mechanisms. Further manipulation

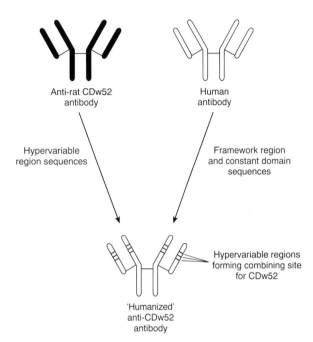

Fig. 19.4 Genesis of a 'humanized' recombinant anti-CDw52 antibody.

of immunoglobulin structure by site-directed mutagenesis allows the substitution of amino acid residues both in the antigen-binding site, to alter the affinity or specificity of binding, and in the constant domains, to enhance or eliminate the various physiologically relevant functions of the antibody.

19.1.5 Phage display libraries

To bypass hybridoma technology and the need for animal immunization, antibodies are being built in bacteria by mimicking features of immune selection (Clackson *et al.* 1991). A random combinatorial library of the rearranged heavy (V_H) and light (V_L) chain genes from immunized animals is joined to a gene encoding a phage coat protein. Phages therefore display on their surface the coat protein fused with diverse scFv antibody fragments. Phages bearing the desired antibodies are then selected, for example, by adsorbing on the immobilized antigen.

There are four key advantages of the phage display technique over conventional hybridoma techniques.

1. As many as 10 million different antibodies can be generated and screened in a single experiment, which is about 10 thousand times as many as are produced in a typical hybridoma experiment.

Thus, the likelihood of finding desirable antibodies is high.

2. Cloned antibody genes are obtained, and can be joined to the gene for an effector protein (e.g. a toxin) to create a bifunctional fusion protein. This obviates the need for purifying antibodies and effector proteins separately and chemically cross-linking them to generate antibody conjugates.

3. Combinatorial libraries of human antibody genes can be prepared, giving human antibodies for clinical use.

4. Production costs are low compared with mammalian cell production techniques.

The steps involved in constructing and screening a phagemid library from the lymphocytes of an immunized individual have several steps in common with the cloning of hybridoma antibody genes, as illustrated in Fig. 19.5. Total mRNA is isolated from the cells and the heavy and light chain variable region genes are reverse transcribed to cDNA and amplified using the polymerase chain reaction (PCR). PCR is a powerful tool for amplifying selected DNA fragments by using specific primers. It is also a convenient and rapid way of cloning individual genes or members of a gene family. Only limited sequence information is necessary for cloning a gene by this approach. A large number of antibody sequences are available and can be found in databases. Conserved regions at both amino and carboxyl termini of the variable domain of heavy (V_H) and light chains (V_L) have been identified. Nucleotide sequences encoding these regions are designed as primers for the amplification of immunoglobulin genes either from a repertoire of B cells or from selected hybridoma cells. The V_H and V_L cDNAs, which represent only a small fraction of the total cDNA, is amplified using pairs of primers that are specific for the amino and carboxyl termini of V_H and V_L. The V_H and V_L DNAs are then assembled into single-chain Fv (scFv) DNA using an oligonucleotide that encodes a flexible linker with the sequence of $(Gly_4Ser)_3$.

The recombinant phages contain phagemid DNA encoding a specific antibody scFv gene and display one or more copies of scFv as fusion proteins on their tips. At this point, phage-displayed scFv that bind to a specific antigen can be selected or enriched by 'panning' against the antigen. Recombinant phages are incubated with antigen-coated plates and non-bound phage are discarded. The bound phages can be eluted and amplified in *E. coli*. Several rounds of panning may be necessary to enrich the antigen-positive phages.

Phage DNA encoding desirable scFv can be ligated in frame with DNA encoding effector molecules (e.g. toxins and cytokines) to produce bifunctional single-chain fusion proteins. Other forms of antibodies can be amplified using their corresponding primers and expressed in *E. coli* systems, including Fd (just the V_H domain), Fv (V_H and V_L non-covalently linked), and Fab (V_H linked to CH1 domain and the paired light chain) fragments.

19.2 Tumour-associated antigens

19.2.1 The tumour cell surface

The plasma membrane of normal cells is a mosaic consisting of different glycoproteins and glycolipids, which are partially embedded in a fluid lipid bilayer. Some membrane molecules serve a transport function, others are involved in cell to cell contact, and many act as receptors for growth and differentiation factors. Some of these molecules are shared by many cell types while others have a more restricted distribution, occasionally being limited to a single cell type or even being only transiently expressed at a particular stage of cell maturation.

When a normal cell becomes malignant, it continues to express many of the cell surface molecules that are characteristic of its normal counterpart. However, these normal molecules can be expressed in abnormal amounts. The malignant cell can also express surface molecules that are not produced by the parent cell, for example, viral antigens or antigens normally expressed only during embryological development. Although these antigens may not be tumour specific, they can often be highly selective for particular types of tumour cells (see Chapter 16).

When a malignant tumour cell is injected into an animal of another species, the animal produces a mixture of antibodies against those cell surface components that it recognizes as foreign. The immunogenic determinants (epitopes) of glycoproteins can be structures formed by either the amino acid residues or by the carbohydrate side chains. Only the carbohydrate component of glycolipids tends to be antigenic however, since the lipid component is sequestered within the membrane bilayer.

Some truly tumour-specific antigens that are recognized by the human immune system have

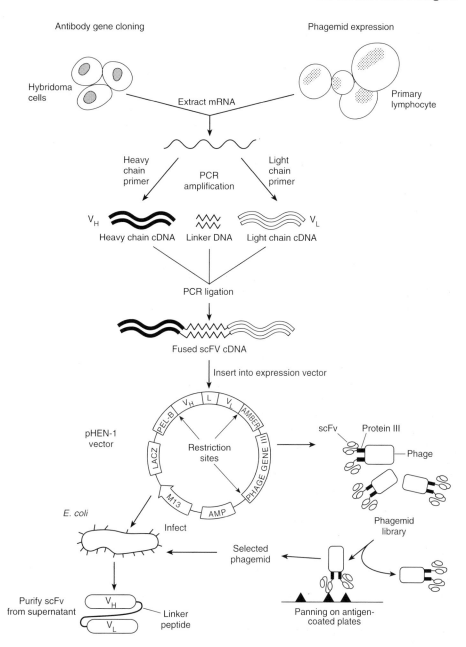

Fig. 19.5 Recombinant antibody techniques.

been characterized. Point mutations in the tumour suppressor gene p53 contribute to malignant transformation of epithelial cells and mutant p53 proteins express antigenic epitopes that are not found in any normal cells. Peptides from mutant p53 proteins become associated with MHC class I antigens on the tumour cell surface and can elicit specific cytotoxic T cell responses. Several other tumour-specific peptides recognized by cytotoxic T cells have also

been described (reviewed by Finn 1993). It is unclear at present whether these tumour-specific markers are expressed in sufficient numbers on tumour cells to provide a basis for antibody-based therapy.

19.2.2 Target antigens

It is the rule rather than the exception that a monoclonal antibody against a tumour-associated antigen binds to some normal cells in addition to the target cell. The normal tissue may express either the same antigen as the tumour cell or a molecule structurally related to that recognized by the antibody. This is not a serious problem for tumour imaging provided that the normal cells have an anatomical distribution that does not obscure the image of the tumour cells. For therapy, however, binding to normal cells reduces the amount of antibody that reaches the tumour and also increases the risk of damage to normal tissues.

Antibodies that react with normal tissues may still be used for therapy in a number of situations. Firstly, this is possible if the normal tissue is not life sustaining; for example, tumours of lymphoid origin can be attacked using antibodies against antigens on T or B lymphocytes because the healthy lymphoid cells that are killed by the treatment are soon replaced by new cells, which emerge from the bone marrow. In clinical trials with immunotoxins against the normal B lineage markers CD19 and CD22 in lymphoma patients, killing of both normal and malignant B lymphocytes was achieved with no apparent immunosuppressive sequelae. Secondly, the normal tissue may express the target antigen at a much lower density than the malignant cells and so escape damage. For example, leukaemic cells induced by human T cell leukaemia virus, HTLV-1, have 10- to 100-fold more surface receptors for interleukin-2 than do normal T lymphocytes. Similarly, malignant cells often proliferate more rapidly than normal cells and so express a relatively high level of the transferrin receptor and other molecules needed for cell division. Lastly, anatomical

barriers can sometimes prevent the antibody from gaining access to the normal tissue bearing the target antigen. An example of this is the carcinoembryonic antigen (CEA) which is often expressed by colon carcinoma cells. CEA is also found on the luminal epithelial cells of the gut but anti-CEA antibody injected intravenously rarely traverses the gut wall to reach the normal cells. Trail and colleagues (1993) were able to cure xenografted human colon carcinomas in rats using a chemotherapeutic drug, doxorubicin, conjugated with the anti-Le^y antibody BR96 with no toxic side effects, despite expression of Le^y on normal rat gut epithelium.

Tumour-associated antigens can arise in a number of different ways (Fig. 19.6). CEA is one example of an 'oncofetal' antigen that is normally associated with fetal cells of the same cellular lineage as the tumour cell, and reflects the tendency of malignant cells to become more primitive. A second type of tumour-associated antigenic determinant is found on molecules that are structural variants of normal cellular products. The p97 antigen associated with melanoma is structurally related to serotransferrin and lactotransferrin. Mutant proteins in other tumours can result from random mutations in the DNA of a cell after exposure to chemical carcinogens or ionizing radiation. Thus, each individual rodent fibrosarcoma induced by exposure to 3-methylcholanthrene has a different unique antigen. Cells transformed by some oncogenic viruses synthesize mutant proteins that are apparently related to the normal products of certain cellular genes (protooncogenes). Of these, a number are expressed at the cell surface, for example, the truncated avian

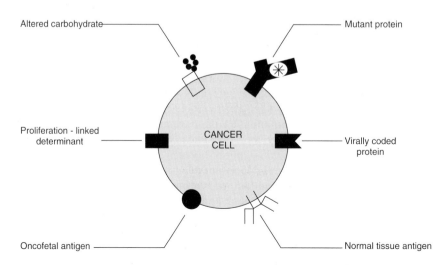

Altered carbohydrate — Mutant protein

Proliferation - linked determinant — CANCER CELL — Virally coded protein

Fig. 19.6 Target antigens. Oncofetal antigen — Normal tissue antigen

epidermal growth factor (EGF) receptor on cells transformed by avian erythroblastosis virus (see Chapters 9 and 11). One of the most extensively studied human tumour markers is the protein product of the *erb*B2 oncogene, p185^{HER2}, a member of the epidermal growth factor receptor superfamily of receptor tyrosine kinases (see Chapter 11). P185^{HER2} serves as an autocrine receptor for a growth factor secreted by breast carcinoma cells. Amplification of the *erb*B2 oncogene and overexpression of the p185^{HER2} protein are closely associated with poor prognosis in breast cancer. Antibodies to p185^{HER2} exert antitumour effects by a variety of biological mechanisms independent of antibody function (see Section 19.4.1).

A large proportion of monoclonal antibodies that detect tumour-associated antigens recognize unusual carbohydrate portions in glycoproteins and glycolipids. These tumour-associated carbohydrate antigens (TACAs) arise either by precursor accumulation resulting from blocked synthesis of a particular side chain, neosynthesis of complex terminal oligosaccharides caused by overexpression of certain glycosyl transferases, or changes in membrane organization or composition that expose previously cryptic (masked) carbohydrate epitopes. Changes in carbohydrate expression on the cell surface may also reveal cryptic peptide antigens, such as the epitopes in the protein core of human milk mucin recognized by the antitumour antibody SM3. Human tumours that display characteristic glycolipid structures include melanoma (GD3), Burkitt's lymphoma (GB3), Hodgkin's disease (asialo GM2 and Gg3), and gastrointestinal adenocarcinomas (Le^a). The structure and function of TACAs has been reviewed by Hakomori (1991). Mounting evidence suggests that TACAs play a pivotal role in tumour progression and metastasis by serving as adhesion molecules between tumour cells, extracellular matrix components, and endothelial cells. GM3 and sialyl Le^x mediate adhesion between melanoma and colorectal carcinoma cells, respectively, and endothelial cells. Antibodies to these structures inhibit metastasis in animal models (Hakomori 1991).

The emerging functions of TACAs are an example of the increasing convergence of tumour immunology and cancer biology. Molecular structures originally described as tumour 'antigens' on the basis of their ability to elicit an immune response and bind to antibodies are now revealed as tumour cell receptors mediating important events in malignant progression. Indeed, the most selective tumour markers are those whose function is most closely associated with neoplastic transformation, such as autocrine growth factor receptors, raising hopes that new discoveries in cancer cell biology will uncover more specific tumour target molecules for antibody-mediated therapy.

19.2.3 Problems of targeting to tumour associated antigens

Only a proportion of the cells in a tumour have the capacity for self renewal and are truly malignant. In some diseases, such as chronic myelocytic leukaemia, these clonogenic malignant cells represent a small proportion of the tumour mass. Although the bulk of cells that carry the target antigen can be successfully imaged using antibodies, in therapy it is imperative that the antibodies reach and kill the clonogenic subpopulation. However, it has proved difficult to identify these rare cells and demonstrate that they also bear the target antigen. In the heterogeneous tumour cell population, some cells express only low amounts of the target antigen and may escape being killed because less antibody binds to them. If these cells are clonogenic, the tumour will regrow. Moreover, as tumour cells continue to proliferate, mutant malignant cells that lack the target antigen frequently emerge. Thus, there are foci of cells within the primary tumour and its metastatic progeny that cannot be recognized by the antibody. This is a serious obstacle to successful imaging or therapy which can sometimes be countered by using 'cocktails' of monoclonal antibodies that recognize several different tumour-associated antigens.

The cells of a tumour that express high levels of the target antigen may also evade being coated by antibody in a number of ways. Firstly, antibodies are not distributed evenly in solid tumour masses for three reasons.

1. The dense packing of tumour cells and fibrous tumour stroma present a formidable physical barrier to macromolecular transport and, combined with the absence of lymphatic drainage, create an elevated interstitial pressure in the tumour core that reduces extravasation and fluid convection.

2. The distribution of blood vessels in most tumours is disorganized and heterogeneous, so that some tumour cells are separated from extravasating antibody by large diffusion distances.

death to cells?
from immune response

3. All of the antibody entering the tumour may become adsorbed in perivascular regions by the first tumour cells encountered, leaving none to reach tumour cells at more distant sites.

Secondly, some antigens, which are loosely associated with the cell membrane, are shed from the tumour cell surface. The antigen in the circulation can then form complexes with the antibody and this greatly reduces the quantity of antibody that actually reaches the tumour cells. Local antigen shedding may not cause major problems if direct binding of the antibody to tumour cells is not required. For example, tumour imaging with radiolabelled antibodies may be enhanced as a result of the presence of a large amount of soluble antigen in the tumour interstitium. Thirdly, the host's immune system may raise its own innocuous 'enhancing' antibodies against the tumour-associated antigen which then coat the malignant cells and 'mask' the antigen from the murine monoclonal antibody.

A possible solution to all of these problems would be to target the endothelial cells of the tumour vascular bed rather than the tumour cells themselves. This 'vascular targeting' approach is discussed in Section 19.5.7.

19.3 Tumour imaging

19.3.1 Principles

Tumour imaging is a procedure that allows the clinician to identify both primary and secondary sites of

tumour growth in a patient and to estimate the overall tumour burden without recourse to surgery. An antitumour antibody labelled with a radioactive isotope, usually iodine-131 (^{131}I) or indium-111 (^{111}In), is injected into the patient intravenously and, after allowing the antibody time to localize within the tumour, the patient is scanned using a radiation detector called a gamma camera. A computer compiles an image of the radioactivity detected in the patient's body and colour codes it according to the intensity of the radiation. Zones of high radioactivity in regions of the body that are not expected to accumulate the antibody or its metabolites indicate the possible presence of a tumour. This is illustrated in Figs 19.7 and 19.8. In combination with other clinical evidence, these results can help determine the most appropriate form of surgical, radiological, or chemotherapeutic treatment.

The principle of radioimmunodetection (RAID) of tumours was first demonstrated by experiments in which tumour-bearing animals were injected with radiolabelled polyclonal antibodies directed against malignant cells. The concentration of antitumour antibodies in the tumour typically reached levels up to four times higher than those in miscellaneous normal tissues. The absolute amount of radioactivity associated with tumour increased in the first few hours after injection, reflecting the time taken by the antibody to get out of the bloodstream and to diffuse to the site of the tumour. Maximal specific uptake by tumour is generally reached between one and four days after injection. Most of the anti-

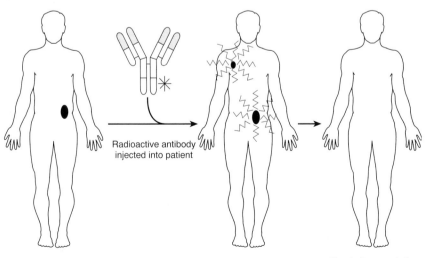

Fig. 19.7 The principle of radioimmuno-localization.

Patient with primary tumour

Radioactive antibody injected into patient

Metastasis detected

Surgical removal of primary tumour and metastasis

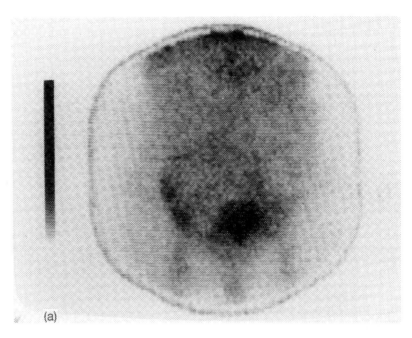

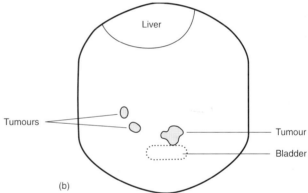

Fig. 19.8 Tumour imaging in a patient. Ovarian tumours in a patient localized by a monoclonal antibody H17E2 labelled with ^{123}I. This antibody recognizes a placental-type alkaline phosphatase associated with ovarian tumours of epithelial origin.

body that is not cleared remains in the blood and extravascular compartment. Consequently, there is background radiation, particularly in blood-rich organs such as the liver and spleen. Tumours in these sites are not easy to detect unless the image is corrected for background radiation.

19.3.2 Clinical studies

The first clinical study using radioimaging to detect tumour tissues was reported by Goldenberg *et al.* in 1978. Patients were injected with ^{131}I-labelled anti-CEA antibodies and were then scanned after an interval of 24–72 hours. To correct the image for the non-specific background radiation, a subtraction technique was used. Before injection of ^{131}I antibody and scanning, patients were injected with technetium-99m (^{99m}Tc), either bound to human serum albumin or free as pertechnetate, ^{99m}TcO$_4$. After computer subtraction of the ^{99m}Tc image from the ^{131}I image, areas of specific antibody uptake were highlighted.

Radioimmunodetection has now become established as a valuable diagnostic procedure through the development of higher affinity immunoconjugates, improvements in radiochemistry, and more sensitive detection systems. Almost 200 clinical trials have been reported since 1978. Many investigators have reported excellent specificity and sensitivity for tumour detection, including the visualization of occult tumour deposits that were not visible using standard radiographic methods (Larson *et al.* 1994). In 1992, 'Oncoscint', an ^{111}In-labelled anticolorectal carcinoma antibody, became the first diagnostic radiopharmaceutical to be approved by the US Food and Drug Administration. Figure 19.8 shows an example of tumour imaging in a patient. Results of trials with ^{111}In and ^{99m}Tc immunoconjugates have been particularly impressive. In an authoritative review, McKearn (1993) reported over 70 per cent sensitivity and specificity in 300 colorectal cancer patients imaged before surgery with ^{111}In immunoconjugates. Fully 97 per cent of deposits subsequently confirmed by surgery and/or histopathology were successfully imaged, including some lesions that were not detected by computerized tomography (CT) scans. ^{99m}Tc-labelled antibodies were even more powerful, displaying 95 per cent sensitivity and 90 per cent specificity in 141 patients with colorectal cancer.

Despite the sensitivity of present radioimaging techniques, some tumours still remain undetected. The amount of radioisotope that reaches tumour sites is small, as a rule 0.001–0.1 per cent of the injected dose per gram of tumour, and so small tumour masses are poorly resolved. In practice, the tumours that are routinely diagnosed have diameters of at least 0.5–1 cm, but metastatic microfoci, which may be more relevant to the long-term survival of the patient, are unlikely to be detected. Even the larger tumours may escape detection if they express a low level of the target antigen or are poorly vascularized. A further problem is that intravenously injected antibody cannot normally penetrate sanctuary sites in the body such as the brain, although direct 'intrathecal' injection into the cerebrospinal fluid is a promising alternative in patients with brain tumours.

Another problem with radioimaging is that areas of high radioactivity that are free of tumour are detected. These false positives occur when immune complexes formed in the blood are trapped by the liver and when free ^{131}I released from the antibody is eliminated from the bloodstream predominantly into the kidneys, urinary bladder, stomach, and intestine. Accumulation of iodine by the thyroid gland is usually blocked by coadministering Lugol's iodine or potassium iodide. Subtraction of the background radiation does not always eliminate false positives. The radiation emitted by ^{99m}Tc has a lower energy than that of ^{131}I and penetrates tissue more poorly resulting in the appearance of 'halo' effects in the image of the ^{131}I radioactivity after subtraction.

19.3.3 Strategies to improve tumour imaging

The sensitivity of tumour detection is improved by using radionuclides with better imaging characteristics than ^{131}I and by better methods for removing background radiation. ^{131}I has too high an energy for optimal imaging with current gamma cameras; radiation with an energy of 0.2–0.4 MeV is most suitable. Further, its half-life is rather long (8 days) so that the patient's normal tissues are exposed excessively to radioactivity and the decay process also produces potentially harmful β-particles. ^{131}I has been superseded by other isotopes of iodine (^{123}I) and by radionuclides that have shorter half-lives, better energy characteristics, and emit no β-particles (Table 19.1). The radioactive metal ions of ^{111}In, ^{99m}Tc, and gallium (^{67}Ga) can now be stably coupled to antibodies by means of chelating molecules. Current chelation chemistry techniques permit easy and efficient attachment of ^{111}In to antibodies with relatively low binding in the liver, and diminished *in vivo* transchelation, which results in transfer of the radioisotope to non-specific serum proteins and subsequent accumulation in normal tissues (Larson *et al.* 1994). Similar methods have been developed for yttrium-90 and ^{99m}Tc. The short half-life (6 hours) of ^{99m}Tc minimizes whole-body irradiation and small antibody fragments (e.g. scFv) can penetrate tumour masses rapidly enough for successful imaging in this shorter time frame (Yokota *et al.* 1992).

Background radiation caused by the residue of circulating radiolabelled antibody can be cleared in a number of days. First, synthetic lipid vesicles called 'liposomes' coated with anti-mouse immunoglobulin bind mouse monoclonal antibodies in per-

Table 19.1 Isotopes for imaging

Isotope	Energy of principle γ emission (MeV)	Half-life (hours)	Method of coupling to antibodies
^{131}I	0.36	192	Direct halogenation
^{123}I	0.16	13	
^{111}In	0.17–0.25	67	Chelation
^{67}Ga	0.09	78	
^{99m}Tc	0.14	6	

ipheral blood and accelerate their clearance, probably because liposome particles are rapidly removed by cells of the reticuloendothelial system. Second, clearance can be enhanced by the injection of a second antibody directed against radiolabelled antibody. Lastly, the use of F(ab')₂, Fab fragments, or scFv antibodies may improve tumour discrimination since antibody fragments are cleared from the circulation much more rapidly than intact Ig. Since these antibody fragments lack the Fc portion, there is less non-specific accumulation of radioactivity by the reticuloendothelial system. An alternative approach to background subtraction depends on the slower rate of loss of radioactivity from tumour tissue as opposed to normal tissue. A series of scans is taken at intervals after injection of the radiolabelled antibody. Zones in the body where the antibody persists show up as 'hot spots' of radiation. This technique avoids the imaging problems associated with the use of a second radionuclide.

An attractive new strategy for decreasing the serum half-life of radionuclides is a two-step approach where a cold bispecific antibody (see Section 19.4.5) recognizing a tumour marker and a radiolabelled hapten is injected and allowed to localize to the tumour for 1–2 days, at which time a low molecular weight radiolabelled hapten is administered in large excess. The hapten will diffuse rapidly throughout the body and clear quickly through the kidneys except where it is bound to the free arm of tumour-bound bispecific antibody. Le Doussal and colleagues (1990) reported encouraging results in animal models and preliminary clinical studies.

The use of single photon emission computerized tomography (SPECT), analogous to CT scanning using X-irradiation, allows a better discrimination between valid and false positive tumour images. The computer constructs images of transverse sections of the patient's body and allows examination of putative tumour sites from several angles. Increasingly sensitive and sophisticated detection systems have significantly improved image interpretation. SPECT images can now be superimposed with other tomographic methods, so radioimmunodetection data can be combined with the anatomical information of CT and MRI (Larson *et al.* 1994). This can resolve equivocal CT or MRI studies or reveal additional occult tumours. Radioimmunodetection plays a complementary role to CT and MRI; for example, RAID is superior to CT for detection of extrahepatic metastases of colo-

rectal carcinoma, whereas CT detected more liver lesions (McKearn 1993).

19.4 Immunotherapy

19.4.1 Mechanisms of tumour cell killing or growth suppression

The goal of antibody-mediated immunotherapy is to treat cancer patients with antitumour antibodies that will bind selectively to tumours and destroy the malignant cells, or stasis or reversal of the neoplastic phenotype, either directly or by stimulating the natural defence mechanisms of the recipient.

There are three main ways in which antibody molecules can suppress tumour cell growth (Fig. 19.9).

Direct growth inhibition Certain antibodies directly interfere with tumour cell proliferation. Examples are blocking antibodies against tumour cell receptors for growth factors. Anti-transferrin receptor antibodies can inhibit tumour growth both *in vitro* and in nude mice. Receptors for mitogenic cytokines, including EGF, IL-2, and PDGF, are frequently up-regulated on certain types of tumour cells (see Chapter 11). Growth factor-induced tumour cell division contributes to neoplastic progression so antibodies that antagonize this process could have great therapeutic value. Unfortunately, since tumour cells commonly secrete growth fac-

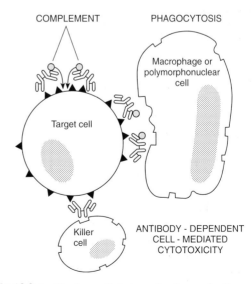

Fig. 19.9 Antibody-mediated mechanisms of cell killing.

tors for which they bear receptors (autocrine effects), complete blocking with antireceptor (or anticytokine) antibodies is difficult to achieve.

Antibodies against Fas and APO-1 induce programmed cell death (apoptosis) in several lymphoid tumours. The mechanism of this effect is unknown, but is probably similar to the physiological process by which proliferative immune responses are regulated. Similarly, induction of 'tumour dormancy' in B-lymphoma cells by anti-idiotype (anti-Id) antibodies is analogous to the delicate regulation of normal B cell immune responses mediated by the idiotype-antiidiotype network.

Anti-p185^{HER2} antibodies inhibit breast tumour growth by several mechanisms including growth factor blockade, induction of terminal differentiation, and increasing sensitivity to *cis*-platinum and TNF-α. *In vivo* antitumour effects can also be demonstrated with antibodies against integrin extracellular matrix receptors or carbohydrate adhesion receptors (see Section 19.2.2). These antibodies inhibit tumour growth or metastasis by interfering with essential interactions between tumour cells and normal host stromal elements.

Complement-mediated cytotoxicity (CDC) Complement is the name given to a series of proteins (C1–C9) present in serum in inactive form. The C1q complement component binds to the Fc part of cell-bound antibody and triggers a cascade reaction in which several of the remaining complement components are activated by proteolytic cleavage. Other complement proteins (C5b–9) then form a 'membrane attack complex' which inserts into the cell membrane and induces lysis.

Antibody-dependent cell-mediated cytotoxicity (ADCC) Several distinct types of defence cells kill antibody-coated cells *in vitro* and it is presumed that they also do this *in vivo*. The effector cells include polymorphonuclear cells (e.g. neutrophils), macrophages, and a type of mononuclear cell called the NK (natural killer) cell which is present in lymphoid tissues but which lacks mature T and B lymphocyte markers (see Chapter 16). All these cells adhere to antibody-coated cells by means of receptors for the Fc portion of the immunoglobulin molecule. Polymorphonuclear cells and macrophages also have receptors for the C3 component of complement. If the antibody is of a type that binds complement, this gives dual recognition, which strengthens the adherence of the effector cell

to the target cell. The various effector cells then kill the target cell by phagocytosis or direct lysis.

The heavy chain subclass of the monoclonal antibody determines which effector systems are activated. With monoclonal antibodies raised in the mouse, IgGs of all major subclasses can elicit cell-mediated cytotoxicity, whereas IgA and IgM cannot. In contrast, IgM is the most powerful activator of complement whereas, IgG2a, IgG2b, and IgG3 fix complement weakly, and IgG1 not at all. The therapeutic effect of an antibody therefore depends on which host defence system is most effective at killing tumour cells. Since IgG heavy chains can now readily be exchanged by recombinant techniques, improved antibodies for immunotherapy should soon emerge. Furthermore, as the short sequences required for activation of each effector system are identified, it may be possible to design hybrid recombinant antibodies that combine optimal CDC and ADCC functions.

19.4.2 Studies in experimental animals

The feasibility of immunotherapy has been demonstrated by several studies in experimental animals. In an early study, Bernstein and his colleagues (1980) showed that up to 3×10^5 leukaemia cells transplanted into mice could be eliminated by intravenous injection of antibody against the Thy1.1 surface antigen expressed by leukaemia cells. When mice carrying 3×10^6 tumour cells subcutaneously were treated in the same fashion, the mice were not cured, apparently for two reasons. Firstly, antigen-positive leukaemia cells coated with antibody were not killed by the host. Secondly, antigen-negative leukaemic cells were detected in the spleen, suggesting that antibody therapy had prevented the spread of antigen-positive tumour cells but that a mutant subpopulation of tumour cells lacking the antigen had escaped. Other studies have tested mouse antibodies against human tumour-associated antigens in mice carrying xenografts of human tumour tissue. In general, significant regression of the transplanted tumour was only observed in animals with small tumour burdens, a situation very different form the clinical situation in human patients with spontaneous tumours and large tumour cell burdens. IgM antibodies were generally ineffective in these *in vivo* studies. Mouse antibodies of the IgG2 and IgG2b subclasses were the most effective and have since been used for phase I clinical trials in humans.

Yefenof *et al.* (1993) found that animals thought to be cured of a mouse B lymphoma by anti-idiotype antibodies in fact harboured dormant tumour cells in their spleens. They subsequently showed that anti-Id and other antibodies against surface IgM on the leukaemia cells were able to induce apoptosis or a reversible dormant, non-cycling state *in vitro* or *in vivo* without activating classical effector mechanisms.

19.4.3 Clinical trials

Trials with mouse monoclonal antibodies have been performed in patients suffering from advanced malignant melanoma and gastrointestinal tumours. However, only tumours of the haemopoietic system, including B cell and T cell leukaemias and lymphomas, have responded well to this treatment and some patients remain disease free after several years.

Miller *et al.* (1982) raised monoclonal antibodies against the idiotypic determinants of the neoplastic cells of a patient with a type of B cell lymphoma called 'follicular lymphoma'. In this form of cancer, a single clone of B cells proliferates and so all the cells of the tumour bear surface Ig with the same idiotype. Since each clone of normal B lymphocytes in the body expresses a molecule with a unique antigen-binding site, the idiotype of the surface Ig of the lymphoma cells provides a unique tumour-specific target antigen. Tumour regression occurred after repeated intravenous infusions of the anti-idiotype monoclonal antibody and continued when treatment was stopped, leading to a complete remission (see Fig. 19.10). The mechanism of this remarkable therapeutic effect is obscure. It is possible that the malignant cells were not killed by the patient's defence systems but that the antibody directly suppressed their proliferation in a manner analogous to that in which anti-idiotypic antibodies normally control the proliferation of cells that produce antibody in response to an antigenic stimulus.

More typically, in therapeutic trials against lymphomas and leukaemias, the infusion of antitumour monoclonal antibodies directed against different lymphocyte-specific antigens induced a rapid decrease in the numbers of circulating tumour cells. These effects usually persisted provided that the level of antibody was maintained by repeated infusions. However, once the antibody was allowed to clear completely, the leukaemic cell counts returned to pretreatment levels or higher. The temporary improvements observed may reflect an inherent limit to the capacity of host effector mechanisms to kill large numbers of tumour cells. It is known, for example, that the capacity of the hepatic reticuloendothelial system to clear antibody-coated tumour cells from the blood can become saturated. The tumour deposits in the lymph nodes may have been more resistant than tumour cells free in the circulation because they were less accessible to the antibody. Alternatively, the lymph nodes may have contained too few effector cells; immunotherapy using monoclonal antibodies relies on the patient being able to destroy the antibody-coated tumour cells and it is likely that the effector systems of a patient with advanced malignant disease will have been compromised either by prior therapy or by the disease itself.

In phase III clinical trials in lymphoma patients in complete remission or with minimal residual disease,

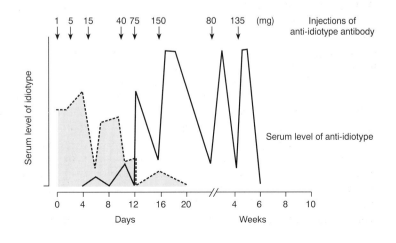

Fig. 19.10 Antibody-mediated immunotherapy of B cell lymphoma. The effect of anti-idiotypic antibody on the level of serum idiotype in a patient with B cell lymphoma (see text). The onset of tumour regression coincided with the antibody-induced clearance of serum idiotype.

anti-idiotype antibodies alone or in combination with interferon-α produced 15–25 per cent complete remissions lasting more than five years (Brown *et al.* 1989). Most other patients had marked temporary remissions curtailed by the emergence of idiotype-negative mutant lymphoma cells, as was seen in previous animals studies. Antitumour effects were not improved by concurrent chemotherapy, so more recent efforts have focused on vaccination of patients in remission after chemotherapy, using monoclonal IgG derived from the patient's own tumour cells along with adjuvants. This approach has the advantage of inducing both humoral and cellular immunity in some patients. In the first excursion of antibody therapy into popular literature, Robin Cook described the dramatic application of idiotype vaccination in his medical thriller *Fever*.

19.4.4 Problems encountered during clinical trials

In addition to the emergence of antigen-negative mutants, several other problems undermining the therapeutic value of the antitumour antibodies arose during clinical trials. These included hypersensitivity reactions to the murine protein in some patients and transient fevers apparently caused by the presence in the circulation of substances released from dying tumour cells. More seriously, patients who were not severely immunosuppressed produced antibodies that bound to and neutralized the injected mouse monoclonal antibodies, thus making further therapy with the antibody pointless. The use of human monoclonal antibodies produced by conventional immunization or by means of genetic engineering ('humanized') should avoid the development of an immune response to the constant domains of a therapeutic antibody. However, anti-idiotypic antibodies, i.e. those that recognize the unique determinants associated with the antigen-binding site of the antibody, may also be generated in patients.

The effectiveness of the antibody treatment was also reduced by the formation of complexes between the infused antibody and target antigens shed from the tumour cell surface. In some patients, this occurred even with target antigens that are not normally shed at high levels because the tumour cell destruction that followed attachment of antibodies and subsequent attack by host effector systems itself tended to raise the systemic level of free antigen.

There is no good solution to the problem of antigen shedding.

Another obstacle encountered in clinical trials was the phenomenon of antigenic modulation. Some cell surface components, when cross-linked by antibodies, are actively internalized by the cell in a matter of minutes or are shed from the cell surface. This reduces the number of molecules of target antigen available for binding by the antibody and may allow the cell to escape killing as the modulated antigen is re-expressed only when antibody is no longer present some days later. Since the cross-linking of target antigens that leads to modulation is a consequence of the bivalency of the antibody molecule, one way to avoid this problem is to use monovalent antitumour antibodies.

19.4.5 Bispecific antibodies

Cytotoxic and helper T lymphocytes are normally activated by antigen only in association with surface antigens of the major histocompatibility complex (MHC) (see Chapter 16). However, T cells can also be activated independently of MHC antigen involvement, by monoclonal antibodies that bind to and cross-link the T cell receptor–CD3 complex or other 'accessory' molecules on the T cell surface (see Chapter 16). Bispecific antibody constructs that combine the activating antibody and an antitumour monoclonal antibody have been created by chemical methods and by hybridoma and recombinant DNA technology. In the first case, bispecific $F(ab')_2$ antibodies are constructed by chemical cross-linking of $F(ab')$ fragments prepared by papain digestion and reduction of the parent antibodies. Alternatively, the two parent hybridomas are fused to form a 'quadroma' which may secrete a bispecific, intact IgG molecule. Bispecific single-chain 'mini-antibodies' have been produced by splicing together two single-chain Fv genes with a short piece of DNA encoding a flexible linker peptide.

These hybrid molecules bring the T cell and the tumour cell into close apposition and activate the effector programme of the T cells (Fig. 19.11). This is called 'effector cell retargeting' because T cells of any specificity are redirected against tumour cells by the bispecific antibody. Because cross-linking of the 'activating' molecule on the T cell is necessary and bispecific antibodies have only a single anti-T cell arm, only those bispecific antibodies that are already bound to tumour cells, and so presented as a multimolecular array, will activate the T cells. Unbound bispecific antibodies in the bloodstream do not cross-link T cell receptors, so inappropriate systemic T cell activation is avoided (Fig. 19.11).

T cells activated by bispecific antibodies produce two distinct types of antitumour activity. Cytotoxic T cells triggered by antibodies against the T cell receptor (TCR) or CD2 lyse tumour cells to which they are bound by secretion of perforin. This process is called 'targeted cytolysis' (Segal *et al.* 1992). Tumour cell death and growth inhibition can also be caused by certain cytokines. Helper T cells activated through a wide range of triggering molecules, including the TCR, CD2, CD3, CD4, or CD28, secrete interferon-γ (IFN-γ) and tumour necrosis factor-α (TNF-α), which are toxic to many tumours. Both of these antitumour mechanisms have been observed in tissue culture assays and in animal models. Secretion of cytotoxic cytokines may be more important than targeted cytolysis *in vivo* for several reasons. Segal and co-workers (1992) found that fewer T cells were required to kill the same number of tumour cells *in vitro* and that tumour cells that lacked the target antigen were also killed. This is

known as a 'bystander effect' and is most important in view of the antigenic heterogeneity and limited accessibility of tumour cells in solid neoplasms (see Section 19.2.3). Furthermore, intratumoural cytokines might activate other local effector cells, such as macrophages and neutrophils, which can also kill tumour cells (Fig. 19.11).

T cells activated with bispecific antibodies have shown good activity and specificity *in vitro* but demonstrate little efficacy against large solid tumours. The best results in animal models were achieved when the tumour cells were restricted to a single body compartment, and so the T cells could be introduced locally. Segal *et al.* (1992) observed marked antitumour effects against ovarian carcinoma restricted to the peritoneal cavity. Targeted T cells are being tested clinically in ovarian carcinoma patients and against brain tumours, where the T cells can be injected intracranially.

Targeted T cells are ineffective against most solid tumours probably because they are unable to bind the tumour endothelium and selectively extravasate at tumour sites. This problem may be overcome in some instances by infusing 'tumour-infiltrating lym-

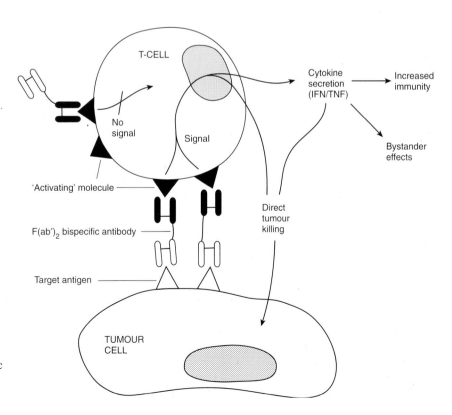

Fig. 19.11 Tumour-specific activation of T cells with bispecific antibodies.

phocytes', T cells that have been recovered from biopsies of the patient's own tumour. These cells appear to have selective homing properties towards the particular tumour from which they were derived. Alternatively, other leukocytes with better broad tumour homing properties, such as monocytes or NK cells, could be activated with bispecific antibodies against appropriate triggering molecules, including CD14 (the monocyte endotoxin receptor) and CD16 (the NK cell–IgG–Fc receptor, Ferrini *et al.* 1992).

Bispecific antibodies have also been used to bring together tumour cells and a variety of soluble anticancer agents (Fig. 19.12). Conventional chemotherapeutic drugs can be localized at the tumour site using antitumourantidrug bispecific antibodies or can be generated *de novo* in tumours from prodrugs using specific enzymes previously localized with bispecific antibodies (Fig. 19.12 and Section 19.5.3). Protein toxins and radiolabelled haptens can also be targeted with bispecific antibodies. The advantage of this approach over direct attachment of the antitumour agent to the antibody (see Sections 19.5 and 19.6) is that non-specific toxicity or background radioactivity in normal tissues can be decreased by allowing the bispecific antibody to clear from these sites before the free drug, toxin, or radionuclide is administered.

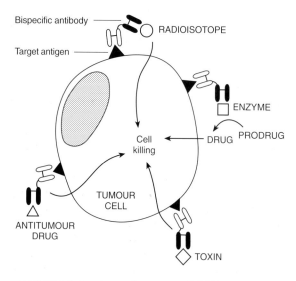

Fig. 19.12 Mechanisms of tumour cell killing with bispecific antibodies.

Bispecific antibody
Target antigen
RADIOISOTOPE
ENZYME
PRODRUG
DRUG
Cell killing
TUMOUR CELL
ANTITUMOUR DRUG
TOXIN

19.5 Targeting of cytotoxic agents

19.5.1 Principles

In general, the anticancer drugs now in clinical use do not discriminate between malignant and normal cells (see Chapter 18). Most exert their effects on dividing cells so that tumour growth is inhibited but the dose of drug that can be used is limited by its toxicity to the normal tissues of the body that need to divide frequently, e.g. gastrointestinal epithelium and the haemopoietic cells of the bone marrow.

The aim of drug targeting is to deliver the cytotoxic drug to the tumour and only expose the rest of the body to a low level of the drug, so preventing harm to normal tissues. Several systems for drug delivery have been explored. The most direct and well-explored approach is to link a low molecular weight drug, radionuclide, or protein toxin of plant or bacterial origin directly to a monoclonal antibody to form a cytotoxic 'immunoconjugate'. Chemotherapeutic drugs have also been targeted in two other ways. The drug can be packaged in liposomes which are then coated with the antitumour antibody, or, as in antibody-directed prodrug therapy (ADEPT), the active drug is released from its inactive prodrug precursor at the tumour site. An antibody–enzyme conjugate is injected and allowed to home to the tumour. Then, non-toxic prodrug, which is metabolized by the targeted enzyme (at the tumour cell surface) to produce fully active drug, is given. Each of these approaches has advantages and limitations and is discussed in the following sections.

19.5.2 Drug conjugates

In early studies, non-covalent complexes made by physically adsorbing chlorambucil to antitumour antibodies were found to kill appropriate tumour cell targets in tissue culture and in mice more efficiently than the free drug or antibody alone. The antitumour effects were later shown to be caused not by drug targeting, but synergism between free drug and antibody after dissociation of the complex. The synergy probably arises because the drug impairs the cell's capacity to repair plasma membrane damage caused by antibody and complement.

To prevent dissociation, covalent bonds have been used to link numerous anticancer agents (e.g. adriamycin, daunomycin, methotrexate, and vindesine) directly to antitumour antibodies. In most cases, the cytotoxicity of the conjugate to target cells *in vitro* exceeded that to cells lacking the target antigen, but the cytotoxic potency of the conjugate was invariably low. These drugs have intracellular sites of action and enter cells by simple diffusion or active transport. Once linked to the antibody, however, they cannot enter the cell by their usual route. Antibody–drug conjugates bind to target antigens on the cell surface, enter the cell in endocytic vesicles, and are degraded by enzymes when the vesicles coalesce with lysosomes. Thus, the low potency of these conjugates may have been because too few drug molecules had originally localized at the cell surface to enter by this route or because drug release by lysosomal enzymes was inefficient.

Much progress has been made in devising ways to accelerate the rate of drug release once internalization has taken place by increasing the susceptibility of the covalent linkage between drug and carrier to hydrolysis. Daunomycin directly linked to albumin is not released by lysosomal enzymes but if a proteinase-sensitive peptide spacer is interspersed between the drug and the carrier, drug release occurs rapidly. Similarly, acid-labile linkages between drug and antibody can improve potency, presumably because the drug dissociates from the conjugate when exposed to the acidic milieu of the lysosome. Trail and colleagues (1993) used an acid-sensitive hydrazone bond to link doxorubicin to a chimeric mouse–human anti-Le^y antibody, BR96. BR96–doxorubicin cured a majority of nude mice and rats bearing established subcutaneous and disseminated Le^y-positive colorectal carcinomas. The superiority of this conjugate over other similar reagents is not fully understood but is probably a result of the novel linker used, which introduced a thioether linkage for high serum stability, and the high density (200 000 molecules per cell) and rapid internalization of the Le^y epitope. The construction and properties of antibody–drug conjugates have been reviewed by Pietersz and McKenzie (1992).

Only about 10 drug molecules can be attached covalently to an antibody molecule without diminishing its antigen-binding capacity. To raise the potency of antibody–drug conjugates, a carrier molecule such as human serum albumin, poly-L-glutamic acid, or dextran can be used. If the carrier molecule is linked to the carbohydrate side chains of the antibody, which occur only in the Fc portion of the IgG molecule, large carriers loaded with doz-

ens of drug molecules can be attached without significantly decreasing antibody-binding affinity. Such conjugates are more effective antitumour agents *in vitro* and *in vivo*. Despite this, the relative weakness of most antibody–drug conjugates had led investigators to seek other means of increasing specific drug delivery to tumours.

19.5.3 Antibody-directed enzyme–prodrug therapy (ADEPT)

One way of increasing the dose of drug at tumour sites is to exploit the amplification effect of enzymatic catalysis. This emerging field has recently been reviewed by Senter and colleagues (1993). The ADEPT approach evolved out of a large body of research in the pharmaceutical industry on pharmacologically inactive drug precursors, or prodrugs. Chemists had designed a wide range of prodrugs intended to be selectively activated at tumour sites, but similarities between neoplastic and normal tissues made it difficult to find tumour-associated enzymes for specific prodrug activation. A solution to this problem is to use antibodies to deliver specific enzymes to the tumour cell surface. ADEPT is a multistep procedure whereby an antitumour antibody–enzyme conjugate is injected and allowed to home to the tumour for 24–48 hours. During this period, levels of unbound conjugate in the circulation and normal organs drop towards baseline, so that systemically administered prodrug is primarily activated by tumour-bound enzyme.

The ADEPT approach has several advantages (Fig. 19.13). Firstly, efficient internalization of conjugates by tumour cells (essential for immunotoxins and drug conjugates) is not required; indeed, non-internalizing membrane antigens are preferable targets for ADEPT. Secondly, enzymatic activation results in a large number of drug molecules generated per conjugate molecule, perhaps many thousands. Lastly, because active drug is generated in the tumour interstitial space (as opposed to intracellularly, as with drug conjugates), it can diffuse freely through surrounding tumour tissues and kill tumour cells that did not bind the original antibody–enzyme conjugate (a bystander effect).

Several enzymes have been used in ADEPT protocols in preclinical animal models (Senter *et al.* 1993). An alkaline phosphatase–anticarcinoma antibody conjugate displayed significant activity against human colon and lung carcinoma xenografts in nude

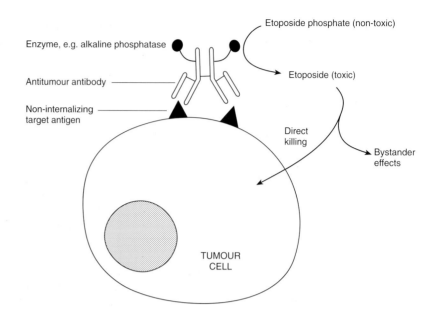

Fig. 19.13 Antibody-directed enzyme–prodrug therapy (ADEPT).

mice when combined with the prodrug etoposide phosphate (Fig. 19.13). Phosphorylation renders etoposide too hydrophilic to pass through lipid bilayers, so the prodrug cannot enter and kill cells. Phosphorylated prodrugs derived from mitomycin C, doxorubicin, and phenol mustard produced similar antitumour effects with the same antibody–alkaline phosphatase conjugate, illustrating the potential of ADEPT for combination chemotherapy with mechanistically distinct anticancer agents using a single antibody-based reagent.

Alkaline phosphatase is not a suitable enzyme for ADEPT in the clinic because it is present in many healthy human tissues, so toxic amounts of phosphorylated prodrug could become activated before reaching the tumour (Senter *et al.* 1993). Bagshawe and co-workers (1988) used the bacterial enzyme carboxypeptidase G2 for the activation of the glutamic acid derivative of benzoic acid mustard. Pronounced antitumour activity was seen, even in mice with tumours that were resistant to tolerable doses of benzoic acid mustard, suggesting that enzymatic generation at tumour sites can result in exceptionally high intratumoural drug concentrations. Two problems were observed in this system. The non-mammalian enzyme was highly immunogenic in patients, so immunosuppressive therapy might also be required. Although optimal tumour enzyme levels were achieved after 24 hours, sufficient conjugate remained in the bloodstream to activate toxic

amounts of prodrug for several days. Sharma and her colleagues (1990) solved this problem by injecting an anti-enzyme antibody after 24 hours, prior to prodrug administration. The antibody neutralized enzyme activity in the blood but also to some extent, in the tumour, but, if the anti-enzyme antibody was derivatized with galactose it was cleared so quickly by liver galactose receptors that it did not reach any extravascular sites and so cleared only the unbound, circulating conjugate.

19.5.4 Liposomes

Liposomes are lipid vesicles of varying size and structural complexity within which a range of polar, non-polar and amphipathic drugs can be encapsulated. Encapsulation protects the drug from metabolic degradation and protects normal tissues from non-specific drug toxicity. However, because of the tendency of their lipid bilayers to interact with cellular surfaces, liposomes are taken up extremely rapidly by phagocytic cells in the blood. This limitation precluded the original liposomes for cancer therapy, but renewed interest now centres on modified liposomes with greatly prolonged plasma half-lives. Papahadjopoulos and his colleagues (1991) produced sterically stabilized 'stealth' liposomes by grafting on to the lipids a highly water-soluble polymer, polyethylene glycol (PEG). The presence of PEG in the lipid bilayer exerts long-range repulsion between liposomes and cell membranes, thus allowing the stealth liposomes to avoid the reticuloendothelial system and persist in the circulation with half-lives of 12–24 hours, rather than 30 minutes.

Apart from short circulation times and reticuloendothelial system uptake, liposomes have two additional limitations as drug delivery agents. Firstly, even the smallest liposomes, single unilamellar vesicles, or SUVs, are 90 nm in diameter and so only extravasate readily in tissues with discontinuous endothelium, such as liver and spleen. Small 'stealth' liposomes cross vascular barriers more easily, probably because they do not aggregate or fuse with endothelial cell membranes. Some tumours produce angiogenic cytokines that also increase vascular permeability and recent reports indicate that stealth liposomes preferentially accumulate in the tumour interstitium. None the less, it is likely that liposomes will be most effective against liver tumours and hepatic metastases from other primary sites. Secondly, liposomes have no inherent target-cell specificity. Many investigators have sought to impart such binding selectivity by coupling antibodies to liposomes to form 'immunoliposomes' (Wright and Huang 1989). Acylated (lipophilic) antibodies can be introduced directly into the bilayer during liposome formation or thiolated antibodies can be cross-linked to the polar head of fatty acid molecules with heterobifunctional reagents. Alternatively, liposomes can be derivatized with Protein A or biotin and subsequently bound to antibodies of the appropriate isotype (see Section 19.1.2) or cross-linked to any biotinylated antibody with streptavidin. Immunoliposomes show good target-cell specificity and drug delivery *in vitro* (Wright and Huang 1989), and, in mice, stealth immunoliposomes loaded with doxorubicin were capable of eradicating small lung tumours (Ahmad *et al.* 1993).

19.5.5 Radionuclides

The radionuclide most commonly used for therapy is ^{131}I, which, in addition to emitting γ-radiation that is useful for radioimaging, emits high energy β-particles, which can penetrate tissues to a distance spanning many cell diameters. This is important for two reasons. Firstly, the radioisotope does not need to be internalized to kill the cell. Secondly, the emissions can kill 'bystander' cells that surround the targeted cell, allowing the destruction of neighbouring malignant cells that do not bear the target antigen and of cells in poorly vascularized tumours. Other β-emitters which could be useful for radiotherapy include phosphorous-32 and yttruim-90.

Two groups of investigators have carried out successful clinical trials with ^{131}I-labelled antibodies. Press and his colleagues (1993) exploited advances in tumour imaging (see Section 19.3.3) and bone marrow transplantation to devise an effective therapeutic regimen for patients with advanced B cell lymphoma. Patients were first injected with monoclonal antibodies against the B cell markers CD20 or CD37 which were labelled with trace amounts of ^{131}I. The dose of radiation absorbed by the tumours and normal tissues was estimated from gamma camera images and biopsies. Only those patients whose tumours received significantly greater irradiation than the liver, lungs, or kidney were eligible for infusion with therapeutic doses of the same antibodies labelled with much higher levels of ^{131}I. The pretreatment imaging procedure thus allowed the investigators to restrict the trial to those patients (about 40 per cent of the total) whose tumours expressed high levels of target antigens and were readily accessible to intravenously administered conjugate. In addition, the optimal dose of antibody could also be determined before treatment. Press *et al.* (1993) calculated that the amount of antibody required to saturate tumour-binding sites would also result in bone marrow toxicity, so samples of the patients' own bone marrow were frozen and reinfused after therapy. Using this aggressive approach, these investigators obtained complete remissions in over 80 per cent of cases and over half of those treated remained disease free up to four years (Press *et al.* 1993).

Kaminski and his colleagues (1993) adopted a slightly different approach to radioimmunotherapy of B cell lymphoma. They treated 10 patients with ^{131}I–anti-CD20 using a much lower dose of the radionuclide. There was no bone marrow suppression at this dose, so bone marrow transplantation was not required. Patients with a favourable distribution of labelled antibody were selected by a similar preimaging procedure to Press *et al.*, but more efficient delivery of the radioconjugate to tumour cells was achieved by presaturating the competing CD20 antigen on more accessible normal B cells in the blood and spleen with a large excess of cold anti-CD20 antibody (Kaminski *et al.* 1993). Four patients with bulky, chemotherapy-resistant disease had complete remissions, but it likely that the unlabelled anti-CD20 antibody was at least partially responsible for these remarkable antitumour effects. Unconjugated anti-CD20 antibody alone caused regressions of a human B lymphoma xenograft in nude mice, perhaps through an inhibitory or apoptotic signalling pathway (see Section 19.4.1). CD20 is a part of the B cell antigen receptor complex that regulates growth and differentiation.

In contrast to the impressive results in lymphoma patients, the ^{131}I-labelled anti-TAG72 antibody CC49 produced no objective tumour responses in 15 colorectal carcinoma patients (Murray *et al.* 1994). This disappointing result reflects the poor permeation of solid epithelial tumour masses by large antibody molecules (see Section 19.2.3) so the CC49 antibody has now been genetically engineered as a single-chain Fv (scFv) fragment that displays markedly improved penetration of large solid tumours (Yokota *et al.* 1992).

Radionuclides also irradiate normal tissues as they circulate through the body in conjugated form and as metabolites. For effective use, the antibody–radionuclide conjugate should localize well within the tumour and not be retained within normal tissues. The recent improvements in methods for tumour imaging offer ways in which non-specific irradiation during therapy can be minimized. A general approach to increase the dose of radiolabelled antibody that localizes in tumour, and to reduce the exposure of uninvolved tissues to radiation, is to administer the antibody to the patient by routes allowing either more direct or more complete access to the tumour than the intravenous route. Regional therapy is possible for neoplasms that are localized in discrete body regions such as the cerebrospinal space (neuroblastoma) or in the peritoneum (ovarian carcinoma). In patients with ovarian carcinoma treated with radiolabelled monoclonal antibody to HMFG antigen, the intraperitoneal route of administration gave consistently higher uptake of radionuclide by ascitic tumour cells than the intravenous route. The intravenous route gave better uptake by solid tumour deposits in the peritoneum because the antibody was unable to reach the deposits except through the vasculature supplying the tumour. Extensive studies have shown that antibody localization to lymph nodes is enhanced by intralymphatic administration. Finally, infusion through the carotid artery may be exploited for the radiotherapy of intracranial malignancies such as gliomas, which are not readily reached by antibodies in the general circulation. It should be noted, however, that there is no ready alternative to systemic therapy in the case of widespread metastatic disease.

Alpha-particles may be more effective cytotoxic agents since they dissipate more energy than β-particles in a path length of only one or two cell diameters, and therefore have an exceedingly powerful cytotoxic action. Possible candidates for targeting include astatine-211 and bismuth-212. An alternative is to target atoms of a non-radioactive isotope of boron (^{10}B) to cells. When this nuclide is subsequently irradiated with low energy thermal neutrons, it undergoes nuclear fission liberating a high-energy α-particle *in situ*. Unfortunately, thermal neutrons penetrate tissue so poorly that this approach to targeting seems to have limited application.

19.5.6 Immunotoxins

Bacterial toxins (e.g. diphtheria toxin, *Pseudomonas* exotoxin) and the plant toxins, ricin and abrin, are extremely potent; a single molecule appears to be sufficient to kill a cell if it enters the cytoplasm. These toxins have a similar molecular architecture, each consisting of two polypeptide chains, A and B, joined by a single disulphide bond, and they bind to virtually all cells of higher animals by means of the B chain. The membrane-bound toxin is taken into the cell by endocytosis and the A chain is then translocated across the membrane of the endocytic vesicle into the cytoplasm where it inactivates the cell's machinery for protein synthesis (Fig. 19.14).

There are three main ways in which toxins have been linked to antibodies to create 'immunotoxins' that are specifically cytotoxic.

The first, and by far the most widely used way to form immunotoxins, is to attach the isolated A chain of the toxin directly to the antibody. Alternatively, instead of the A chain, use can be made of one of the naturally occurring single chain ribosome-damaging proteins (e.g. saporin) whose action on ribosomes is identical to that of ricin A chain. It is necessary to join the antibody and the A chain by means of an introduced disulphide bond to allow for release of the A chain from the antibody by endogenous thiols. A-chain release is necessary in order to inhibit ribosomal protein synthesis. A-chain immunotoxins are almost wholly selective in their toxic effect upon target cells in tissue culture. The main problem with this type of immunotoxin is that the toxicity to target cells varies greatly depending on the antigenic determinant recognized, the type of target cell, and its stage in the cell cycle. The reasons underlying these differences are not understood but are presumed to reflect the pathway by which the A-chain immunotoxin enters the cell and the influence of the metabolic status of the cell upon that process. A decade of development during the 1980s resulted in second generation A chain-type immunotoxins. These immunotoxins employ stronger cross-linkers to prevent premature release of toxin A chain, are made from non-glycosylated toxins to prevent hepatic entrapment and hepatotoxicity, and have improved purity. Second generation immunotoxins show substantially increased antitumour activity in animal models, commonly inducing cures of established ascitic tumours and subcutaneous tumour nodules up to 7 mm in diameter (Vitetta *et al.* 1993).

The second way to prepare an immunotoxin is to link the intact toxin to the antibody. These immunotoxins have the advantage that they are consistently highly toxic to cells with the appropriate antigens, but suffer from poor specificity because the toxin moiety can bind to non-target cells. These constructs, therefore, tend to be highly poisonous to animals. One way to diminish non-specific toxicity is to synthesize 'blocked' ricin immunotoxins in which the galactose-binding sites of the toxin have been blocked using affinity labels made of a chemically reactive group coupled to a galactose-containing oligosaccharide. An anti-CD19-blocked ricin immunotoxin killed greater than 99.99 per cent of CD19-positive human B lymphoma cells *in vitro* and significantly prolonged the survival of SCID mice bearing human lymphoma xenografts in the peritoneal cavity, ovaries, brain, bone marrow, muscle, and lymph nodes (Shah *et al.* 1993).

The third, and the most recent, method for forming immunotoxins is by making recombinant bifunctional fusion proteins. The genes for the antibody are spliced together with the gene for the toxin and expressed in *E. coli* as a single molecule (Pastan and Fitzgerald 1991). The toxin moieties used to date are bacterial toxins (CRM-45, DAB-486, or PE-40) which have been truncated to remove their cell binding sites. The targeting moieties have included antibody scFv and a variety of growth factors (e.g. IL-2, IL-6, GM-CSF, EGF) whose receptors are up-regulated on tumour cells. Recombinant immunotoxins are highly stable in the blood because they contain

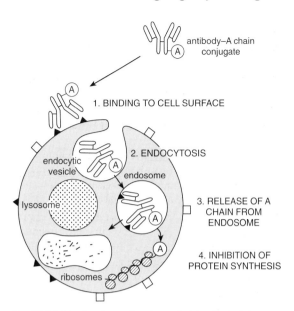

Fig. 19.14 Mechanism of action of ricin A chain immunotoxins.

no reducible disulphide bonds and can be relatively cheaply produced by large-scale culture of recombinant bacteria. Such immunotoxins have similar or superior antitumour activity in nude mouse models to biochemically prepared immunotoxins (Pastan and Fitzgerald 1991).

The results of the first phase I clinical trial of immunotoxins were published in 1987. By 1993, 377 patients had been treated with 11 different immunotoxins in 15 phase I/II trials (Vitetta *et al.* 1993). Phase I/II clinical trials are carried out in patients with advanced, bulky disease who have failed all currently available therapies. As a consequence, few if any clinical responses are expected; the primary purpose is to examine drug toxicity and determine the maximum tolerated dose. Indeed, 95 per cent of drugs in current use for cancer therapy produced less than 5 per cent response rates in phase I trials. Immunotoxins have proved remarkably potent against lymphomas and leukaemias: 41 out of 237 (over 17 per cent) of patients achieved partial or complete remissions. Ricin A chain, blocked ricin, saporin, and truncated DT have all been used to prepare effective immunotoxins against these relatively accessible tumours. By contrast, very poor response rates are characteristic of trials in solid tumour patients. Of 140 patients with melanoma or carcinoma of the colon, breast, or ovary, less than 3 per cent responded to immunotoxin therapy, primarily because of inaccessibility of the cells to immunotoxins.

The side effects of immunotoxin therapy are different from those of conventional therapy or of treatment with radioactive or drug conjugates, in that there is no damage to rapidly dividing normal tissues, such as gut epithelium, hair follicles, and bone marrow. Blocked ricin and PE immunotoxins are hepatotoxic. Ricin A chain immunotoxins cause reversible myalgias and, to a dose-limiting degree, a vascular leak syndrome reminiscent of one of the side effects of IL-2 therapy (Vitetta and Thorpe 1993). Free ricin A chain apparently induces endothelial cell rounding, giving rise to intercellular gaps, increased vascular permeability, and systemic oedema.

Another problem is that immunotoxins evoke an immune response in patients unless they are immunosuppressed by prior therapy or by their disease. This limits the duration of treatment to approximately one week before antibody responses negate the benefit of the therapy.

The ultimate goal of immunotoxin therapy is to treat patients with minimal residual disease with cocktails of immunotoxins within optimized clinical regimens, as an adjuvant therapy in combination with aggressive chemotherapy.

19.5.7 Vascular targeting

Radiolabelled antibodies, drug conjugates, and immunotoxins have proved far more effective against leukaemias and lymphomas than against carcinomas and other solid tumours, both in animal models and clinical trials. The principal reason for this is the relative inaccessibility of some malignant cells in solid tumours to antibody-sized molecules. There is a low absolute uptake of antibodies into solid tumours; commonly as little as 0.01 per cent of the injected dose homes to each gram of tumour in clinical studies. Antibodies that do enter the tumour mass fail to permeate evenly through the parenchyma for several interrelated reasons, as discussed in Section 19.3.

To circumvent these problems, an attractive approach originally proposed by Denekamp (1984) would be to target the endothelial cells of the tumour vascular bed, rather than the tumour cells themselves. Tumour endothelial cells are freely accessible to intravenously administered antibodies and, being untransformed, are unlikely to give rise to antigen-negative mutants. There is also an in-built amplification effect because thousands of tumour cells rely on each capillary loop for oxygen and nutrients (Denekamp 1984). For vascular targeting to succeed, antibodies specific or selective for tumour endothelial cells are required. Nutrition of growing tumours is maintained by constant growth of new blood vessel sprouts, or angiogenesis. During angiogenesis, endothelial cells must *migrate* towards the source of the angiogenic stimulus and *proliferate* to form the new vascular bed, so endothelial cell migration and proliferation markers could be selectively up-regulated on tumour endothelial cells. Two such molecules, endosialin and endoglin (a receptor for TGF-β), have been characterized.

Although vascular targeting has several theoretical advantages over conventional approaches, this superiority had not, until recently, been tested *in vivo* because tumour endothelial cell markers in experimental animals had not been discovered. Burrows and Thorpe (1993) developed a mouse vascular targeting model using transfectant tumour cells. A neuroblastoma cell line was transfected with the mouse IFN-γ gene. When grown in nude mice, the tumour cells secreted IFN-γ which activated endothelial cells within the tumour mass to express MHC class II antigens. In animals treated with an anti-class II–ricin A chain immunotoxin, all tumour endothelial cells were killed and large solid tumours became blackened and necrotic through loss of blood supply. In contrast, an immunotoxin against the tumour cells had only minor effects (Burrows and Thorpe 1993). These studies illustrate the potential of vascular targeting and increasing research interest now centres upon the search for more specific tumour endothelial cell antigens and development of clinically relevant animal models.

19.6 Bone marrow transplantation

A number of malignant diseases, including leukaemia and lymphoma, respond to high dose chemotherapy and whole-body irradiation. This treatment is not more widely adopted because it destroys the haemopoietic stem cells of the patient's bone marrow. The limited treatment with drugs and radiation that can be given to the patient may not eradicate all tumour cells and frequently the patient relapses. Furthermore, repeated treatment with suboptimal doses of chemotherapy encourages the outgrowth of multidrug-resistant tumour cells. If higher and potentially curative doses of radiochemotherapy are to be used, the bone marrow of the patient must be reconstituted after treatment (see Chapter 17).

There are two ways to do this. In autologous bone marrow transplantation, a sample of the patient's own marrow is removed before therapy and later reimplanted on completion of the treatment. With diseases such as leukaemia or lymphoma, the marrow is infiltrated with malignant cells and so it is imperative to clear the marrow of these cells before it is returned to the patient. The alternative method, allogeneic bone marrow transplantation, is to give the patient normal bone marrow from another individual. In this case, the donor and recipient must be matched for histocompatibility antigens in order to reduce the risk of provoking graft versus host disease (GVHD), a life-threatening complication that results from the attack of host cells by T lymphocytes in the allograft. GVHD is a common occurrence even with closely matched donors and recipients. The solution to this problem is to remove or kill the T lymphocytes in the marrow of the donor before it is infused into the patient.

Bone marrow purging is performed to eliminate malignant cells from autologous marrow grafts or T lymphocytes from allogeneic marrow grafts while leaving the haemopoietic stem cells intact. This has been made possible by using antibodies recognizing antigens that are present on malignant cells or T lymphocytes but are absent from the stem cells. Three approaches have been used clinically: complement-mediated cytolysis, immunotoxins, and magnetic removal of T cells or tumour cells coated with antibody-conjugated magnetite-containing microspheres. Typically, 99.9 per cent or more of the unwanted cells can be removed using these procedures.

Two main problems have arisen with T cell purging. Firstly, the extensive depletion of T cells from allogeneic marrow results in a higher incidence of graft failure or rejection after transplantation. The reasons for this are unclear. Some T cells may need to be present in the marrow to suppress residual host immunity or to elaborate lymphokines needed for successful grafting. Secondly, there is evidence that depleting marrow grafts of T cells increases the risk of leukaemic recurrence. It is not clear whether specific T cell subsets are responsible for these problems. By choosing antigens restricted to various T cell subsets, the appropriate combinations of immu-

notoxins could selectively eliminate the subsets that promote GVHD without impairing the beneficial properties of other T cells in the marrow.

It is unclear whether the procedures will be of value in the treatment of other malignant diseases in which there is bone marrow involvement. To be successful, intense radiochemotherapy must eradicate all the clonogenic tumour cells in the patient's body or reduce them to a number that can be contained by the patient's immune and other defence mechanisms when they recover from the effects of the treatment. Other diseases that are responsive to radiochemotherapy and in which benefit might be expected from more intense treatment are lymphoma, oat cell carcinoma of the lung, carcinoma of the breast, testis, and ovary, and paediatric malignancies such as Wilms' tumour. The emergence of recombinant haemopoietic growth factors as readily available pharmaceuticals now permits oncologists to use much higher (supralethal) doses of chemotherapy followed by 'rescue' with autologous bone marrow cells in combination with r.GM-CSF or other cytokines.

19.7 Conclusion

Monoclonal antibodies have revived earlier optimism for the prospect of treating cancer by immunotherapy. Antitumour monoclonal antibodies and their conjugates with cytotoxic agents have been evaluated in patients whose tumours are resistant to conventional forms of therapy. The main value of such trials has been to ascertain the side effects of the therapy and to identify the inherent limitations to these novel pharmacological agents. The true therapeutic value may only emerge when trials are performed with antibody constructs made to improved design in patients with disease at a less advanced stage.

The principle of using antibody molecules as carriers of cytotoxic agents with no inherent tumour cell specificity is being extended to other biologically active molecules such as interleukins, interferons, and inducers of cell differentiation. Further developments in hybridoma technology and genetic engineering will allow the manipulation of the structures of therapeutically important immunoglobulins, polypeptide hormones, toxins, and enzymes, and the creation of novel antibody molecules with characteristics desirable for cancer therapy in humans. Improvements in the effectiveness of targeting are likely to stem from a better understanding of the behaviour of antibody-based agents in animals and the physiological barriers to their movement and action. Furthermore, advances in our understanding of the fundamental processes that

determine tumour growth and metastasis at the molecular level should provide new and possibly more suitable targets for antibody-mediated therapy.

References and further reading

Ahmad, I., *et al.* (1993). Antibody-targeted delivery of doxorubicin entrapped in sterically stabilized liposomes can eradicate lung cancer in mice. *Cancer Research,* **53**, 1484–8.

Bach, J. F., Fracchia, G. N., and Chatenoud, L. (1993). Safety and efficacy of therapeutic monoclonal antibodies in clinical therapy. *Immunology Today,* 421–5.

Bagshawe, K. D., *et al.* (1988). A cytotoxic agent can be generated selectively at cancer sites. *British Journal of Cancer,* **58**, 700–3.

Burrows, F. J. and Thorpe, P. E. (1993). Eradication of large solid tumors in mice with an immunotoxin directed against tumour vasculature. *Proceedings of the National Academy of Sciences, USA,* **90**, 8996–9000.

Chen, S.-Y., *et al.* (1994). Intracellular antibodies as a new class of therapeutic molecules for gene therapy. *Human Gene Therapy,* **5**, 595–601.

Denekamp, J. (1984). Vasculature as a target for tumour therapy. *Progress in Applied Microcirculation,* **4**, 28–38.

Ferrini, S., *et al.* (1992). Targeting the T or NK lymphocytes against tumour cells by bispecific monoclonal antibodies: role of different triggering molecules. *International Journal of Cancer,* **7** (Suppl.), 15–18.

Finn, O. J. (1993) Tumor-rejection antigens recognised by T lymphocytes. *Current Opinion in Immunology,* **5**, 701–8.

Hakomori, S. (1991). Possible functions of tumor-associated carbohydrate antigens. *Current Opinion in Immunology,* **3**, 646–53.

Harlow, E. and Lane, D. (1988). *Antibodies—a laboratory manual.* Cold Spring Harbor Laboratory, New York.

Kaminski, M. S., *et al.* (1993). Radio-immunotherapy of B-cell lymphoma with ^{131}I-anti-

B1 (anti CD20) antibody. *New England Journal of Medicine,* **329**, 459–65.

Larrick, J. W., *et al.* (1992). Therapeutic human antibodies derived from PCR amplification of B-cell variable regions. *Immunological Reviews,* **130**, 69–85.

Larson, S. M., *et al.* (1994). Overview of clinical radioimmunodetection of human tumors. *Cancer,* **73** (Suppl.), 832–35.

LeDoussal, J. M., *et al.* (1990). Targeting the Indium 111-labeled bivalent hapten to human melanoma mediated by bispecific monoclonal antibody conjugates. *Cancer Research,* **50**, 3445–52.

McKearn, T. J. (1993). Radioimmunodetection of solid tumors. *Cancer,* **71** (Suppl.), 4302–13.

Murray, J. L., *et al.* (1994). Phase II radioimmunotherapy trial with ^{131}I-CC49 in colorectal cancer. *Cancer,* **73**, 1057–66.

Papahadjopoulos, D., *et al.* (1991). Sterically stabilized liposomes: improvements in pharmacokinetics and antitumor therapeutics efficacy. *Proceedings of the National Academy of Sciences, USA,* **88**, 11460–4.

Pastan, I. and Fitzgerald, D. J. (1991). Recombinant toxins for cancer treatment. *Science,* **254**, 1173–7.

Pietersz, G. A. and McKenzie, I. F. C. (1992). Antibody conjugates for the treatment of cancer. *Immunological Reviews,* **129**, 57–80.

Press, O. W., *et al.* (1993). Radiolabeled antibody therapy of B-cell lymphoma with autologous bone marrow support. *New England Journal of Medicine,* **329**, 1219–24.

Riethmuller, G., *et al.* (1993). Monoclonal antibodies in cancer therapy. *Current Opinion in Immunology,* **5**, 732–9.

Segal, D. M., *et al.* (1992). Targeting of anti-tumor responses with bispecific antibodies. *Immunobiology*, **185**, 390–402.

Senter, P. D., *et al.* (1993). Generation of cytotoxic agents by targeted enzymes. *Bioconjugate Chemistry*, **4**, 3–9.

Shah, S. A., *et al.* (1993). Anti-B4-blocked ricin immunotoxin shows therapeutic efficacy in four different SCID mouse tumour models. *Cancer Research*, **53**, 1360–7.

Sharma, S. K., *et al.* (1990). Inactivation and clearance of an anti-CEA carboxypeptidase G2 conjugate in blood after localization in a xenograft model. *British Journal of Cancer*, **61**, 659–62.

Trail, P.A., *et al.* (1993). Cure of xenografted human carcinomas by BR96-doxorubicin immunoconjugates. *Science*, **261**, 212–15.

Vitetta, E. S. and Thorpe, P. E. (1991). Immunotoxins. In *Biologic therapy of cancer* (ed. V. T. DeVita, jun., S. Hellmann, and S. A. Rosenberg), pp. 482–95, J.B. Lippincott Company, New York.

Vitetta, E.S., *et al.* (1993). Immunotoxins: magic bullets or misguided missiles? *Trends in Pharmacological Sciences*, **14**, 148–54.

Winter, G. and Milstein, C. (1991). Man-made antibodies. *Nature*, **349**, 293–9.

Wright, S. and Huang, L. (1989). Antibody-directed liposomes as drug-delivery vehicles. *Advanced Drug Delivery Reviews*, **3**, 343–89.

Yefenof, E., *et al.* (1993). Cancer dormancy: isolation and characterization of dormant lymphoma cells. *Proceedings of the National Academy of Sciences, USA*, **90**, 1829–33.

Yokota, T., *et al.* (1992). Rapid tumour penetration of a single-chain Fv and comparison with other immunoglobulin forms. *Cancer Research*, **52**, 3402–8.

20

Cytokines and cancer

FRANCES R. BALKWILL

20.1 Cytokines and the cytokine network

Cytokines are important components of cellular communication in multicellular organisms. Together with hormones and neurotransmitters, they coordinate interactions between cells, particularly over a short range. Cytokines play a major role in orchestrating the immune response where they act in a complex, overlapping, but tightly controlled, network. Cytokines also participate in the control of growth and development in the embryo, and in later life they participate in wound healing and inflammation. Some cytokines are a vital component of non-specific host responses against virus infection.

The term 'cytokine' embraces well over one hundred short-acting, transiently produced polypeptides whose main characteristics are listed in Table 20.1. Interleukins (ILs) 1–18 (and counting), interferons (IFNs), tumour necrosis factors (TNFs), colony-stimulating factors (CSFs), growth factors, chemokines, and many other proteins whose name ends in 'factor' can be called cytokines. Most cytokines have a range of activities but many have been named after the first activity that identified them. Thus, these names do not necessarily describe their most important functions *in vitro* or *in vivo*. For instance,

an interleukin may not control just communication between leucocytes and an interferon will have many other properties apart from inducing an antiviral state in cells. The cytokine IL-6 was first identified as a B cell differentiation factor but is now known to act in haemopoietic, endocrine, hepatic, and neural systems as well.

Production of cytokines is tightly controlled at several levels; transcription, translation, secretion, and, sometimes, activation of precursor. Moreover, the active protein can be rapidly neutralized by binding to soluble receptors, causing internalization of the receptors into the cell, and extracellular degradation. With such complex control, it is not surprising that inappropriate cytokine production is thought to be involved in the pathogenesis of some autoimmune and malignant diseases, and acute and chronic infections.

20.1.1 Cytokine receptors

Most cytokines bear little resemblance to each other at the level of DNA and amino acid, but some three-dimensional structural homology is seen. This is reflected in the fact that cytokine receptors form distinct families whose members include several hormones as well. Studies on cytokine receptor protein structure and amino acid sequence have identified at least four distinct receptor groups. The immunoglo-

Table 20.1 Characteristics of cytokines

Low molecular weight (8–70 kDa) polypeptides

Monomers, heterodimers, homodimers, or trimers

Intercellular signalling molecules

Control tissue development and repair, immunity, and inflammation

Bind to specific receptor complexes on cell surface

Receptors form distinct families

Interact in a complex network

Multiple and redundant activities

Aberrant production contributes to disease

bulin superfamily includes receptors for IL-1α and -1β, M-CSF, and platelet-derived growth factor (PDGF). Its members are characterized by three domains in the extracellular portion of the molecule, and a common three-dimensional structure of two β sheets held together by a disulphide bond. The cysteine residues involved in formation of this disulphide bond are highly conserved and occur in almost the same location in all family members.

The largest receptor family, usually called the haemopoietin or cytokine receptor superfamily, comprises the IL-2β and -γ receptors and those for IL-3, -4, -5, -6, -7, -9, -11, leukaemia inhibitory factor (LIF), G- and GM-CSF, prolactin, growth hormone and erythropoietin. These receptors are all type 1 membrane glycoproteins, with their N-termini outside the plasma membrane and a single hydrophobic transmembrane domain. The major region of homology occurs in the extracellular, ligand-binding domain, and is contained within a stretch of about 210 amino acids. There are four common cysteine residues located in the N-terminal half of the molecule, and a Trp–Ser–X–Trp–Ser motif located just above the transmembrane domain. These features are found in all members except IL-7, which lacks two of the cysteine residues, and the growth hormone receptor, which lacks the Trp–Ser–X–Trp–Ser motif. The IL-6 receptor also has an N-terminal immunoglobulin-like domain.

The TNF receptor superfamily is distinct from the above and, apart from the two receptors that bind both TNF-α and -β, includes nerve growth factor receptor, CD30 and CD40, Fas, and some viral proteins, which, in their soluble form, can bind TNF. The cysteine-rich extracellular portion is folded into a repeating domain structure. Members of this superfamily have cysteine residues at particular posi-

tions in the primary structure. Other amino acids such as tyrosine, glycine, and proline are also at conserved positions.

Chemokines are small inflammatory cytokines that are best known for their ability to attract lymphocytes, macrophages, and neutrophils. Receptors for chemokines such IL-8, MIP-1α, and GRO belong to the rhodopsin superfamily of seven transmembrane G-protein receptors. Ligand binding to these receptors is complex with multiple cytokines binding to a single receptor and multiple cytokines binding to a specific ligand. The β-adrenergic receptor is also a member of this family.

Many cytokine receptors are complexes, consisting of a 'private' ligand-binding molecule, which is specific for an individual cytokine, and a 'public' signal transducer, which is shared by several cytokines. For instance IL-6, LIF, oncostatin M, and IL-11 all use a public signal transducer, gp130, and the IL-2 receptor γ is also involved in IL-4 and IL-7 signal transduction. The general characteristics of such receptors are described in Table 20.2. It is now clear that the pleiotropy and redundancy of cytokines can be explained on the basis of the molecular structures of cytokine receptors.

20.1.2 Control of the cytokine network

The most distinctive, and often confusing, characteristics of cytokines are the number of different actions an individual cytokine can have, at least *in vitro*, their apparent redundancy in activity; and their ability to interact with one another. These interactions cannot at present be called a cascade because there is little evidence that cytokines act in a particular temporal sequence. A more appropriate term would seem to be a cytokine network. Cytokine production and the induction of other members of the network is very tightly regulated. The major ele-

Table 20.2 General characteristics of some cytokine receptors

'Private' ligand-binding receptor

'Public' signal transducer

Cytokine induced homo- or hetero-dimerization

Activation of Jaks and Stats

Induction of ras–MAP kinase cascade

Activation of cytoplasmic and/or nuclear transcription factors

ments of control that have been identified so far are listed in Table 20.3.

These levels of control may vary from cytokine to cytokine. However, the general principle is that cytokines induce the transient, tightly controlled, and local production of other cytokines or their inactive precursors. Control at the level of receptor expression includes the shedding of receptor molecules from the cell surface to form soluble receptors, which may also be generated *de novo* by alternate splicing of the receptor mRNA. The biological function of these cytokine-binding proteins is not clear, but they circulate at nanogram levels in the blood. At least one cytokine family, IL-1α and -1β, also contains a receptor antagonist. This polypeptide is closely related to the two active forms of the cytokine, binds to the receptor, but does not transmit a signal. The differential regulation of the receptor antagonist and functional cytokines make it likely that it represents another level of control of the cytokine network.

20.1.3 Actions of cytokines on cell growth, death, and differentiated function

As described above, individual cytokines generally show a number of actions *in vitro*, but there is a high degree of redundancy in these. All cytokines control cell growth, death, and survival in some way, but their actions on differentiated function appear to be more distinct. Some of the *in vitro* actions of cytokines are described in Table 20.4.

The overall result of exposure to a cytokine *in vitro* or *in vivo* is highly dependent on the context in which the cell receives the signal. A good example of this would be the effect of TNF-α on endothelium. A spectrum of activities has been recorded, ranging from stimulation of growth, induction of

Table 20.3 Control of the cytokine network

Cytokines regulate the production of other cytokines
Cytokines transmodulate cytokine receptors
Cytokine action generally local
Strict and complex controls of transcription and translation
Post-translational modification intracellularly and extracellularly
Transient induction
Soluble forms of cytokine receptors
Receptor antagonists
Alleles may be associated with levels of production

Table 20.4 Some in vitro actions of cytokines

Proliferation (including stimulation of haemopoietic colony formation)
Survival
Cytostasis
Apoptosis
Differentiation
Effects on metabolism
Motility
Adhesion to other cells
Adhesion to basement membrane
Protease/protease inhibitor secretion
Control of Th1/Th2 pathways
Generation of specific and non-specific cytotoxic cells
Regulation of antibody production
Phagocytosis
Resistance to virus infection
Production of other cytokines/cytokine receptors
Activation of osteoclasts

procoagulant activity, and alterations in surface antigen expression, to changes in morphology, cytostasis, or induction of apoptosis (see Glossary). The outcome of TNF-α binding to its receptors on endothelial cells is dependent on the dose of cytokine, the proliferative state of the cells, and the presence of other cytokines.

The multiplicity and redundancy of actions *in vitro* has made it difficult to determine the *in vivo* function of an individual cytokine and the reason for the existence of so many different cytokine molecules. The powerful technique of homologous recombination, with the ability to eliminate individual cytokine genes, has been important in clarifying these questions. There are now strains of 'knockout' mice with specific deficiencies for cytokines such as IL-2, IL-4, TGF-β, TGF-α, IFN-γ, lymphotoxin, LIF, and some cytokine receptors, e.g. IFN-γ and TNFRp55. While defects in these mice vary in severity, some generalizations can be made.

It would appear that few cytokines are essential for normal fetal development, and none appear to be essential for T cell development, apart from lymphotoxin, which appears to be central to the development of peripheral lymphoid organs. Mice unable to make this cytokine lack lymph nodes and Peyer's patches but show normal CD4:CD8 ratios in blood. Mice defective in TGF-β show a range of autoimmune phenomena and overexpress several cytokines, confirming the down-regulatory role of this cytokine in the network. At the other extreme, mice deficient in TGF-α are normal apart from wavy whiskers and hair associated with disorganized hair follicles, and are able to repair wounds normally. Mice deficient in IL-2 have a 40-fold increase in circulating IgG1 and those deficient in IL-4 are unable to make IgE. LIF knock-out mice appear normal apart from a retarded growth rate and decreased numbers of haemopoietic stem cells, but are infertile as a result of a failure of ovarian implantation. It appears that uterine expression of this cytokine (originally identified as a factor that inhibited differentiation of leukaemia cells) is necessary on the fourth day of gestation for implantation of the embryo. Mice deficient in either IFN-γ or one of its receptors have increased susceptibility to intracellular parasites, defective macrophage nitric oxide production, and decreased macrophage class II MHC. Several different types of cytokine knock-out mice develop inflammatory bowel disease in later life. This suggests that a range of subtle immune deficiencies might result in disease at the site of major antigenic challenge in the body.

20.1.4 Current concept of the cytokine network

Cytokines can thus be viewed as components of an intercellular signalling language, with the action of an individual cytokine being contextual. Many actions of individual cytokines are redundant, but one or more actions are unique and thus have ensured the survival of the protein during vertebrate evolution.

20.2 Cytokine networks in cancer

Whether used as therapy or produced locally during the development of a cancer, cytokines can act on tumour cells, tumour stroma and the host. Cytokines influence many aspects of tumour cell biology, including proliferation, survival and death, motility, surface antigen expression, and cell–cell or cell–matrix interactions. They may also control neovascularization, extracellular matrix synthesis, leucocyte infiltration, stromal cell proliferation, and local immune response. Finally, the cytokine context of a tumour can affect local nutritional balance, systemic metabolism, and host

immune status (see Table 20.5). Imbalances in the cytokine network are to be expected in tumours where there is genetic damage to cytokine ligands and/or receptors. In addition, many components of cytokine pathways have been identified as proto-oncogenes or tumour suppressor genes.

20.2.1 The endogenous cytokine network in ovarian cancer

One of the tumours in which the cytokine network is being examined is human epithelial ovarian cancer. This tumour microenvironment is rich in mRNA for growth factors, pro-inflammatory cytokines, and chemokines, but weak in lymphocyte-associated cytokines. Potential autocrine loops exist for several cytokines including IL-1, IGF-1, M-CSF, GM-CSF, and TFN-α. Receptors for at least two cytokines, IL-4 and IFN-γ are expressed in the absence of ligand. The cytokine mRNA profile of ovarian cancer cell lines is similar apart from the chemokines RANTES, MIP-1α, and MIP-1β, which are expressed in biopsies, but rarely detected in cell lines, suggesting that their role may be in tumour/stroma communication. Cytokines whose expression is maintained in the epithelial tumour cells after tissue culture or xenotransplantation may contribute to key survival/growth loops and may be targets for therapy. The redundancy of the network would suggest that targeting a single endogenous cytokine may prove ineffective. However, a combination of cytokines and inhibitors, delivered systemically or locally, could provide a greater degree of specificity whether the desired result is apoptotic tumour cell death; destruction of the tumour vasculature;

Table 20.5 Activities endogenous cytokines in tumours may influence

Cell proliferation
Cell viability/death
Cell motility
Surface antigen expression
Angiogenesis
Extracellular matrix synthesis
Immune response
Nutritional balance
Systemic metabolic state
Systemic immune state

induction of a tumour-specific host immune resopnse; or, optimally, a combination of all three.

20.2.2 Functional significance of local cytokines

As described in Table 20.5, the local cytokines could influence many aspects of tumour cell behaviour and orchestrate communication with the stroma. Defining the roles of individual cytokines is, however, difficult. The action of individual cytokines is contextual, the response of a cell or tissue being dependent on a variety of factors such as cytokine concentration, proliferative and nutritional status of the cell/tissue, and the presence of other cytokines. Thus, an individual cytokine may signal growth, differentiation, movement, cytostasis, or death depending on the context in which the cell/tissue 'reads' its message. *In vitro* studies with single cell populations and cytokines may have little significance to the *in vivo* reality. Three ways in which this information can be obtained are apparent: the use of animal models; the correlation of endogenous cytokines with other parameters such as infiltrating cells, stromal support elements, and extracellular matrix; and the prognostic significance of levels of various cytokines and their receptors.

Animal studies Animal studies suggest that TNF plays a role in tumour invasion and spread in ovarian cancer. In one animal model, injection of TNF generates many elements of solid tumour stroma around small clusters of tumour cells. Free-floating tumour cells become solid intraperitoneal tumours with connective tissue, fibroblast, and blood vessel support. In addition, transfection of TNF into tumour cells, can, in some cases, enhance their invasive capacity, as can pretreatment of tumour cells before IV injection. There is some experimental evidence that chemokines such as MCP-1 can alter the host cell content of tumours. Transfection of the gene for this chemokine into a murine transplantable tumour results in increased macrophage infiltration and tumour growth inhibition, which is proportional to MCP-1 production by individual lines. Conversely, a role for macrophages in tumour cell growth and viability is suggested by an experiment in which Chinese hamster ovary (CHO) cells were transfected with IL-10. The cells lost tumorigenicity both in nude and SCID mice in an IL-10 dose-dependent manner. Histological examination revealed that CHO wild-type tumours were substantially infiltrated with macrophages, but CHO–IL-10 tumours were virtually macrophage free. Cell populations from murine transplantable tumours have been transfected with a number of other cytokine genes. Local expression of cytokines that are capable of stimulating an immune or inflammatory response, particularly IL-2, IL-4, IP-10, and IL-12, discourages tumour cell growth. In experiments where mice are injected with wild-type and/or transfected tumour cells expressing high levels of the cytokines, a profound inhibitory effect on tumour development is found, and in rare cases, most notably with IL-12 transfectants, animals become resistant to rechallenge by the wild-type tumour. The effect of an individual cytokine is often dependent on the cell line transfected, probably reflecting the cytokine context into which the gene has been introduced. This is particularly true after transfecting TNF, where the results range from enhanced invasiveness through to no effect to inhibition of tumour growth, depending on the cell line. These experiments provide information that can be related to the action of endogenous cytokines, particularly in their control of tumour cell populations. Although the introduced cytokine is continually expressed at high levels that probably overwhelm any endogenous network, the experiments demonstrate the power of manipulating local cytokine networks.

Inactivation of individual cytokine genes in mice by targeted recombination has been a powerful tool for elucidating individual components of cytokine networks. These mice could provide useful information on the role of cytokines in malignant progression, particularly if crossed with oncogene transgenic, or suppressor gene knock-out, mice.

Cytokine-directed processes Matrix metalloproteases (MMPs) and their inhibitors are important elements in the control of extracellular matrix synthesis and breakdown in tumours. Their production and activation is controlled by cytokines such as TNF and TGF-β. We have compared the localization and activity of the type IV collagenase, MMP-9, and its inducer, TNF, in ovarian cancer biopsies. Cells with the morphological appearance of infiltrating macrophages showed high expression of MMP-9 mRNA. Similar cells also stained positive for TNF protein and expressed TNF mRNA. Quantitative zymography on single tissue sections of the biopsies revealed levels of enzyme that were significantly higher than found in breast or bowel cancer biopsies. Only the occasional tumour-associated macrophage expresses TNF in the latter two cancers, and overall levels of TNF are appreciably lower. We were unable to find a direct correlation between levels of TNF mRNA expression and levels of MMP-9 when *in situ* hybridization results were compared with zymography of tissue sections, but this probably reflects the complexity of the control of the two systems. However, in co-cultures of tumour cells and macrophages there was also evidence for the involvement of TNF in the stimulation of MMP-9 release. The evidence that links TNF with MMP-9, taken together with our experiments using an MMP inhibitor in ovarian cancer xenografts (see below) suggests the following hypothesis. We propose that the 'normal' response of the host to a tumour is to encapsulate. The tumour cells, however, 'recruit' stromal cells to produce proteases that destroy their attempts at walling the tumour off.

Another activity of endogenous cytokines may be to control influx of host cells into tumours. We have found that *in situ* expression in ovarian cancer biopsies of mRNA for the chemokines MCP-1 and RANTES correlates both the CD8+ T lymphocyte and the CD68+ macrophage infiltrate.

Prognostic significance of local cytokines In general, high levels of cytokine or receptor are associated with a poor prognosis, or advanced malignancy. For instance, levels of TNF mRNA as measured by *in situ* hybridization, positively correlated with tumour grade in a study of 40 biopsies of serous ovarian carcinoma. Radioreceptor assays on membrane preparations from 72 biopsies revealed that EGFR expression and residual disease were significant correlates of high risk of progression. Interestingly, omental metastases tended to have higher levels of EGFR compared with the corresponding primary tumour. Patients with PDGFR-α-expressing tumours had a shorter survival compared with those patients with negatively staining tumours. In advanced ovarian cancer, low levels of M-CSF in ascitic fluid were associated with longer overall survival. Only residual disease after cytoreductive therapy had greater prognostic significance. Local cytokines also have potential to systemically influence a number of homeostatic processes and immune responses. For instance, a

correlation was found between biologically active IL-6 in ascitic fluid and reactive thrombocytosis in a group of patients with advanced disease.

The angiogenic cytokine VEGF is produced by tumour cells and stroma and its expression often correlates with the degree of vascularization and grade of malignancy. Its receptors, KDR and flt are mainly expressed by the tumour endothelium. Abundant levels of VEGF were found by immunoassay in the ascites of patients with epithelial ovarian cancer. Malignant epithelium was identified as one source of the VEGF. In breast cancer, *in situ* hybridization was used to show the presence of high levels of VEGF mRNA in tumour cells in comedotype ductal carcinoma *in situ*, infiltrating ductal carcinoma, and metastatic ductal carcinoma. Flt and KDR were strongly expressed in endothelial cells of small capillaries adjacent to malignant tumour cells. In a study involving 103 primary breast cancers, VEGF expression, assessed by immunohistochemistry, was found to correlate with an increment in microvascular density. Morever, the relapse-free survival rate of VEGF-rich tumours was significantly worse than the VEGF-poor tumours. Expression of VEGF and KDR are higher in metastatic than in non-metastatic human colon cancers, as assessed by immunohistochemistry. The increased expression correlated with the extent of neovascularization and proliferative index of tumour cells. VEGF mRNA expression was significantly increased in 26 of 27 hypervascular renal cell carcinoma tissues, when compared with adjacent normal kidney tissues. Even small tumours, when hypervascular, overexpressed VEGF mRNA.

Cytokines as cancer markers In some advanced cancer, cytokines and/or their soluble receptors are found in blood or ascitic fluid. Once again, high levels of cytokines or receptors are associated with a poor prognosis or advanced malignancy. For instance, serum levels of TNF-α were significantly higher in patients with head and neck cancer compared with controls with benign disease. Serum levels of the α component of the IL-2 receptor were elevated in patients with non-Hodgkin's lymphoma compared with control subjects, and these levels were related to tumour stage. In patients with colorectal cancer, serum IL-6 levels were increased compared with controls, and were highest in patients with liver or lung metastasis. Serum IL-8 levels were also elevated in colorectal cancer, and showed significant differences according to histological type, being lower in well-differentiated adenocarcinomas compared with other types. As with IL-6, serum IL-8 levels were significantly higher in patients with liver or lung metastasis.

20.3 Cytokine treatment of cancer

20.3.1 Exogenous cytokines in the treatment of cancer

In the last fifty years, the emphasis of cancer therapy has been directed to agents that destroy rapidly dividing cells, generally by interfering with DNA synthesis. It is now clear that malignant disease is also characterized by unscheduled cell survival and aberrant stromal interactions. Hence, new targets for therapy include the extracellular matrix, tumour stroma, cell motility, adhesion molecules, neovascularization, and signal transduction pathways. These are all areas in which cytokines could have an impact. The paradigm for cytokine therapy is IFN-α, the first cytokine to be made by genetic engineering.

20.3.2 Interferon-α

The antitumour activity of IFN-α seen in experimental animals has been confirmed in clinical trials over the last 15 years, although the types of tumour that respond to IFNs could not have been predicted from preclinical studies. In clinical trial so far, IFN-α has been most effective in the heamatological malignancies. The high activity of several IFN-α preparations in hairy cell leukaemia, a relatively uncommon leukaemia, was confirmed world-wide, although superior agents for treatment have now emerged. In a majority of hairy cell leukaemia patients, IFN-α normalized peripheral blood cell counts, and cytogenetic improvement in the bone marrow was seen after several months of therapy. Similar findings have been reported in chronic myelogenous leukaemia (CML), a multilineage haematological malignancy characterized by a reciprocal translocation between chromosomes 9 and 22 to form the chimeric *bcr–abl* oncogene. In an analysis of 190 patients treated with partially purified IFN-αs or recombinant IFN-α, 74% had normal peripheral blood smears (haematological remission) with 53% of those patients in remission achieving cytogenetic remission in the bone marrow. Approximately 30% of the total population achieved durable remission with a risk of relapse largely confined to the first

three years. In an Italian study, over 300 patients were randomized to receive recombinant IFN-α or chemotherapy with hydroxyurea. IFN-α prolonged the time to disease progression compared with chemotherapy and improved survival. In a UK trial, the median survival of 293 IFN-α treated patients was 61 months compared with the 41 months of those receiving chemotherapy. There are some data that suggest that responses are as good with lower doses as they are with doses that cause significant toxicity, and further trials are underway to confirm this.

Other tumours of the myeloid system that are partially differentiated, such as polycythemia vera and disorders involving high platelet counts, may respond to this cytokine. IFN-α caused a rapid and selective lowering of the platelet count in over 80% of patients with essential thrombocytaemia. Normalization of bone marrow histology occurred in about half the patients who had normal blood smears. Multiple myeloma is another haematological malignancy in which IFN-α has activity during remission induction, although response rates are worse than those seen with conventional therapy (mean response rate of 209 patients, 23.4%). However, IFN-α may be useful as maintenance therapy, since maintenance chemotherapy does not delay relapse. Following standard induction therapy, patients receiving IFN-α had an increased relapse-free survival (26 months versus 14 months) and the median duration of survival increased marginally, although this was lost on follow-up. In two other studies, maintenance IFN-α increased remission but in a third study it showed no effect. In many studies of IFN-α in myeloma, there is evidence that those patients with IgA or Bence–Jones myeloma respond best.

Several studies have shown that IFN-αs have antitumour activity in low grade 'favourable histology' lymphoma, achieving a response rate of about 25%. IFN-α produced objective responses in patients with carcinoid and malignant endocrine pancreatic tumour, AIDS-related Kaposi's sarcoma, and in a small minority of patients with renal cell carcinoma and melanoma. IFN-α had anti-angiogenic activity in animal models and this may account for its action in Kaposi's sarcoma. Other evidence of this action comes from the dramatic regression of life-threatening pulmonary haemangiomas in children receiving IFN-α. However, results of IFN-α therapy in solid tumours are, in general, disappointing, although slowly proliferating variants of renal cell carcinoma and melanoma will undergo regression, with response rates generally between 10 and 15%. There is some evidence that IFN-α works best against melanoma in an adjuvant/low tumour load setting. The trials so far suggest that very low doses over a long period, or very high doses over a short period, are less effective than moderately high doses for a period of approximately one year. The most persuasive results come from a randomized control study of 287 patients receiving high dose, 20MU/m²/day Iv for one month and 10MU/m²/day SC for 48 weeks, IFN-α for deep or regionally metastic melanoma. Control patients received no therapy, only close observation. With a median follow-up time of 6.9 years, a significant prolongation of relapse-free survival (from 1 to 1.7 years, p = 0.002) and overall survival (from 2.8 to 3.8 years, p = 0.02) was observed in the treated group compared with the control group. The effect on relapse rate was most pronounced early in the treatment interval and the treatment was of most benefit to node-positive patients. IFN-α is, in fact, the first agent to show a significant benefit in a randomized trials with high-risk melanoma patients.

20.3.3 Mechanisms of IFN-α action against human cancer

IFN-αs therefore have antitumour activity in a limited number of human cancers, mainly those of haematological origin. Activity is generally seen in slow-growing tumours. As was found in the animal models, continuous dosage is more effective than intermittent, and responses are slow, being maximal at 12 months or longer. It seems likely that IFN-α will act best at early stages of a cancer and that its activity in advanced cancer will be negligible. Dose–response relationships are still not entirely clear but clinical efficacy is generally seen at doses of 2–5 MU (equivalent to 2–5 μg per m² per day, or three times weekly).

Current evidence would suggest that IFN-α acts as a negative regulator in responsive cancers, not as an immunomodulator of a host–cancer response. In this respect, it can be considered a prototype tumour supressor protein, repressing the malignant phenotype in some cancers that are capable of differentiation. One way that it may act is by down-regulating response to autocrine growth/survival factors. In a myeloma cell line, for instance, IFN-α down-regulated expression of receptors, especially gp80, for the autocrine growth factor, IL-6. IFN-α can also

induce other tumour supressor proteins such as the protein kinase that phosphorylates the eukaryotic peptide chain initiation factor; the IFN regulatory proteins IRF-1 and IRF-2; and a latent endoribonuclease, Rnase L. It is of interest that some of the proteins encoded by oncogenic viruses can inhibit the action of these IFN-inducible regulators. There is evidence that some tumour cells may be deficient in IFN-α production. Cells from some patients with non-Hodgkin's lymphoma, chronic, and acute lymphocytic leukaemia are unable to make IFN-α, an ability that is restored at remission. This deficiency may lie in the loss of genes in p21–22 from chromosome 9, where the IFN gene cluster lies, and may be secondary to the loss of the nearby retinoic acid receptor. However, in cell lines derived from some malignant melanomas, a deficiency in IFN-α secretion had a more specific cause. There was a failure of IFN-α gene activation at the promoter level because of disruption of a *trans*-acting IFN-α gene transcription factor. Other potential targets for IFN-α action include tumour blood vessels, tumour cell signal transduction pathways, as well as components of the extracellular matrix and cellular adhesion molecules. It is likely that optimal activity will be achieved by combining IFN-α with other tumour supressors such as retinoids, or with specific antagonists of autocrine growth/survival factors.

20.3.4 Interferon-γ

In many respects, the clinical results with IFN-γ have been disappointing in most of the clinical trials reported so far. The immunomodulatory role of this cytokine in both macrophage and T cell responses is well defined and although, more recently, its role in TH1 immunosuppressive responses has been identified, other properties, particularly macrophage activation, made this a promising candidate for clinical trial. However, in the majority of advanced cancers, results are, at best, similar to those obtained with IFN-α. Two small trials have suggested efficacy of a low immunomodulatory dose in renal cell carcinoma and malignant melanoma patients, but was not effective in patients with a large tumour burden. Similarly, local administration of higher doses in refractory ovarian cancer were able to induce responses in patients with microscopic or small (< 5 mm) tumours, but not patients with a larger tumour volume. IFN-γ injected intraperitoneally has been demonstrated to increase tumour-associated glycoprotein (TAG-72) and carcinoem-bryonic antigen (CEA) expression on tumour cells *in vivo*, suggesting a potential role for its use as an adjuvant in enhancing monoclonal antibody binding to human carcinoma cell populations.

More recent studies, described below, suggest that local intratumoural induction of IFN-γ is a crucial mechanism in the antitumour activity of the hetero-dimeric cytokine, IL-12. Thus, the lack of activity of IFN-γ in clinical trials may be related to the method of delivery. Certainly it is true that optimal dose, routes, and schedules have not yet been determined.

A large European multicentre phase II trial of intraperitoneal IFN-γ in patients after chemother-apy with persistent residual disease at second-look laparotomy has recently been conducted. A dose of 20 MUm^2 was administered twice per week for 3–4 months. Thirty-one per cent of patients responded to therapy (23%, complete response, 8% partial response), with fever being the most common clin-ical adverse reaction. Both young age and tumour burden were predictive factors of response, with fig-ures of 52, 35, and 16% response in patients less than 50 years, between 50–59 years, and more than 60 years, respectively.

20.3.5 Tumour necrosis factor, TNF

The historical background of TNF and laboratory preclinical data generated great interest in the use of this cytokine in clinical cancer trials, particularly as the recombinant purified cytokine had tumour necrosing activity against syngeneic murine trans-plantable tumours. However, TNF was less active against human tumours growing subcutaneously in nude mice, except when injected directly into the tumour. This observation led to the use of TNF in a xenograft model of ovarian cancer where it could be given locally. Intraperitoneal (IP) TNF therapy of the ascitic tumour led to a modest doubling of mouse survival time. TNF eradicated the ascites, but, surprisingly, had promoted the development of solid intraperitoneal tumours with a well-devel-oped stroma, much evidence of neovascularization, and a histopathological resemblance to human ovar-ian cancer. As described above, these and other ani-mal experiments from several labs suggested that TNF might encourage tumour invasion and stroma formation.

Maybe not surprisingly, in general, the results of clinical trials of recombinant TNF have been disap-pointing. The toxicity of systemic administration was considerable, and response rates were below 1 per cent. When given locally, however, results have been more interesting. In a similar fashion to the observations in ascitic xenograft models of ovarian cancer, TNF has been shown to eradicate ascites in patients with advanced cancer. This is achieved in spite of the fact that ascitic fluid contains high levels of several cytokines and their soluble receptors, including soluble TNF receptors. The treatment appears to be palliative, with no evidence of increased survival. Another palliative treatment of great interest is the use of a high dose (three times the maximally tolerated systemic dose) of TNF with IFN-γ pretreatment and melphalan (a chemothera-peutic drug) in isolated limb perfusion. Response rates in excess of 90 per cent have been recorded in patients with melanoma and sarcoma, and ampu-tation avoided. In such circumstances TNF appears to induce haemorrhagic necrosis owing to a selective destruction of the tumour, but not normal, vascula-ture in the affected limb. The apparent sensitivity of the tumour vasculature for high dose TNF may lead to other therapeutic strategies that will target TNF to the tumour endothelium.

These clinical results illustrate the paradoxical nature of this cytokine. When given systemically below the maximally tolerated dose, TNF induces considerable toxicity with no clinical benefit. When given locoregionally, it is less toxic, can eradicate ascites, and seems to be selectively toxic for tumour endothelium. However, the cytokine is present in a minority of host cells in a range of tumours and is expressed by tumour cells in ovarian cancers. It is not inconceivable that TNF antagonists would be of use in early disease whereas the cytokine itself may be of use to eradicate advanced solid tumours or ascitic disease.

20.3.6 Interleukin-2

After preclinical studies showed that this cytokine had antitumour activity, particularly when adminis-tered with *ex vivo* IL-2-activated killer lymphocytes (LAK), high dose IL-2 plus chemotherapy was administered to patients. Some of these patients received autologous LAK cells which had been acti-vated *ex vivo* with IL-2 after plasmapheresis. This approach was associated with life-threatening toxi-city which necessitated close monitoring in intensive care units. More recent trials have concentrated on continuous infusion of IL-2 alone or with autologous activated cells, other cytokines, or chemotherapy. A survey of the US experience with 788 patients illustrates the current status of IL-2 trials. Responses were detected in 18 per cent of melanoma, 8 per cent of renal cell carcinoma, and 1 per cent of colorectal cancer patients. There was no overall difference in survival between those patients receiving IL-2 alone or in combination. However, the median duration of responses for all trials was only 4.4 months with overall survival of approximately 30 per cent at one year. Within this large study there were undoubtedly a small number of useful and sustained clinical responses, and trials such as these have led to successful licence applications for IL-2 in the treatment of renal cell carcinoma and melanoma. However, the relatively high toxicity (primarily vascular leakage syndrome) suggests the necessity of identifying the subgroup of patients most likely to benefit from IL-2 treatment.

20.3.7 Interleukin-12

Although this cytokine is only just entering clinical trial, the results in animal tumour models have been more promising and wide ranging than those obtained with any other cytokine tested so far. IL-12 is a heterodimeric cytokine, the product of two independent genes, that was originally known as cytotoxic lymphocyte maturation factor and natural killer cell stimulatory factor. It is produced by monocytes and possibly B cells, and acts on T and NK cells. Its most important activity is to stimulate uncommitted T cells to differentiate into IL-2 and IFN-γ-producing TH1 cells, with a resulting cell-mediated immune response. In addition, IL-12 transiently augments NK and LAK activity and proliferation. In animal models of *Leishmaniasis*, *Listeria*, and lymphocytic choriomeningitis virus infections, the therapeutic activity of IL-12 is thought to be a result of promotion of TH1 responses and a T cell-independent stimulation of macrophage activity. IL-12 causes tumour stasis, tumour regression, increased mouse survival times, and occasionally cure of disease in a range of transplantable murine tumour models. Activity has also been noted in experimental metastasis models. As IL-12 is not active against transplantable tumours in nude mice, and mice cured of their tumours are specifically resistant to rechallenge

with the same tumour line, its action is considered to be T cell dependent. Endogenously generated IFN-γ is also important, as IL-12 is much less active in mice treated with antibodies to IFN-γ. However, IFN-γ therapy does not mimic the action of IL-12. These data suggest that a network of endogenous cytokines is induced by IL-12 in the tumour microenvironment and has direct and indirect effects on the tumour.

20.3.8 Colony-stimulating factors, CSFs

The translation of basic research on the growth of haemopoietic stem cells (see Chapter 12) into a licensed recombinant cytokine therapy has been remarkable. Although the growth of bone marrow progenitors in soft agar was first studied in 1965, the cytokines regulating their growth were only cloned in the 1980s. Two of these, G-CSF (cloned in 1985) and GM-CSF (cloned in 1986) were available commercially as an adjunct to myelosuppressive chemotherapy only five years later in 1991. Their advent in the clinic offered a new technique of supportive care. Both cytokines induced a peripheral leucocytosis in normal volunteers at doses as low as 3 µg/kg/day and were well tolerated. GM-CSF at doses above 30 µg/kg/day may induce dose-limiting toxicity. Both of these cytokines have proved effective at reducing treatment-related toxicities. G-CSF, for instance, in a randomized, placebo-controlled trial of patients receiving high dose chemotherapy for lymphoma, decreased the period of severe neutropenia, hospitalization for fever, the use of parenteral antibiotics, and overall hospital stay. In a similar trial of patients receiving high dose chemoradiotherapy and autologous bone marrow transplant (ABMT), GM-CSF accelerated peripheral blood neutrophil recovery, decreased post-ABMT hospital stay, and decreased the number of infections.

It is, however, not clear whether CSFs have any other clinical benefit. There is little evidence that they increase response rate or survival and it is not certain whether the potential to increase dose will result in clinical benefit. Indeed, there are reports that GM-CSF may be an autocrine growth and survival factor in several malignancies in addition to those of haemopoietic origin. Other potential clinical applications of these cytokines include failure of marrow engraftment, burns, diseases of abnormal neutrophil function, and chronic infections.

20.3.9 Future directions for cytokine therapy

As we understand more of the local cytokine environment of tumours, and of the local action of cytokines, methods for targeting cytokines to the tumour site become of prime importance. Prompted by encouraging laboratory studies, there are a range of clinical cancer trials, planned or underway, using cytokine gene directed therapy. Several approaches are being followed, all with the aim of provoking powerful local inflammation and generating systemic and specific immune responses to the tumour. The cytokines IL-2, IL-4, GM-CSF, and IL-12 are most frequently used in such protocols. Proposals include transfection of the relevant gene into autologous or allogeneic tumour cells or stromal components *ex vivo* . Other approaches use cell-specific promoters to direct the gene *in vivo*, with direct injection, viral, or liposomal vectors being used for delivery.

Cytokine gene therapy is not the only option. Slow release delivery systems for cytokine protein may also be effective and provoke useful biological responses, as a recent study on GM-CSF microspheres showed.

The redundancy of the network detailed above would suggest that targeting a single endogenous cytokine will prove ineffective. However, a combination of cytokines and inhibitors, delivered systemically or locally, could provide a greater degree of specificity whether the desired result is apoptotic tumour cell death, destruction of tumour vasculature, induction of a tumour-specific host immune response, or, optimally, a combination of all three.

References and further reading

Balkwill, F.R. (1992). Tumour necrosis factor and cancer. *Progress in Growth Factor Research*, **4**, 121–37.

Balkwill, F. R. (1994). Cytokine therapy of cancer. The importance of knowing the context. *Eur. Cytokine Netw.*, **5**, 379–85.

Browning, J. L., Ngam-ek, A., Lawton, P., De Marinis, J., Tizard, R., Chou, E. P. *et al.* (1993). Lymphotoxin β, a novel member of the TNF family that forms a heteromeric complex with lymphotoxin on the cell surface. *Cell*, **72**, 847–56.

Brunda, M. J. (1994). Interleukin-12. *Journal of Leukocyte Biology*, **55**, 280–8.

Brunda, M. J., Luistro, L., Warrier, R. R., Wright, R. B., Hubbard, B. R., Murphy, M. *et al.* (1993). Antitumor and antimetastatic activity of interleukin 12 against murine tumours. *Journal of Experimental Medicine*, **178**, 1223–30.

Burke, F., Naylor, M. S., Davies, B., and Balkwill, F. (1993). The cytokine wall chart. *Immunology Today*, **14**, 165–70.

Cosman, D., Lyman, S. D., Idzerda, R. J., Beckmann, M. P., Park, L. S., Goodwin, R. G. *et al.* (1990). A new cytokine receptor superfamily. *Trends in Biological Sciences*, **15**, 265–70.

Demetri, G. (1993). Beyond supportive care: what are the next questions in the use of hemopoietic cytokines with cytotoxic chemotherapy? *Blood*, **82**, 2278–80.

Dillman, R. O., Church, C., Oldham, R. K., West, W., Schartzberg, L., and Birch, R. (1993). Inpatient continuous-infusion interleukin-2 in 788 patients with cancer. *Cancer*, **71**, 2358–70.

Engelhard, M., and Brittinger, G. (1994) Clinical relevance of granulocyte-macrophage colony-stimulating factor. *Seminars in Oncology*, **21**; 1–4

Gutterman, J. U. (1994). Cytokine therapeutics: lessons from interferon-α. *Proceedings of the National Academy of Sciences, USA*, **91**, 1198–205.

Heaney, M. L. and Golde, D. W. (1993). Soluble hormone receptors. *Blood*, **82**, 1945–8.

Kelvin, D. J., Michiel, D. F., Johnston, J. A., Lloyd, A. R. Sprenger, H., Oppenheim, J. J., and Weng, J. M. (1993). Chemokines and serpentines: the molecular biology of chemokine receptors. *Journal of Leukocyte Biology*, **54**, 604–12.

Kirkwood, J. M., Strawderman, M. H., Ernstoff, M. S., Smith, T. J., Borden, E. C., and Blum, R. H. (1996). Interferon Alfa-2b adjuvant therapy of high-risk resected cutaneous melanoma: the Eastern Cooperative Oncology Group Trial EST 1684. *Journal of Clinical Oncology*, **14**, 7–17.

Kishimoto, T., Taga, T., and Akira, S. (1994). Cytokine signal transduction. *Cell*, **76**, 253–62.

Kondo, M., Takeshita, T., Higuchi, M., Nakamura, M., Svdo, T., Nishikawa, S., and Sugamara, K. (1994). Functional participation of the IL-2 receptor γ chain in IL-7 receptor complexes. *Science*, **263**, 1453.

Lengyel, P. (1993). Tumor-suppressor genes: news about the interferon connection. *Proceedings of the National Academy of Sciences, USA*, **90**, 5893–5.

Metcalf, D. (1993). Hematopoietic regulators: redundancy or subtlety? *Blood*, **82**, 3515–23.

Miyajima, A., Mui, A. L.-F., Ogorochi, T., and Sakamak, K. (1993). Receptors for granulocyte-macrophage colony-stimulating factor, interleukin-3, and interleukin-5. *Blood*, **82**, 1960–74.

Oppenheim, J. J., Zachariae, C. O. C., Mukaida, N., and Mutsushima, K. (1991). Properties of the novel proinflammatory supergene "intercrine" cytokine family. *Annual Review of Immunology*, **9**, 617–48.

Sims, J. E., March, C. J., and Cosman, D. (1988). cDNA expression cloning of the IL-1 receptor, a member of the immunoglobulin superfamily. *Science*, **241**, 585–9.

Smith, C. A., David, T., Anderson, D., *et al.* (1990). A receptor for tumor necrosis factor defines an unusual family of cellular and viral proteins. *Science*, **248**, 1019–23.

Tahara, H., Zeh, H.J., III, Storkus, W.J ., Pappo, I., Watkins, S. C., Gubler, U., Wolf, S. F., Robbins, P. D., and Lotze, M. T. (1994). Fibroblasts genetically engineered to secrete interleukin 12 can suppress tumor growth and induce antitumor immunity to a murine melanoma *in vivo*. *Cancer Research*, **54**, 182–9.

Taverne, J. (1993). Transgenic mice in the study of cytokine function. *International Journal of Experimental Pathology*, **74**, 525–46.

Tepper, R. I., Pattengale, P. K., and Leder, P. (1989). Murine interleukin-4 displays potent anti-tumor activity *in vivo*. *Cell*, **57**, 503–12.

Urabe, A (1994). Interferons for the treatment of hematological malignancies. *Oncology*, **51**, 137–41.

Vedantham, S., Gamliel, H., and Golomb, H. M. (1992). Mechanism of interferon action in hairy cell leukemia: a model of effective cancer biotherapy. *Cancer Research*, **52**, 1056–66.

21

Screening and chemoprevention

JACK CUZICK

Screening is aimed at selecting a small group of individuals, who are likely to benefit from some form of treatment, from a larger population to reduce the morbidity and mortality from some disease, which for our present purpose is cancer. Screening can take several forms, can be aimed at different populations, and can have different goals. Very often it is a multistage process in which individuals positive at one stage are referred on to a more invasive or intensive procedure to see if cancer is present. There are several pitfalls in the evaluation of the efficacy of screening modalities and it is vitally important that screening should do more good than harm, since one is approaching a healthy population and asking them to undergo a medical procedure, as opposed to the usual clinical paradigm in which an unwell patient approaches the doctor and actively seeks advice and treatment.

Since screening can only identify individuals in need of treatment, alone it cannot affect the course of cancer. It is the subsequent treatment that aims to do this. In most cases this is surgical, but when an increased risk of developing cancer is found and/or precancerous lesions that may recur are detected, there is increasing interest and activity in the use of agents to arrest the development of cancer. Chemoprevention is an intervention aimed at preventing cancer by the use of some anticancer substance, and may be an appropriate action for individuals identified during screening to be at high risk of cancer or to have precursor lesions. It is a rapidly developing area and includes many aspects unrelated to screening.

In this chapter I review some general considerations relevant to screening for any disease, and then examine the role of screening for a number of specific cancers.

The key issues in screening are the existence of a safe, acceptable test that discriminates well between those in need of treatment and those that are not; sufficient knowledge of the natural history of the disease to know at which stage early detection is likely to be important for reducing mortality and morbidity, and choice of the population to be screened. Other issues such as the age range, screening interval, and follow-up procedures are also important and can have a large impact on the cost of screening. These issues are discussed in greater detail below with the possible methods for evaluating screening programmes. A perfect screening test would detect all lesions destined to become cancer at a stage before they become untreatable, but would not refer for further investigation and treatment any abnormality not destined to become invasive cancer. In practice, this is never achieved and one is usually prepared to tolerate a considerable amount of overtreatment for the safety and peace of mind that the treatment of any suspicious lesions brings.

21.1 Types of screening tests

Screening tests can be divided according to the type of abnormality they aim to detect. Many are aimed at early detection of the cancer itself. These can never reduce the incidence of disease, but may reduce mortality and morbidity associated with advanced disease. For example, a reduction in breast cancer mortality has been clearly demonstrated in women over the age of 50 who have been screened by mammography, and this is owing to the fact that, at least in some women, early detection permits the surgical removal of the lump *before* it has metastasized, so that the chances of cure are high. However, this example also illustrates the limitations of screening tests aimed at early detection, since some breast cancers metastasize at a very early stage before they are detectable by mammography; for these women, slightly earlier detection of their cancers by mammography is probably of little benefit.

Other screening methods aim to detect precancerous lesions. The classic example is cervical cytology. Here the goal is to detect precursor lesions before they become invasive, so that removal carries an almost 100 per cent cure rate. In this case a major problem is knowing which lesions are likely to become cancerous if left untreated so as to avoid overtreatment of benign lesions with no malignant potential.

These two examples illustrate the need to understand the natural history of the cancer under consideration. Screening can only be effective if lesions are detected at a time when effective treatment is still possible and in this respect the ability to detect precancerous lesions is a key feature. The use of mammography is thought to reduce mortality from breast cancer by about 30 per cent, whereas estimates of the mortality reduction associated with regular cervical smears is nearer to 80–90 per cent. However, screening can only be cost effective and

generally acceptable to the population if treatment, especially invasive and unpleasant treatment, is restricted as much as possible to those lesions that are destined to become malignant if left untreated. The benign to malignant ratio in biopsies following a mammographically detected abnormality is well below one in European centres, whereas far more preinvasive cervical intraepithelial neoplasia (CIN) lesions are treated than would ever become cancer. It is also worth remembering that because breast cancer is so much more common in the Western world, mammographic screening still has a greater potential for overall mortality reduction, even though the test is less effective.

A third form of screening, which is becoming increasingly common, is genetic testing. This field will develop enormously in the future as more cancer-associated genes are found (see Chapters 4, 9, and 10). At the moment it is limited to rare cancer family syndromes such as familial adenomatous polyposis (FAP), where genetic testing can indicate which family members carry a mutation with almost 100 per cent penetrance for colon cancer. Similar tests can now be performed on families with a rare gene (*BRCA1*) predisposing to breast cancer (and ovarian cancer in some families). Some genetic changes, such as the Li–Fraumeni syndrome (a mutation in the *TP53* gene), are also clearly linked to a high risk of many cancers, and screening for this mutation imposes a severe challenge since identified carriers must then be screened regularly. Future work will make similar tests available for other cancers that run in families and eventually allow one to test for sporadic or somatic mutations in the general population that increase the risk of cancer. This is already leading to difficult ethical problems. Who should be tested and who has the right to know the results of such tests? Genetic screening will lead to a very different form of programme as it will involve whole families, require intensive follow-up of individuals testing positive, and mean the use of chemopreventive agents or prophylactic surgical removal of the organs at risk.

21.2 Safety and acceptability

Safety and acceptability are also important issues when considering the introduction of a screening test. The demands are far greater than in a therapeutic setting, since the number of screenings needed to save one life is usually measured in the thousands.

Thus even a low complication rate can seriously affect the risk–benefit ratio. Not only problems occurring at the initial screen, but also any untoward effects associated with the further investigation of false positives, need to be assessed. An example is screening for bowel cancer by faecal occult blood testing. Here the initial procedure is certainly safe (although not necessarily acceptable), but when rehydrated faecal samples are assayed, the positivity rate approaches 10 per cent and all of these individuals may have to be referred for colonoscopy, a relatively major procedure.

Acceptability is a larger issue, which partly relates to safety but also includes issues of inconvenience and cost, such as test frequency. To a large extent, acceptability is based on prevailing social perceptions. For example, any kind of screening for bowel cancer, which requires collection of faecal material or endoscopic viewing of the bowel, will have to overcome certain taboos. A large element in achieving this will be the ability to persuade patients that the test truly protects them from cancer. This cannot be claimed until convincing large trials are completed, so the problems are particularly acute at the early stages of development of a new test. However, social taboos can be overcome, as evidenced by the high rate of attendance that is now achieved in Britain and Scandinavia following an invitation for a cervical smear or a mammogram, where embarrassment, fear, and discomfort were initial barriers. Education of the public and profession about the benefits and goals of screening can make a large impact on the compliance rates and ultimately on the effectiveness of a screening programme.

21.3 Who should be screened?

The population chosen for screening is crucial to its success. A key issue in deciding if screening is appropriate is the amount of disease present in the population offered screening. In public health terms this means that population screening has the potential for doing the most good if directed at the major cancers. For the developed world the common cancers arise in the lung, bowel, breast, prostate, stomach (especially in Japan), ovary, and bladder. For developing countries the priorities are different. For example, cervix cancer would have the highest priority in many places, liver cancer would be important in Africa and the south-east coast of China, and

oesophageal cancer would rate high in parts of China, south-east Africa, and around and to the east of the Caspian Sea.

While focusing on the common cancers is helpful in deciding which sites are good candidates for screening, this is of little help unless an effective screening test exists. Less common cancers can be appropriate targets if highly effective but simple means of screening exist, as for example in cervix cancer. Some modalities are only suitable for high risk populations. For example, regular screening for bladder cancer by urine cytology is appropriate for workers in the dyestuff or rubber industry where the risk is increased because of exposure to chemicals known to cause bladder cancer. However, it would not be cost effective if applied to the general population. In other cases it might be appropriate to screen the general population once, but only apply repeated screening for a high risk subgroup identified at the initial screen. An example of this would be to offer a single sigmoidoscopy around age 60 to the entire population to screen for precursors to bowel cancer and to reserve further screening at regular intervals for individuals with large or other high risk adenomas. At the other extreme is screening of the entire (male/female) population within a given age range at regular intervals . The two procedures for which this has become established practice are cytological examination of cervical smears in women aged 20–65 every 3–5 years and mammographic imaging of the breast in women aged 50–65 every 2–3 years.

21.4 Evaluation of screening

21.4.1 Evaluating the test

Screening tests are usually evaluated in terms of sensitivity, specificity, and positive predictive value. These quantities are computed from a 2×2 table, which classifies whether disease was present or not according to whether the test was positive or negative. The basic quantities are shown in Fig. 21.1. Sensitivity indicates what proportion of individuals with disease were positive on the test, while specificity gives the proportion of individuals without the disease who tested negative. Sensitivity and specificity do not depend on the prevalence of disease. A measure that also reflects this is the positive predictive value. This is defined as the probability of having disease given that the test was positive. The negative predictive value, which gives the probabil-

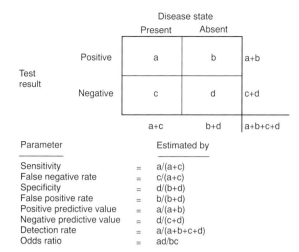

Test result		Disease state		
		Present	Absent	
	Positive	a	b	a+b
	Negative	c	d	c+d
		a+c	b+d	a+b+c+d

Parameter		Estimated by
Sensitivity	=	a/(a+c)
False negative rate	=	c/(a+c)
Specificity	=	d/(b+d)
False positive rate	=	b/(b+d)
Positive predictive value	=	a/(a+b)
Negative predictive value	=	d/(c+d)
Detection rate	=	a/(a+b+c+d)
Odds ratio	=	ad/bc

Fig. 21.1 Parameters used for evaluating a screening test. The values of a, b, c, and d are the number of screened individuals in a given category.

ity of being disease free given that the test was negative, is also sometimes used. Sometimes false positive rates and false negative rates are given. These are just the proportions of the total population that are falsely classified as positive or negative, respectively, although the rates are sometimes misused. The detection rate is the proportion of the total population who are truly positive.

Implementation of these measures is often difficult. A major problem is that unless the entire population offered screening receives a full diagnostic work-up, the total number of people who have the disease is not known. When a number of screening tests are applied simultaneously, their relative sensitivities can be determined from the number of diseased individuals among those who were positive on any test. Alternatively, cancers arising within a given interval after screening (usually one or two years) can be used as a surrogate for false negative tests. Another problem is how to decide what constitutes disease being present, especially when screening for precursor lesions. Also, when a multistep screening process is applied, it may be difficult to decide at what stage the test is positive, although both of these problems can be overcome by careful recording and reporting.

21.4.2 Effectiveness of screening

The measures indicated above can be used to evaluate the validity of the screening test, but they do not provide information about the effectiveness of screening in reducing mortality. Such 'process measures' need to be augmented by measures that directly assess the benefits of screening in terms of the reduction in morbidity and mortality, before a test can be recommended. There are several potential pitfalls in carrying out these analyses.

21.4.3 Potential biases

By far the most difficult part of any cost–benefit assessment is an evaluation of the effectiveness of the screening intervention. Because any specific cancer is relatively rare over a 5–10 year period, a large number of subjects need to be screened to provide enough cancers for useful comparisons. Naive analyses are subject to serious biases, which have not always been appreciated. The most important of these are lead time bias and length bias. Lead time bias refers to the fact that early detection of disease will give the appearance of better survival in screen-detected cases compared with symptomatically detected cases, even when screening has no effect on the natural history of disease. In this circumstance screening is actually detrimental to the patient who is given a death sentence and cancer label sooner, but whose disease course is unchanged. This appears to be the case for lung cancer screening by chest X-ray. In a less extreme form, where screening does some good, the apparent benefits can be exaggerated by this bias. However, it should be remembered that the effects of these biases are dependent on the treatments currently available and new more effective treatment may make earlier detection more important.

A different bias, leading to similarly exaggerated apparent benefits of screening, is known as length bias. This is a little more subtle but is a result of the fact that more slowly growing cancers, which have a better prognosis, are more likely to be detected by screening. The reason for this is that because of their slower growth, the time interval of potential preclinical detection by screening is longer, so that their chances of being detected by screening are greater. Thus, good prognosis cancers are preferentially detected by screening. An extreme form of this bias occurs when cancers are detected by screening that would not become apparent during the lifetime of the individual. This is a major problem in screening for prostate cancer.

21.4.4 Case–control studies

These biases indicate that it is inappropriate to judge screening methods by comparing the survival times of screen-detected and symptomatic cases. What is needed is to analyse two populations, one of which receives screening and the other of which does not, and so serves as a control group. One method of doing this is to invite an entire population for screening and then compare the cancer rates of those who accept screening against those who do not. This is usually done on a case–control basis by comparing the screening histories of people who developed or died from cancer with randomly selected (age and sex matched) controls who did not develop cancer. While this approach is much better than the comparison of survival times in screen-detected versus symptomatic cases, it still suffers from the serious bias that the cancer risk among individuals who chose to accept screening is often different from those who refuse it, even when screening has no effect. The use of case–control studies to evaluate screening is complicated and attempts to correct this and other biases by using a third control population in an unscreened area can help to overcome these problems. These issues are discussed in greater detail by Moss (1991).

21.4.5 Randomized trials

The only truly reliable way of assessing screening procedures (or almost any medical intervention) is by means of a randomized trial. For this a population suitable for screening is identified, but only a randomly chosen proportion (often one-half) is offered screening. Random allocation is done at the individual level or in small units such as household, or for very large trials, by medical practice. The cancer mortality (and incidence for screening methods designed to detect precancerous lesions) is then compared between the two randomized groups without regard to actual compliance. Low compliance will make such trials impossible and this is usually the key issue in obtaining a proper evaluation.

21.4.6 Intermediate end-points

Because of the large size of the populations studied and long follow-up time needed to evaluate screening properly, there has been much interest in using short-term, intermediate end-points for evaluation. These include detection rates for precancerous and cancerous lesions and characteristics of the cancers detected such as size and grade. The rate of occurrence of 'interval cancers' in the period following a screen showing no abnormalities can also be used. These markers are very useful for deciding if a screening modality has promise and for tuning the finer parameters of a screening programme, such as the screening interval and age group to be offered screening. However, they can be unreliable as the only method of evaluation and need to be underpinned by clearly established mortality reductions in randomized trials. Further discussion of the use of intermediate markers in evaluating screening programmes can be found in Duffy et al. (1991).

21.4.7 Screening programmes

Once a safe, effective, and acceptable screening test is found, further efforts are needed to create a cost-effective screening programme. The costs of a screening programme depend on the frequency with which the test is offered, the age range over which screening takes place, and the policy for referral for additional tests. Less tangible costs in terms of anxiety, time, and personal expense consumed in attending a screening clinic also need to be considered. Effectiveness depends on a high compliance rate, quality control of the screening test, and appropriate treatment and follow-up for individuals found to have positive results. Regular monitoring and audit of a programme is essential to assure that goals are met and cancer mortality is being reduced. Case–control studies looking at the screening history of individuals dying from (or in some cases developing) the cancer of interest are an important part of this process. Ultimately, bottom line figures such as cost or number of screens required per life-year saved, need to be computed to put screening programmes into perspective and to allow comparisons between screening programmes for different cancers, screening for other diseases, and other medical interventions such as kidney transplants, etc.

21.5 Screening for specific cancers

In the following sections we review possible screening methods in various sites. Some of these are accepted and form the basis of national programmes, while others are at different stages of evaluation. New, innovative methods are constantly being developed, but there is only space to indicate cursorily a few of these here. As screening is of no use without treatment, I comment briefly on the further actions that may be taken when positive results are found. These may (increasingly so in the future) include chemoprevention, and some of the directions in this field are also noted. Our remarks in this area are limited and do not include a large body of basic developmental work on chemoprevention aimed at the general population (De Palo *et al.* 1992). Likewise, the larger issue of primary prevention of cancer, which includes many other cancer-avoidance methods, is only touched upon.

21.5.1 Cervix cancer

The universally accepted screening method for preventing cervix cancer is cytological examination of cervical scrapes that have been smeared on to slides and stained by Papanicolou's method. This procedure has a long history. In 1928 Papanicolou published a report indicating that cervix cancer could be diagnosed from exfoliated cells. Working with Traut, he developed this into a screening test in the 1930s and they published their definitive work in 1943. The war delayed initial attempts at implementation but the subsequent slow acceptance of the approach meant that large-scale field trials did not begin until the 1960s. These were turned into organized screening programmes in the Nordic countries (except Norway) during the 1960s and already by the mid-1970s large reductions in incidence and mortality were seen in these countries (except Norway) (Fig. 21.2; Hakama 1982; Laara *et al.* 1987). Screening programmes have been less well organized in other countries and the benefits in terms of national trends have been less clear.

'Pap smear' screening is designed to detect precancerous lesions. The nomenclature for these lesions varies with country and continues to change. In Britain the degree of dyskaryosis (disturbance of normal cell structure and arrangement, see Chapter 1) is reported with the grades borderline, mild, moderate, severe, and potentially invasive. A roughly similar system exists in the US based on the degree of dysplasia. This system is mirrored by a histopathological classification of biopsies based on the depth of cervical intraepithelial neoplasia (CIN) which has grades 1, 2, and 3 according to whether the lesion is confined to the lower one-third, two-thirds, or greater depth of epithelium. The corre-

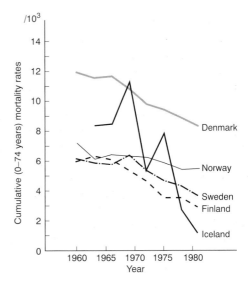

Fig. 21.2 Trends in cumulative mortality rates from cervical cancer in Nordic countries, 1960–82 (Läärä *et al.* 1987).

spondence between cytology and histology is by no means perfect and much confusion arises when the terms are used interchangeably. In particular, low grade cytological abnormalities are associated with a wide range of underlying lesions when biopsied and assessed by histology. Recently, a new system, the Bethesda classification, has been introduced (NCI Workshop 1989) which scores lesions as high grade squamous intraepithethial lesions (HGSIL), which is roughly CIN 2/3; low grade squamous intraepithelial lesions (LGSIL), roughly CIN 1; and atypical squamous cells of undetermined significance (ASCUS), which relates to lesser changes. This system is meant to be used both for cytology and histology but the poor correlation between the two raises doubts as to whether this is helpful.

Unfortunately, the efficacy of this method has never been evaluated by means of a randomized trial. However, following pioneering work by Clarke and Anderson (1979) in Canada, several case–control studies have been undertaken around the work and these have been collated and synthesized in an important paper (IARC Working Party 1986). The main results are summarized in Table 21.1 and the implications for a screening programme are shown in Table 21.2. Compared with unscreened women, the reduction in cancer incidence afforded by screening women aged 20–64 every five years was

Table 21.1 Geometric mean relative protection against cervical cancer in women with two or more previously negative smears participating in centrally organized screening programmes

Months since last negative smear	Relative protection[1] (No. of cases)	95% Confidence limits
0–11	15.3 (25)	10.0 to 22.6
12–23	11.9 (23)	7.5 to 18.3
24–35	8.0 (25)	5.2 to 11.8
36–47	5.3 (30)	3.6 to 7.6
48–59	2.8 (30)	1.9 to 4.0
60–71	3.6 (16)	2.1 to 5.9
72–119	1.6 (6)	0.6 to 3.5
120+	0.8[2] (7)	0.3 to 1.6
Never screened	1.0 (reference group)	

[1] A large relative protection corresponds to a larger benefit of screening, e.g. a relative protection of 10 means that the odds of developing cancer in the stated interval is one-tenth that of an age-matched woman who was never screened.

[2] Based on figures from Aberdeen and Iceland only.

From IARC Working Party (1986).

estimated to be 84 per cent, and this increases to 91 per cent if screening is undertaken every three years. Little additional gain is achieved by screening more often. These results refer specifically to the protection afforded by regular negative smears, and as such evaluate the test, but not the entire programme, since some patients with abnormal smears still go on to develop cancer. Thus, the results in Table 21.2 are, to some extent, optimistic, even if full compliance were achieved. However, they do make clear that the screening interval used is less critical than the need to achieve a high compliance and to assure abnormal cytological findings are properly followed up.

Case–control studies offer an important way of continually monitoring screening programmes, not only to assess the relative protection in the years following a negative smear, but also to evaluate other potential weaknesses such as low compliance, failure to follow-up adequately women with positive smears, development of cancer in women who have had abnormal smears that subsequently became normal without intervention, and adequacy and correct reading of smears in women who subsequently developed cancer.

Successful as it has been, screening by cytology is not without its problems. It is very tedious and labour intensive, and requires subjective judgements. Work on automating the reading of smears has been

Table 21.2 Effect of different screening policies on incidence rates of cervical cancer in women aged 20–64

Screening programme	Cumulative rate/10^5 women	% Reduction in incidence	Number of tests	Number of cases prevented/10^5 tests
No screening	1575			
Screening every five years:				
Ages 20–64	258.6	84	9	146
Ages 25–64	287.8	82	8	161
Ages 35–64	480.9	70	6	182
Screening every year ages 20–34, then every five years ages 35–64	233.4	85	21	64
Screening at ages 25, 26, and 30, then every five years	275.4	83	9	144
Screening every three years:				
Ages 20–64	138.9	91	15	96
Ages 25–64	161.8	90	13	109
Ages 35–64	354.9	78	10	122
Screening every year ages 20–34, then every three years ages 35–64	132.0	92	25	59
Screening at ages 25, 26, and 29, then every three years	157.4	90	14	101
Screening every year ages 20–64	105.2	93	45	33

From IARC Working Party (1986).

ongoing for over thirty years (Banda-Gamboa *et al.* 1992) and computer-assisted systems are beginning to become available. These systems are only able to highlight areas needing more careful (human) analysis and are currently limited to performing a double check on smears read as normal by human technicians.

At a more basic level, there is much interest in applying tests for the human papillomavirus (HPV) in a screening context. Numerous case–control studies have shown very high odds ratios associated with HPV infection (Table 21.3; Muñoz and Bosch 1992) and it has been clearly demonstrated that certain types of papillomavirus (types 16, 18, 31, 33, 35, 45, 51, 52, 56) are more related to cancer and high grade CIN than other low risk genital types (6, 11, 42, 43, 44). The oncogenic role of the high risk types, especially HPV-16, is also supported by much laboratory research.

One role for HPV testing may lie in its use as a second level screen for women with borderline or mild abnormalities on cytology. Only about 20–30 per cent of these women actually have high grade CIN in need of immediate treatment. Initial studies (Cuzick *et al.* 1992, 1994; Bavin *et al.* 1993) have suggested that testing for high risk types of HPV on the smear material by PCR may be useful in deciding which women should be referred immedi-

ately and which can be followed by cytological surveillance. Some representative results are shown in Table 21.4 which suggest that this test may be helpful in some, but not all cases, and the chain of types included in the test is an important variable.

The larger question of the role of HPV testing as part of primary screening is also of interest. By using PCR technology, HPV testing can be performed on the cells left over from a smear and the technique is automatable and potentially very cheap. Studies by Reid *et al.* (1991) and Cuzick *et al.* (1994) have shown that HPV testing for high risk disease has a much higher pick up rate for CIN 2/3 than cytology, and that the positive predictive value for CIN 2/3 is around 40–50 per cent, which is similar to that for moderate dyskaryosis, which is already routinely referred for further colposcopic investigation. However, large trials will be needed to evaluate properly the role of HPV testing within a screening programme, and these have yet to be done. It seems likely, however, that HPV testing and cytology will prove complementary and the best approach will involve a combination of the two methods.

Other approaches to cervical screening include cervicography (Stafl 1981; Tawa *et al.* 1988; Szarewski *et al.* 1991), which attempts to mimic the view seen on colposcopy by a photograph that can be taken by a nurse and later reviewed by the

Table 21.3 Case–control studies of HPV status and invasive cervix cancer

Study	No. cases (% positive)	No. controls (% positive)	OR (95% CI)	Method and type
Hong Kong (Donnan *et al.* 1989)	30 (37)	17 (6)	9.3 (1.0–84.1)	Southern HPV-16
Uganda (Schmauz *et al.* 1989)	34 (50)	23 (4)	22.0 (5.1–104.3)	Southern HPV-16, -18
Latin America (Reeves *et al.* 1989)	721 (47)	1225 (18)	4.0 (3.3–5.0)	FISH HPV-16, -18
Pakistan (Anwar *et al.* 1991)	80 (69)	30 (10)	19.8 (5.8–66.8)	ISH HPV-16, -18
Japan (Anwar *et al.* 1991)	82 (68)	26 (19)	9.0 (3.2–25.7)	ISH HPV-16, -18
China (Peng *et al.* 1991)	101 (35)	146 (1)	32.9 (7.7–141.1)	PCR HPV-16, -33
Columbia (Muñoz and Besch 1992)	87 (72)	98 (13)	15.6 (6.9–34.7)	PCR Manos-consensus
Spain (Muñoz and Besch 1992)	142 (69)	130 (5)	46.2 (18.5–115.1)	PCR Manos-consensus

HPV = human papillomavirus; Southern = Southern blot bybridization; FISH = filter *in situ* hybridization; ISH = *in situ* hybridization; PCR = polymerase chain reaction; OR = odds ratio; CI = confidence interval.

Table 21-4 Positive predictive value for CIN 2/3 of HPV testing and degree of dyskaryosis in asymptomatic women who had an abnormal cervical smear

	HPV testing		Cytology	
Type	True positive/ All positive (%)	Dyskaryosis	True positive/ All positive (%)
HPV-16	39/42 (93)	Severe	29/38 (76)
HPV-18	6/9 (67)		
		Moderate	
HPV-31	14/20 (70)		
HPV-33	11/16 (69)	Mild	12/31 (39)
HPV-35	2/4 (50)		

A total of 73 of the 133 women in this study had CIN 2/3 (from Cuzick *et al.* 1994).

gynaecologist. Initial results suggest a high sensitivity but poor specificity for high grade lesions. Feulgen staining for acid-label DNA (Partington *et al.* 1991), infrared spectroscopy (Wong *et al.* 1991), and increased activity of the enzymes 6-phosphogluconate dehydrogenase and glucose 6-phosphate dehydrogenase (Jonas *et al.* 1992) have been suggested as screening techniques, but they have not been investigated in any detail.

A long-term strategy is vaccination against HPV, but this approach is still in its early stages. At present the only approach to primary prevention is to limit exposure to HPV by reducing the number of sexual partners and/or use of the condom. There have been attempts at chemoprevention of cervix cancer by treating CIN. Because most cervix cancer has a squamous cell origin, topical retinoids have been applied (Romney *et al.* 1985). Also, because of the viral involvement, interferons (which have an effect on skin cancer; see Chapter 20) have also been used. Studies of high dose treatment with vitamins C and E, β-carotene, and folic acid of low grade lesions are also being carried out.

21.5.2 Breast cancer

The most fully investigated method for early detection of breast cancer is mammography. This method is aimed at early detection of invasive cancer and so is limited by the fact that this may still be too late to affect survival. As a result, moderate benefits of the

order of a 30 per cent reduction in mortality are expected from this approach. However, because breast cancer is so common (about 1 in 11 women in the Western world) a benefit of this magnitude is well worth having and would amount to a larger reduction in the death toll from cancer in the Western world than the complete eradication of cervix cancer.

Gershon-Cohen advocated the use of X-ray screening as a test for breast cancer in the 1930s (Gershon-Cohen and Colcha 1937). However, it was not until 1964 that the first randomized trial of mammography was conducted by the Health Insurance Plan (HIP) in New York City (Shapiro *et al.* 1982). Four annual mammograms were offered to 31 000 randomly selected women aged 40–64 and the remaining 31 000 unscreened women served as a control group. Clinical palpation of the breast was also undertaken at each visit in the screened group. Since then other randomized trials have been mounted in Canada, Sweden, and Scotland, and non-randomized studies have been performed in Holland, Italy, and the UK. Subsets of these data have been reviewed by Hurley and Kaldor (1992), Nystrom *et al.* (1993), and Elwood *et al.* (1993). There is a consensus that mammography is effective in women aged over 50 and the studies overall suggest that 2–3 yearly screening can reduce breast cancer mortality by about 30 per cent in this age group (Fig. 21.3). There is considerable controversy about the value of mammography at ages 40–49, however, and several studies to date have failed to show a significant benefit (Fig. 21.3). There are at least three mutually non-exclusive possible reasons for this: (i) breast cancer is less frequent in this age group and to date the available data and short follow-up do not rule out the possibility of a 10–20 per cent mortality reduction, (ii) the lead time gained by screening is shorter in younger women so that screening must be done annually to have an effect, and (iii) the breast is more dense in premenopausal women, making imaging more difficult and limiting its application.

While the first point must be accepted, there is mounting evidence that the remaining two points are valid. Using Swedish data, Tabar *et al.* (1992) have shown that for women under 50 the rate of cancer in the year following screening drops only to about half that in an unscreened population, whereas in older women the rates were about 20 per cent of control rates for the first two years

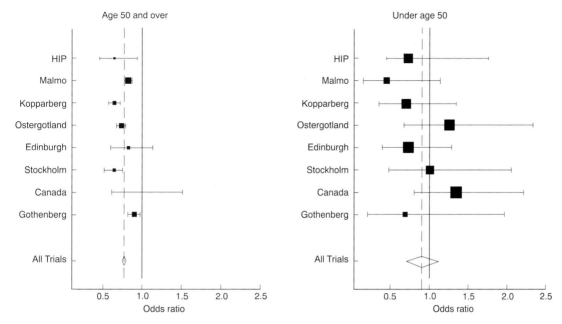

Fig. 21.3 Mortality reduction in randomized trials of mammographic screening for breast cancer according to age at first screening.

after screening and rose to about one-half only after three years. Additionally, intermediate end-points such as the ratio of cancers detected at the first (prevalent) screen divided by the expected annual incidence rate are lower in younger women (Table 21.5). Overall the lower rates of disease and the poorer performance of the test make mammography a less viable proposition in younger women than in women aged over 50 years.

The most discrepant results in young women are the better survival in the HIP study and poorer sur-

vival in the Canadian study. One reason put forward for this is the additional screening by physical examination. In the HIP study this was given annually to the screened population along with mammography, while in the Canadian study both groups had an initial physical examination. However, other studies suggest that with currently available equipment, physical examination adds little to the detection rates achieved by mammography, so the role of physical examinations remain unclear.

Breast self examination (BSE) has also been recommended as a way of detecting cancers earlier. Although widely recommended, the evidence for efficacy is minimal (Ellman *et al.* 1993; Gastrin *et al.* 1994) and the only reported randomized study, which comes from Russia (Semiglazov *et al.* 1993), showed that it led to an increase in the biopsy rate without any reduction in cancer mortality. A problem with BSE is that it is difficult to teach women how to do it well and, unless it does improve survival, the anxiety generated by the recommended monthly exam may more than outweigh any benefits.

Ultrasound has been considered for breast screening but appears to be too expensive and lack sensitivity, but because it can be done safely at short intervals, it is used in follow-up and may have a

Table 21.5 Prevalence to incidence ratios in screening populations by age for breast cancer

Age group	Study		
	Two counties, Sweden Tabar *et al.* (1992)	Florence, Italy Paci and Duffy (1991)	Nijmegen, Netherlands[1] Peer *et al.* (1994)
40–49	1.99	0.74	1.16
50–59	2.50	2.42	3.72
60–69	3.52	3.36	
70–74	4.06	3.36	4.67

[1] Prevalence to interval cancer rate for women aged <50, 50–69, 70+.

role in young women who have a family history or dense breasts that are opaque to radiology. The possibility of using MRI for breast screening has also been raised, especially in dense breasts, but this is extremely expensive and has yet to be validated. Genetic testing for breast cancer is also a future possibility and one rare but highly penetrant gene (*BRCA1*) has already been identified. Because the results of a test on one person affect the risk of cancer in other family members, complicated ethical issues arise when considering this form of screening.

Breast cancer prevention Because current methods of screening for breast cancer are early detection procedures, which have a limited but important effect on mortality, there has been a major interest in trying to prevent breast cancer. Prevention programmes have mostly used a family history of breast cancer to find high risk individuals, but it is possible to use features on the mammogram to do this as well. Wolfe (1976) originally proposed this, and several studies have shown that the extent of high density areas on a mammogram is a strong predictor of risk of developing disease (Oza and Boyd 1993). This may prove an important additional use of mammography.

One approach to prevention is to try to reduce dietary fat intake (Howe *et al.* 1990; Boyd *et al.* 1992), but it is not clear if this needs to be done as early as during adolescence, or whether it will prove acceptable to the population. Another approach has been to try to make breast cancer prevention a beneficial side effect of some other hormonal manipulation such as oral contraception. Oral contraceptives reduce ovarian cancer by about 50 per cent and the combined pill may also reduce endometrial cancer, but they appear to lead to a small increase of breast cancer, at least in young people (UK National Case–Control Study Group 1989). Pike and colleagues (Spicer *et al.* 1994) are working on new methods of contraception which may also reduce breast cancer risk, but these are at very early stages of development.

The area of chemoprevention that has generated the most interest and activity is the use of tamoxifen to try to prevent disease in high risk women (Cuzick *et al.* 1986). Tamoxifen has been used for over 20 years to treat breast cancer and has been shown to be effective in this context (EBCTCG 1992) as well as having a low side-effect profile (Powles *et al.* 1994), although it does lead to an increase in endo-

metrial cancer (Fornander *et al.* 1993). Large trials are underway in the US, Italy, and the UK (with centres in Europe and Australia) to explore the use of tamoxifen as a chemopreventive agent.

21.5.3 Colorectal cancer

The screening method that has received the most attention for colorectal cancer is the use of a guaiac impregnated slide to test for small amounts of blood in a stool sample. The goal of the test is to detect cancers at an early stage when they are still treatable and the very good survival of Dukes stage A cancers (better than 90 per cent at five years) compared with colorectal cancer overall (approximately 30 per cent at five years) suggests that this could be successful. The test actually detects haem but will react positively to any peroxidase and is not very specific. It detects blood from any lesion in the bowels as well as reacting to a number of foods (red meat, fresh fruits and vegetables with peroxidase activity, e.g. tomatoes) and aspirin-induced gastrointestinal bleeding. Dietary restriction before testing or retesting has been used to try to minimize false positives. The sensitivity of the test is also an area for concern (Ahlquist *et al.* 1993) and it can be affected by vitamin C supplementation. The issue of whether or not to rehydrate samples before testing is also important. Rehydration improves sensitivity but at the expense of a large number of false positive tests. In one trial conducted in Minnesota the positivity rate for rehydrated tests was almost 10 per cent (Mandel *et al.* 1993) leading to many unnecessary referrals for colonoscopy. In that study a mortality reduction of 33 per cent for colorectal cancer has been found for annual occult blood testing, but it is unclear whether the results can be attributed to any selective value of screening, or are merely due to the fact that 38 per cent of this group received a colonoscopy at some stage as a result of a positive test. It is possible that similar reductions in mortality could be achieved by colonoscopy and polyp removal in 38 per cent of any population. Further trials are ongoing in Denmark, Sweden, and the UK (Table 21.6) and they should eventually provide a measurement of potentially neoplastic polyps.

New occult blood tests are being developed to attempt to improve on the test (Haemoccult II) currently in use. These include an immunological test specific for human haemoglobin (Hemeselect) and a more sensitive guaiac based test (Haemoccult–

Table 21.6 Controlled trials of screening by Haemoccult

Location and reference	Number completing test (% of total)	Sample rehydrated	Positivity rate (%)	PPV for cancer (%)	Number of cancers detected at 1st screen	No. Interval cancers	Sensitivity (%)
Nottingham, UK (Hardcastle *et al.* 1989)	27,651 (53)	No	2.3	10.2	75	36	67
Funen, Denmark (Kronborg *et al.* 1989)	20,672 (67)	No	1.0	17.7	38	36	52
Gothenburg, Sweden (Kewenter *et al.* (1994)	4,436 (67)	No	1.9	4.8	4	14	22
	16,911 (62)	Yes	5.1	5.0	43	8	84
Minnesota, US (Colon cancer relatives) (Ahlquist *et al.* 1993)	12,312 (57)	No	3.8	4.2	20	40	33
Minnesota, US (Mandel *et al.* 1993)	~4,300 (76)	No	2.4	5.6	—	—	81[1]
	~20,000 (76)	Yes	9.8	2.2	—	—	92[1]

[1]False negatives only include cancers diagnosed within one year of negative test.
PPV = Positive predictive value.

SENSA) which detects haem-derived porphyrins, so that it can detect degraded de-ironed haems as well as the intact haem detected by Haemoccult II (St. John *et al.* 1993). These have yet to be evaluated in prospective randomized trials.

Another approach to colorectal cancer screening is based on the work of Morson (1976) who proposed that most cancers arise from pre-existing adenomas. Adenomas are precancerous growths that occur throughout the bowel and have the same subsite distribution as cancers, but occur at a younger age. Thus a better strategy to control colon cancer may be to detect and remove adenomas, since the transition time from an adenoma to a carcinoma is thought to be very long (of the order of 10–25 years), implying that screening need only be carried out very infrequently. Also, since one is now preventing cancer rather than detecting it early, the potential for mortality reduction is much greater.

Faecal occult blood testing detects some adenomas, although the sensitivity is low. Another approach, based specifically on this idea, is to use flexible 60-cm sigmoidoscopy as a screening tool. This is far less expensive or traumatic than complete colonoscopy and approximately 60 per cent of colorectal cancers occur in the region accessible by this instrument. To date there is limited evidence on its efficacy. Selby *et al.* (1992) have shown, in a case-control study, that mortality caused by cancers within reach of the rigid sigmoidoscope (approximately within 20 cm of the anus) was reduced by 60 per cent for at least 10 years (Table 21.7) and similar results have been reported in a

smaller study by Newcomb *et al.* (1992). Several studies have suggested that endoscopic surveillance of the bowel greatly reduces colon cancer rates, but a direct demonstration that screening by sigmoidoscopy reduces mortality will require a large randomized trial. Such a trial has been proposed by Atkin *et al.* (1993). They argue that most of the benefit of sigmoidoscopy would accrue from a single screening test and only a small group of individuals (about 3–5 per cent in most series) would need colonoscopy and

Table 21.7 Most recent screening sigmoidoscopy in case subjects and controls, before the diagnosis of fatal cancer within reach of the rigid sigmoidscope in the case subjects

Years before diagnosis	Case subjects (*N* = 261)	Controls (*N* = 868)	Odds ratio
	No. (%)		
1–2	4 (1.6)	27 (3.1)	0.41 (0.14–1.22)
3–4	5 (2.0)	20 (2.3)	0.74 (0.27–2.01)
5–6	5 (2.0)	30 (3.5)	0.44 (0.17–1.15)
7–8	1 (0.4)	22 (2.5)	0.11 (0.01–0.83)
9–10	1 (0.4)	21 (2.4)	0.12 (0.02–0.93)
Multiple	7 (2.6)	90 (10.3)	0.22 (0.10–0.47)
1–10	23 (8.8)	210 (24.2)	0.41 (0.25–0.69)
>10 years or never	238	658	1[1]

From Selby *et al.* (1992).
[1] Reference category.

further surveillance. A key issue is at what age this single screen should take place. Ideally, this should be after most adenomas have appeared, but few of the cancers have developed. Figure 21.4 shows that this window of opportunity is probably between ages 55 and 65.

The genetic alterations leading to colon cancer (see Chapter 4) are better understood than for any other cancer. Mutations in the *APC* gene on chromosome 5q22 lead to polyposis coli (and cancer if untreated) when inherited, and somatic mutations are also found in sporadic adenomas and cancers (Ichii *et al.* 1993). Mutations in the *APC* gene appear to act at a very early stage leading to the development of adenomas. Several other genes including K-*ras*, *DCC*, *MCC* are related to colon cancer. Genes on chromosome 2 (*COCA1* for colon cancer gene 1) and chromosome 3 are related to a colon cancer family syndrome known as hereditary non-polyposis colon cancer (HNPCC). Tests based on detecting mutations in DNA in exfoliated cells in stools by PCR are at an early stage of development.

There are several important leads for the chemoprevention of colon cancer. Aspirin and other non-steroidal anti-inflammatory drugs (NSAIDs) have been shown to protect against cancer in several case-control studies, and another NSAID, known as sulindac, has been shown to be capable of causing small adenomas to regress. However, no reduction in colorectal cancer has been seen yet in a prospective double-blind, randomized study of aspirin in American physicians after five years of follow-up (Gann *et al.* 1993). Chemoprevention with NSAIDs, β-carotene, vitamin D, and calcium has

been suggested, as well as dietary modifications to increase the consumption of fibre, reduce fat intake, and increase the consumption of fresh fruit and vegetables. Studies looking at the effect of these interventions on small adenomas are under way.

21.5.4 Prostate cancer

Screening for prostate cancer provides a dilemma unique among cancer sites. The disease is exceedingly common but many cancers are indolent and are asymptomatic at the time of death from another cause. Indeed, autopsy studies have shown that about 10 per cent of men aged 50 who died from other causes have a focus of invasive disease and this increases to at least 40 per cent in 80-year old men (Fig. 21.5). Thus, while death from prostate cancer is common, being only second to lung cancer in men in many Western countries, the true incidence is much higher, and the as yet unsolved problem is how to discriminate aggressive disease with lethal potential from indolent cancers that are likely to remain asymptomatic for the remainder of the patient's lifetime.

Nevertheless, prostate cancer is a significant public health problem and an obvious target for screening. Three screening modalities are currently in use. Digital rectal examination involves palpation of the prostate to detect increased size. A blood test is also available which measures the level of prostate-specific

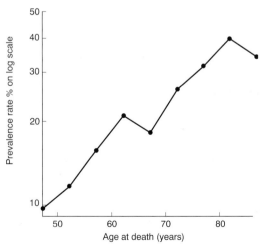

Fig. 21.5 Age–prevalence curve for latent prostatic carcinoma in autopsy specimens of men dying from other causes (adjusted for area effects) (Breslow *et al.* 1977).

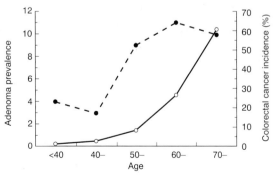

Fig. 21.4 Distal adenomas detected at screening by sigmoidoscopy versus colorectal cancer incidence (Atkin *et al.* 1993).

antigen (PSA), a glycoprotein produced only by (benign or malignant) prostate cells. A third method is transrectal ultrasonography, which, because of its cost, is usually reserved as a second stage screen in individuals who are positive for one of the first two tests, although many clinical algorithms for combining these tests exist. PSA is well established as a tumour marker in patients with prostatic cancer, but its use as a screening test has generated much controversy. A typical cut-off for positivity is 4 ng/ml and levels above this are very common at older ages (Table 21.8). There is little doubt that this test is relatively specific for prostate disease but it is unable to distinguish benign from malignant lesions unless higher cut-off levels are used and even less able to distinguish aggressive cancers from slowly growing ones.

When a screening test is positive, the next step is a transurethral prostatic resection to obtain a biopsy. This can distinguish benign from malignant disease, but malignant cases then usually go on to a radical prostatectomy with or without radiotherapy. This is a major operation with some mortality and high morbidity, often including incontinence and impotence. To date, no trials have been completed to show if prostate screening has any effect on mortality, although a large trial is underway in the US (Prorok *et al.* 1991). Basic questions regarding the value of radical surgical and radiotherapy treatment in early disease have also not been established and randomized trials are urgently needed.

Prostate cancer is now the most common cancer in men in the US and there has been a large recent increase in incidence. However, mortality is little changed and the most striking increases in incidence are seen at older ages (Lu-Yao and Greenberg 1994). Figure 21.6 shows that mortality is unrelated to incidence rates in different parts of the US and suggests that the increases are owing to increased utilization of screening. These observations raise doubts about the value of currently available screening methods and the results of randomized trials are awaited with much interest.

The use of the 5-α reductase inhibitor finasteride to prevent prostate cancer is currently under evaluation. This drug has an established place in treating benign prostatic hypertrophy and Ross and Henderson (1994) have pioneered its development

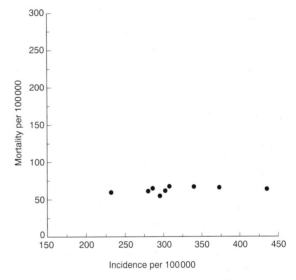

Fig. 21.6 Age-adjusted incidence and mortality rates for prostate cancer in nine Surveillance, Epidemiology and End Result (SEER) areas for white men aged 50–79, 1983–9 (Lu-Yao and Greenberg 1994).

Table 21.8 Serum PSA concentrations and the incidence of prostate cancer as a function of age in 1653 men

Age group (years)	Number of men (%)	Serum PSA level			
		4.0–9.9 ng/ml		≥10.0 ng/ml	
		Number (%)	Number with cancer/ Number with biopsy (%)	Number (%)	Number with cancer/ Number with biopsy (%)
50–59	629 (38)	12 (2)	2/11 (18)	4 (1)	1/3 (33)
60–69	737 (45)	53 (7)	8/40 (20)	15 (2)	12/15 (80)
70–79	264 (16)	39 (15)	9/32 (28)	10 (4)	4/8 (50)
80–89	23 (1)	3 (13)	0/2 (0)	1 (4)	1/1 (100)
All	1653	107 (6)	19/85 (22)	30 (2)	18/27 (67)

From Catalona *et al.* (1991)

as a chemopreventive agent. It works by blocking the intraprostatic conversion of testosterone to the much more potent androgen dihydrotestosterone (DHT). Finasteride appears to have few side effects and reduces PSA levels, but as yet there are no data on its ability to prevent prostate cancer. A large trial to evaluate this is being planned in the US (Kramer *et al.* 1993).

21.5.5 Melanoma

The incidence of melanoma is increasing at a faster rate than any other cancer in many Western countries, presumably because of the fashion for a suntan and the greater exposure to sunlight. Details as to which types of sun exposure are harmful are not clear, but there is some evidence that excessive burning during childhood may be particularly associated with increased risk. Skins that burn easily and people with fair or red hair are at increased risk. It is also well established that having lots of naevi (moles) or 'dysplastic' or 'atypical' naevi are also major risk factors and the inherited 'atypical mole syndrome' increases the risk by about 10-fold.

The only available screening modality is early recognition of melanoma, and the 10-year survival rate for early thin lesions (less than 0.76 mm) is very good (about 90 per cent) whereas thicker lesions (greater than 4 mm) have a much poorer prognosis (about 30 per cent). Because it has the very highest rate of melanoma in the world, Australia has taken the lead in promoting screening. Methods used include public education, free skin examinations at the beach or in city centres, and teaching people with high risk skin types or many naevi how to recognize a melanoma. Regular examination of people with the atypical mole syndrome by a dermatologist is also carried out, but one of the most important aspects of this may be to teach these people how to recognize malignant changes or new malignant lesions. None of these approaches have been subjected to serious scientific evaluation and at present it is difficult to confidently ascribe benefit to any of them. The use of psoralen-based sunscreens constitutes a form of chemoprevention that appears to be effective for non-melanoma skin cancer. Its value for melanoma is still unclear.

21.5.6 Ovarian cancer

Screening for ovarian cancer is still at a research stage. Two methods, transabdominal/transvaginal ultrasonography and a blood test for the tumour marker CA-125, have been most actively studied.

Ultrasound screening involves looking for enlarged ovaries. Its main problem is a lack of specificity since most enlarged ovaries are caused by benign cysts. Campbell *et al.* (1989) did a screening study on 5479 volunteers aged above 40 recruited by media publicity. They used transabdominal ultrasound annually for up to three years and 326 (5.9 per cent) women were found to be positive and referred to a surgeon for laparotomy/laparoscopy. Five of these women were found to have primary ovarian cancer (all stage I) and an additional four had metastatic cancer in the ovary from a primary in the breast or colon. The positive predictive value per test was about 1.4 per cent, which is too low when the next stage involves abdominal surgery. The false positive rate on the first screen was 3.5 per cent, dropping to 1.8 per cent and 1.2 per cent on subsequent screens. To improve the specificity, transvaginal colour Doppler ultrasound has been used to image blood flow. Blood vessel formation is thought to be a good discriminant between cancer and benign cysts and early reports indicate that the test can substantially reduce the false positive rate (Bourne *et al.* 1993), although it is still unclear whether this will be enough to make population screening viable.

Another approach is to measure serum CA-125. This is a tumour marker that has an established place in monitoring tumour burden, response to treatment, and recurrence in women with established ovarian cancer. CA-125 is produced normally in the embryonal Mullerian duct and coelomic epithelium and is raised in about 80 per cent of women with ovarian cancer, but can also be elevated when benign ovarian cysts, endometriosis, or cancers of the colon, breast, or pancreas are present, as well as in pregnancy. Using a cut-off of 30 U/ml for serum CA-125, Jacobs *et al.* (1993) have reported a false positive rate of about 1.4 per cent in a study of 22 000 asymptomatic postmenopausal women aged over 45, and a sensitivity of 60 per cent. Better specificity can be obtained by requiring both ultrasound and CA-125 to be positive and in this study the false positive rate was reduced to 1.4 per 1000 when ultrasound was used as a second stage screen (Fig. 21.7). Only one of 19 true positive patients was lost in this manner. Concern has been raised about the low sensitivity of this approach (60 per cent) and Bourne *et al.* (1994) suggested that a lower threshold for CA-

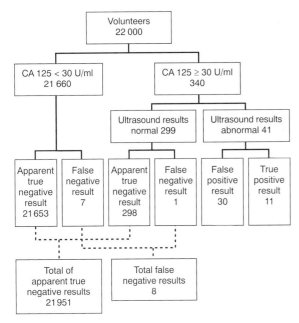

Fig. 21.7 Summary of study findings in 22 000 postmenopausal volunteer women participating in a screening programme for ovarian cancer (Jacobs *et al.* 1993).

125 should be used (they suggest 20 U/ml). However, gains in sensitivity by this approach will be at the expense of specificity. Other serum markers such as CA 15-3, PLAP, HMFG1, and HMFG2 may help to refine the diagnosis, but since the next step is abdominal surgery very high positive predictive values (above 10 per cent at least) are needed for a screening test to be viable. One way of easing the burden is to focus screening on high risk women (currently only those whose mother or sister has developed the disease), but even here randomized trials are necessary to obtain reliable assessments. Questions regarding the appropriate age and interval at which to screen are even less well understood.

Use of oral contraceptives reduces the risk of ovarian cancer by about 50 per cent, presumably because ovarian function is suppressed. This is a substantial achievement, but as yet no coordinated effort has been undertaken to try to prevent ovarian cancer by this or any other means (except surgical removal in very high risk women).

21.5.7 Stomach cancer

Because of its high incidence and mortality, screening for gastric cancer by barium X-ray is already a national programme in Japan. The aim is to screen everyone over the age of 40 every year in order to detect cancer at an earlier stage. In Miyagi Prefecture almost three million tests were performed between 1960 and 1988 and the test was positive in about 10 per cent of cases leading to a recommendation for gastroscopy. The positive predictive value is reported to be 1.7 per cent (Hisamichi *et al.* 1991). No randomized trials have been reported, but indications of effectiveness have been seen in time trends of mortality, cohort studies, and case–control studies (see Hisamichi *et al.* 1991). The results from a case–control study in Miyagi Prefecture are shown in Table 21.9 (Fukao *et al.* 1987) and suggest a substantial benefit in the year following screening, but little benefit subsequently. Potential biases exist in all these analyses since the incidence of stomach cancer is falling in Japan and compliers may have a different risk than non-compliers.

Table 21.9 Optimal interval for screening for stomach cancer

Time since last negative result (years)	Number of cases of advanced cancer	Number of controls	Relative protection	95% Confidence interval
1	132	220	2.92	2.09–4.08
2	40	31	1.36	0.80–2.32
3	23	18	1.37	0.70–2.67
4	16	9	0.99	0.42–2.32
Never screened	156	89	1[1]	
Total	367	367		

From Fukao *et al.* (1987).

[1] Reference category.

Another approach to stomach cancer prevention is screening for *Helicobacter pylori* infection and eradication by antibiotic therapy. *Helicobacter pylori* causes chronic active gastritis which can progress to chronic atrophic gastritis, which is thought to be one of the early steps in gastric carcinogenesis. Several epidemiological studies have linked *Helicobacter pylori* to stomach cancer (De Koster *et al.* 1993) and studies are ongoing in Venezuela to examine the effect of intensive treatment of *H. pylori* infection on stomach cancer incidence, although work in this area is still at an early stage. Population screening is not viable in Western countries, but stomach cancer is still very common in South America, eastern Europe, and parts of Asia and the possibility that screening can reduce mortality should be more fully investigated there.

Dietary modification is another possible approach to stomach cancer prevention. A high consumption of salt and salted foods are established risk factors and consumption of fresh fruits and vegetables appears to be protective, and so dietary modification of these intakes would seem wise. Chemoprevention trials with vitamin C have also been suggested in individuals with intestinal metaplasia or as an adjuvant following *H. pylori* eradication. Dietary supplementation of vitamins C, E, and β-carotene has also been recommended in high risk areas.

21.5.8 Oesophageal cancer

Oesophageal cancer is relatively rare in most parts of the world but there are pockets of very high risk, notably northern China, south and east of the Caspian Sea, and southern and eastern Africa. In Linxian, Henan Province, China, screening for precursor lesions by oesophageal balloon cytology has been undertaken in over 12 000 normal individuals aged 40–69. Cancer was detected in 2 per cent of the population and some degree of dysplasia was found in another 29 per cent. This latter population was invited to join a trial of dietary supplementation, and a non-significant 8 per cent reduction in oesophageal/upper stomach cancer was observed (Li *et al.* 1993). In parallel, a dietary intervention involving 30 000 individuals aged 40–69 was carried out in four Linxian communities. The group receiving β-carotene, vitamin E, and selenium had a significant 13 per cent reduction in overall cancer mortality and a 21 per cent reduction in stomach cancer, but oesophageal cancer was only reduced by a non-signifi-

cant 5 per cent (Blot *et al.* 1993). This result is encouraging for the use of these supplements in areas where the diet is severely deficient. However, it is less likely to be of value in the Western world where intakes are substantially higher.

21.5.9 Nasopharyngeal cancer

This cancer is very rare in most of the world but is important in a few places, notably south-eastern China and in Eskimos where it appears to be related to infection with Epstein–Barr virus. Serological tests for the virus have been undertaken (Zeng *et al.* 1982; Chen *et al.* 1989), but with present methodology, this does not seem to be useful, even in high risk populations.

21.5.10 Neuroblastoma

Neuroblastoma is the second most common malignancy in children and accounts for about 10 per cent of childhood cancer. In Japan, neonates are screened by looking for elevated levels of the catecholamine metabolites vanillylmandolic acid (VMA) and homovallic acid (HVA) in urine at ages 3 and 6 months. Sensitivity is about 80 per cent and about 1 in 8500 infants tested turn out to have neuroblastoma. Prognosis appears to be much improved by early detection (Sawada *et al.* 1991; Sawada 1992) but there is no evidence of reduced incidence rates at older ages or a decrease in mortality. It is possible that the cases picked up by screening are of a different variety which would regress spontaneously and are not related to the more aggressive tumours that arise in children aged over one year (Murphy *et al.* 1991). A randomized trial is needed to see if overall mortality is actually reduced.

21.5.11 Lung cancer

Several relatively small studies have examined the use of chest X-rays and sputum cytology as a method of early diagnosis of lung cancer. While the studies have shown evidence of earlier detection, this has not had any effect on mortality (Prorok *et al.* 1991) and detection may still be too late to affect the natural history. However, as lung cancer is the commonest cancer world-wide, even a small benefit would be useful, and a trial of chest X-rays large enough to detect a 10 per cent reduction in mortality (which would have been missed on previous studies), is now ongoing in the US (Prorok *et al.* 1991). In view of the enormity of the lung cancer problem, detection of cancer-associated markers in sputum would seem a useful area for future research.

About 90 per cent of lung cancer can be attributed to smoking and reduction of tobacco intake is clearly the most important preventive measure. A large prospective randomized study of dietary supplementation with β-carotene and vitamin E in smokers has been undertaken in Finland. After 5–8 years of follow-up the results have proved negative and, surprisingly, β-carotene was found to be associated with a significant 18 per cent *increase* of lung cancer (Heinonen and Albanes 1994).

21.5.12 Bladder cancer

Bladder cancer screening by cytology is routinely offered to occupationally exposed workers in the rubber and dyestuff industries. Some pilot work has been done in north Africa in high risk areas where schistosomiasis is endemic. Infection with this parasite is often associated with the late development of bladder cancer. Haematuria has also been suggested as a screening test. Neither of these tests are very specific and a greater positive predictive value needs to be achieved before screening and the attendant invasive follow-up investigations can be contemplated in the general population.

21.5.13 Liver cancer

Chronic carriers of hepatitis B virus surface antigen are at a greatly increased risk of liver cancer. Both of these are common in south-eastern China and tropical Africa. A possible approach to screening for liver cancer is first to look for chronic carriers, who are then screened for an increased level of α-fetoprotein which is a tumour marker for liver cancer. Further investigation by ultrasound could be useful in detecting small cancers that are surgically resectable. Such an approach has been suggested by Sun *et al.* (1988). However, prevention by vaccination against hepatitis B may be a better prospect and field trials of vaccination shortly after birth are ongoing in several high risk areas.

21.6 The need for DNA sequencing in epidemiology

We are rapidly coming to an end of what we can learn about the causes of cancer by simply asking patients questions about previous exposures. More detailed and precise measures of exposures and

genetic traits are needed if real progress is to be made. Over the next decade this may well become the main focus of epidemiology as the interactions between inherited traits and DNA damage caused by exposure to carcinogens are explored to pinpoint the stages of cancer development.

One small but important entry into this field relates to the role of the human papillomavirus (HPV) to cervix cancer. Molecular biology techniques such as the polymerase chain reaction (PCR) have already revolutionized our ability to detect HPV DNA reliably in the small amount of material in cervical smears, and to develop a taxonomy of the carcinogenic risk associated with sequence variation even within a single type is important in determining its pathogenicity. To study this, it is necessary to sequence moderate sized segments (several hundred base pairs) of the HPV DNA in a few hundred isolates of HPV from both high grade and low grade disease. This needs to be done for the major oncogene types and represents sequencing several hundred kilobases of DNA, which is only feasible with an automated machine.

Furthermore, there is accumulating evidence that the patient's genetic make-up (in the form of HLA types) determines response to HPV infection. The most interesting region appears to be DR, which, because of its extreme polymorphism is best typed by direct sequencing of PCR products of patient DNA. Again this will involve several hundred kilobases of DNA.

These projects are only the beginning of what can be done. Sequencing the breast cancer gene (*BRCA1*) in early onset non-familial cases is another major project. Also, looking for mutations in the many genes associated with colon cancer, especially hMSH2 and hMSH1 on chromosomes 2 and 3, is likely to produce important new results.

21.7 Conclusion

It must always be remembered that screening has the potential to do harm as well as good, and it is essential that the benefits be clearly established to outweigh the risks before screening programmes are introduced. At present this has only been done for cervical screening and for mammographic breast screening in women aged 50 or more. The balance also looks very positive for infrequent (once in a lifetime) bowel screening by sigmoidoscopy, but this needs to be demonstrated in a large randomized trial. Serious problems still exist in terms of high false positive rates for ovarian screening, and a similar problem of detecting cancer that is not likely to be fatal exists for prostate cancer. Until these problems are minimized, or at least fully evaluated in well-designed prospective randomized trials, these modalities cannot be recommended for routine use. Approaches to other cancers require even more

development and should be restricted to specialized high risk groups in the developed Western world.

Chemoprevention is at an even earlier stage of development and all methods under current consideration (tamoxifen, other manoeuvers to affect hormones (fenasteride), synthetic retinoids, antioxidants) must be proven in randomized trials before they can be recommended for use, even in high risk populations.

References and further reading

Ahlquist, D. A., Wieand, H. S., Moertel, C. G., McGill, D. B., Loprinzi, C. L., O'Connell, M. J., *et al.* (1993). Accuracy of fecal occult blood screening for colorectal neoplasia. A prospective study using Hemoccult and HemoQuant tests. *Journal of the American Medical Association*, **269**, 1262–7.

Alexander, F. E., Anderson, T. J., Brown, H. K., Forrest, A. P. M., Hepburn, W., Kirkpatrick, A. E., *et al.* (1994). The Edinburgh randomised trial of breast cancer screening: results after 10 years of followup. *British Journal of Cancer*, **70**, 542–8.

Andersson, I., Aspegren, K., Janzon, L., Landberg, T., Lindholm, K., Linell, F., *et al.* (1988). Mammographic screening and mortality from breast cancer: the Malmo mammographic screening trial. *British Medical Journal*, **297**, 943–8.

Anwar, K., Inuzuka, M., Shiraishi, T., and Nakakuki, K. (1991). Detection of HPV DNA in neoplastic and non-neoplastic cervical specimens from Pakistan and Japan by non-isotopic *in situ* hybridization. *International Journal of Cancer*, **47**, 675–80.

Atkin, W. S., Cuzick, J., Northover, J. M. A., and Whynes, D. K. (1993). Prevention of colorectal cancer by once-only sigmoidoscopy. *Lancet*, **341**, 736–40.

Banda-Gamboa, H., Ricketts, I., Cairns, A., Hussein, K., Tucker, J. H., and Husain, N. (1992). Automation in cervical cytology: an overview. *Analytical Cellular Pathology*, **4**, 25–48.

Bavin, P. J., Giles, J. A., Deery, A., Crow, J., Griffiths, P. D., Emery, V. C., and Walker, P. G. (1993). Use of semi-quantitative PCR for human papillomavirus DNA type 16 to identify women with high grade cervical disease in a population

presenting with a mildly dyskaryotic smear report. *British Journal of Cancer*, **67**, 602–5.

Blot, W. J., Li, J. Y., Taylor, P. R., Guo, W., Dawsey, S., Wang, G. Q., *et al.* (1993). Nutrition Intervention Trials in Linxian, China: supplementation with specific vitamin/mineral combinations, cancer incidence, and disease-specific mortality in the general population. *Journal of the National Cancer Institute*, **85**, 1483–92.

Bourne, T. H., Campbell, S., Reynolds, K. M., Whitehead, M. I., Hampson, J., Royston, P., *et al.* (1993). Screening for early familial ovarian cancer with transvaginal ultrasonography and colour blood flow imaging. *British Medical Journal*, **306**, 1025–9.

Bourne, T. H., Campbell, S., Reynolds, K., Hampson, J., Bhatt, L., Crayford, T. J. B., *et al.* (1994). The potential role of serum CA 125 in an ultrasound-based screening program for familial ovarian cancer. *Gynecologic Oncology*, **52**, 379–85.

Boyd, N. F., Cousins, M., Lockwood, G., and Tritchler, D. (1992). Dietary fat and breast cancer risk: the feasibility of a clinical trial of breast cancer prevention. *Lipids*, **27**, 821–6.

Breslow, N., Chan, C. W., Dhom, G., Drury, R. A. B., Franks, L. M., Gellei, B., *et al.* (1977). Latent carcinoma of prostate at autopsy in seven areas. *International Journal of Cancer*, **20**, 680–8.

Campbell, S., Bhan, V., Royston, P., Whitehead, M. I., and Collins, W. P. (1989). Transabdominal ultrasound screening for early ovarian cancer. *British Medical Journal*, **299**, 1363–7.

Catalona, W. J., Smith, D. S., Ratliff, T. L., Dodds, K. M., Coplen, D. E., Yuan, J. J. J., *et al.* (1991). Measurement of prostate-specific antigen in serum as a screening test for prostate cancer. *New England Journal of Medicine*, **324**, 1156–61.

Chen, J. Y., Chen, C. J., Liu, M. Y., Cho, S. M., Hsu, M. M., Lynn, T. C., *et al.* (1989). Antibody to Epstein–Barr virus-specific DNase as a marker for field survey of patients with nasopharyngeal carcinoma in Taiwan. *Journal of Medical Virology*, **27**, 269–73.

Clarke, E. A. and Anderson, T. W. (1979). Does screening by "PAP" smears help prevent cervical cancer? *Lancet*, **ii**, 1–4.

Cuzick J., Wang, D. Y., and Bulbrook, R. D. (1986). The prevention of breast cancer. *Lancet*, **ii**, 83–6.

Cuzick, J., Terry G., Ho, L., Hollingworth, T., and Anderson, M. (1992). Human papillomavirus type 16 DNA in cervical smears as a predictor of high-grade cervical intraepithelial neoplasia. *Lancet*, **339**, 959–60.

Cuzick, J., Terry, G., Ho, L., Hollingworth, T., and Anderson, M. (1994). Type-specific human papillomavirus DNA in abnormal smears as a predictor of high-grade intraepithelial neoplasia. *British Journal of Cancer*, **69**, 167–71.

De Palo, G., Sporn, M., and Veronesi, U. (Eds.) (1992). *Progress and perspectives in chemoprevention of cancer*. Serono Symposia Publications, Vol. 79. Raven Press, New York.

De Koster, E., Buset, M., Nyst, J.-F., and Deltenre, M. (1993). Gastric screening prospects. *European Journal of Cancer Prevention, **2**, 263–8.

Doll, R. and Peto, R. (1976). Mortality in relation to smoking: 20 years' observations on male British doctors. *British Medical Journal*, **2**, 1525–36.

Donnan S. P. B., Wong F. W. S., Ho, S. C., Lau, E. M. C., Takashi, K., and Estève, J. (1989). Reproductive and sexual risk factors and human papilloma virus infection in cervical cancer among Hong Kong Chinese. *International Journal of Epidemiology*, **18**, 32–6.

Duffy, S. W., Tabar, L., Fagerberg, G., Gad, A., Grontoft, O., South, M. C., and Day, N. E. (1991). Breast screening, prognostic factors and survival—results from the Swedish two county study. *British Journal of Cancer*, **64**, 1133–8.

Early Breast Cancer Trialists' Collaborative Group (EBCTCG) (1992). Systemic treatment of early breast cancer by hormonal, cytotoxic, or immune therapy. *Lancet*, **339**, 1–15, 71–85.

Ellman, R., Moss, S. M., Coleman, D., and Chamberlain, J. (1993). Breast self-examination programmes in the trial of early detection of breast cancer: ten year findings. *British Journal of Cancer*, **68**, 208–12.

Elwood, J. M., Cox, B., and Richardson, A. K. (1993). The effectiveness of breast cancer screening by mammography in younger women. *Online Journal of Current Clinical Trials*, document 32, para. 1–195.

Fornander, T., Hellstrom, A. C., and Moberger, B. (1993). Descriptive clinicopathologic study of 17 patients with endometrial cancer. *European Journal of Cancer*, **85**, 1850–5.

Frisell, J., Eklund, G., Hellstrom, L., Lidbrink, E., Rutqvist, L. E., and Somell A. (1991). Randomized study of mammography screening: preliminary report on mortality in the Stockholm trial. *Breast Cancer Research and Treatment*, **18**, 49–56.

Fukao, A., Hisamichi, S., and Sugawara, N. (1987). A case control study on evaluating the effect of mass screening on decreasing advanced stomach cancer (in Japanese). *Journal of the Japanese Society of Gastroenterology Mass Survey*, **75**, 112–16.

Gann, P. H., Manson, J. E., Glynn, R. J., Buring, J. E., and Hennekens, C. H. (1993). Low-dose aspirin and incidence of colorectal tumors in a randomised trial. *Journal of the National Cancer Institute*, **85**, 1220–4.

Gastrin, G., Miller, A. B., To, T., Aronson, K. J., Wall, C., Hakama, M., *et al.* (1994). Incidence and mortality from breast cancer in the Mama program for breast screening in Finland 1973–1986. *Cancer*, **73**, 2168–74.

Gershon-Cohen, J. and Colcher, A. E. (1937). Evaluation of roentgen diagnosis of early carcinoma of the breast. *Journal of the American Medical Association*, **108**, 867–71.

Hakama, M. (1982). Trends in the incidence of cervical cancer in the Nordic countries. In: *Trends in cancer incidence: causes and practical implications* (ed. K. Magnus), pp. 279–92. Hemisphere Publishing Corporation, Washington.

Hardcastle, J. D., Chamberlain, J., Sheffield, J., Balfour, T. W., Armitage, N. C., Thomas, W. M., *et al.* (1989). Randomised, controlled trial of faecal occult blood screening for colorectal cancer. *Lancet,* **i**, 1160–4.

Heinonen, O. P. and Albanes, D. (1994). The effect of vitamin E and beta carotene on the incidence of lung cancer and other cancers in male smokers. *New England Journal of Medicine,* **330**, 1029–35.

Hisamichi, S., Fukao, A., Sugawara, N., Nishikouri, M., Komatsu, S., Tsuji, I., *et al.* (1991). Evaluation of mass screening programme for stomach cancer in Japan. In *Cancer screening* (ed. A.B. Miller, J. Chamberlain, N.E. Day, M. Hakama, and P.C. Prorok), pp. 357–70. Cambridge University Press, New York.

Howe, G. R., Hirohata, T., Hislop, T. G., Iscovich, J. M., Yuan, J.-M. Katsouyanni, K., *et al.* (1990). Dietary factors and risk of breast cancer: combined analysis of 12 case control studies. *Journal of the National Cancer Institute,* **82**, 561–9.

Hurley, S. F. and Kaldor, J. M. (1992). The benefits and risks of mammographic screening for breast cancer. *Epidemiologic Reviews,* **14**, 101–30.

IARC Working Party (1986). Screening for squamous cervical cancer: Duration of low risk after negative results of cervical cytology and its implication for screening policies. *British Medical Journal,* **293**, 659–64.

Ichii, S., Takeda, S., Horii, A., Nakatsuru, S., Miyoshi, Y., Emi, M., *et al.* (1993). Detailed analysis of genetic alterations in colorectal tumors from patients with and without familial adenomatous polyposis (FAP). *Oncogene,* **8**, 2399–405.

Jacobs, I., Davies, A. P., Bridges, J., Stabile, I., Fay, T., Lower, A., *et al.* (1993). Prevalence screening for ovarian cancer in postmenopausal women by CA 125 measurement and ultrasonography. *British Medical Journal,* **306**, 1030–4.

Jonas, S. K., Benedetto, C., Flatman, A., Hammond, R. H., Micheletti, L., Riley, C., *et al.* (1992). Increased activity of 6-phosphogluconate dehydrogenase and glucose-6-phosphate dehydrogenase in purified cell suspensions and single cells from the uterine cervix in cervical intraepithelial neoplasia. *British Journal of Cancer,* **66**, 185–91.

Kramer, B. S., Brawley, O. W., Nayfield, S., Johnson, K., Greenwald, P., and Ford, L. G. (1993). NCI studies in primary prevention of breast and prostate cancer. *Cancer Research, Therapy and Control,* **3**, 203–11.

Kewenter, J., Brevinge, H., Engaras, B., Haglind, E., and Ahren, C. (1994). Followup after screening for colorectal neoplasms with fecal occult blood testing in a controlled trial. *Disease of Colon and Rectum,* **37**, 115–19.

Kronborg, O., Fenger, C., Olsen, J., Bech, K., and Sondergaard, O. (1989). Repeated screening for colorectal cancer with fecal occult blood test. A prospective randomized study at Funen in Denmark. *Scandinavian Journal of Gastroenterology,* **24**, 599–606.

Läärä, E., Day, N. E., and Hakama, M. (1987). Trends in mortality from cervical cancer in the Nordic countries: association with organised screening programmes. *Lancet,* **i**, 1247–9.

Li, J. Y., Taylor, P. R., Li, B., Dawsey, S., Wang, G-Q., Ershow, A. G., *et al.* (1993). Nutrition Intervention Trials in Linxian, China: multiple vitamin/mineral supplementation, cancer incidence, and disease-specific mortality among adults with esophageal dysplasia. *Journal of the National Cancer Institute,* **85**, 1492–8.

Lorincz, A. T., Reid, R., Jenson, A. B., Greenberg, M. D., Lancaster, W., and Kurman, R. J. (1992). Human papillomavirus infection of the cervix: relative risk associations of fifteen common anogenital types. *Obstetrics and Gynaecology,* **79**, 328–37.

Lu-Yao, G. L. and Greenberg, E. R. (1994). Changes in prostate cancer incidence and treatment in USA. *Lancet,* **343**, 251–4.

Mandel, J. S., Bond, J. H., Church, T. R., Snover, D. C., Bradley, M. G., Schuman, L. M., and Ederer, F. (1993). Reducing mortality from colorectal cancer by screening for fecal occult blood. *New England Journal of Medicine,* **328**, 1365–71.

Miller, A. B., Baines, C. J., To, T., and Wall, C. (1992a). Canadian National Breast Screening Study: 1. Breast cancer detection and death rates among women aged 40 to 49 years. *Canadian Medical Association Journal,* **147**, 1459–76.

Miller, A. B., Baines, C. J., To, T., and Wall, C. (1992b). Canadian National Breast Screening

Study: 2. Breast cancer detection and death rates among women aged 50 to 59 years. *Canadian Medical Association Journal*, **147**, 1477–88.

Morson, B. C. (1976). Genesis of colorectal cancer. *Gastroenterology*, **5**, 505–25.

Moss, S. M. (1991). Case control studies of screening. *International Journal of Epidemiology*, **20**, 1–6.

Muñoz, N. and Bosch, F. X. (1992). HPV and cervical neoplasia: review of case control and cohort studies. In *The epidemiology of human papillomavirus and cervical cancer* (ed. N. Munoz, F.X. Bosch, K.V. Shah, and A. Meheus), Vol. 119, pp. 251–61. IARC, Lyon.

Murphy, S. B., Cohn, S. L., Craft, A. W., Woods, W. G., Sawada, T., Castleberry, R. P., *et al.* (1991). Do children benefit from mass screening for neuroblastoma? *Lancet*, **337**, 344–5.

National Cancer Institute (NCI) Workshop (1989). The 1988 Bethesda system for reporting cervical/vaginal cytological diagnoses. *Journal of the American Medical Association*, **289**, 1049–51.

Newcomb, P. A., Norfleet, R. G., Storer, B. E., Surawicz, T. S., and Marcus, P. M. (1992). Screening sigmoidoscopy and colorectal cancer mortality. *Journal of the National Cancer Institute*, **84**, 1572–5.

Nyström, L., Rutqvist, L. E., Wall, S., Lindgren, A., Lindqvist, M., Rydén, S., *et al.* (1993). Breast cancer screening with mammography: overview of Swedish randomised trials. *Lancet*, **341**, 973–8.

Oza, A. M. and Boyd, N. F. (1993). Mammographic parenchymal patterns: a marker of breast cancer risk. *Epidemiologic Reviews*, **15**, 196–208.

Paci, E. and Duffy, S. W. (1991). Modelling the analysis of breast cancer screening programmes: sensitivity, lead time and predictive value in the Florence district programme (1975–1986). *International Journal of Epidemiology*, **20**, 852–8.

Partington, C. K., Sincock, A. M., and Steele, S. J. (1991). Quantitative determination of acid-labile DNA in cervical intraepithelial neoplasia. *Cancer*, **67**, 3104–9.

Peer, P. G. M., Holland, R., Hendriks, J. H. C. L., Mravunac, M., and Verbeek, A. L. M. (1994). Age-specific effectiveness of the Nijmegen population-based breast cancer-screening program: assessment of early indicators of screening effectiveness. *Journal of the National Cancer Institute*, **86**, 436–41.

Peng, H. Q., Liu, S. L., Mann, V., Rohan, T., and Rawls, W. (1991). Human papillomavirus types 16 and 33, herpes simplex virus type 2 and other risk factors for cervical cancer in Sichuan Province, China. *International Journal of Cancer*, **47**, 711–16.

Powles, T. J., Jones, A. L., Ashley, S. E., O'Brien, M. E. R., Tidy, V. A., Treleavan, J., *et al.* (1994). The Royal Marsden Hospital pilot tamoxifen chemoprevention trial. *Breast Cancer Research and Treatment*, **31**, 73–82.

Prorok, P. C., Byar, D. P., Smart, C. R., Baker, S. G., and Connor, R. J. (1991). Evaluation of screening for prostate, lung, and colorectal cancers: the PLC Trial. In *Cancer screening* (ed. A.B. Miller, J. Chamberlain, N.E. Day, M. Hakama, and P.C. Prorok), pp. 300–20. Cambridge University Press, New York.

Ransohoff, D. F. and Lang, C. A. (1991). Screening for colorectal cancer. *New England Journal of Medicine*, **325**, 37–41.

Reeves, W. C., Brinton, L. A., Garcia, M., Brenes, M. M., Herrero, R., Gaitan, E., *et al.* (1989). Human papillomavirus infection and cervical cancer in Latin America. *New England Journal of Medicine*, **320**, 1437–41.

Reid, R., Greenberg M. D., Lorincz, A. T., Jenson, A. B., Laverty, C. R., Husain, M., *et al.* (1991). Should cervical cytologic testing be augmented by cervicography or human papillomavirus deoxyribonucleic acid detection? *American Journal of Obstetrics and Gynecology*, **164**, 1461–71.

Romney, S. L., Dwyer, A., Slagle, S., Duttagupta, C., Palan, P. R., Basu, J., *et al.* (1985). Chemoprevention of cervix cancer: Phase I–II: A feasibility study involving the topical vaginal administration of retinyl acetate gel. *Gynecological Oncology*, **20**, 109–19.

Ross, R. K. and Henderson, B.E . (1994). Do diet and androgens alter prostate cancer risk via a common etiologic pathway? *Journal of the National Cancer Institute*, **86**, 252–4.

Sawada, T. (1992). Past and future of neuroblastoma screening in Japan. *American Journal of Pediatrics Hematology and Oncology*, **14**, 320–6.

Sawada, T., Matsumura, T., Matsuda, Y., and Kawakatsu, H. (1991). Neuroblastoma: studies in Japan. In *Cancer screening* (eds. A.B. Miller, J. Chamberlain, N.E. Day, M. Hakama, and P.C. Prorok), pp. 325–36. Cambridge University Press, New York.

Schmauz, R., Okong, P., de Villiers, E. M., Dennin, R., Brade, L., Lwanga, S. K., and Owor, R. (1989). Multiple infections in cases of cervical cancer from a high-incidence area in tropical Africa. *International Journal of Cancer*, **43**, 805–9.

Selby, J. V., Friedman, G. D., Quesenberry, C. P., and Weiss, N. S. (1992). A case control study of screening sigmoidoscopy and mortality from colorectal cancer. *New England Journal of Medicine*, **326**, 653–7.

Semiglazov, V. F., Sagaidak, V. N., Moiseyenko, V. M., and Mikhailov, E. A. (1993). Study of the role of breast self-examination in the reduction of mortality from breast cancer. *European Journal of Cancer*, **29A**, 2039–46.

Shapiro, S., Venet, W., Strax, P, Venet, L., and Roeser, R. (1982). Ten-to-fourteen year effect of screening on breast cancer mortality. *Journal of the National Cancer Institute*, **69**, 349–55.

Spicer, D. V., Ursin G., Parisky, Y. R., Pearce, J. G., Shoupe, D., Pike, A., and Pike, M. C. (1994). Changes in mammographic densities induced by a hormonal contraceptive designed to reduce breast cancer risk. *Journal of the National Cancer Institute*, **86**, 431–6.

Stafl, A. (1981). Cervicography: a new method for cervical cancer detection. *American Journal of Obstetrics and Gynecology*, **39**, 815–25.

St. John, D. J. B., Young, G. P., Alexeyeff, M. A., Deacon, M. C., Cuthbertson, A. M., Macrae, F. A., and Penfold, J. C. (1993). Evaluation of new occult blood tests for detection of colorectal neoplasia. *Gastroenterology*, **104**, 1661–8.

Sun, T., Yu, H., Hsia, C., Wang, N., and Huang, X. (1988). Evaluation of sero-survey trials for the early detection of hepatocellular carcinoma in area of high prevalence. In *Screening for gastrointestinal cancer* (ed. J. Chamberlain and A.B. Miller), pp. 81–6. Hans Huber, Bern

Szarewski, A., Cuzick, J., Edwards, R., Butler, B., and Singer A. (1991). The use of cervicography in a primary screening service. *British Journal of Obstetrics and Gynaecology*, **98**, 313–17.

Tabar, L., Fagerberg, G., Duffy, S. W., Day, N. E., Gad, A., and Gröntoft, O. (1992). Update of the Swedish two-county program of mammographic screening for breast cancer. *Radiologic Clinics of North America*, **30**, 187–209.

Tawa, K., Forsythe, A., Cove, J. K., Saltz, A., Peters, H. W., and Watring, W. G. (1988). A comparison of the papanicolaou smear and the cervigram: sensitivity, specificity, and cost analysis. *Obstetrics and Gynecology*, **71**, 229–35.

UK National Case–Control Study Group (1989). Oral contraceptive use and breast cancer risk in young women: subgroup analyses. *Lancet*, **i**, 973–82.

Wolfe, J. N. (1976). Risk for breast cancer development determined by mammographic parenchymal pattern. *Cancer*, **37**, 2486–92.

Wong, P. T. T., Wong, R. K., Caputo, T. A., Godwin, T. A., and Rigas, B. (1991). Infrared spectroscopy of exfoliated human cervical cells: evidence of extensive structural changes during carcinogenesis. *Proceedings of the National Academy of Sciences, USA*, **88**, 10988–92.

Zeng, Y., Zhang L. G., Li, H. Y., Jan, M. G., Zhang, Q., Wu, Y. C., *et al.* (1982). Serological mass survey for early detection of nasopharyngeal carcinoma in Wuzhou City, China. *International Journal of Cancer*, **29**, 139–41.

22

Some conclusions and prospects

ROBIN A. WEISS

22.1 Understanding carcinogenesis

It is evident from the foregoing chapters that we are gaining major insight into the nature of cancer. The excitement in this field derives from the realization that a finite, analysable set of genes is involved in carcinogenesis. These are the genes called oncogenes and tumour suppressor genes (see Chapter 9). Their identification has brought together seemingly distinct areas of cancer research such as chemical and radiation carcinogenesis (see Chapters 6 and 7), oncogenic viruses (see Chapter 8), chromosome anomalies (see Chapter 10), and growth factors (see Chapter 11). While it is possible that oncogenes may also underlie some of the specific inherited predispositions to cancer (see Chapter 4), they have been chiefly identified in association with the mutation and rearrangement of genes during carcinogenesis; in other words cancer is usually the result of genetic changes in somatic cells.

The somatic mutation hypothesis of cancer has a venerable pedigree. The notion that carcinogenesis involves genetic change dates from the turn of the century when Boveri identified chromosomes as the repository of genetic material and speculated on chromosome imbalance in cancer. The link between mutation and cancer was first drawn by Muller in 1927, who demonstrated the mutagenicity of ionizing radiation in fruit flies (radium and X-rays were already known to cause cancer). Later, Auerbach showed that a carcinogenic chemical, mustard gas, also induced mutations, and it now appears that the great majority of chemical carci-

nogens or their active metabolites are mutagens (see Chapter 6).

Thus the concept that certain stages in carcinogenesis, in particular initiating events, were mutational has been firmly embedded in our thinking about cancer for many decades. But this gave no indication as to which genes became altered, or indeed whether the same genes were regularly affected. It was thought that the accumulation of mutations might allow otherwise recessive traits to appear, by removing the action of some of the very large number of genes involved in cellular control processes. The recent studies of oncogenes has focused attention on just 20 out of the 50 000 or so genes in the human genome.

The repeated identification of the same set of genes—whether captured by retroviruses, or revealed by DNA transfection, DNA amplification, or chromosome rearrangement—indicates that these genes are of major importance in understanding cancer. Moreover, oncogenes are active genes, and tend to be expressed in a dominant manner. Mutation may cause overexpression of a normal protein or normal levels of expression of an altered protein, but in each case the gene products contribute positively to the neoplastic phenotype. Oncogenes challenge the earlier assumption that deletion of active genes led to cancer, that normality is dominant, and that cancer is recessive.

Carcinogenesis is, of course, a much more complicated, multistep process than the activation or mutation of a single oncogene (see Chapters 1 and 6). Mutated oncogenes are not clearly dominant over their normal alleles, and expression of several different oncogenes may act synergistically in producing the malignant phenotype (see Chapter 9). Moreover, some somatic cell hybrids between normal and malignant cells have a normal phenotype. Nevertheless, the evidence that identifiable proteins encoded by oncogenes contribute to neoplastic transformation is a major step forward in our understanding of cancer, and suggests new means of treatment by blocking the function of such proteins.

The oncogene concept contrasts with theories that gene deletion leads to cancer. However, this does appear to be the case for tumour suppressor genes, sometimes called antioncogenes. These genes have mainly been identified through rare, familial, inherited predispositions to cancer, among which are the genes for familial retinoblastoma, *RB1*, familial breast cancer (BRCA1 and BRCA2) and p53 (Li-Fraumeni syndrome). Tumour suppressor genes encode proteins that are necessary to prevent uncontrolled cell proliferation, whereas the proteins of oncogenes actively promote such growth. Thus specific genes may be involved in carcinogenesis either by stimulating cell growth or by failing to restrain cell growth, or by failing to induce apoptosis.

In general, oncogenes may be thought of as dominant, because a single gene will give rise to a protein acting to stimulate growth. In contrast, tumour suppressor genes tend to be recessive, because one must lose the function of both copies in a diploid cell to release the cell from its control. In heritable predisposition to cancers, only one good copy of a tumour suppressor gene is inherited in the first place, so that a mutation in the remaining one may lead to cancer (see Chapter 4). Recent investigations of non-heritable tumours suggest that both copies may be lost in the malignant clone. For example, many sporadic colon carcinomas have chromosome deletions around the same locus that determines familial polyposis coli.

New insight into viral carcinogenesis (Chapter 8) also points to the interaction of tumour suppressor genes. For example, the protein encoded by one of the transforming genes of human papillomavirus actually binds to and inactivates the protein encoded by the cell's retinoblastoma gene. The net result is the same as losing the gene, because its protein is no longer present in a biologically active form sufficient to restrain cell proliferation.

The somatic mutation hypothesis of cancer presupposes the clonal origin of the cells comprising the malignant population. Clearly, a mutation or genetic change occurring in one cell can only be passed on to that cell's linear descendants, i.e. its derivative clone. By and large, where cancers have been amenable to analysis, clonality has been upheld. For example, there is a polymorphism for an enzyme coded by an X-linked gene which happens to be relatively common in black people. Following inactivation of one or other X chromosome early in female development, each cell will express only one form of the enzyme. Thus normal tissues display a fine mosaic of cells expressing one or other enzymatic form (see Chapter 4). Fialkow's studies show that the malignant cells in a tumour usually express one form of the enzyme only, demonstrating the clonal derivation of the tumour cells after X chromosome inactivation has taken place.

Other evidence also points to a clonal evolution of tumour cells at early stages of carcinogenesis. In chronic granulocytic leukaemia, a chromosome translocation (the 'Philadelphia' chromosome) involving the *abl* oncogene (see Chapters 9, 10, and 12) is present in the majority of apparently normal and premalignant cells of the blood, indicating that a clonal stem cell carrying the translocated chromosomes has populated almost all the bone marrow before malignancy appears. Experimental chemical carcinogenesis in mouse skin indicates that a *ras* gene is mutated in codon 12 in premalignant stages of papillomatosis (see Chapters 6 and 9), again indicating clonality.

It is not clear, however, that all premalignant changes are clonal in origin. Pathologists frequently recognize 'field changes' in tissues that look abnormal and from which a malignant tumour may emerge (see Chapter 1). For example, cancer of the stomach frequently arises in patches of stomach epithelium that have undergone intestinal metaplasia, in which the tissue resembles the epithelium of the intestine rather than the stomach, and this observation has been used in early screening for stomach cancer in Japan where this tumour is common. We do not know exactly what triggers metaplasia and whether such altered patches of epithelium are clonal in origin.

In concluding a discussion on the genetic basis of carcinogenesis one should mention that the clonal nature of the cancer in which mutations in a single cell lead to a malignant cell population is not universally accepted. An epigenetic view of cancer was long held by the radiotherapist, Sir David Smithers, and more recently by Dr Harry Rubin. 'Cancer is no more a disease of cells than a traffic jam is a disease of cars', wrote Smithers in 1962, continuing, 'A lifetime study of the internal combustion engine would not help anyone to understand our traffic problems. A traffic jam is due to a failure of the normal relationship between driven cars and their environment and can occur whether they themselves are running normally or not'.

This is an attractive argument, but a deceptive one. The body's environment can be of crucial importance in allowing tumours to develop. Many remain dependent on hormones (see Chapters 14 and 15) and growth factors (see Chapter 11), and possibly the host immune system (see Chapter 16). Local interactions between cells also remain important to all but the most anaplastic tumour cells. Thus the cancer 'seed' requires fertile 'soil' in which to proliferate, as is shown by the relative inefficiency of the process of metastasis (see Chapter 2). Although thousands of tumour cells may be released from a primary tumour, only a very small number will develop into secondary tumours. Nevertheless, the interaction of tumour cells with the host environment is an elective or permissive process of stimulation and response in which an essential lesion always exists in the tumour cell itself. This after all is the basis of surgery, radiotherapy, and chemotherapy (see Chapters 17 and 18) directed to the elimination of the tumour. Drug resistance following chemotherapy is another example of clonal evolution and progression of tumours in which genetic changes within the malignant cell (for example gene amplification) determine the response to and escape from therapy.

Smithers based his views on observations that human tumours, particularly embryonal tumours occurring early in childhood, may occasionally regress spontaneously, and he concluded that the malignant phenotype was reversible. Certainly tumour cells differ from normal cells in subtle ways, such as arrested differentiation (see Chapter 12) in which less malignant behaviour may develop if the tumour cells can be made to follow a normal cell maturation pathway. Indeed, there has recently been increased emphasis in introducing so called biological response modifiers into cancer therapy. But the natural history of tumour progression (see Chapter 6) unfortunately promotes the selection of subclones with greater malignant potential.

Is there any experimental evidence for the reversibility of malignancy, as one might expect if carcinogenesis were a non-genetic phenomenon? There are some suggestive findings that merit more detailed investigation. For example, in leopard frogs, isolated nuclei from Lucke carcinoma cells (a kidney tumour induced by a herpesvirus) have been introduced into activated, enucleated frog eggs. Following nuclear transplantation, a small proportion of the nuclei allowed the development of tadpoles with normal, differentiated tissues, but it has not been unequivocally demonstrated that these nuclei came from tumour cells rather than from the stroma. Mouse teratocarcinomas containing pluripotential embryonal carcinoma cells have been the subject of extensive study, as these cancer cells can differentiate into many types of apparently normal cells. The introduction of such cells into the embryonic blastocyst allows incorporation into the inner cell mass, and hence into the embryo. Using genetic markers, it has been shown that the embryonal carcinoma cells contribute to most of the normal tissues of the mouse, although such mice have a higher frequency of teratocarcinoma. It has also been found that the descendants of embryonal cell lines can form a normal germ line, but this remains to be confirmed with fully malignant teratocarcinoma cells. Similarly, crown gall tumours in tobacco plants, which are induced by transfer of a bacterial plasmid, can give rise to normal tissues and to whole plants. Thus, heritable normal behaviour can be restored to certain pluripotent cancer cells by transplantation into, or cultivation in, a suitable environment.

These experiments suggest that the cancer phenotype is not inexorably irreversible but do not refute the somatic mutation hypothesis. The chromosome changes in many tumour cells, the mutagenic properties of most carcinogens, and the alteration of specific genes in oncogenesis, strongly suggest that carcinogenesis involves genetic changes in the cells that become malignant. In addition, activated oncogenes introduced into the germ line of mice cause a genetic predisposition to cancer.

22.2 Prospects for prevention and screening

One of the biggest problems in attempting to reduce the incidence of cancer is that of changing the life style of the people at risk. In the 30 years since it became firmly established that cigarette smoking is causally linked to lung cancer, little progress has been made in reducing cigarette smoking or in stopping new cohorts of youngsters acquiring this addictive habit. Dietary factors (see Chapter 3) may be equally important, though less clearly defined, in human carcinogenesis, particularly in the digestive tract itself, and changing patterns of cancer are evident, such as the decrease of stomach cancer and rise of colorectal cancer. It is difficult to change dietary habits, though the availability of fresh or frozen vegetables in all seasons and the increasing recognition of the importance of dietary fibre is leading to better health.

With occupational cancers caused in part by industrial exposure, it is much easier to prevent access to the carcinogens once they have been identified. The recognition of β-naphthylamine as a bladder carcinogen (see Chapter 6) soon led to protection of workers who were exposed to this chemical in the rubber and dye industries. Similar measures have been undertaken to reduce exposure to asbestos and related carcinogenic fibres.

One of the brightest prospects for prevention arises from the recognition of microbes as important environmental carcinogens for human cancer (see Chapter 8). As shown in Chapter 3 (Table 3.10), 5–15 per cent of cancers in the US are listed as being possibly attributable to infection, chiefly by viruses. Across the world, this percentage is likely to be higher, as the prevalence of oncogenic viruses has been relatively low in the Western world.

Carcinoma of the uterine cervix is becoming the most common cancer of women, especially in South America. Two strains of human papillomavirus (HPV-16 and HPV-18) appear to be causally linked to flat cervical warts and neoplasia. It is interesting to note that these agents were not isolated *in vitro* as infectious viruses; rather, they have been identified through molecular genetic techniques so that the viral genes have been cloned before virus isolation. Cervical cancer is a disease easily curable by minor surgery if recognized at an early stage before invasion of the subepithelial tissue of the cervix has taken place. Furthermore, the cancer, as well as preneoplastic dysplasia, can be recognized by direct inspection (colposcopy) and by the examination of cervical smears. The advantages of regular screening for cervical cancer are proven in reducing cancer

mortality and morbidity. Yet the costs of preventive screening as a public health measure are considerable and to date the awareness of its value is largely restricted to those women least at risk of developing the disease. With the identification of the incriminating virus, the possibility of developing immunizing vaccines is being actively pursued, although for human papillomaviruses this approach is still in its infancy.

Preventive immunization does appear to be effective in the transmission of hepatitis B virus (HBV). The virus is prevalent in Africa and Asia. It is associated with primary liver cancer, a rare tumour in the West, but ranking sixth in cancer mortality world-wide. Dietary aflatoxins (see Chapter 7) may also play a role in human liver cancer, and there is evidence that HBV and aflatoxin act synergistically. HBV is typically transmitted perinatally. Protection from infection can be achieved with preparations of pooled antibody to HBV surface antigen administered postnatally, following some weeks later with vaccination with surface antigen itself, manufactured by recombinant DNA methods. Trials in Taiwan and Japan suggest that the cycle of maternal transmission to infants can be broken by these measures, and this promises a dramatic reduction in the incidence of liver cancer in 40–60 years time.

There is intensive research on vaccines to other viruses, such as Epstein–Barr virus (EBV) and human T cell leukaemia virus type 1 (HTLV-1), but much development is still required before vaccines can be given preliminary trials. Infection by EBV is ubiquitous, and of the two malignancies associated with EBV, a major risk factor for one, Burkitt's lymphoma, may be malaria. Given the high morbidity and mortality of malaria itself, this is the disease that must be tackled. With EBV, however, it is undifferentiated nasopharyngeal carcinoma (NPC) that causes at least 50 times more premature deaths than those from Burkitt's lymphoma.

NPC is prevalent among Chinese living in southern China and throughout south-east Asia. Like most cancers, NPC is multifactorial in causation, with evidence of a slight heritable predisposition (increased risk with certain HLA haplotypes) and evidence of dietary nitrosamines or nickel salts early in life as well. But the presence of EBV genomes in the tumour cells and of raised antibody levels to viral antigens in NPC patients implicates the virus as having the major causative role, and gives hopes for future prevention.

Like cervical carcinoma, NPC is readily treatable if recognized at an early stage in its growth. Early diagnosis is being introduced in China by mass screening for serum IgA specific to an EBV antigen. The IgA can be recognized in a drop of blood from a pin-pricked ear lobe, blotted on to paper. Since EBV IgA is elevated at an early stage of NPC growth, healthy subjects with elevated IgA are then investigated for carcinoma *in situ* and are treated curatively at this stage by simple surgery or radiotherapy. The mass screening for EBV IgA in the communes of southern China promises to be the most effective scheme of preventing cancer deaths.

The identification of a new human herpes virus (HHV-8 or KSHV) associated with Kaposi's sarcoma and primary effusion lymphomas, especially in immunodeficient individuals, provides a further lead for screening and eventually a vaccine. Similarly, the identification of *Helicobacter pylori* playing an aetiological role in gastric cancer and gut-associated lymphomas may lead to control through antibiotics and immunization.

22.3 Prospects for new treatment

Modern methods of cancer treatment have been reviewed in Chapter 17, 18, and 19. Surgical removal and radiotherapy remain the major treatments for solid tumours, although chemotherapy plays an increasingly important role. The newer physical methods of imaging, employing computerized tomography (CT) and magnetic resonance imaging (MRI), are proving of great importance not only for diagnosis, but for conformational radiotherapy planning too. Immunological methods of imaging with radiolabelled antibodies (see Chapter 19) are still in a primitive state compared with CT and NMR but may one day prove to be of greater use for detecting small tumours, especially metastases where the nature of the primary tumour is already known.

There have been very considerable advances in chemotherapeutic treatment (see Chapter 17) especially in leukaemia and in tumours of children and young adults. The major cancers of older patients, such as carcinoma of the breast, stomach, and colon, have been disappointingly refractory to curative chemotherapy.

Much discussion of alternative treatment modalities is devoted to immunological mechanisms (see Chapter 16) and immunological vehicles of targeting cytotoxic agents or toxins to the tumour (see Chapter 19). Monoclonal antibodies that bind to the surface of tumour cells but not to haemopoietic stem cells are already proving to be clinically useful in 'cleansing' bone marrow in autologous transplantation. It remains to be seen whether immunological targeting will be successful in tackling solid tumours *in vivo*, but it seems well worth the current investment in this field.

As with more conventional chemotherapy, a problem with immunologically targeted therapy is the likelihood of resistant clones emerging, especially as tumour cells are known to modulate the expression of cell surface antigens. Perhaps the development of new radionuclides emitting α-particles will be of most promise with antibody treatment; such nuclides may kill all cells within a short range of the targeted antibodies and the need to translocate antibody or toxin across the cell membrane is obviated. However, as related in Chapter 19, there is a need for more research into appropriate radionuclides for conjugation with monoclonal antibodies.

Where expression of surface antigen is a necessary part of the malignant phenotype, there is more hope for immunotherapy, as cells that express the antigen can be killed, and cells that cease to express it should lose their malignancy. The overamplified expression of receptors for epidermal growth factor in many squamous cell carcinomas (see Chapter 11) may also be appropriate targets for immunotherapy. In the next few years, much effort will be made to develop drugs or other reagents that directly and selectively block the function of oncogene products.

An area of basic research that is rapidly being applied to cancer therapy is that of locally acting growth and differentiation factors, called cytokines (Chapter 20). These proteins are produced by one cell type and usually act as 'paracrine' factors stimulating the proliferation, differentiation, or degeneration of other, neighbouring cells that express specific receptors. The best known cytokines are the interleukins (IL-1 to -6) affecting lymphoid cells, and the specific growth factors for myeloid cells. Interferon is classified as a cytokine.

A few years ago, great publicity was given to the potential of interferons as antitumour therapy. Interferons were originally discovered as endogenous antiviral agents, but they can promote terminal differentiation or arrest the growth of certain tumour cells too. Now that abundant interferon has become available through gene cloning, it is apparent that most cancers are unresponsive and, further, that high doses of interferon are extremely unpleasant and toxic for the patient. Therefore a disillusionment has set in that has perhaps been exacerbated by the overenthusiastic claims for interferon before it could be tested in appropriate clinical trials. Yet amid this disappointment, one rare kind of malignancy, hairy cell leukaemia, is responding well to interferon in giving a complete response (regression) in the majority of patients, and interferon has become the preferred means of treatment for these patients. We do not understand why this leukaemia is so sensitive to interferon.

Another cytokine, tumour necrosis factor (TNF), took the place of interferon in the media as the 'magic cure-all' for cancer. Like interferon, the gene encoding TNF has been cloned so that large amounts of this factor can be manufactured in bacteria. TNF is naturally produced in small amounts by macrophages in response to bacterial endotoxins. It is identical to a protein known as cachectin, which is thought to play a role in the wasting of normal tissues (cachexia) seen in many advanced cancer patients. Certain animal tumours are cured by TNF administration but preliminary clinical trials on human malignancy have been disappointing. If it promotes cachexia TNF may do more harm than good, but like interferon it is hoped that some human tumours will be eliminated by this biological product.

Currently, immunological control is enjoying a renaissance in considering tumour treatment, through the agency of another cytokine, interleukin-2 (IL-2). Reports suggest that interleukin-2 may also be of value in stimulating the host immune T cell response to some tumours. This locally acting factor promotes the growth of T lymphocytes. By extracting tumour-infiltrated lymphocytes and amplifying the numbers in culture by IL-2, re-inoculation may help to arrest the growth of the malignant tissue.

22.4 Prospects for gene therapy

22.4.1 Introduction

Gene therapy denotes the placement and expression of genes in human tissues as a means of treatment.

Gene therapy was originally conceived as a means of replacing defective genes with normal or 'wild-type' alternatives in diseases resulting from inherited single gene disorders. Thus enzyme deficiencies, haemophilia, or cystic fibrosis might be corrected by providing genes that provide the proteins to permit normal functions to take place. While research looks promising for a number of single gene disorders, most clinical trials using gene therapy are for cancer treatment.

The approaches to cancer gene therapy are broader than gene therapy aimed to correct inherited gene disorders (Fig. 22.1). While corrective or replacement gene therapy in cancer is being attempted, genes are also being employed to make malignant cells appear more 'foreign' or recognizable to the immune system. A third approach is to

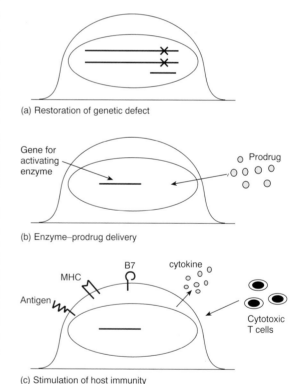

(a) Restoration of genetic defect

(b) Enzyme–prodrug delivery

(c) Stimulation of host immunity

Fig. 22.1 Approaches to gene transfer into tumour cells. (a) Introduction of corrective genes, e.g. wild-type *p53*, or antisense to K-*ras*. (b) Introduction of enzymes activating systemically administered prodrugs. (c) Introduction of cytokine or immune genes to attract cytotoxic T lymphocytes into the tumour.

provide genes that encode enzymes that will selectively convert prodrugs to cytotoxic drugs in the tumour. Finally, genes that can help to protect normal tissues from conventional cytotoxic drugs are being targeted to the most sensitive tissues, such as stem cells, to permit the administration of higher dose drugs.

None of these approaches to cancer treatment has yet advanced beyond exploratory phase I or II clinical trials and many inherent obstacles to successful treatment remain to be overcome. In this section the promise and problems of gene therapy for cancer are reviewed together with the means of gene delivery, since they have not been introduced in earlier chapters.

22.4.2 Corrective gene therapy

As already discussed cancer, is a disease that involves gene changes in cells (Chapters 4 and 10). While several different genes may contribute to the malignant phenotype of the cancer cell, restoring just one of them to normal function may prevent the expression of malignancy. Where the loss of a tumour suppressor gene, such as the retinoblastoma gene or p53, leads to cancer, its replacement could lead to regaining growth control in those cells that take up and express the new gene. Where a mutant oncogene is actively promoting uncontrolled growth, such as K-*ras*, the expression of antisense RNA through gene therapy might inhibit gene expression or translation of the mRNA and thus help to arrest cell proliferation.

The introduction of wild-type tumour suppressor genes or antisense constructs for oncogenes into tumour cells in culture has been demonstrated to restore normal growth control. It is doubtful, however, whether all the malignant cells could be targeted *in vivo* to ensure that the tumour would not continue to grow from the cells that had escaped receiving or expressing the corrective gene. The enthusiasts for this approach to cancer gene therapy are optimistic that improved methods of gene delivery will effectively cover the vast majority of malignant cells. The few remaining cells might then be controlled by the immune system. However, cancer is a clonal disease, and any cell that did not receive the corrective gene, or did not express it, or in which the gene later mutated to a non-functional state would still have the potential to give rise to new tumour growth. For this reason corrective gene ther-

apy is unlikely to provide curative treatment although it might conceivably delay tumour growth.

The clonal nature of cancer proliferation and progression thus places much more stringent constraints on corrective gene therapy than in its use to treat inherited deficiencies. To correct, say, haemophilia A, a relatively small proportion of cells secreting clotting factor VIII, even from an ectopic site, may be all that is required to alleviate the major symptoms of the disease, provided that sufficient clotting factor is present in the blood plasma. Similarly, in cystic fibrosis, if as few as 10 per cent of the epithelial cells lining the lung express the normal cell membrane chloride channels encoded by the cystic fibrosis gene, normal lung function may be largely restored. Where quantitative protein levels need to be more precise, gene therapy presents a greater problem. For example, in β-thalassaemia, an important aspect of the syndrome is the production of normal levels of α-haemoglobin which are toxic when too little β-haemoglobin is produced. Thus, corrective gene therapy will need to be controlled quantitatively as well as qualitatively. But corrective cancer gene therapy has the further limitation that individual cancer cells escaping the therapeutic gene are likely to emerge and grow during tumour progression. In addition, our methods of gene delivery *in vivo* (see below) are still woefully inadequate.

22.4.3 Immunological gene therapy

The aim of immunological gene therapy is to engender an enhanced immune response to the tumour cells leading to their destruction by cytotoxic T cells. Immunological therapy is most likely to be effective for those tumours that express antigens that elicit some immune responses in any case. Malignant melanoma has attracted the most attention because cytotoxic T cells (CTLs) specific to MAGE, tyrosinase, and ganglioside antigens occur in metastatic melanoma (see Chapter 16). Clear cell carcinoma of the kidney is another possible cancer target.

The gene therapy approach to 'therapeutic vaccination' is being explored by a number of methods to enhance the recognition and destruction of tumour cells by cytotoxic T lymphocytes. Firstly, by introducing genes into tumour cells that secrete immune cytokines, CTLs can be attracted to infiltrate tumour tissue and become activated there.

Interleukin-2 (IL-2), IL-12, and interferon-γ are being tested both in tumour models and in clinical trials as a gene delivery of cytokine therapy (see Chapter 20).

Secondly, cell surface molecules that enhance immune responses can be expressed in tumour cells through gene delivery. Many tumours do not express, or down-regulate major histocompatibility (MHC) antigens. By making these cells express class I or II MHC antigens, bearing tumour antigenic peptides, CTLs may act directly to kill the tumour cells. Class II MHC molecules are naturally expressed on antigen-presenting cells of the immune system such as macrophages and dendritic cells. Gene transfer of class II MHC into tumour cells converts them into antigen-presenting cells to enhance cell-mediated immunity within the tumour. Other cell surface molecules that augment the primary interaction between MHC antigens and T cell receptors are CD28 on T cells and B7 on antigen-presenting cells; again gene transfer of B7 into tumour cells can enhance CTL responses to them.

Thirdly, xenogenization ('making foreign') of tumour cells by entirely foreign antigens may stimulate the immune system to recognize natural cellular antigens too, so that the non-treated tumour cells are also destroyed by CTLs. This notion was first tested by infecting tumour cells with viruses such as the avian paramyxovirus, Newcastle disease virus. Now xenogenization is being accomplished by foreign gene transfer.

Immune therapy of tumours by gene transfer of cytokines, auxiliary molecules of immune cells, or foreign antigens will only have a lasting effect if it stimulates systemic immune responses against resident tumour cells, even at distant sites. Thus the cytokine gene therapy being attempted for melanoma involves transferring cytokine genes into cultured melanoma cells and reinoculating them (after γ-irradiation to prevent their own growth) into the patient. The hope, based on studies of malignant melanoma in mice, is that the patient's natural immunity will be stimulated to attack the resident, metastatic tumour cells throughout the body in a systemic way.

22.4.4 Prodrug gene therapy

One of the most promising applications of gene therapy is to deliver genes for enzymes that activate otherwise innocuous prodrugs into cytotoxic compounds locally in the tumour. This method is sometimes known as gene-directed enzyme–prodrug therapy (GDEPT) or gene–prodrug activation therapy (GPAT).

The first prodrug to be tested for cancer gene therapy was ganciclovir. It was developed as an antiviral drug for herpe viruses such as herpes simplex virus and cytomegalovirus. Ganciclovir is an analogue of the nucleoside thymidine. It is converted into a monophosphate by herpesvirus thymidine kinase (TK) but not by cellular TK enzymes. Once the monophosphate, analogous to thymidine monophosphate (TMP) is formed, cellular enzymes rapidly convert it into the triphosphate (TTP) which becomes incorporated into DNA in place of TMP. However, ganciclovir TP acts as a chain terminator so that DNA replication is arrested and the cells in which this occurs eventually die. The prodrug is already licensed for use in herpes infections as it kills cells actively replicating herpesviruses, and, because it is harmless until phosphorylated, uninfected cells are spared.

By introducing the gene for herpesvirus TK into tumour cells, those cells also become susceptible to the cytotoxic effects of activated ganciclovir. This approach has been tried with limited success with a number of tumours, including a clinical trial on patients suffering from glioblastoma, a malignant form of brain tumour. Other prodrug–enzyme combinations under investigation are bacterial cytidine deaminase converting 5-fluorocytidine into the cytoxic 5-fluorouracil (5FU), and bacterial nitroreductase converting a nitrogen mustard compound known as CB1954 into a highly toxic alkylating agent. The nitroreductase–CB1954 combination has been used for its demonstrated ability to kill cells when the enzyme itself is targeted to tumours by conjugation with monoclonal antibody (see Chapter 19). Direct delivery of the gene is a promising alternative.

A major limitation of prodrug–gene therapy is again that not all tumour cells will take up and express the gene for the enzyme that converts the prodrug into its active form. Hence it will be important that the activated drugs exhibit what is called a 'bystander effect', that is, that they diffuse into and affect neighbouring cells. Activated ganciclovir has good bystander effect provided the tumour cells express gap junctions, as the triphosphate does not diffuse across membranes. CB1954 and 5FU also exhibit bystander effects and a further advantage of CB1954 is that it is cytotoxic for non-proliferating cells, whereas ganciclovir is only active in S-phase cells. A number of new prodrug–enzyme combinations will doubtless be developed soon. Which, if any, prove to be genuinely efficacious as a new means of cancer chemotherapy remains to be determined from clinical trials.

22.4.5 Gene therapy delivery and targeting

Genes can be delivered to human cells and tissues in viral vectors, in liposomes, and as DNA (Table 22.1). Direct, *in vivo* introduction of genes is more difficult to achieve with high efficiency than the insertion of genes into cells '*ex vivo*' followed by re-inoculation of the cells into the patient. The latter method is preferred for target cells such as haemopoietic progenitor cells. These cells can be enriched through their expression of CD34 antigen, and it is sometimes possible to introduce a selectable marker alongside the therapeutic gene. For cancer application, consideration is being given to introducing a gene conferring multidrug resistance to haemopoietic cells to spare them during conventional chemotherapy.

Liposomes encapsulating the DNA for the cystic fibrosis (*CF*) gene has been successfully applied *in vivo* to the nasal epithelium, which then transiently expresses the CF chloride channel proteins. The next trials will be to see whether inhalation of CF–liposomes through a nebulizer will successfully deliver the gene to the lungs, a primary target for CF gene therapy. Previously, adenovirus vectors bearing the *CF* gene have delivered it to the lung epithelium, but current adenovirus vectors have proved to be allergenic.

Plasmid DNA is taken up well into skeletal muscle by intramuscular injection. Muscle tissue has little extracellular space, and the DNA inoculated into the large volume cytoplasm of muscle fibres migrates to the numerous nuclei in this syncytial tissue. This method of gene delivery looks most promising for 'DNA vaccination', but its use in cancer gene therapy is likely to be more restricted. More fancy ways of delivering DNA have been devised and are already in experimental use. DNA attached to colloidal gold can be 'shot' into cells at high velocity. Conjugates of DNA with polylysine and adenovirus fusion protein aid attachment and internalization.

Among the viral vectors (Table 22.1), retroviruses have been the most developed experimentally to date. Retroviral vectors based on Moloney murine leukaemia virus carry the therapeutic gene in place of viral genes. The viral packaging proteins for the vector DNA are supplied *in trans* in specially constructed packaging cell lines, adapted so that the 'helper' genome mRNAs providing the packaging proteins cannot themselves be incorporated into the vector particles (Fig. 22.2). The Moloney virus can only infect and integrate into proliferating cells, as dissolution of the nuclear membrane during mitosis is necessary for the preintegration viral core complex to gain access to host chromosomes. The present generation of retroviral vectors, therefore, can only be targeted to proliferating cells. However, for cancer gene therapy this might be turned to advantage, for example by targeting genes for prodrug-activating enzymes to the proliferating tumour cells or to endothelial cells of tumour neovasculature, thus protecting the non-dividing endothelium elsewhere in the body.

Other viral vectors can infect non-proliferating cells. Herpes simplex virus can carry large DNA inserts whereas the coding capacity of the adenovirus-associated virus (AAV) vector is limited. Viruses that establish persistent 'infections' are employed in order to maintain the gene in the target cells, but for some applications, e.g. therapeutic vac-

Table 22.1 Delivering cancer gene therapy

Warheads

Genes for cytokines

    Immune recognition antigens

    Enzymes-activating prodrugs

    Tumour suppression

    Apoptosis

    Antisense and ribosyme RNA

    Multiple drug resistance

Missiles

Naked DNA

DNA complexed with membrane fusion reagents

Liposomes

Viral vectors

    Retrovirus

    Adenovirus

    Adenoassociated virus

    Parvovirus

    Herpes simplex virus

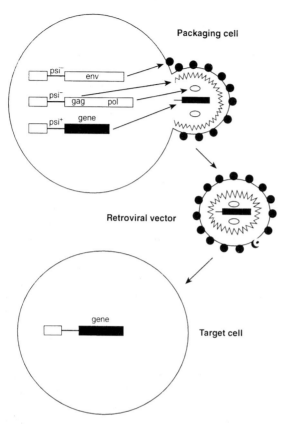

Fig. 22.2 A retroviral packaging cell line. The packaging cell constitutively produces retroviral particles which assemble only those vector genomes containing the psi (Ψ) packaging signal sequence. In the target cell the therapeutic gene carried as RNA in the vector is reverse transcribed to DNA which integrates into chromosomal DNA.

cines, transient gene delivery might be sufficient. There is concern that integrating viruses such as retroviruses and parvovirus may cause harmful insertional mutagenesis. Human parvovirus B19 has a preferential integration site in human chromosome 19, but that specificity depends on a viral protein that is lost in the construction of the parvoviral vector.

When target cells are temporarily cultured *ex vivo* and can be stimulated to proliferate, moderately efficient gene transfer can be effected. For direct delivery *in vivo*, however, a number of other problems arise. It may be difficult to attain a sufficiently high multiplicity of infection to deliver genes to enough target cells. The vectors should not infect the wrong cell types, especially germ cells. Currently, considerable research and development effort is being applied to devising high titre retroviral vectors that show targeting specificity at two stages: firstly, the viral envelope may be engineered to attach to cell surface receptors specifically expressed on the target tissue, e.g. epidermal growth factor receptor or erythropoietin receptor; secondly, the gene in the vector can be placed under a tissue-specific promoter so that it will only be expressed after infection and integration in the appropriate target cell, e.g. a carcinoembryonic antigen promoter for colorectal cancer, or a tyrosinase promoter for melanoma.

Another potential problem for *in vivo* delivery of Moloney-based retroviral vectors is the sensitivity of murine retroviral envelopes to human complement. However, by using human packaging cells and non-murine envelopes surrounding Moloney core proteins, this problem can be avoided. There is likely to be rapid development of several kinds of viral vector for gene therapy to provide safer, more efficacious, and more precisely delivered gene therapy.

22.4.6 Safety and ethics of gene therapy

Government authorities have placed particular emphasis on the safety and ethics of applying gene therapy to humans, by the institution of special bodies such as the Recombinant DNA Advisory Committee (RAC) in the US and the Gene Therapy Advisory Committee (GTAC) in the UK. There are two main reasons why gene therapy raises particular problems for clinical practice. One is that it is a new and unexplored method of treatment for chronic diseases; the other is that there is general concern over genetic manipulation in humans.

The safety issues in gene therapy concern unwanted or deleterious side effects of the treatment. These may arise from the gene itself, which is supposed to be therapeutic, or from the delivery systems. There is concern that the genes may reach the wrong tissues, even eggs and sperm, and thus be passed on to the next generation. In corrective gene therapy, an immune reaction may be elicited to the gene product, if the protein expressed from the gene has not previously been seen by the patient as part of 'self'; this may also apply to enzymes in prodrug therapy. But such immune reactions are more likely to reduce the efficacy of the therapy than be directly harmful.

The delivery systems, especially viral vectors, also have to be carefully monitored. Viral vectors are disabled, so that they are not able to replicate freely in the body's tissues but act once to deliver and express the therapeutic gene. Early versions of vectors in experimental use were not always sufficiently defective, and replication-competent viruses occasionally emerged. Rescue of replicating virus can also conceivably occur by recombination with latent or persistent related viruses in the patient, e.g. adenovirus or herpesvirus. Insertional mutagenesis has already been mentioned, and it might have a carcinogenic effect by activating cellular oncogenes adjacent to the integrated viral promoter. However, it should be borne in mind that many of the conventional treatments for cancer are demonstrably carcinogenic, e.g. radiotherapy and chemotherapy with alkylating agents. The risks of gene therapy are unlikely to be greater; rather it is their novelty that raises concern.

In fact, what is called somatic gene therapy, the delivery of genes to diseased tissue, does not pose really novel ethical issues that have not been raised earlier with the introduction of other kinds of therapy. For example, tissue and organ transplantation introduces complete DNA genomes—the entire human chromosome set—of the donor into the recipient, and live attenuated vaccines such as for polio and measles introduce viruses akin to vectors. In contrast to somatic gene therapy, current public opinion holds that germ line therapy, i.e. the introduction or deletion of genes in germ cells passed on to the next generation, must be avoided. Thus the human equivalent of transgenic or 'knock-out' mice has not been approved, although one day one could possibly envisage applications that might make future generations genetically resistant, say, to developing some of the more prevalent human cancers.

Gene therapy is still in its infancy. It has produced more hype than genuine, realistic hope. Yet some successes are likely to come, and these will include cancer treatment. To date, cancer has represented more than 50 per cent of the clinical trials submitted to RAC and GTAC. It is appropriate at this early stage of gene therapy technology that geneticists and oncologists should proceed with great care and caution.

22.5 Conclusion

Lastly, we should not forget the progress that has been made in recent years in improving palliative treatment, designed not to cure cancer, but to improve the quality of life remaining to the affected individual. Most chronic diseases, such as cardiovascular disease, arthritis, diabetes, etc., are not curable, and we have, perhaps, expected too much of oncologists in hoping for the magic bullet. In the meantime, great advances have been made in symptomatic treatment, pain control, and psychological management. With one-quarter of deaths in the Western world attributable to malignant disease, improvements in the care of incurable cancer patients deserves considerable devotion and resources alongside the search for preventive measures and curative treatment.

Cancer is an exciting field of research, for it presents challenging questions in our basic understanding of cell physiology and development, coupled with the prospect of helping to alleviate a major source of human suffering and death. The study of cancer is multidisciplinary, involving scientists and clinicians in many different specialities. To ensure further progress in combating cancer we must practice what we preach, and be open to the new leads that the cross-fertilization of multidisciplinary research affords.

References and further reading

Bridgewater, J., Springer, C., Knox, R., Minton, N., Michael, P., and Collins, M.K.L. (1995). Expression of the bacterial nitroreductase enzyme in mammalian cells renders them selectively sensitive to killing by the prodrug CB1954. *European Journal of Cancer*, 31A(13–14): 2362–70.

Caruso, M., Panis, Y., Gagandeep, S., Houssin, D., Salzmann, J.L., and Klatzmann, D. (1993). Regression of established macroscopic liver metastases after *in situ* transduction of a suicide gene. *Proceedings of the National Academy of Sciences, USA*, **90**, 7024–8.

Cosset, F. L., Takeuchi, Y., Battini, J.-L., Weiss, R. A., and Collins, M. K. L. (1995). High titer packaging cells producing recombinant retroviruses resistant to human serum. *Journal of Virology,* **69,** 7430–6.

Culver, K. W. and Blaese, R. M. (1994). Gene therapy for cancer. *Trends in Genetics,* **10,** 174–8.

Freeman, S. M., Abboud, C. N., Whartenby, K. A., Packman, C. H., Koeplin, D. S., Moolten, F. L., and Abraham, G. N. (1993). The "bystander effect": tumor regression when a fraction of the tumor mass is genetically modified. *Cancer Research,* **53,** 5274–83.

Harris, J. D., Gutierrez, A. A., Hurst, H. C., Sikora, K., and Lemoine, N.R. (1994). Gene therapy for cancer using tumour-specific prodrug activation. *Gene Therapy,* **1,** 170–5.

Heller, H., Davey, B., and Bailey, L. (ed.) (1989). *Reducing the risk of cancers.* Hodder & Stoughton, London.

Lever, A. M. L. and Goodfellow, P. N. (ed.) (1995). Gene therapy. *British Medical Bulletin,* **51,** 1–242.

Mulligan, R. C. (1993). The basic science of gene therapy. *Science,* **260,** 926–31.

Sun, W. H., Burkholder, J. K., Sun, J., Culp, J., Turner, J., Lu, X. G., *et al.* (1995). *In vivo* cytokine gene transfer by gene gun reduces tumor growth in mice. *Proceedings of the National Academy of Sciences, USA,* **92,** 2889–93.

Vessey, M. P. and Gray, M. (ed.) (1987). *Cancer risks and prevention.* Oxford University Press, Oxford.

Vile, R.G. and Hart, I.R. (1993). Use of tissue-specific expression of the herpes simplex virus thymidine kinase gene to inhibit growth of established murine melanomas following direct intratumoral injection of DNA. *Cancer Research,* **53,** 3860–4.

Glossary

α-particle The nucleus of the helium atom (charge of $+2$) and mass 4.

abl An oncogene originally discovered in the Abelson strain of murine leukaemia virus. This virus causes pre-B cell tumours, whereas a related feline virus isolate causes sarcomas. The cellular *abl* gene is important in chronic granulocytic leukaemia of humans. The gene product displays tyrosine protein kinase (q.v.) activity.

acentric chromosome A chromosome lacking a centromere and, hence, incapable of attaching to the spindle at mitosis; consequently these chromosomes are randomly distributed between daughter cells at mitosis.

actin A cytoskeletal protein family found in all cell types. In muscle cells it is involved in the contractile function of the tissue.

active immunization Induction of a state of immunity by administering antigen.

acute leukaemia A tumour of the reticuloendothelial system that usually runs a rapid course from disease onset to death.

adduct The addition product between two molecules, e.g. a carcinogen (or its metabolite) and a nucleic acid in DNA.

adenocarcinoma A malignant tumour of glandular epithelium.

adenoma A solid, benign glandular tumour.

adjuvant A substance that increases the immune response to an antigen given at the same time.

affinity Used herein for the degree of binding or interaction, e.g. between a ligand and its receptor, or between an antigen and an antibody specific for that antigen. One can speak of high or low affinity receptors or antibodies.

aflatoxin A toxic food contaminant produced by fungi of the genus *Aspergillus*.

alkylating The process of attaching alkyl (usually methyl or ethyl) groups to a chemical structure such as a DNA base.

allele Alternative form of a gene found at the same locus of a chromosome: short for allelomorph.

alloantigen Antigens that exist in alternative forms that distinguish one individual of a species from another.

allogeneic Genetically dissimilar.

allogeneic graft (allograft) Graft between genetically dissimilar individuals of the same species.

amino acid One of twenty molecules used as the "building blocks" of a protein.

anaplasia Loss of differentiated characters (dedifferentiation).

anastomosis The surgical reuniting of the severed ends of a tubular structure such as gut or a major blood vessel.

anchorage independent growth Growth (cell division) in suspension in a liquid or semi-solid medium, without attachment to a solid substrate. This form of growth is a property of many tumours.

androgens Steroid hormones secreted mainly by the testis; maintain male characteristics.

aneuploidy The presence of extra chromosomes or the absence of chromosomes, so that the karyotype is neither haploid (q.v.) nor an exact multiple thereof.

angiogenesis New growth of blood vessels.

antibody A globular protein produced by animals in response to an antigen (q.v.) and which binds specifically to the antigen.

antigen A molecule that is capable of stimulating the formation of antibodies (q.v.).

antioncogene *see* tumour suppressor gene.

antisense oligonucleotide Synthetic nucleotide fragments (generally 15–20 bases in length) complementary to RNA or DNA sequences used to inhibit specifically the transcription or translation of a gene.

apoptosis Programmed cell death, which maintains total cell numbers within physiologically appropriate ranges. Apoptosis is an active form of cell suicide that sometimes requires new gene expression for its initiation and that often culminates in a characteristic set of biochemical and morphological events. These include genomic DNA cleavage by endonucleases, chromatin condensation (pyknosis), nuclear fragmentation, proteolysis of cytoskeletal and other proteins, plasma membrane blebbing, and cell shrinkage; the macromolecular components of cells are thus degraded so that their constituent subunits can be recycled in the body.

aromatic amines Polycyclic compounds consisting of hydrocarbon ring structures with at least one nitrogen-containing amine group.

ascites Accumulation of serous fluid in the peritoneal cavity.

attenuated virus A virus whose pathogenicity is reduced by passage outside its natural host.

autocrine Self stimulation of a cell through production of both a factor and its specific receptor.

autophosphorylation A process by which a protein has the ability to add phosphate groups to amino acids within the protein (*see also* protein kinase).

autosome Any chromosome that is not a sex chromosome.

auxotroph An organism (e.g. a bacterium) capable of synthesizing from simple nutrients all the complex biochemical compounds needed for its own growth.

axilla The armpit, which contains the majority of the lymph nodes draining the breast and arm.

axon Process of a nerve cell that carries impulses from the nerve body to a nerve or other target cell.

B cell B lymphocyte: the immune cells of the lineage that makes antibodies.

base The purine or pyrimidine component of nucleotides (q.v.).

base change (in nucleotides) *See* mutation.

benign tumour Tumour that does not invade or metastasize; an absolute distinction from malignant tumours is not possible (*see* Chapter 1).

bracken The fern *Pteridium aquilinum*.

Burkitt's lymphoma A tumour in humans of mature immunoglobulin-producing B lymphocytes.

burst forming unit-erythroid (BFU-E) A colony of immature and mature red blood cells growing in a semi-solid medium.

bypass The rerouting of the normal contents of a tubular structure, such as the bile duct or bowel where an inoperable blockage is present.

c-onc The cellular gene corresponding to a viral oncogene and sharing close DNA sequence homology. It is thought that the virus 'picked up' the cellular gene by chance.

cannula A hollow needle.

carcinogen A chemical substance, or physical agent such as X-ray irradiation or ultraviolet irradiation, that causes cancer.

carcinogenesis Process of tumour induction and development.

carcinoma A malignant tumour of epithelium.

carrier A host with an asymptomatic infection who serves as a source of infection to others.

casein kinase Serine/threonine kinase that phosphorylates many oncogene proteins.

cDNA A complementary (copy) DNA transcribed (q.v.) from an RNA template by the enzyme RNA-dependent DNA polymerase (reverse transcriptase).

centimorgan (cM) A measure of distance between two genes based on the frequency with which they are inherited together.

centromere Constricted portion of chromosome at which the chromatids (q.v.) are joined. It may be central (metacentric), off centre (submetacentric), or near one end (acrocentric).

chemical repair Conversion of a free radical to a stable molecule (usually by hydrogen atom transfer).

chemotaxis Response of cells or organisms to chemical stimuli: attraction towards is positive and repulsion negative chemotaxis.

chorioallantois Embryonic membrane formed by the fusion of the wall of the allantoic sac to the chorion. It underlies the porous egg shell in birds.

choriocarcinoma Cancer of uterus derived from placental tissue.

chromatid One of the two spiral filaments joined at the centromere (q.v) which make up a chromosome and which separate in cell division, each going to a different pole of the dividing cell and each becoming a chromosome of one of the two daughter cells.

chromatin A complex of fibres in the cell nucleus, made up of DNA, histones and other proteins. During cell division the chromatin condenses into coils to form chromosomes (q.v.)

chromosome A structure in the nucleus made up of a linear strand of DNA associated with histones, RNA, and other proteins. In cell division the material (chromatin) becomes compactly coiled and clearly visible either after staining or by special microscopic techniques. Each organism of a species has a specific number (diploid number) of chromosomes in its somatic cells, e.g. 46 in humans.

chromosome mapping Assignment of a gene or other DNA sequence to a particular position on a specific chromosome.

cirrhosis Fibrous repair in response to damage in the liver.

***cis* activation** Stimulation of transcription by a DNA sequence on the same chromosome.

class (of antibody) Antibody class is determined by differences in the structure of the constant part of the molecule. Different classes have different biological functions.

clastogenic Giving rise to or inducing breakages, e.g. in chromosomes.

clonal chromosomal aberrations Structural chromosome defects or chromosomal gains observed in at least two cells within a tumour, or chromosomal losses observed in at least three cells within a tumour.

clone (*noun*) A collection of cells, organisms, nucleic acid sequences, etc. that are all derived from the same ancestor and are thus more or less identical; a population of cells derived from a single cell by division, and so usually presumed to contain the same genetic information subject to the occurrence of mutations.

clone (*verb*) To make a clone of nucleic acid sequence by genetic manipulation, replicating the desired sequence in a microorganism, or to isolate single cells.

codon A sequence of three nucleic acids or bases in DNA that together specify the encoded amino acid. Thus a sequence of DNA codons specifies the amino acid sequence of the encoded protein.

collagenase Enzyme that digests collagen.

colony-stimulating factor (CSF) A group of proteins that stimulate the proliferation and differentiation of haemopoietic cells growing as colonies in a semi-solid medium; e.g. M-CSF (q.v.), G-CSF (for granulocytes), GM-CSF (q.v.), multi-CSF, etc.

colostomy Artificial external opening of large bowel.

colposcopy Examination of the uterine cervix with a magnifying lens.

complement A group of serum proteins that can be activated by cell-bound antibody (q.v.) to lyse antibody-coated cells.

complete carcinogen An agent, usually a chemical compound, that is able to induce cancer alone, i.e. without the need for subsequent treatment by a tumour-promoting agent.

conization Removal of a cone of tissue from the uterine cervix.

connective tissue (mesenchyme) Supporting tissues, made up of mesenchymal cells, collagen fibres, and interstitial substances. Bone, cartilage, fatty tissue, and blood vessels are specialized forms of connective tissue.

conserved sequence A DNA seqeunce that has remained virtually unchanged throughout evolution.

contigs An arrangement of overlapping cloned DNA sequences representing a region of the genome (q.v.)

contrast medium X-ray dense material for delineating internal structure.

cosmid A large plasmid (q.v.) used as a vector (q.v.) for cloning (q.v.) medium length (about 4050 kb) DNA sequences.

CRE Cyclic-AMP response element; an upstream regulatory transcription signal.

CREB A family of genes encoding transcription factors with leucine repeats that bind as dimers to the CRE.

cystic lesion A cyst is a fluid-containing sac, usually with a thin wall.

cytochrome (P450) Iron-containing, electron–accepting molecule involved in oxidation-reduction reactions requiring energy, in this case the oxidative metabolism of carcinogens. P450 defines the characteristic absorption wavelength of a particular cytochrome on which these reactions are dependent.

cytokine Generally a low molecular weight protein involved in cell regulation. Cytokines are secreted transiently, and generally locally, during embryogenesis, tissue remodelling and repair, immunity, and inflammation. Cytokines interact in a complex network where induction of one cytokine results in the production of other members of the network; binding of one cytokine to its cell surface receptor can alter expression of other cytokine receptors, and they can up-regulate or down-regulate each others' action.

cytolytic Lysing (killing) cells.

cytopathic Damaging cells, often leading to their death.

cytoskeleton The network of insoluble, multifunctional filaments (e.g. actin, vimentin, cytokeratin) remaining after extraction of cells in detergent.

cytotoxicity Cell killing.

deletion The removal of a segment of a chromosome or gene from a coding or non-coding region.

dielectric relaxation time The time required for the molecules in a medium to readjust following passage of radiation.

diethylstilboestrol A powerful, synthetic oestrogen.

differentiation antigen Molecule detected by an antibody on or in one cell type which is associated with state of maturation or position in a developmental lineage.

differentiation Process of development of new characters in cells or tissues.

diploid Having twice the haploid number of chromosomes. Normal human somatic cells are diploid, having 46 chromosomes (23 pairs).

direct repeats DNA-binding sites that consist of sequences that are duplicated on the same strand of DNA in the same orientation.

DNA fingerprinting A pattern of DNA sequences, e.g. tandem repeat sequence (q.v.), unique to an individual.

dominant An allele that manifests its effects in heterozygotes (q.v.), i.e. when present in a single dose, as well as in homozygotes. A characteristic determined by a dominant allele.

dominant negative effect When the presence of a mutant gene protein interacts with the product from the normal allele of that gene and abrogates the gene's normal function.

double minutes Pairs of small acentric chromosomes that often carry amplified genes.

down-regulation The decrease in the number of available (exposed) cell surface receptors following interaction with the specific factor that binds to the particular receptor.

downstream By convention a nucleotide sequence is read from the 5′ end to the 3′ end, or from the beginning to the end in terms of coding potential, then one designates those sequences more 3′ or more 'endward' as being downstream.

downstream promotion An insertional mutagenic event (q.v.) involving specifically a sequence that promotes gene transcription (hence 'promoter'). For this effect, the promoter must be located before the 5′ end (beginning) of the gene; the promoter is thus 'upstream' and it promotes the transcription of the gene elements that are 'downstream' (or toward the 3′ end).

ectoderm Outer of the three primary germ layers in animal embryos, which develops mainly into epidermis, nervous tissue.

electrophilic Literally, 'electron loving'. Applied to electron-deficient chemical compounds that carry a net positive charge and are attracted to chemicals with an excess of electrons, with which they bond covalently.

embolus Blood clot, tumour cells, or other particles in bloodstream.

endocrine Stimulation by factor produced at one site, e.g. specific cells in a gland, and acting at a distant site.

endocytosis The process by which molecules bound to the cell surface are internalized by the cell.

endoderm Innermost of the three primary germ layers in the animal embryo which gives rise to the lining of the gut from pharynx to rectum and derivatives from it such as liver, pancreas, etc., and the respiratory epithelium.

endoscope Optical instrument, passed through an orifice, e.g. mouth, anus, for visualizing internal organs.

endothelium Cells lining blood vessels.

enhancer Eukaryotic promoter element that increases the transcriptional activity of a gene; may be upstream or downstream of the gene, or even inserted within the gene. Equally efficient in either orientation.

enhancer insertion An insertional mutation (q.v.) involving specifically a sequence that enhances (increases) the level of gene transcription (hence 'enhancer').

epidermal growth factor (EGF) A factor originally described for its mitogenic activity for epidermal cells. It is growth promoting for other cells as well.

epigenetic mechanisms Regulating expression of gene activity but not involving alterations in gene structure.

epithelium Tissue-specific surface or glandular cells.

epitope A structural region of an antigen (q.v.) that is recognized by an antibody (q.v.) molecule.

epoxide A derivative of an aromatic (ring structured) molecule in which an oxygen molecule forms a bridge across an opened double bond between two carbon atoms.

epoxide hydrase An enzyme that utilizes an epoxide substrate, breaks open the oxygen bridge, and adds one molecule of water to form a diol derivative.

erbA A gene sequence originally found in an avian erythroblastosis virus as part of a fusion to *erbB* (q.v.). It may not be an oncogene *per se*.

erbB An oncogene originally found in two isolates of avian erythroblastosis leukaemia virus. It represents part of the gene for the receptor for epidermal growth factor (EGF, q.v.).

erythroblastosis A leukaemia of red blood cell precursors.

erythrocyte Most mature red blood cell from which the nucleus has been extruded (in mammals).

erythropoietin A growth factor that stimulates the proliferation and differentiation of erythrocyte precursor cells.

ets An oncogene originally found in an avian mye-loblastosis virus (strain E26) fused to the *myb* oncogene (q.v.). Now known to encode a class of transcription factors.

eukaryote Higher organisms whose cells are complex, containing nuclei and other organelles.

exocrine Secreting externally; exocrine glands deliver their secretions to an epithelial surface through ducts.

exon The parts of a gene sequence that are found in the messenger RNA (transcript) molecule which will be used for producing (translating) the protein product of the gene. Parts of the gene not found in the transcripts are known as introns (q.v.).

expression vector A plasmid-like DNA construct containing genes that can be transcribed and translated when introduced into an appropriate host cell. Vectors may be constructed with constitutively active or inducible promoters.

faecal occult blood The presence of small amounts of blood in faeces not detectable with the naked eye, which may be an indicator of colonic cancer.

familial polyposis coli Inherited condition where multiple polyps (small benign tumours) of the colon and rectum develop and which predisposes to colon cancer. The gene involved is known as *APC*.

fes An oncogene originally found in a feline sarcoma virus (Gardner-Arnstein strain). The gene product displays tyrosine protein kinase (q.v.) activity.

fgr An oncogene originally found in a feline sarcoma virus (Gardner-Rasheed strain). Its gene product has tyrosine protein kinase (q.v.) activity.

fibrosis Formation of scar tissue.

filling defect A region of an X-ray or scan with absence of medium or isotope often owing to the presence of tumour.

fms An oncogene originally found in a feline sarcoma virus (McDonough strain). Its product displays tyrosine kinase (q.v.) activity. This gene may be related or identical to the gene encoding the receptor for macrophage colony-stimulating factor (q.v.).

fos An oncogene originally found in two murine osteosarcoma viruses. Its product is found in the nucleus and is more abundant in cells responding to growth factor stimulation, and in amnion and mature monocytes.

fps An oncogene originally found in two avian sarcoma viruses (strains Fujinami and PRCII). Its product displays tyrosine protein kinase (q.v.) activity.

frameshift mutation A mutation in which, by addition or deletion (other than in multiples of three) of nucleic acids, the reading frame of the triplet code is disrupted. All downstream codons are thereby altered and as a rule no functional protein is produced.

free radical An unstable molecular fragment caused by breakage of a chemical bond in a molecule.

gene A region of DNA that encodes a protein. The sequence of bases forms a code in which three bases (a triplet) specify a particular amino acid.

gene activation Generally meant to imply that a dormant gene has been 'turned on' so that messenger RNA is made (transcribed).

gene amplification A mutation event whereby a gene is found in greater than the normal number of copies. Amplification generally involves very long stretches of chromosomes (i.e. many genes) and may occur so that the genes are amplified in number many times. (*See also* homogeneously staining regions and double minutes.)

gene cloning Making many copies of a single isolated gene by inserting it into bacteria or other cells.

gene expression The process by which the information encoded by a gene is converted into a protein. In clinical genetics, the way in which a gene is expressed in a given individual.

gene library A collection of fragments of DNA cloned into bacteria or viruses. DNA that is cloned directly from the genome of an organism is known as a genomic library, whereas DNA that is transcribed from messenger RNA from a particular organism or tissue is known as a cDNA library.

gene therapy Replacing a defective gene with a normal gene in somatic cells or in germ cells.

genetic code The sequence of DNA nucleotides (q.v.) that determines the amino acid sequence of the translated protein. The genetic code is 'read' in triplets of bases called codons (q.v.)

genetic marker An allele of a gene that follows standard Mendelian segregation and so can be used to study linkage in families or associations with a characteristic within populations.

genome The total genetic material of an organism.

genome project An international research programme aimed at mapping all the genes in a genome (q.v.), e.g. yeast, human.

genomic footprinting A method of determining whether DNA-binding sites are occupied by proteins either *in vitro* or *in vivo*.

genotoxin An agent that is toxic through its ability to damage DNA. At high levels of damage, this is lethal for the cell.

genotype The genetic constitution of an individual, usually at a particular locus. *See also* phenotype.

germ (cell) line Cells that give rise to the sperm or egg (ovum) which transmit genes from one generation to another and are thus potentially immortal. All other cells are somatic and die with the individual. Only mutations in the germ cell line can be passed on to future generations. Also used to designate unaltered gene configurations.

glucocorticoids Steroid hormones secreted by the adrenal cortex for the control of carbohydrate metabolism; they also have anti-inflammatory properties and kill certain types of lymphocytes.

glycolipid A lipid molecule having a covalently attached oligosaccharide (q.v.).

glycoprotein A protein molecule having a covalently attached oligosaccharide (q.v.).

glycosaminoglycan A polysaccharide component of a mucoprotein (q.v.).

gonadotrophins Hormones secreted by the anterior lobe of the pituitary (q.v.).

granulocyte White blood cell (various maturation stages include the neutrophils and polymorphonuclear cells) involved in the defence system against foreign matter.

granulocyte/macrophage colony-stimulating factor (GM-CSF) A factor that stimulates the proliferation and differentiation of precursor cells of the granulocyte and macrophage lineages. Note that these two lineages share a common precursor cell, one that is already more differentiated than the haemopoietic stem cell (known as the CFUs or pluripotential stem cell) that gives rise to all the blood cells.

Ha-*ras* An oncogene originally found in two mouse sarcoma viruses (strains Harvey and BALB). Its product is an enzyme catalysing guanosine triphosphate (GTP). It is a member of a multigene family (Ki-*ras*, N-*ras*, q.v.), members of which are often found in mutated form in tumours.

haematuria Blood in the urine.

haemoccult test A clinical biochemical test that detects the presence of blood in the faeces.

haemopoietic Blood cell forming (also called haematopoietic).

half-life The time taken for half a given quantity of a chemical (e.g. radioisotopes, proteins, nucleic acids) to degrade or decay. Short half-lives reflect an unstable chemical.

haploid Having one copy of each chromosome, as in the gametes. The human haploid chromosome number is 23.

helix–loop–helix Domain occurring in some proteins that regulate transcription; composed of two α-helical regions separated by a β turn. Such proteins generally bind to DNA as dimers.

hemicorporectomy Surgical removal of lower half of the body.

hemizygous Having only one copy of a given genetic locus (or of a number of loci in the case of deletions or loss of whole chromosomes).

heteroantiserum Antiserum raised in one animal species against cells or molecules of another.

heterozygous Having different alleles at a given locus on homologous chromosomes.

histocompatibility genes Genes that determine susceptibility or resistance to tissue or tumour transplants.

histones Highly basic proteins usually associated with DNA in chromatin (q.v.).

histopathology The study and diagnosis of disease by microscopy.

HLA The major histocompatibility system of humans. It is a complex genetic region coding for two major classes of cell surface determinants involved in the control of immune function. There are also other genes in the region, in particular controlling certain of the complement components.

homogeneously staining region (HSR) Region of a chromosome staining with an intermediate intensity throughout its length and without the normal pattern of light and dark bands.

homologous chromosomes Chromosomes that carry genes governing the same characteristics and that pair during meiosis (q.v.) (the cell division which produces eggs and sperm). Individuals receive one member of a homologous pair of chromosomes from their father and the other member from their mother.

homozygous Having the same allele at a given locus on homologous chromosomes.

hormone A specific chemical substance produced by cells and carried to other cells or organs, often in the blood, to produce a specific effect at a distance.

hybridization, nucleic acid *See* Northern and Southern blotting/hybridization.

hybridoma A hybrid tumour cell created by the fusion of two or more cells of different type. The term is commonly used to refer to monoclonal antibody-producing cells formed by fusion of a sensitized B lymphocyte and a myeloma (q.v.) cell.

hydrophilic Literally, 'water loving'. Describes property of a substance preferentially found in water extracts as opposed to lipids.

hydrophobic Literally, 'water fearing'. Describes property of a substance preferentially found in lipid extracts (such as membranes) as opposed to water.

hyperdiploid Having more than the diploid number of chromosomes.

hyperplasia Increase in number of cells in response to stimulus—a reversible process.

hypertrophy Increase in size of cell or tissue.

hypodiploid Having fewer than the diploid number of chromosomes.

IL-1 Interleukin-1. A factor produced by monocytes, involved in immune response reactions of antigen presentation by monocytes to T lymphocytes.

IL-2 Interleukin-2. T lymphocyte growth factor (previously called TCGF).

IL-3 Interleukin-3. A factor that stimulates growth of early multilineage haemopoietic cells.

immunogen A substance that stimulates an animal to produce antibodies (q.v.).

immunoglobulin An antibody (q.v.) molecule.

immunotherapy A form of therapy in which the host's immune system is activated or augmented, e.g. by the use of antitumour antibodies (q.v.).

immunotoxin A hybrid protein molecule, formed by the conjugation of an antibody and a toxic protein, capable of binding to cells bearing surface antigens recognized by the antibody and made with the intention of killing the cells selectively.

infectious mononucleosis A disease characterized by an imbalance of the immune cells in the body and a massive proliferation of T cells (q.v.).

inflammation Tissue response to infection or damage.

initiation The primary step in tumour induction caused by a carcinogen.

insertional mutagenesis A mutation caused by the insertion of new genetic material into a normal gene or sequences surrounding it. The term is generally used in relation to integrations of retroviruses (q.v.) into chromosomal DNA, although it applies to other inserted material, including DNA sequences moved from one chromosomal site to another ('transposition').

insulin A hormone produced by B cells of the pancreas. It is concerned with the regulation of carbohydrate, fat, and protein metabolism. A deficiency of insulin causes diabetes.

integration Insertion of viral DNA within a host chromosome. First applied to integration of phage DNA in the bacterial chromosome.

integrin Cell transmembrane heterodimeric protein that mediates cell–cell and/or cell–substratum adhesion.

interferon A group of proteins produced by cells in response to viral infection and other stimuli. Their effects are complex and include antiviral actions exerted at various stages.

interleukin Substance produced by a cell of the immune system which acts on other cells (*see also* IL-1, IL-2, IL-3).

internal mammary lymph nodes Deeply located lymph nodes that drain the breast and arm found at the sides of the sternum (breast bone).

intravenous urogram X-ray of urinary tract after injection of radio-opaque material, which is concentrated in the kidney.

intron The parts of a gene sequence that are not found in the messenger RNA (transcript) molecule that will be used to produce the protein product of the gene. Introns are removed from the initial RNA copy of the gene by a process known as splicing (q.v.).

inversion A chromosomal aberration that arises when two breaks occur in the same chromosome and the region between the breaks is reinserted after a 180° rotation resulting in a reversed gene order.

inverted repeats DNA-binding sites that consist of sequences that are inverted and duplicated on the opposite strand of DNA.

ionization potential Energy required to liberate a non-nuclear electron from an atom or molecule.

isochromosome A chromosomal aberration in which one of the arms of a chromosome is deleted and the other arm is duplicated. The two arms of an isochromosome are therefore of equal length and contain the same genes.

isogenic genetically identical.

isogenic graft (isograft) Graft between genetically identical individuals, e.g. between identical twins.

isotope One or two or more atoms having the same atomic number but different mass, e.g. ^{123}I and ^{131}I are radioactive isotopes of iodine.

jun An oncogene originally found in an avian sarcoma virus, S17. Forms a complex with the oncogene *fos* to become a transcription factor, known as AP-1.

Kaposi's sarcoma A tumour, possibly arising from endothelial cells, often found as skin lesions, purple or blue in colour.

karyotype The chromosome complement analysed and set out according to size, shape, and banding patterns of each chromosome.

keratinocyte Major epithelial cell type of the skin or epidermis, which contains large quantities of cytoskeletal proteins of the cytokeratin family.

Ki-*ras* An oncogene originally identified in a mouse sarcoma virus (Kirsten strain). It is a member of a multigene family (Ha-*ras*, N-*ras*, q.v.), members of which are often found in mutated form in tumours. Its product is an enzyme catalysing guanosine triphosphate (GTP).

kilobase (kb) 1000 bases (nucleotides) of single-stranded DNA or RNA; kilobase pairs (kbp) for double-stranded DNA; conversion factor to daltons depends on the exact base composition but, in general, average values of 345 daltons and 330 daltons per nucleotide of RNA and DNA, respectively, give reasonable estimates. Thus, 10 kb = 3.45×10^6 daltons (RNA) or 3.30×10^6 daltons (single-stranded DNA). To estimate coding potential from an RNA molecule, assuming an average of 110 daltons per amino acid, use 1 kb (RNA) = 37 kilodaltons (protein).

kilodalton (kDa) 1000 daltons, where a dalton is the standard unit of atomic mass very nearly equal to that of a hydrogen atom. The molecular weight of a protein is based on the atomic weights of the individual elements.

kinase An enzyme that transfers phosphate groups to a protein at serine, threonine, and/or tyrosine residues.

kit An oncogene originally found in a feline sarcoma virus (strain HZ4).

L-*myc* An oncogene identified by gene amplification (q.v.) in a lung carcinoma. Member of the *myc* multigene family of nuclear transcription factors.

laparotomy Surgical incision in flank or abdomen, usually for operations on abdominal contents.

LET (linear energy transfer) Rate of energy loss to the surrounding medium, in a radiation track (unit: keV/μm).

leucine zipper A protein sequence of five leucine residues each separated by six residues. It mediates dimer formation via a coiled-coil of parallel α helices and is normally adjacent to a basic DNA-binding domain. Found in a family of genes including many oncogenes with transcriptional activity.

leucosis A proliferative disease of leucocytes.

leukaemia A malignant disease of the blood-forming organs leading to the overproduction of neoplastic white blood cells or their precursors, in the blood and bone marrow.

leukoerythroblastic anaemia An anaemia in which immature red cells and increased numbers of white cells are present in the blood.

library A collection of DNA clones representing either all expressed genes, a cDNA (q.v.) library, or a whole genome (q.v.), a genomic library.

life span study An ongoing epidemiological study, e.g. of excess cancer incidence in atomic bomb survivors from the Japanese cities of Hiroshima and Nagasaki.

ligand The substance with which a receptor acts specifically to form a complex, at least transiently.

ligase An enzyme that joins together two fragments of double-stranded DNA.

linkage map A map of the relative positions of gene loci on a chromosome deduced from the frequency with which they are inherited together.

linkage The presence of two or more genes on the same chromosome causing a tendency of alleles of these genes to be inherited together. Linkage occurs only when the genes are sufficiently close to one another on the same chromosome. Can be used to search for coinherited genetic characters.

lipid bilayer Description of the membranes of cells, including the plasma membrane, of two apposed layers each containing lipid molecules.

liposome A synthetic lipid vesicle.

locus (plural, **loci**) Position of a gene on a chromosome.

loss of heterozygosity (LOH) The situation pertaining when one allele of a chromosome has been lost; sometimes the remaining allele is reduplicated. Usually large segments of chromosomes undergo this process simultaneously, leaving a long stretch of DNA that is homozygous at all alleles along its length.

LTR A structure found at both ends of the provirus DNA of a retrovirus (q.v.), hence 'long terminal repeat'

lymphangiogram X-ray of lymphatic vessels.

lymphocyte White blood cell of the T or B lineage.

lymphokine Substance produced by lymphocytes which acts on other cells (*see also* interleukin).

lymphoma A solid tumour of T or B lymphocytes, e.g. in the lymph nodes, thymus, or spleen.

lysosome The cellular organelle that degrades molecules that have been taken into a cell by endocytosis (q.v.).

macrophage White cell found in all tissues, which can ingest and break down antigens.

macrophage/monocyte colony-stimulating factor (M-CSF) A factor that stimulates the growth and differentiation of cells of the macrophage/monocyte (q.v.) lineage. Also known as colony-stimulating factor 1 (CSF-1).

malignant tumour Tumour that is capable of invading surrounding tissues and of metastasizing.

mammography X-ray of breast.

MAP kinases Mitogen-activated serine/threonine kinases, also known as extracellular signal-related kinases (ERKs); highly conserved sequences that are activated by signal transduction pathways.

marker chromosome Abnormal or rearranged chromosome that was used as a characteristic feature, but now defined as one in which no part can be identified by conventional cytogenetics.

mastectomy Surgical removal of breast.

megabase (Mb) Unit of length of DNA equivalent to 1 million nucleotides (q.v.).

megakaryocyte White blood cell that undergoes nuclear division without cell division, leading to a multinucleated cell. It shatters to produce the subcellular entities known as platelets (q.v.) that participate in wound healing.

meiosis Two successive cell divisions from a diploid cell, in which the chromosomes are duplicated only once so that each of the new daughter cells has only half the diploid chromosome number, e.g. in the formation of gametes (sperm and ova).

MEN 2A/2B Multiple endocrine neoplasia syndromes, including thyroid carcinomas and benign tumours of the adrenal medulla (phaeochromocytoma).

mesenchyme *See* connective tissue.

mesoderm The germ layer lying between ectoderm (q.v.) and endoderm (q.v.). It gives rise to an epithelial component (epithelium of genital and most of urinary system), striated muscle including heart, and mesenchyme (connective tissue, cartilage, bone, smooth muscle, and blood cells).

met An oncogene originally identified by transfection (q.v.) of DNA from a human osteosarcoma (q.v.) cell line treated with a chemical carcinogen (q.v.). Known to be the receptor for hepatocyte growth factor (scatter factor).

metaphase The phase of mitosis or meiosis in which the condensed chromosomes attached to the spindle fibres can line up on an equatorial plate between the two poles of the cell.

metaplasia Abnormal alteration in the structure of cells.

metastasis A secondary tumour arising from cells carried to a distant site from a primary tumour.

microsome (-al) Subcellular membranous particles with membrane-bound enzyme activities, derived from the endoplasmic reticulum, in cell fractionation procedures.

microtome A cutting device that produces thin sections of tissue for microscopic examination.

mineralocorticoids Steroid hormones secreted by the adrenal cortex for the maintenance of ion balance, especially Na^+ ions.

mitogen A compound capable of causing cells to divide.

mitosis Process of cell division.

modal chromosome number The number of chromosomes per cell that is found most frequently even in a mixed cell population.

modified radical mastectomy Surgical treatment for breast cancer involving removal of breast, overlying skin, small pectoral muscle, and the axillary lymph nodes.

molecular excitation A change in the electronic configuration of an atom or molecule (accompanied by absorption of energy).

molecular mass (M$_r$) The relative molecular weight of a protein based on its *in vitro* properties as calculated, for example, by its migration through a gel separation system, where charge, tertiary structure, and post-translational modification may influence the pattern of migration. This value is distinct from the true molecular weight based on the individual atomic weights of component elements.

monoclonal Derived from a single cell.

monocyte Similar cell to the macrophage but found in the blood. Both cells assist in immune responses.

monosomy The presence of only one member of a chromosome pair.

mos An oncogene originally found in a mouse sarcoma virus (Moloney strain). Its gene product has serine protein kinase (q.v.) activity.

mucoprotein Protein-polysaccharide complexes that are major components of mucins.

mutagen A chemical or physical agent that causes changes in the structure of DNA (mutations).

mutagenesis Effecting a heritable change in a nucleic acid.

mutagenicity The capacity of an agent (e.g. a chemical) to cause DNA mutation.

mutation A heritable change in the genetic material. Mutations in the broadest sense include any change, from a single base pair change in the DNA to substantial deletions or rearrangements of the DNA even involving major parts or the whole of chromosomes, and including chromosome translocations.

mutation frequency The ratio of mutated cells to normal cells following, for example, radiation (expressed either as per cell irradiated or per cell surviving).

myb An oncogene originally found in two avian myeloblastosis (myeloid leukaemia) viruses. Its product is found in the nucleus, and it is a transcription factor. The gene has been activated by adjacent insertion of retroviruses (q.v.) in several rodent myeloid leukaemias.

myc An oncogene originally found in four avian 'myelocytoma' viruses. Its product is found in the nucleus and appears to be a DNA-binding protein with transcriptional activity. It is a member of a multigene family (including L-*myc* and N-*myc*, q.v.).

myeloid Literally, 'of the bone marrow'. However, in speaking of myeloid leukaemia, one is denoting cells of the granulocytic or monocytic lineages.

myeloma A plasma cell tumour.

myxoid Mucinous.

N-*myc* An oncogene identified by gene amplification (q.v.) in a neuroblastoma (q.v.). Member of the *myc* (q.v.) multigene family.

N-*ras* An oncogene originally identified as a gene amplified in a human neuroblastoma (q.v.) and subsequently in other tumour types. It is a member of a multigene family (Ha-*ras*, Ki-*ras*, q.v.), members of which are often found in mutated form in tumours.

nasopharyngeal carcinoma Carcinoma of the squamous epithelium of the postnasal space.

natural killer (NK) cells Cells that are believed to kill, non-specifically, tumour and virus-infected cells.

necrosis Tissue death.

neonatal thymectomy Removal of the thymus at birth, leaving the animal without functioning T cells.

neoplasia Tumour growth.

neoplasm Tumour.

neu An oncogene originally identified by transfection (q.v.) of DNA from a rodent neuroblastoma. Known to be a member of the epidermal growth factor receptor family; also called *ERBB2* and *HER2*.

neuroblastoma A malignant tumour of neural crest origin. It may arise in any site containing sympathetic nervous tissue but is most commonly found in and around the adrenals.

neuroendocrine system A system of cells widely distributed throughout the body, which produces regulatory peptides. One group acts as hormones on distant organs, or on cells locally. A second group is produced at nerve endings and acts as neurotransmitters.

neurotransmitter A substance released from the axon terminal (nerve ending) of a nerve cell on excitation which stimulates or inhibits a target cell.

NGF Nerve growth factor.

Northern blotting/hybridization A technique wherein RNA is fractionated according to size by electrophoresis in agarose-formaldehyde gels and then the RNA is transferred ('blotted') onto nitrocellulose paper. The RNA is then fixed to the paper by baking and then can be identified by using specific nucleic acid sequences ('probes', these may be RNA or DNA) of a particular gene or part of a gene ('hybridization'). This technique allows identification of genes being expressed (i.e. transcribed into RNA), quantitation of levels expressed, etc.

nucleotide The unit component of a nucleic acid comprising a base (q.v.), a sugar, and a phosphate group.

oestrogens Steroid hormones secreted by the ovary; maintain female characteristics.

oligosaccharide A structure composed of three or more sugar residues covalently attached to protein in glycoproteins (q.v.) and glycolipids (q.v.).

oncogene Literally, a gene causing cancer. Oncogenes were identified by their presence in cancer-causing viruses, where their function is critical for viral transforming properties.

ORF Open reading frame.

osteolytic Bone destroying.

osteosarcoma A malignant tumour of bone composed of proliferating spindle cells that directly form tumour osteoid.

P450 A class of enzymes involved in oxygenating various compounds, the mono-oxygenases or mixed function oxidases.

p53 A tumour suppressor gene that is mutated in about 70 per cent of human cancers. Has pleiotropic effects, including transcriptional activation and transcriptional repression, and is involved in promoting cell growth and inducing apoptosis in specific cases.

palliation Treatment to ease symptoms.

PAP test Named after Papanicolaou who devised a staining method for cells shed (or scraped) from the surface of epithelial tissues; particularly used for the routine screening of uterine cervix for cancer cells.

papilloma A benign tumour usually on a surface, with a frond-like structure.

para-aortic Alongside the aorta.

paracentesis Puncture or tapping of a fluid-filled space with a hollow needle to draw off the contained liquid.

paracrine Stimulation of a cell through interaction with a substance produced by a neighbouring cell.

parasitism A relationship in which one member (the parasite) benefits at the cost of the other (the host). (*See also* symbiosis.)

partial hepatectomy Surgical removal of part of the liver.

particle accelerators Machines that emit pulses or continuous beams of high energy particulate radiation (cyclotrons, van de Graff accelerators, Betatrons, etc.).

passive immunization Immunity acquired by receiving immune cells or antibody.

PDGF Platelet-derived growth factor (q.v.).

penetration Passage of a virus from outside to inside the host cell.

phagocytosis The process by which large particles or cells are engulfed by cells of the reticuloendothelial system (q.v.), such as macrophages.

phenotype The combination of characteristics expressed by a particular cell or organism.

phorbol ester A variety of compounds originally isolated from plants that are active as tumour-promoting (q.v.) agents in multistep carcinogenesis assays.

phosphorylation The process of addition of phosphate groups to a protein (*see also* protein kinase).

physical mapping A linear map of the location of genes on a chromosome as determined by physical detection of overlaps between cloned DNA fragments (contigs q.v.) rather than by linkage (q.v.) analysis.

pituitary gland (hypophysis) A small gland at the base of the brain with two main lobes, anterior (adenohypophysis) and posterior (neurohypophysis). The anterior lobe produces hormones that control secretion in sex glands, thyroid, adrenal, etc. The posterior lobe secretes other hormones that are formed in specialised nerve cells in the hypothalamus. These hormones influence blood pressure, water balance, etc.

plasma cell A fully differentiated B lymphocyte synthesizing and secreting antibody (q.v.).

plasma The fluid component of blood.

plasmid Small circular double-stranded DNA up to 200 kb that can replicate independently and be transferred from one organism (or cell) to another.

platelet A subcellular component of the blood formed from megakaryocytes (q.v.) concerned with blood clotting; releases mitogens at the site of the wound.

platelet derived growth factor (PDGF) A factor in platelets (q.v.) that is mitogenic for cells at the site of a wound (e.g. endothelial cells, q.v.). Part of the gene for PDGF has been captured by a simian sarcoma virus in which it is known as *sis* (q.v.).

pleural effusion Fluid in the pleural space (surrounding the lungs) in abnormal amounts.

point mutation Substitution of a single nucleotide base within a DNA molecule.

polyclonal Derived from more than one cell.

polycyclic hydrocarbons A class of organic chemicals consisting of carbon and hydrogen molecules arranged in a series of linked ring structures.

polymerase chain reaction (PCR) A relatively new molecular biological technique whereby one or two small oligonucleotides (*c.* 15–25 bases long) of a known sequence are used as a 'primer' to drive a reaction containing a DNA molecule with the primer sequence, excess single nucleotides of A, T, C, and G, and polymerase. The polymerase copies the sequence adjacent to the primer and creates double-stranded DNA. The double-stranded DNA is then heated to separate the strands, and then the polymerase reaction is repeated. This procedure is followed for many cycles (up to 50–60 times), giving many thousands of copies of the sequence adjacent to the primer from the DNA used as a 'template'. In the case of using two primers, one is using oligonucleotides known to be found at the ends of the DNA of interest such that the intervening sequence is the one that is amplified. One can also use polyT oligonucleotides to amplify up the cDNA (complementary DNA) formed from a small amount of messenger (poly A-containing) RNA.

polymorphism The occurrence of two or more alleles for a given locus in a population where at least two alleles appear with frequencies of more than 1 per cent.

polyp A tumour projecting from a surface, usually epithelial.

preclinical disease Disease detected in individuals without symptoms.

prednisolone A powerful, synthetic glucocorticoid.

primer (oligonucleotide primer) A short DNA sequence used to initiate the synthesis of DNA, as in a polmerase chain reaction (q.v.).

probe Generally a single strand of labelled DNA (usually with a radioactive marker). The probe binds to single-stranded RNA or DNA which has a complementary sequence. The hybrids can then be isolated from mixtures, or detected by autoradiography or other methods. Nowadays, probes can also be made from RNA.

progestins Steroid hormones secreted by the ovary during the menstrual cycle and pregnancy.

promoter A DNA sequence found at the 3′ end of the gene that contains the start site for transcription and other regulatory sequences; orientation dependent.

promoter insertion An insertional mutagenic (q.v.) event involving specifically a sequence that promotes gene transcription (hence 'promoter'). *See also* downstream promotion.

promotion Stages following initiation; may be caused by specific non-carcinogenic promoting agents.

prostaglandins A group of compounds of similar structure found in the prostate (hence the name) but now known to be widely distributed in the body and affecting blood vessels, nervous system, uterus, etc.

protease Protein-digesting enzyme.

protein kinase An enzyme that adds phosphate groups to amino acids (generally serine, threonine, and tyrosine); the process is known as phosphorylation (q.v.).

protein kinase C A serine and threonine protein kinase (q.v.) important in the cell's response to growth factor stimulation.

protooncogene The normal cellular counterpart of a gene identified as causing a tumour (c-*onc* and v-*onc*, q.v.).

proviral integration The incorporation of the retroviral DNA provirus into the cellular genome. Generally occurs at random sites.

provirus The intracellular double-stranded DNA form of the retrovirus genome, either free or integrated.

proximate metabolite/carcinogen The carcinogen or its metabolite which undergoes metabolic or spontaneous conversion to a further derivative, the ultimate metabolite/carcinogen, which binds to the target macromolecule, usually DNA.

pseudodiploid Diploid (q.v.) chromosome number but with numerical or structural chromosome abnormalities.

pseudogene A gene thought to be permanently inactive. Many lack introns (q.v.) compared with related genes that are active. May have arisen by gene duplication events.

radiation fractionation Exposure to radiation over two or more periods separated by intervals of time.

radioimaging A technique that uses radioactive substances to visualize sites within the patient's body, e.g. the sites of tumour.

radionuclide An atom that undergoes spontaneous decay with the release of radiation. Radionuclides can be used for the radioimaging (q.v.) or therapy of cancer.

radioprotector A chemical substance that reduces the biological effects of radiation.

radon A chemically inert radioactive gas: a product of radium disintegration.

raf An oncogene originally identified in a murine sarcoma virus (strain 3611). Its product has protein kinase (q.v.) activity. Also know as *mil*.

RB1 Tumour suppressor gene involved in the formation of retinoblastomas (q.v.)

RBE (relative biological efficiency or effectiveness) The ratio of absorbed doses of two different types of radiation required to give the same level of effect.

receptor A structural molecule that binds to a specific factor (e.g. hormone, vitamin, antigen, etc.). These may be found at the cell surface (cell surface receptor, membrane receptor) or within the cytoplasm (cytosolic receptor).

receptor translocation Movement of a receptor from one part of the cell (e.g. the cell surface) to another site in the cell. This may be called internalization if the complex is taken inside the cell.

recessive An allele that is expressed only when present in the homozygous or hemizygous state (compare with dominant).

recessive mutation A mutation that is not expressed in the phenotype if it is balanced by a corresponding normal gene on the homologous chromosome, i.e. it is expressed only when both homologous genes are affected or if one is deleted.

recombinant DNA (gene splicing) DNA (genes) from different sources, e.g. bacterial, yeast or mammalian, can be cut into fragments and ligated to form hybrid DNA. This can be inserted into another organism, e.g. bacterial DNA carrying a human gene can be inserted into bacteria which then produce proteins coded for by the human gene.

recombination Process of exchange of genetic information between two homologous chromosomes, presumed to occur through breakage of both chromosomes at homologous sites followed by reunion after exchange. Also can occur between other RNA or DNA molecules (as with viruses).

rel An oncogene originally found in an avian reticuloendotheliosis (q.v.) virus.

reporter genes Genes that encode proteins/enzymes whose expression/activity can be easily measured so that the activity of the promoter can be determined in cells under different conditions.

response elements Binding sites for transcription factors in the promoters of genes.

restriction enzymes (restriction endonucleases) These enzymes isolated chiefly from prokaryotes recognize a specific sequence usually about four to six base pairs long within double-stranded DNA and cut the DNA specifically at a precise distance from that site only. Different enzymes recognize different sequences as a rule; there are several examples of enzymes isolated from different sources that cleave within the same target sequences. They are known as isoschizomers.

restriction fragment length polymorphisms (RFLPs) Restriction enzymes (q.v.) cut samples of DNA consistently into fragments of different lengths. If individuals differ in the distribution of sequences recognized by the enzymes, the DNA is cut into different sized fragments. These consistent minor variations in length can be used to map genes to specific chromosomes and help to trace genetic diseases in families.

ret A transmembrane receptor protein kinase oncogene associated primarily with thyroid neoplasms.

reticuloendothelial system 'Defence cells'. A diffuse system of phagocytic cells involved with the clearance of foreign proteins, immune complexes, large particles, and cells from the bloodstream.

reticuloendotheliosis A proliferative disease of reticuloendothelial cells.

retinoblastoma Malignant tumour of retinal cells, usually arising in children less than 5 years of age. In familial inheritance, a germ line mutation of the *RB1* gene is found.

retroperitoneal Lying behind the peritoneum.

retrovirus A member of a family of viruses sharing several physicochemical properties including the type of organization of the RNA genome and an enzyme (known as reverse transcriptase) which makes a DNA copy of the genome (provirus, q.v.) to become incorporated into the chromosomal DNA of the infected host cell.

reverse transcriptase An enzyme, RNA-dependent DNA polymerase, encoded by retroviruses. In the viral life cycle, the enzyme carried in the virus particle facilitates the synthesis of a DNA copy of the viral RNA genome. It then makes a second DNA strand complementary to the first and also degrades the viral RNA (template). Used in laboratory procedures to prepare complementary DNA copies (cDNA) of other RNAs.

reversion (reverted) The process by which a mutation is corrected, by 'back mutation' to the original (wild-type) DNA sequence. The reverted cell (or virus, etc.) now has a normal phenotype.

ribosomes Cellular particles at which proteins are synthesized.

risk factors Environmental or inherited influences that increase the chance of cells progressing from a normal to neoplastic phenotype.

RNA splicing A maturation process that removes internal sequences from polyribonucleotide chains (splicing, q.v.).

RNA-dependent DNA polymerase *See* reverse transcriptase.

ros An oncogene originally found in an avian sarcoma virus. Its product has tyrosine protein kinase (q.v.) activity.

salvage pathway A biochemical pathway in the synthesis of DNA that reutilizes pre-existing nucleic acids and their precursors rather than synthesizing them *de novo* from single carbon units.

sarcoma A malignant tumour of mesenchyme.

Schwannoma Tumour of the nerve sheath.

screening The testing of a normal population to detect clinical or preclinical disease.

sequencing A technique for establishing the structure of DNA by recognizing the order of the nucleotides (q.v.) or of protein by the order of its amino acids.

serum The fluid left after blood has clotted owing to substances released from platelets; some plasma proteins have been removed.

signal transduction Used in reference to the process by which the interactions between a growth factor and its specific receptor at the cell surface generate a signal that is transmitted to the cell nucleus as a stimulus to proliferate.

sis An oncogene originally found in a simian sarcoma virus. The gene is part of the cellular gene encoding platelet-derived growth factor (PDGF, q.v.).

sister chromatid exchange Exchange of genetic material between individual sister chromatids (q.v.).

ski An oncogene originally found in an avian carcinoma virus. Its product is found in the nucleus of cells.

somatic Refers to cells that are not part of the germ line and so their genetic complement is not passed from parent to offspring.

Southern blotting/hybridization A technique wherein DNA is fractionated according to size by electrophoresis in agarose gels (the DNA may be precut using restriction endonucleases, q.v.), and then the DNA is transferred ('blotted') on to nitrocellulose paper. The DNA is then fixed to the paper by baking and may then be identified by using specific nucleic acid sequences ('probes'; these may be RNA or DNA) of a particular gene or part of a gene ('hybridization'). The double-stranded DNA in the gel is treated with alkali before blotting; this provides single-stranded nucleic acid which can then bind covalently ('anneal') to the probes. The technique allows identification of the size of a gene, a map of restriction enzyme sites, gene amplification, gene deletion, gene rearrangement, etc.

specificity (of antibody or cells) The ability to distinguish between different antigens.

splicing An event that removes specifically the sequences of the non-coding parts of a gene (introns, q.v.) from the initial RNA molecule complementary in sequence to the gene. This is part of the 'processing' of the RNA molecule to its active form (the messenger RNA transcript) used to produce the gene product.

squamous Scaly or flattened, usually applied to epithelium.

src An oncogene originally found in an avian sarcoma virus. Its product has tyrosine protein kinase (q.v.) activity.

stem cell Precursor cell capable of growing and differentiating in response to a stimulus.

stilboestrol A powerful, synthetic oestrogen.

symbiosis 'Living together': an association of two organisms that confers mutual benefit.

synergism (synergy) Two or more compounds whose effects are additive or more than additive.

syngeneic graft Graft between individuals that have been inbred until their genetic similarity allows acceptance of grafts between members of the strain, e.g. between mice of an inbred strain.

synteny When genes are found in an identical linear relationship to other genes from one species to another, they are called syntenic, and the conservation of linear relationship is called synteny.

T cell T lymphocytes: a group of cells responsible for cell-mediated immunity.

tandem repeat sequence Multiple copies of a short DNA sequence lying in series along a chromosome; used in physical mapping (q.v.) and linkage mapping (q.v.) and also in DNA fingerprinting (q.v.) because each person's pattern of tandem repeats is likely to be unique.

targeting The directing of substances such as drugs or toxins to target cells by attaching them to carriers, such as antibodies (q.v.), that bind to the target cell specifically.

telomere Each of the extremities of a chromosome. There are numerous repeated sequences that are lost progressively with cell ageing.

terminal differentiation Progression of cells through successive differentiative stages from undifferentiated to fully differentiated and culminating in growth arrest.

testosterone The main male sex hormone, secreted by the testis.

tetraploid Having four times the haploid number of chromosomes.

***trans* activation (transactivation)** Modulation of gene transcription by the product of a locus from another chromosome.

transcription A base-pairing process that copies one nucleic acid into a complementary polynucleotide chain.

transcription factors Proteins that regulate the rate of gene transcription by RNA polymerase II. They usually, but not always, bind directly to DNA at sites in the gene promoter and recruit proteins that control transcriptional initiation (initiation factors).

transduction The process by which a virus genome recombines with other nucleic acids leading to the capture of new sequences or genes. The new material is 'transduced'.

transfect To introduce foreign DNA into a cell by experimental means so that the DNA integrates into the genome and is expressed in its new host cell. Transfection, the process.

transformation A word used in many ways. In this book, it means a change of morphological appearance of a cell ('morphological transformation') generally by a virus, chemical carcinogen, physical reagent, or even some unidentified ('spontaneous') event.

transforming growth factor (TGF) A factor that can cause a reversible change in normal cell phenotype such that cells grow into colonies in semi-solid media (anchorage-independent growth). TGF-β requires EGF to produce this phenotype whereas TGF-α can work alone.

transgenic Transferring a gene across species or strain barriers. In modern usage, animals carrying a gene introduced artificially during the early embryonic stage and now incorporated into the genome. The newly incorporated gene is called a transgene.

translation A term describing the process whereby the triplet code sequence of a messenger RNA molecule is used to produce a specific order (chain) of amino acids that form a protein.

translocation A chromosomal aberration in which part of one chromosome joins on to another chromosome. A reciprocal translocation refers to the transfer of material between two chromosomes.

transmembrane Something spanning the membrane. Generally in regard to plasma membrane; e.g. a protein found external to, within, and internal to the plasma membrane.

triplet code The code by which a sequence of three nucleic acids (bases) specifies one amino acid. Each triplet thus forms one codon.

triploid Having three times the haploid number of chromosomes.

trisomy The presence of three chromosomes of one type.

truncation Literally, 'a shortening'. In the context of this book, it means that a gene has been shortened by some event and thereby the protein product of the gene is smaller.

tumour promoter An agent capable of providing later steps in multi-step carcinogenesis systems whereby an initiated (preneoplastic) cell is converted to a neoplastic one (*see* initiation and promotion). Generally a specific tumour promoter is required for a particular initiating agent.

tumour suppressor gene Genes whose normal role is to regulate cell division in a negative fashion (leading to cell growth arrest) and, following mutation or loss of one or both alleles, may have the effect of allowing cells to progress through cell divisions in an unrestricted fashion.

tyrosine kinase A family of proteins with protein kinase (q.v.) activity for tyrosine residues. The protein products may be found as transmembrane receptors or non-membrane receptors.

ultimate metabolite/carcinogen *See* proximate metabolite/carcinogen.

upstream By convention a nucleotide sequence is read from the 5′ end to the 3′ end, or from the beginning to the end in terms of coding potential, then one designates those sequences more 5′ or more 'towards the beginning' as being upstream.

urothelium The epithelial cells lining the urinary tract.

v-*onc* An oncogene identified in a virus (*see* oncogene).

vector A DNA molecule, usually derived from a virus or bacterial plasmid (q.v.), which acts as a vehicle to introduce foreign DNA into host cells for cloning (q.v.) and then to recover it.

Western blot A technique similar to Northern or Southern blotting (q.v.) but used to separate and identify proteins.

Wilms' tumour Childhood tumour arising from renal tissue.

xenograft Graft between individuals of different species.

yes An oncogene originally found in two avian sarcoma viruses. Its product has tyrosine protein kinase (q.v.) activity.

Index